Handbook of Nephrology

Handbook of Nephrology

Edited by Bianca Keaton

hayle
medical

New York

Hayle Medical,
750 Third Avenue, 9th Floor,
New York, NY 10017, USA

Visit us on the World Wide Web at:
www.haylemedical.com

ISBN: 978-1-63241-665-0

Cataloging-in-Publication Data

Handbook of nephrology / edited by Bianca Keaton.
    p. cm.
Includes bibliographical references and index.
ISBN 978-1-63241-665-0
1. Nephrology. 2. Kidneys--Diseases. I. Keaton, Bianca.
RC902 .H36 2019
616.61--dc23

Table of Contents

Preface

The purpose of the book is to provide a glimpse into the dynamics and to present opinions and studies of some of the scientists engaged in the development of new ideas in the field from very different standpoints. This book will prove useful to students and researchers owing to its high content quality.

Nephrology is the branch of medicine dealing with the study of kidneys. It is concerned with the prevention, diagnosis and treatment of kidney diseases. Maintaining a healthy diet is an effective way to prevent kidney diseases. Nephrologists are physicians whose expertise lies in the diagnosis and treatment of kidney diseases. Some common kidney diseases are kidney stones, acute renal failure and chronic kidney disease. Blood urea nitrogen and other clinical urine tests are some of the commonly preferred tests to evaluate kidney diseases. Dialysis and renal transplantation are two of the most common and effective ways to treat kidney diseases. This book is compiled in such a manner, that it will provide in-depth knowledge about the theory and practice of nephrology. Different approaches, evaluations, methodologies and advanced studies on nephrology have been included in it. Students, researchers, experts and all associated with this field will benefit alike from this book.

At the end, I would like to appreciate all the efforts made by the authors in completing their chapters professionally. I express my deepest gratitude to all of them for contributing to this book by sharing their valuable works. A special thanks to my family and friends for their constant support in this journey.

Editor

Effects of pretransplant peritoneal vs hemodialysis modality on outcome of first kidney transplantation from donors after cardiac death

Xiajing Che[1†], Xiaoqian Yang[1†], Jiayi Yan[1†], Yanhong Yuan[1], Qing Ma[1], Liang Ying[2], Minfang Zhang[1], Qin Wang[1], Ming Zhang[2*], Zhaohui Ni[1*] and Shan Mou[1*]

Abstract

Background: The effect of pretransplant peritoneal dialysis (PD) or hemodialysis (HD) modality on outcomes of kidney transplantation (KT) for end-stage renal disease (ESRD) is debatable. We evaluated the outcomes these modalities in KT from donor after cardiac death (DCD).

Methods: A cohort of 251 patients on HD, PD or pre-emptive who underwent first KT from DCD between January 2014 and December 2016 were prospectively analyzed to compare for outcomes on recovery of renal function, complications as well as patient and graft survival. The patients were followed till August 2017. Data on 104 HD and 98 PD were available for final comparative outcome analysis, 5 pre-emptive were analyzed as the control group.

Results: Both HD and PD group patients were well matched for demographic and baseline characteristics. The follow-up period was 12.5 (3.0, 22.0) months in HD and 12.0 (6.0, 20.0) months in PD patients. Post-transplant renal functions between the two groups showed no differences. Among PD patients, 16 (16.3%) suffered delayed graft function, versus 19 (18.3%) in HD, with no statistical differences ($p = 0.715$). Complications of acute rejection, infections were comparable between the groups. The patient survival, graft survival and death-censored graft survival were similar for HD and PD after adjusting for other multiple risk factors.

Conclusions: Our results indicate that outcome of first KT from DCD is not affected by pretransplant dialysis modality of PD or HD in aspects of recovery of renal function, complications as well as patient and graft survival.

Keywords: Dialysis modality, Donor after cardiac death (DCD), Hemodialysis (HD), Outcomes of kidney transplantation, Peritoneal dialysis (PD)

Background

Peritoneal dialysis (PD), hemodialysis (HD) and kidney transplantation (KT) are three main renal replacement therapies for end-stage renal disease (ESRD) and KT with advances in technology and immunosuppressants is preferred for the recovery of renal function and the improvement of life quality [1, 2]. The availability of donor kidney has restricted the transplant and dialysis is essential while waiting for KT.

While awaiting KT, 30–40% of patients can be effectively treated by PD which is far away from the actual 11% and many suitable PD candidates are treated with HD [3]. Controversies on pretransplant dialysis modality continues with reported increased risks of early graft failure in PD patients [4]. Recent studies show equivalent outcomes for PD and HD [5–7]. Yet, other studies indicate better outcome of PD for patient survival, graft function as well as the delayed graft function (DGF) [8–13].

* Correspondence: drmingzhang@126.com; profnizh@126.com;
shan_mou@shsmu.edu.cn
†Xiajing Che, Xiaoqian Yang and Jiayi Yan contributed equally to this work.
²Transplantation Center of Ren Ji Hospital, School of Medicine, Shanghai Jiao Tong University, 160 Pujian Road, Shanghai 200127, China
¹Department of Nephrology, Molecular Cell Laboratory for Kidney Disease, Renji Hospital, School of Medicine, Shanghai Jiao Tong University, 160 Pujian Road, Shanghai 200127, China

More studies are needed to clarify the identical or even better function of PD compared with HD. Therefore, we conducted this prospective cohort study to compare the effects of pretransplant HD vs PD on outcomes of renal function, post-transplant complications, graft as well as patient survival of first KT from Donor after cardiac death (DCD).

Methods

Study population

This was a prospective cohort study of ESRD (defined as eGFR< 15 ml/min/1.73 m^2) patients who received their first kidney transplantation from DCD between January 2014 and December 2016 in renji hospital affiliated to School of Medicine of Shanghai Jiaotong University, a hospital at Pudong New District, Shanghai, China. During the transplantation, the technical issues that may affect the outcome of transplant like organ transplantation, preservation as well as surgical operation were all performed by same transplant team in our hospital. DCD was defined as awaiting cardiac arrest after withdrawal of life-supporting treatment in the intensive care unit.

Patients above 18 years of age who had been on the same dialysis modality (hemodialysis or peritoneal dialysis) for at least 3 months without a switch or underwent transplantation before the initiation of dialysis (pre-emptive kidney transplantation, PKT) were included. Patients who were living donor transplant, second KT or multiple organ transplants and lost to follow-up were excluded. Follow-up was terminated on August 2017. Finally data on 104 HD and 98 PD group met the inclusion criteria and were included for comparative outcome analysis. 5 PKT patients were analyzed as the control group (Fig. 1).

The protocol of this study was reviewed and approved by the Ethics Committee of Renji hospital, and patients were included only after signing informed consent.

Data source

Donor variables included age, gender, BMI, blood group, percentage of hypertension, mean time of intensive care unit(ICU) stay, HLA mismatching, estimated glomerular filtration rate (eGFR) and the causes of death. The baseline variables of recipients in two groups of patients on hemodialysis or peritoneal dialysis included age, gender, body mass index (BMI), blood group, duration time on pretransplant dialysis, post-transplant hospital stay and follow-up time, preoperative medical condition, percentage of anti-hypertensive drugs required, percentage

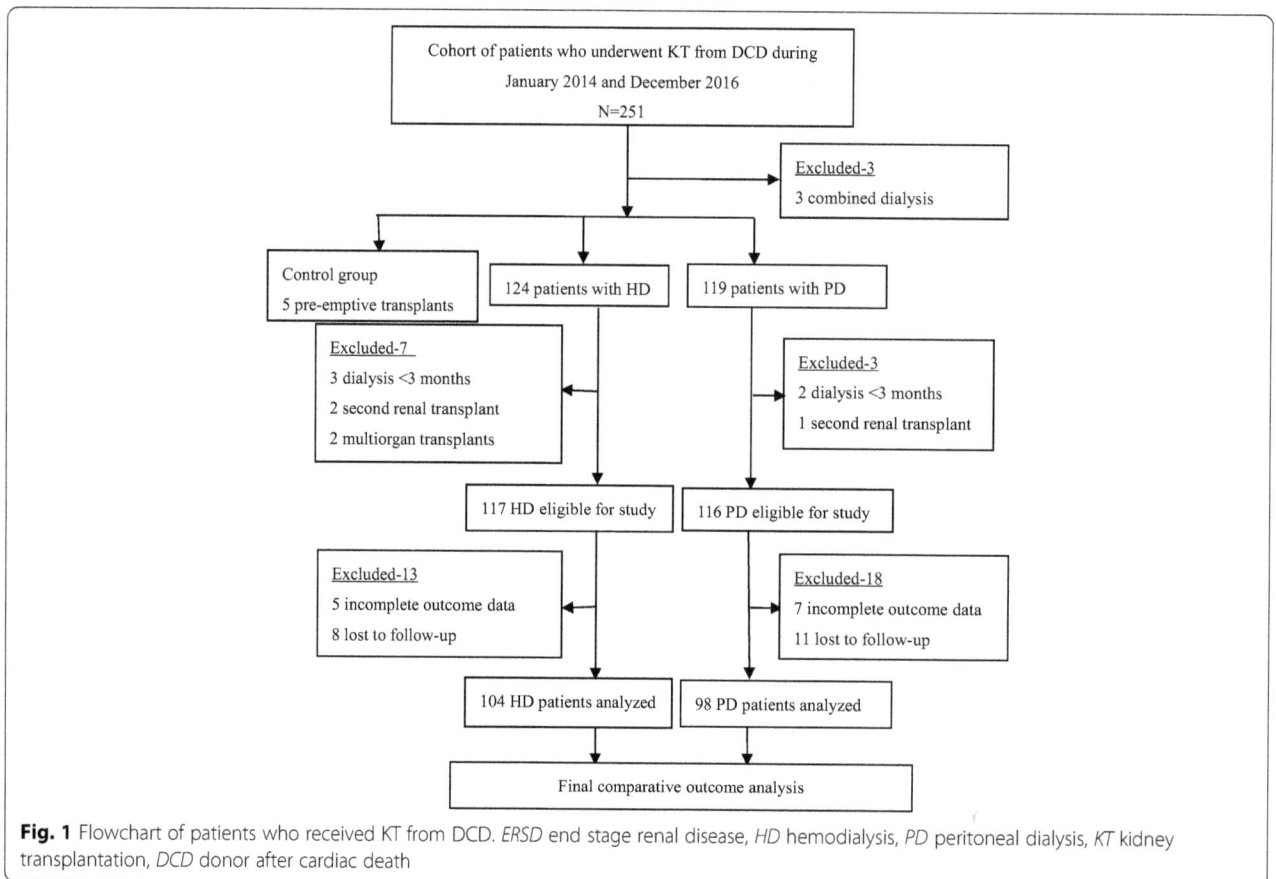

Fig. 1 Flowchart of patients who received KT from DCD. *ERSD* end stage renal disease, *HD* hemodialysis, *PD* peritoneal dialysis, *KT* kidney transplantation, *DCD* donor after cardiac death

Effects of pretransplant peritoneal vs hemodialysis modality on outcome of first kidney transplantation...

3

of hepatitis B virus (HBV) infection, native kidney diseases, pretransplant urinary volume, percentage of anuric patients and immunosuppresion therapy. The laboratory parameters of white blood cell count, creatinine, cholesterol, triglyceride of both donors and recipients were collected. The percentage of neutrophilic granulocyte and lymphocyte, haemoglobin, serum urea nitrogen, serum uric acid, serum albumin, alanine aminotransferase (ALT), blood glucose, serum potassium, serum sodium, parathyroid hormone, serum calcium, serum phosphate, low-density lipoprotein (LDL), high-density lipoprotein (HDL), and lymphocyte subtypes were also obtained from recipients. Among which the eGFR was estimated using the chronic kidney disease epidemiology collaboration (CKD-EPI) equation which was calculated according to the gender, the serum creatinine, the age and the race.

Post-transplant variables included renal function (serum creatinine, 24 h urine volume and the eGFR), haemoglobin, serum albumin, cholesterol, triglyceride, serum calcium and serum phosphate. The postoperative complications during hospitalization of delayed graft function (DGF), acute rejection (AR) and surgical complications including the urinary-fistula, hydronephrosis and hematoma after tranplantation were recorded. The infective complications including viral infection(cytomegalovirus, JC virus, BK virus, varicella zoster virus), fungal infection as well as bacterial infection(tuberculosis, urinary tract infection, acute bacterial pneumonia, gastrointestinal infection) were recorded during hospitalization and the whole follow-up time.

Table 1 Demography and Clinical Characteristics of ESRD patients on pretransplant pre-emptive, HD or PD who received KT from DCD

Characteristics	PKT group (n = 5)	HD group (n = 104)	PD group (n = 98)	p-value
Age(years)	36.2 ± 10.1	42.4 ± 9.7	39.5 ± 11.6	0.053
Male, n (%)	4(80.0)	65(62.5)	56(57.1)	0.437
BMI (kg/m^2)	22.1(20.2,26.1)	21.2(18.9,23.6)	21.5(19.9,23.8)	0.470
Blood group (A:B:AB:O)	2:2:0:1	27:26:13:38	27:29:8:34	0.706
Duration on dialysis (months)	0(0,0)	15.5(6.0,36.0)	24.0(6.0,36.0)	0.583
Hospital stay (days)	17.0(12.5,19.5)	20.0(15.0,26.0)	18.5(15.0,29.0)	0.337
Follow-up time (months)	19.0(10.5,35.0)	12.5(3.0,22.0)	12.0(6.0,20.0)	0.961
Preoperative medical condition, n (%)				
Diabetes mellitus	0(0)	13(12.5)	6(6.1)	0.121
Cardiovascular disease	0(0)	5(4.8)	2(2.0)	0.490
Hypertension	5(100)	91(87.5)	90(91.8)	0.313
Antihypertensive agents, n (%)	5(100)	76(73.1)	75(76.5)	0.572
HBV (+)	0(0)	9(8.7)	8(8.2)	0.900
Cause of end-stage renal disease, n (%)				0.188
Glomerulonephritis	4(80)	68(64.8)	64(66.0)	
Diabetes	0(0)	5(4.8)	1(1.0)	
Hypertensive nephrosclerosis	0(0)	2(1.9)	1(1.0)	
Polycystic kidney disease	1(20)	6(5.7)	1(1.0)	
Chronic pyelonephritis	0(0)	1(1.0)	2(2.1)	
Others	0(0)	2(1.9)	6(6.2)	
Unknown	0(0)	21(20.0)	22(22.7)	
Pretransplant urinary volume (ml/24 h)	2000(1750,2000)	200(100,500)	500(100,1000)	0.073
Anuric patients (%)	0(0)	19(18.3)	18(18.4)	0.986
Immunosuppresion therapy, n (%)				0.310
St + FK + MMF	5(100)	97(93.3)	95(96.9)	
St + CyA	0(0)	2(1.9)	0(0)	
St + CyA + MMF	0(0)	5(4.8)	3(3.1)	

P-value, between hemodialysis and peritoneal dialysis group

ERSD end stage renal disease, HD hemodialysis, PD peritoneal dialysis, PKT pre-emptive kidney transplantation, KT kidney transplantation, DCD donor after cardiac death, BMI body mass index, HBV hepatitis B virus, St steroids, FK tacrolimus, MMF mofetil mycofenolate, CyA cyclosporine A

The DGF was defined as the requirement for dialysis in the first week after transplantation, or serum creatinine level increased, remained unchanged, or decreased by less than 10% per day immediately after surgery [14, 15]. All patients with biopsy-proven acute rejection and those with features of antibody-mediated rejection, with borderline changes and allograft dysfunction who received treatment for acute rejection were considered to have rejection [14, 15]. The patient, graft and death-censored graft survival were compared between HD and PD groups. The causes of patient mortality and graft failure were recorded. Death-censored graft failure was defined as suffering graft failure without death.

Statistical methods

The statistical analysis was performed by using the SPSS 22 version software. All numeric variables were tested for normality of their distribution. Independent samples t-test and Mann-Whitney U test were respectively used for analyzing data whose distribution are normal and abnormal. Results are described as mean ± standard deviations (SD) for normally distributed data, median and interquartile range (IQR, pp. 25–75) for abnormally distributed data. The Chi square or Fisher's exact tests was utilized to compare the categorical variables between the two groups. The results were expressed in numbers and relative frequencies [n(%)].

The patient and graft survival were calculated from the date of transplantation to the endpoints of the study. The univariate and multivariate analysis were conducted for risk factors for graft failure in HD and PD groups. The univariate analysis was conducted to study the risk factors of patient mortality and graft failure. Variables whose $p < 0.05$ in the univariate analysis or clinical meaningful were enrolled into multivariate analysis. The cox proportional regression models were used to assess the relative risks.

Variables of p values < 0.05 were considered to be statistically significant. All statistical tests were two-tailed.

Table 2 Pretransplant Laboratory Parameters of Kidney Recipients

Laboratory Parameters	PKT group (n = 5)	HD group (n = 104)	PD group (n = 98)	p-value
Serum white blood cell (10^9/L)	6.2 ± 1.4	7.1 ± 1.8	7.1 ± 2.0	0.832
Neut %	62.6 ± 8.2	68.1 ± 7.4	68.8 ± 8.6	0.539
Lymph%	21.6(19.6,31.0)	21.6(17.4,26.2)	20.5(15.8,26.0)	0.168
Haemoglobin (g/L)	101.4 ± 8.9	115.8 ± 19.8	105.1 ± 18.7	< 0.001*
Serum potassium (mmol/L)	3.5(2.9,4.3)	4.3(3.9,4.8)	3.8(3.3,4.3)	< 0.001*
Serum sodium (mmol/L)	140.0(137.5142.0)	139.0(138.0,141.0)	139.0(136.0,141.0)	0.213
PTH (pg/ml)	202.4(149.7707.4)	221.0(87.8431.2)	216.3(134.1469.0)	0.198
Serum calcium (mmol/L)	2.1 ± 0.2	2.4 ± 0.2	2.3 ± 0.2	0.008*
Serum phosphate (mmol/L)	1.8(1.7,3.0)	1.7(1.3,2.3)	1.8(1.3,2.3)	0.864
Serum creatinine (umol/L)	751.0(706.5785.3)	827.2(647.0,1068.0)	1104.1(827.8,1426.7)	< 0.001*
Serum urea nitrogen (mmol/L)	36.1 ± 13.7	18.7 ± 6.6	21.9 ± 6.4	0.001*
Serum uric acid (μmol/L)	533.0(372.5642.0)	346.0(290.3424.5)	408.5(384.8462.5)	< 0.001*
Serum albumin (g/L)	48.9 ± 4.2	48.4 ± 4.4	42.7 ± 4.3	< 0.001*
ALT(U/L)	14.0(7.0,19.4)	14.0(9.7,20.0)	16.0(11.0,20.5)	0.151
Blood Glucose (mmol/L)	4.5(3.3,5.9)	4.4(3.8,4.9)	4.3(3.6,5.0)	0.983
Cholesterol (mmol/L)	4.3 ± 0.9	4.8 ± 1.1	5.1 ± 1.2	0.086
Triglyceride (mmol/L)	1.8(1.2,3.7)	1.6(1.1,2.9)	1.7(1.2,2.6)	0.683
LDL (mmol/L)	2.1(2.0,2.8)	2.5(2.2,3.1)	2.9(2.2,3.6)	0.057
HDL (mmol/L)	1.0(0.9,1.2)	1.1(0.9,1.6)	1.1(0.9,1.4)	0.675
Lymphocyte subtypes(%)				
CD3$^+$(%)	76.3(70.2,84.2)	70.8(62.9, 76.6)	71.0(66.0, 75.9)	0.868
CD4$^+$/CD8$^+$	1.7(1.2,1.9)	1.6(1.2, 2.1)	1.6(1.2, 2.0)	0.766
CD19$^+$(%)	6.8(5.5,11.0)	11.1(7.7, 13.6)	9.5(7.2, 13.8)	0.636
CD16$^+$CD56$^+$(%)	13.1(6.8,18.2)	14.6(9.9, 19.2)	5.6(10.1, 19.5)	0.742

P-value, between hemodialysis and peritoneal dialysis group; *, statistically significant
PKT pre-emptive kidney transplantation, HD hemodialysis, PD peritoneal dialysis, PT parathyroid hormone, ALT alanine aminotransferase, LDL low-density lipoprotein, HDL high-density lipoprotein

Table 3 Demography and Clinical Characteristics of Kidney Donors after Cardiac Death (DCD)

Characteristics	Donated to PKT (n = 5)	Donated to HD (n = 79)	Donated to PD (n = 83)	p-value
Age(years)	42.8 ± 17.0	40.3 ± 13.7	37.7 ± 16.5	0.451
Male, n (%)	5(100.0)	52(65.8)	62(74.7)	0.216
BMI (kg/m^2)	21.8(20.4,26.5)	21.5(19.5,23.0)	21.2(19.8,24.0)	0.972
Blood group (A:B:AB:O)	2:2:0:1	13:20:9:37	18:23:11:31	0.649
Hypertension(%)	2(40.0)	36(41.8)	25(34.4)	0.355
ICU stay	2.0(1.5,21.0)	2.0(1.5,4.0)	2.0(1.0,4.5)	0.510
HLA mismatching				0.098
0–2	3(60.0)	23(29.1)	13(15.7)	
3–4	1(20.0)	8(10.1)	13(15.7)	
5–6	1(20.0)	48(60.8)	57(68.7)	
Serum white blood cell (10^9/L)	12.7 ± 9.0	12.2 ± 5.7	14.6 ± 9.9	0.424
Serum creatinine (umol/L)	64.1(36.5,65.5)	67.5(48.7107.3)	74.0(48.0,95.0)	0.947
Cholesterol (mmol/L)	3.3 ± 1.1	3.2 ± 1.3	3.7 ± 1.6	0.429
Triglyceride (mmol/L)	1.2 ± 0.6	1.4 ± 0.7	1.3 ± 0.8	0.830
eGFR(mL/min/1.73m^2)	110.0(98.0,133.0)	129.4(72.1215.2)	109.5(72.8209.0)	0.930
Cause of death,n (%)				0.179
Cerebrovascular accident	2(40.0)	27(34.6)	28(37.3)	
Trauma	3(60.0)	23(29.5)	26(34.7)	
Cerebral tumor	0(0)	3(3.8)	2(2.7)	
Others	0(0)	3(3.8)	8(10.7)	
Unknown	0(0)	22(28.2)	11(14.7)	

P-value, between hemodialysis and peritoneal dialysis group

PKT pre-emptive kidney transplantation, HD hemodialysis, PD peritoneal dialysis, ICU intensive care unit, eGFR estimated glomerular filtration rate

Results

Baseline clinical characteristics

The baseline information of recipients and donors in HD, PD and PKT group was analyzed. Among them, PKT group was analyzed as the control group. Patients in both PD and HD groups were comparable for demographic and clinical characteristics (Table 1). The pretransplant laboratory parameters in PD group were lower compared with HD group with regard to haemoglobin, serum albumin, serum potassium and serum calcium ($p < 0.05$). On the contrary, the serum creatinine, serum urea nitrogen and serum uric acid were higher in PD group ($p < 0.05$) (Table 2). Donors characteristics was comparable for recipient in both PD and HD groups (Table 3).

Post-transplant renal function outcomes

The post-transplant renal function outcomes of PKT were labeled as control. In view of the HD and PD group, the post-transplant serum creatinine showed no differences throughout the follow-up between the HD and PD groups ($p > 0.05$) (Fig. 2). Pretransplant serum creatinine was higher in PD patients ($p < 0.05$). There was no differences ($p = 0.210$) in serum creatinine reduction to half of baseline in two groups, with 1.0 (1.0, 2.0) d in HD

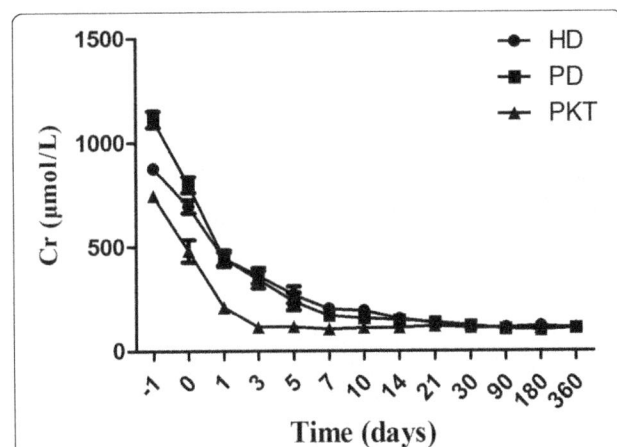

Fig. 2 The serum creatinine from pretransplant to 1 year after transplantation in PD, HD and PKT. The horizontal ordinate refers to the pretransplant time (– 1) as well as post transplantation follow-up time. The baseline serum creatinine level is higher in PD patients compared with HD patients ($p < 0.05$). During the follow-up time, the serum creatinine level had no differences between the HD and PD groups ($p > 0.05$). PKT group was used as the control group. Data were expressed as means±S.E

and 1.0 (1.0, 1.3) d in PD group. The serum creatinine levels at different post-transplant time points reduced statistically compared to pretransplant, which were coherent between the HD and PD groups ($p < 0.001$). There were significant differences in serum creatinine at different time points throughout the follow-up within two groups ($p < 0.001$). The 24-h urinary volume remained similar between the two groups during the follow-up period ($p > 0.05$) (Fig. 3). The mean eGFR at 1 month (68.52 ± 23.72 vs 68.04 ± 28.66, $p = 0.902$), 6 month (68.45 ± 23.15 vs 74.85 ± 22.87, $p = 0.167$) and last follow-up (69.74 ± 24.65 vs 68.54 ± 26.01, $p = 0.737$) were also similar between the two groups (Table 4).

Other laboratory parameters post transplantation

Triglyceride levels at 6 months post transplantation were significantly higher in the PD group [PD: 2.1(1.8,2.5) vs HD:1.6 (1.2,2.1), $p = 0.010$]. At other time points the triglyceride levels were similar in two groups. There were no statistical differences between PD and HD patients in haemoglobin, serum albumin, cholesterol, triglyceride, serum calcium and serum phosphate levels throughout the follow-up period (Table 4).

Post-transplant complications

There were only 2 infective complications in PKT group. For HD and PD group, the hyperacute rejection didn't appear in both groups. The acute rejection rate in HD group [6.7% (7/104)] were similar to PD group [6.1% (6/98)] ($p = 0.860$). There were total 35 patients (17.3%) with DGF, 19 patients (18.3%) in HD and 16 (16.3%) in PD group. Statistically no significant differences ($p = 0.715$).

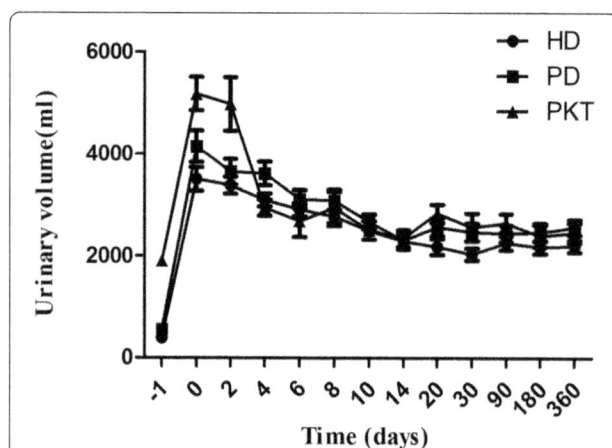

Fig. 3 The urinary volume from pretransplant to 1 year after transplantation in PD, HD and PKT. The horizontal ordinate refers to the pretransplant time (− 1) as well as post transplantation follow-up time. During the whole follow-up period as well as pretransplant time, the urinary volume remained similar between the HD and PD patients ($p > 0.05$).PKT group was used as the control group. Data were expressed as means±S.E

Table 4 Post Kidney Transplant Laboratory Parameters of the Recipients

Characteristics	PKT group (n = 5)	HD group (n = 104)	PD group (n = 98)	P-value
Haemoglobin after transplantation at different time (g/L)				
1 month	115.6 ± 14.6	108.0 ± 20.1	103.7 ± 22.8	0.210
6 months	129.4 ± 10.1	125.3 ± 21.7	133.5 ± 20.8	0.059
The last follow-up	135.0 ± 17.8	125.2 ± 28.9	126.2 ± 26.6	0.817
Serum albumin after transplantation at different time (g/L)				
1 month	46.5 ± 2.0	42.3 ± 4.4	41.6 ± 5.3	0.394
6 months	46.9 ± 2.0	44.9 ± 3.4	45.3 ± 4.0	0.537
The last follow-up	46.1 ± 3.3	43.6 ± 5.2	43.6 ± 5.6	0.951
Cholesterol after transplantation at different time (mmol/L)				
1 month	4.9 ± 1.1	4.9 ± 1.4	4.8 ± 1.1	0.477
6 months	4.4 ± 0.5	4.8 ± 0.9	5.2 ± 0.9	0.064
The last follow-up	4.0 ± 0.8	4.8 ± 1.1	4.9 ± 1.0	0.655
Triglyceride after transplantation at different time (mmol/L)				
1 month	2.3(1.1,4.4)	1.8(1.5,2.6)	2.0(1.5,2.8)	0.533
6 months	1.5(1.1,3.0)	1.6(1.2,2.1)	2.1(1.8,2.5)	0.010*
The last follow-up	1.1(1.0,2.8)	1.6(1.1,2.3)	1.9(1.2,2.5)	0.106
Serum calcium after transplantation at different time (mmol/L)				
1 month	2.4(2.3,2.5)	2.3(2.2,2.4)	2.3(2.3,2.4)	0.374
6 months	2.4(2.2,2.7)	2.5(2.3,2.6)	2.4(2.4,2.7)	0.950
The last follow-up	2.4(2.2,2.5)	2.5(2.3,2.5)	2.4(2.3,2.6)	0.899
Serum phosphate after transplantation at different time (mmol/L)				
1 month	0.7(0.4,0.9)	0.6(0.5,0.8)	0.7(0.5,0.9)	0.291
6 months	0.9(0.9,1.2)	1.0(0.8,1.1)	0.9(0.8,1.1)	0.138
The last follow-up	0.9(0.9,1.1)	1.0(0.8,1.1)	0.9(0.8,1.1)	0.079
eGFR after transplantation at different time (mL/min/1.73m²)				
1 month	63.1 ± 13.8	68.5 ± 23.7	68.0 ± 28.7	0.902
6 month	58.0 ± 8.7	68.5 ± 23.2	74.9 ± 22.9	0.167
The last follow-up	57.0 ± 10.3	69.7 ± 24.7	68.5 ± 26.0	0.737

P-value, between hemodialysis and peritoneal dialysis group; *, statistically significant
PKT pre-emptive kidney transplantation, HD hemodialysis, PD peritoneal dialysis

Surgical and infective complications throughout the hospitalization and follow-up period were did not differ between two groups (Table 5).

Patient mortality and graft failure

There were no death and graft failure in PKT group. There were total 7 deaths, 4 in the HD and 3 in the PD group. The patient survival rate between two groups showed no significant differences ($p = 1.000$). There were 13 graft failure, 7 in HD and 6 in PD group, and causes of graft failure were statistically different between two groups ($p < 0.001$). The graft survival rates were similar

Table 5 Post Kidney Transplant Complications

Complications	PKT group (n = 5)	HD group (n = 104)	PD group (n = 98)	P-value
Delayed recovery of graft function, n (%)	0(0)	19(18.3)	16(16.3)	0.715
Acute rejection, n (%)	0(0)	7(6.7)	6(6.1)	0.860
Surgical complications, n (%)				
Urinaryfistula	0(0)	1(1.0)	1(1.0)	1.000
Hydronephrosis	0(0)	6(5.8)	4(4.1)	0.820
Hematoma	0(0)	4(3.8)	4(4.1)	1.000
Infection, n (%)				
Cytomegalovirus	0(0)	21(20.2)	20(20.4)	0.970
JC virus	0(0)	13(12.5)	13(13.3)	0.871
BK virus	0(0)	17(16.3)	15(15.3)	0.840
Varicella zoster virus	0(0)	0(0)	1(1.0)	0.485
Fungal infectio	0(0)	4(3.8)	5(5.1)	0.927
Tuberculosis	0(0)	2(1.9)	0(0)	0.498
Urinary tract infection	1(20.0)	7(6.7)	11(11.2)	0.263
Acute bacterial pneumonia	1(20.0)	17(16.3)	12(12.2)	0.406

P-value, between hemodialysis and peritoneal dialysis group
PKT pre-emptive kidney transplantation, HD hemodialysis, PD peritoneal dialysis

between the two groups (p = 0.860). The death-censored graft failure i.e. graft failure without death (3 in each of HD and PD group) was not different between the two groups (p = 1.000) (Table 6).

The cox proportional hazards model showed pretransplant dialysis modality (HD and PD) had no correlation with patient survival or graft failure or death-censored graft survival After adjusting for other related multiple risk factors, the PD patients had similar rates of graft failure compared with HD in multivariate cox proportional hazards analysis (Table 7). When separately analyzed for HD and PD groups, the surgical complications in HD

patients were independent stimulating factors of graft failure and DGF was an independent factor inversely correlated with graft survival in PD patients (Table 8).

Discussion

Up to 30–40% of patients are can be effectively treated by PD, far away from current 11% [16] and many suitable PD candidates are treated with HD [17]. The use of PD is lower than HD owing to the aging of dialysis population, comorbidity and social conditions that make home PD difficult. More studies are needed to

Table 6 The Patient and Graft Survival Rates throughout Follow-up Time and the Causes of Graft Failure

Characteristics	PKT group (n = 5)	HD group (n = 104)	PD group (n = 98)	p-value
Transplatation outcomes, %(n)				
Patient survival	100.0(5/5)	96.2(100/104)	96.9(95/98)	1.000
Graft survival	100.0(5/5)	93.3(97/104)	93.9(92/98)	0.860
Death-censored graft survival	100.0(5/5)	97.1(101/104)	96.9(95/98)	1.000
Causes of graft failure, % (n)				< 0.001*
Acute rejection	0(0/0)	0(0/7)	28.6(2/7)	
Severe infection	0(0/0)	28.6(2/7)	57.1(4/7)	
Primary failure	0(0/0)	0(0/7)	14.3(1/7)	
Surgical complications	0(0/0)	57.1(4/7)	0(0/7)	
Others	0(0/0)	14.3(1/7)	0(0/7)	

P-value, between hemodialysis and peritoneal dialysis group; *, statistically significant
PKT pre-emptive kidney transplantation, HD hemodialysis, PD peritoneal dialysis

Table 7 The Univariate and Multivariate Analysis for Effects of HD vs PD and Other Factors on Outcomes of Non-preemptive Kidney Transplantation

Death	Univariate analysis			Multivariate analysis		
	P	RR	95%CI	P	RR	95%CI
HD vs PD	0.977	1.02	0.23-4.57	0.977		
Younger recipient age	0.071	1.07	0.99-1.16	0.062		
Male (vs female)	0.134	0.29	0.06-1.47	0.109		
Smaller BMI	0.100	1.08	0.99-1.18			
Shorter dialysis duration	0.828	1.00	0.98-1.03	0.828		
DGF	0.126	3.23	0.72-14.43			
Surgical complications	0.224	3.73	0.45-30.97			
Acute rejection	0.499	2.07	0.25-17.23			
Infection	0.123	3.64	0.71-18.75			

0 1 2 3 4 5

Graft failure	Univariate analysis			Multivariate analysis		
	P	RR	95%CI	P	RR	95%CI
HD vs PD	0.808	0.87	0.29-2.60	0.637		
Younger recipient age	0.322	1.03	0.98-1.08	0.124		
Male (vs female)	0.015	0.20	0.06-0.74	0.048	0.27	0.07-0.99
Smaller BMI	0.882	0.99	0.86-1.14			
Shorter dialysis duration	0.839	1.00	0.98-1.02	0.381		
DGF	<0.001	7.50	2.45-22.93	0.005	5.27	1.64-16.96
Surgical complications	0.002	7.70	2.10-28.16	0.038	4.18	1.08-16.21
Acute rejection	0.283	2.28	0.51-10.30			
Infection	0.352	1.68	0.57-5.00			

0 1 2 3 4 5

Death-censored Graft failure	Univariate analysis			Multivariate analysis		
	P	RR	95%CI	P	RR	95%CI
HD vs PD	0.690	0.72	0.15-3.58	0.613		
Younger recipient age	0.646	0.98	0.91-1.06	0.174		
Male (vs female)	0.062	0.13	0.02-1.11	0.327		
Smaller BMI	0.016	0.63	0.43-0.92	0.010	0.53	0.33-0.86
Shorter dialysis duration	0.622	0.99	0.95-1.03	0.246		
DGF	0.003	24.52	2.87-209.91	0.011	16.69	1.90-146.57
Surgical complications	0.003	13.10	2.38-72.08	0.006	19.63	2.30-167.43
Acute rejection	0.377	2.63	0.31-22.54			
Infection	0.741	0.75	0.14-34.10			

0 1 2 3 4 5

HD hemodialysis, *PD* peritoneal dialysis, *P* p value, *RR* relative risk, *CI* confidence interval, *BMI* body mass index, *DGF* delayed graft failure

clarify the identical or even better function of PD compared with HD.

Our results indicated both the immediate and long-term renal function, the serum creatinine and urine output, were similar between the HD and PD, consistent with other studies [6, 11]. In our study, the baseline serum creatinine was higher in PD than HD patients. The HD just before the transplantation could have lowered the serum creatinine. In contrast, PD lowers creatinine in moderate ways and high baseline serum creatinine in PD patients doesn't mean it is inferior to HD in creatinine reduction. This could be the reason why both groups had similar renal function after transplantation.

We had no significant differences in the incidence of AR, which is in line with recent studies [3, 6, 11, 12]. This may be due to the availability of and rational novel immunosuppressive protocols nowadays. Our study shows similar incidence of DGF in both PD and HD patients, as reported by others [6, 10]. We also found that DGF was inversely associated with the graft survival and death-censored graft survival regardless of dialysis modality. The DGF is associated with greater risk of patient death in addition to graft and death-censored graft failure [18]. Ischemic-reperfusion of donated kidney caused by post-ischemic acute tubular necrosis and interstitial inflammation results in DGF [19]. The PD patients has lower

Table 8 Univariate and Multivariate Analysis for Effects of Factors on Graft Failure of Kidney for Non-preemptive Transplantation According to Dialysis Modality

	Univariate analysis			Multivariate analysis		
	P	RR	95% CI	P	RR	95% CI
Graft failure in HD						
Younger recipient age	0.731	0.99	0.92–1.06	0.947		
Male (vs female)	0.100	0.25	0.05–1.30	0.290		
Smaller BMI	0.761	1.02	0.89–1.17			
Shorter dialysis duration	0.211	0.96	0.91–1.02	0.250		
DGF	0.017	6.23	1.40–27.85	0.588		
Surgical complications	< 0.001	26.12	5.70–119.80	< 0.001	26.12	5.70–119.80
Acute rejection	0.629	0.044	–			
Infection	0.472	0.55	0.11–2.83			
Graft failure in PD						
Younger recipient age	0.071	1.06	0.99–1.15	0.105		
Male (vs female)	0.084	0.15	0.02–1.29	0.112		
Smaller BMI	0.420	0.88	0.64–1.20			
Shorter dialysis duration	0.373	1.01	0.99–1.04	0.962		
DGF	0.010	9.39	1.72–51.29	0.010	9.39	1.72–51.29
Surgical complications	0.700	0.05	–	0.708		
Acute rejection	0.036	6.15	1.12–33.67			
Infection	0.058	7.96	0.93–68.11			

HD hemodialysis, PD peritoneal dialysis, P p value, RR relative risk, CI confidence interval, BMI body mass index, DG delayed graft failure

incidence of DGF in comparison with the HD [9, 11, 12]. This could be due to better hydration status and preservation of residual renal function (RRF) in PD patients [13]. Additionally, the PD patients has less oxidative stress which can exacerbate ischemic-reperfusion injury in kidney compared with HD patients [20].

Our results shows similar patient, graft and death-censored graft survival rate in PD and HD groups, consistent with most other studies [5, 6, 12]. Earlier, in a large cohort study of 22,776 patients concluded a higher rate of early graft failure (during the first 3 months after KT) in PD, possibly due to higher incidence of early graft thrombosis [18]. While the long-term graft failure and patient mortality remained similar. Some studies report PD had better patient survival, better quality of life, better nutritional status and fewer blood transfusions [9–11]. The differences might be associated with the different sample size and the follow-up time.

Some of the limitations of our study could be a single-center and inclusion of first transplantation from DCD only may not be applicable to all renal transplantations. In addition, the study variables of donors were incomplete, with some statistically analysis based on the less data compared to recipients. Besides, the pre-emptive kidney transplantation group in the cohort had only 5 patients, with people too less to be statistically comparative analyzed, finally simply summarized and displayed as the control

group. And the follow-up period was not long enough, with further study and investigations to go on.

Conclusions

The choice of dialysis modality, HD or PD, prior to kidney transplantation had no influences on the patient, graft and death-censored graft survival. The immediate and long-term complications after transplantation, and renal function between the two groups were similar. Thus we can conclude that PD is equally good with potential for wider applicability as pretransplant modality of dialysis.

Abbreviations
ALT: Alanine aminotransferase; AR: Acute rejection; BMI: Body mass index; CyA: Cyclosporine A; DCD: Donor after cardiac death; DGF: Delayed graft function; eGFR: Estimated glomerular filtration rate; ESRD: End-stage renal disease; FK: Tacrolimus; HBV: Hepatitis B virus; HD: Hemodialysis; HDL: High-density lipoprotein; ICU: Intensive care unit; KT: Kidney transplantation; LDL: Low-density lipoprotein; MMF: Mofetil mycofenolate; P: p value; PD: Peritoneal dialysis; PKT: Pre-emptive kidney transplantation; PTH: Parathyroid hormone; RR: Relative risk; SD: Standard deviations; St: Steroids

Funding
This work was supported in part by the National Natural Science Foundation of China (81573748, 81770668). The study was sponsored by the Program of Shanghai Academic Research Leader (16XD1401900) as well as by a grant ([2017]485) from the Shanghai Leadership Training Program in 2017. The funding bodies did not contribute to the design of the study, collection, analysis, and interpretation of data, and in manuscript writing.

Authors' contributions

We thank all of the authors at the Ren Ji Hospital in Shanghai, China for their work. SM, XJC, XQY and JYY proposed the research idea and designed the study. XJC, XQY, JYY, YHY, QM, LY, MFZ, QW participated in data acquisition. XJC, XQY and JYY made substantial contributions to the analysis of data and were major contributors in writing the manuscript. XJC, SM, ZHN and MZ co-reviewed and revised the manuscript. All authors read and approved the final manuscript.

Competing interests

The authors declare that they have no competing interests.

References

1. Czyżewski L, Sańko-Resmer J, Wyzgał J, et al. Assessment of health-related quality of life of patients after kidney transplantation in comparison with hemodialysis and peritoneal dialysis. Ann Transplant. 2014;19:576–85.
2. Hourmant M, Garandeau C. The evolution of kidney transplantation over the last 20 years. Presse Med. 2011;40:1074–80.
3. Li PK, Chow KM, Van de Luijtgaarden MW, et al. Changes in the worldwide epidemiology of peritoneal dialysis. Nat Rev Nephrol. 2017;13:90–103.
4. Sezer S, Karakan S, Özdemir Acar FN, et al. Dialysis as a bridge therapy to renal transplantation: comparison of graft outcomes according to mode of dialysis treatment. Transplant Proc. 2011;43:485-7.
5. Kramer A, Jager KJ, Fogarty DG, et al. Association between pre-transplant dialysis modality and patient and graft survival after kidney transplantation. Nephrol Dial Transplant. 2012;27:4473–80.
6. Prasad N, Vardhan H, Baburaj VP, et al. Do the outcomes of living donor renal allograft recipients differ with peritoneal dialysis and hemodialysis as a bridge renal replacement therapy? Saudi J Kidney Dis Transpl. 2014;25:1202–9.
7. Neretljak I, Mihovilović K, Kovacević-Vojtusek I, et al. Effect of pretransplant dialysis modality on incidence of early posttransplant infections in kidney recipients. Acta Med Croatica. 2011;65(Suppl 3):58–62.
8. Issa N, Lankireddy S, Kukla A. Should peritoneal dialysis be the preferred therapy pre-kidney transplantation? Adv Perit Dial. 2012;28:89–93.
9. Tang M, Li T, Hong LA. Comparison of transplant outcomes in peritoneal and hemodialysis patients: a meta-analysis. Blood Purif. 2016;42:170–6.
10. Molnar MZ, Mehrotra R, Duong U, et al. Dialysis modality and outcomes in kidney transplant recipients. Clin J Am Soc Nephrol. 2012;7:332–41.
11. Lópezoliva MO, Rivas B, Pérezfernández E, et al. Pretransplant peritoneal dialysis relative to hemodialysis improves long-term survival of kidney transplant patients: a single-center observational study. Int Urol Nephrol. 2014;46:825–32.
12. Song SH, Lee JG, Lee J, et al. Outcomes of kidney recipients according to mode of Pretransplantation renal replacement therapy. Transplantation Proc. 2016;48:2461–3.
13. Domenici A, Comunian MC, Fazzari L, et al. Incremental peritoneal Dialysis Favourably compares with hemodialysis as a bridge to renal transplantation. Int J Nephrol. 2011;2011:204216.
14. Nagaraja P, Roberts GW, Stephens M, et al. Influence of delayed graft function and acute rejection on outcomes after kidney transplantation from donors after cardiac death. Transplantation. 2012;94:1218–23.
15. Wu WK, Famure O, Li Y, et al. Delayed graft function and the risk of acute rejection in the modern era of kidney transplantation. Kidney Int. 2015;88:851–8.
16. Giuliani A, Karopadi AN, Prieto-Velasco M, et al. Worldwide experiences with assisted peritoneal Dialysis. Perit Dial Int. 2017;37:503–8.
17. Mendelssohn DC. A skeptical view of assisted home peritoneal dialysis. Kidney Int. 2007;71:602–4.
18. Snyder JJ, Kasiske BL, Gilbertson DT, et al. A comparison of transplant outcomes in peritoneal and hemodialysis patients. Kidney Int. 2002;63:1423–30.
19. Siedlecki A, Irish W, Brennan DC. Delayed graft function in the kidney transplant. Am J Transplant. 2011;11:2279–96.
20. Vostálová J, Galandáková A, Strebl P, et al. Oxidative stress in patients on regular hemodialysis and peritoneal dialysis. Vnitr Lek. 2012;58:466–72.

2

Incidence of glomerulonephritis and non-diabetic end-stage renal disease in a developing middle-east region near armed conflict

Alaa A Ali[1], Dana A Sharif[2], Safa E Almukhtar[3], Kais Hasan Abd[4], Zana Sidiq M Saleem[4] and Michael D Hughson[1*] (iD)

Abstract

Background: Estimates of the incidence of glomerulonephritis (GN) and end-stage renal disease (ESRD) in an Iraqi population are compared with the United States (US) and Jordan.

Methods: The study set consist of renal biopsies performed in 2012 and 2013 in the Kurdish provinces of Northern Iraq. The age specific and age standardized incidence of GN was calculated from the 2011 population. ESRD incidence was estimated from Sulaimaniyah dialysis center records of patient's inititating hemodialysis in 2017.

Results: At an annual biopsy rate of 7.8 per 100,000 persons in the Kurdish region, the number of diagnoses (2 years), the average age of diagnosis, and annual age standardized incidence (ASI)/100,000 for focal segmental glomerulosclerosis (FSGS) was $n = 135$, 27.3 ± 17.6 years, ASI = 1.6; and for all glomerulonephritis (GN) was $n = 384$, 30.4 ± 17.0 years, ASI = 5.1. FSGS represented 35% of GN biopsies, membranous glomerulonephritis 18%, systemic lupus erythematosus 13%, and immunoglobulin A nephropathy 7%. For FSGS and all GN, the peak age of diagnoses was 35–44 years of age with age specific rates declining after age 45. The unadjusted annual ESRD rate was 60 per million with an age specific peak at 55–64 years and a decline after age 65. The assigned cause of ESRD was 23% diabetes, 18% hypertension, and 12% GN with FSGS comprising 41% of biopsy-diagnosed, non-diabetic ESRD.

Conclusions: The regional incidence of ESRD in Northern Iraq is much lower than the crude incidences of 100 and 390 per million for Jordan and the US respectively. This is associated with low renal disease rates in the Iraqi elderly and an apparent major contribution of FSGS to ESRD.

Keywords: Glomerulonephritis, FSGS, ESRD, Middle-east, Iraq

Background

Chronic kidney disease (CKD) is being diagnosed with increased frequency worldwide [1–3]. Glomerulonephritis (GN) is a major cause of CKD but is estimated to account for only 10% of end-stage renal disease (ESRD) in the West and in the developed countries of Asia where more than 75% of ESRD is attributed to diabetes and hypertension [4, 5]. Many of the larger countries of the Middle-East are unable to collect comprehensive

data on kidney disease, and the incidence of CKD and the extent to which GN or diabetes contributes to ESRD are poorly defined [6].

The regional frequencies of different types of CKD are mainly determined by the proportions of diagnostic categories in biopsy series. These studies have shown that IgA nephropathy (IGAN) is the predominant form of CKD in many European and Asian populations but is rare among persons of African ancestry and, when compared to Europe, is relatively uncommon in the Middle-East [7, 8]. An increased frequency in the diagnoses of focal segmental glomerulosclerosis (FSGS) seems to have begun in the early 1980s in the United

* Correspondence: mhughson@bellsouth.net

[1]Department of Pathology, Shorsh General Hospital, Qirga Road, Sulaimaniyah, Kurdistan, Iraq

Full list of author information is available at the end of the article

States (US) and Brazil and in the 1990s in Singapore and India, and FSGS is now the major cause of nephrotic syndrome in many parts of the world [7, 9–12].

In the US and Australia, biopsy registries from well-defined populations have been used to estimate the incidence of specific types of glomerular diseases [13, 14]. In both countries, GN rates composed largely of IGAN and FSGS increased steadily with age, with the relative risk of GN, diabetes, and hypertension all contributing to a growing population of older ESRD patients.

The Middle-East is often considered a homogeneous region with respect to disease [15]. We question this assumption. Conflict has been a part of Iraqi life for nearly 30 years, and epidemiologic record keeping on non-communicable diseases other than cancer is only beginning to receive attention. This current study used a renal biopsy registry from the largely Kurdish population of Northern Iraq to investigate the incidence of the common forms of GN that might lead to ESRD. We also applied the proposals by Anand et al., [15], on the use and initiation of dialysis services as surrogates for prevalence and incidence of ESRD when regional or national data is not available. The findings are compared to Jordan, the adjacent country having a rigorous collection of nationwide data on ESRD, to assess how the findings in Northern Iraq might contribute to a better understanding about the variability of CKD in the region.

Methods

Data collection and calculation of age specific glomerulonephritis incidence

Study subjects consisted of patients having renal biopsies performed in the Kurdish region of Northern Iraq between Jan 1 2012 to Dec 31, 2013. This was the 2 year period before the large population dislocations caused by the ISIS conflict that began in March 2014. All biopsies were studied by light microscopy in 18 serial sections using hematoxylin and eosin, periodic acid-Shiff, Masson trichrome, and Jones methenamine stains, and by immunofluorescence microscopy with fluorescein conjugated anti-human IgG, IgM, IgA, C3, C1q, and albumin. Selected cases were sent off-site for electron microscopy. The 2011–2012 United Nations Iraq population data [16] and the 2012 Iraqi Cancer Registry [17] was used for estimates of the Kurdistan population in 5 year age ranges from 0 to 65+ years old. Age specific incidence per 100,000 population was calculated for focal segmental glomerulosclerosis (FSGS), membranous glomerulonephropathy (MGN), systemic lupus erythematosus nephritis (SLE), immunoglobulin A nephropathy (IGAN), and all glomerulonephritis (GN). Minimal change disease (MCD) was not included in all GN, because it generally contributes little to the risk of ESRD.

Kurdistan, Olmstead County, Minnesota, and Victoria, Australia standardized glomerulonephritis incidence calculations

The Olmstead County and Victoria studies [13, 14] were chosen for comparisons with Kurdistan, because they provided age standardized incidence rates or enough information that standardized incidence rates could be calculated. The United States (US) 2000 Census [18] was used for age adjustments for Kurdistan and Victoria because this was applied to the Olmsted county data.

Estimates of ESRD incidence in Sulaimaniyah governate; comparison with the kingdom of Jordan

The numbers of patients in 2017 who received dialysis at the regional centers in Sulaimainyah City were tabulated by age. Monthly records were searched for persons dialysed in prior months and for those initiating dialysis. An annual average for all dialysed persons and for persons initiating dialysis was calculated from monthly data. The centers served a catchment area of an estimated 1,310,000 persons having an age distribution similar to that of the rest of the Kurdish region. Crude (unadjusted), age specific, and age adjusted incidence rates were determined. Data from the National Registry of End-Stage Renal Disease of the Kingdom of Jordan was compared with Kurdistan [19].

Results

Analysis of the Kurdistan 2012 and 2013 biopsies

Biopsies of 763 native kidneys were received in the 2-year period, 622 of the biopsies were satisfactory for specific diagnoses that are listed in Table 1. The indicated reasons for the biopsies were nephrotic syndrome 52%, proteinuria and hematuria 31%, hematuria without proteinuria 5%, renal insufficiency 7%, and unspecified 1%.

FSGS was the most frequent diagnosis at 22%, followed by MCD at 13%, and MGN at 11%. SLE, IGAN, crescentic GN, and end-stage chronic glomerulonephritis not otherwise specified (CGN-NOS) represented 8, 5, 4 and 4% of the biopsies respectively. CGN-NOS demonstrated globally solidified glomeruli with non-specific immunofluorescence staining and was thought to largely represent late-stage FSGS. Tubulointerstitial nephritis (TIN) comprised 7% of the biopsies, and chronic kidney disease not otherwise specified (CKD-NOS) was found in 10 cases (1.6%) that had interstitial fibrosis and tubular atrophy but with little inflammation and no glomerular disease. GN that included HUS was diagnosed in 384 biopsies. The age of 66% of GN patients fell between 19 to 41 years old with 24% being ≤14 and 9% being ≥55 years old (Table 2). Overall, the sex distribution was nearly equal, but this varied with disease. SLE was predominantly female (84%), and IGAN predominantly male (61%).

Table 1 2012–2013 renal biopsy diagnoses. Sub-types of diseases are listed

Diagnosis	n	Male	Age (years)	Subtypes (n)
MCD	82	58%	21.5 ± 15.8	IgMN(2), FGGS(4)
FSGS	135	53%	27.3 ± 17.6	Collapsing(2)
MGN	71	46%	37.1 ± 15.0	
SLE	51	16%	30.5 ± 11.8	Class I (3), II(3), III(9), IV(23), V(10), VI(3)
IGAN	28	61%	29.5 ± 17.0	Haas class I(3), II(8), III(7), IV(3), V(3), HSP(4)
Crescentic GN	26	54%	37.1 ± 19.8	Pauci-immune(21); crescentic class(6), mixed class(8), sclerotic class(7). AGBMD(2), ICD(3)
MPGN	12	75%	37.8 ± 20.3	Type 1(11), type2(0), cryoglobulinemia-associated(1)
PSGN	10	80%	18.0 ± 19.5	
Other GN	18	56%	29.9 ± 14.4	MePGN(13), C1qN(2), fibril GN(1), diffuse mesangial sclerosis(1) Obesity-associated glomerulomegaly(1)
CGN-NOS	24	71%	27.2 ± 14.0	
HUS	9	55%	29.0 ± 20.5	D+ (3), APL(1), PP(2)
TIN	46	55%	32.9 ± 20.4	acute pyelonephritis(6)
arteriolosclerosis	52	48%	49.6 ± 15.2	
Amyloidosis AL	2	40%	55.5 ± 0.7	Myeloma(2)
Amyloidosis AA	19	40%	40.2 ± 23.4	RA(4), JRA(3), arthritis(2), SLE (1), FMF(1), asthma(1), bronchiectasis(3), unknown(4).
Myeloma kidney	4	50%	59.3 ± 7.7	
Diabetes	5	40%	47.0 ± 6.4	
Other non-glomerular	28	46%	29.7 ± 14.7	Acute kidney injury(14),basement membrane disease(2) CKD NOS (10), Fabry's(1), scleroderma(1)
total	622	51%	30.2 ± 18.6	

Abbreviations: *MCD* minimal change disease, *FSGS* focal segmental glomerulosclerosis, *MGN* membranous glomerulonephritis (GN), *SLE* lupus nephritis, *IGAN* immunoglobulin A nephropathy, *MPGN* membranoproliferative GN, *PSGN* post-streptococcal GN, *CGN-NOS ESRD* end-stage chronic GN not otherwise specified, *HUS* hemolytic uremic syndrome, *TIN* tubulointerstitial nephritis, *APL* anti-phospholipid syndrome, *PP* postpartum, *C1qN* C1q nephropathy, *MePGN* mesangial proliferative GN (not IGAN or SLE), *fibril GN* fibrillary GN, *IgMN* IgM nephropathy, *FGGS* focal global glomerulosclerosis, *HSP* Henoch-Schoenlein purpura, *AGBMD* antiglomerular basement membrane disease, *ICD* immune-complex disease, *CKD NOS* chronic kidney disease, not otherwise specified, *RA* rheumatoid arthritis, *JRA* juvenile rheumatoid arthritis, *FMF* familial Mediterranean fever

End-stage kidney disease (ESKD) was diagnosed in 78 biopsies (Table 3). The indicated reasons for biopsy was nephrotic syndrome and renal failure in 23 cases, unexplained renal failure with proteinuria in 45 cases, and unexplained renal failure alone 10 cases. Our regional criteria for biopsy does not include confirmation of ESRD, and the diagnosis of an end-stage kidney was largely unanticipated and before dependency on renal replacement therapy was recognized. The majority (55.0%) of these biopsies were end-stage GN. Many of these GN biopsies were categorized as CGN-NOS (30.8%) but also included late-stage FSGS with characteristic segmental lesions (7.7%), SLE class VI (3.8%), Hass class V IgAN (3.8%), and sclerotic class pauci-immune GN (9%). TIN consisted of 16.7% and CKD-NOS 9.0% of ESKD biopsies. The combination of CGN-NOS and late-stage FSGS represented 41% of non-diabetic ESKD biopsies.

Kurdistan population and estimates of age specific and age standardized GN incidence

The estimated population for Kurdistan in 2011 was 4,900,000 persons. This is a young population characteristic of the Middle East with 61% being under 25 years of age (Table 4). The annual crude biopsy rate in Kurdistan for native kidneys including unsatisfactory specimens for the years 2012–2013 was 7.8 per 100,000 (381 biopsies/4,900,000 persons). The age specific incidence for FSGS, MGN, SLE, IgAN, and all GN are shown in Table 5 together with the total US 2000 age standardized incidence for each diagnosis. GN was rare before 15 years of age, and the highest age specific incidence occurred between 35 and 44 years of age in all diagnostic categories. Thereafter, age specific incidence declined for all disease categories and after age 65 returned to rates seen at 15–24 years old (Fig. 1).

Compared to other disease categories, FSGS had higher age specific incidences from childhood to 64 years old and a higher total age adjusted incidence. The peak age specific incidence for the diagnosis of FSGS occurred at 35–44 years of age when it was 2.8/100,000 compared to 2.6/100,000 for MGN. The age standardized incidence of SLE for females was 1.07/100,000 compared to 0.2/100,000 for males. For IGAN the age standardized incidence for males was 0.4/100/000 compared to 0.2/100,000 for females.

Table 2 Age and sex distribution of all glomerulonephritis (without minimal change disease) over the 2 year period 2012–2013

| 2012–2013 | | | | | | | | | |
Age (years)	0–4	5–14	15–24	25–34	35–44	45–54	55–64	65+	Total (male)
FSGS	12 7 M	19 9 M	26 16 M	27 15 M	21 8 M	13 8 M	7 6 M	3 3 M	135 (53%)
MGN	1 M	2 2 M	10 5 M	19 9 M	19 6 M	11 6 M	5 1 M	4 3 M	71 (46%)
SLE		4 1 M	12 3 M	16 0 M	12 2 M	6 2 M		1 0 M	51 (16%)
IGAN	1 0 M	6 2 M	4 1 M	7 7 M	4 3 M	3 2 M	2 1 M	1 M	28 (61%)
Crescentic GN		2 1 M	6 3 M	5 1 M	5 4 M	3 1 M	2 1 M	3 3 M	26 (54%)
MPGN			4 3 M	3 2 M		2 1 M	1 M	2 2 M	12 (75%)
PSGN		8 7 M	1 0 M					1 M	10 (80%)
other GN	2 1 M	1 0 M	4 1 M	5 3 M	4 3 M	1 M	1 M		18 (56%)
CGN-NOS ESRD	1 M	4 2 M	3 M	10 9 M	5 3 M			1 M	24 (71%)
HUS		4 3 M	1 0 M	1 0 M	1 0 M		2 2 M		9 (55%)
Total GN	24 10 M	50 27 M	71 33 M	93 46 M	71 29 M	39 21 M	20 13 M	16 14 M	384 (50%)

Abbreviations: M male, FSGS focal segmental glomerulosclerosis, MGN membranous glomerulonephritis (GN), MPGN membranoproliferative GN, IGAN immunoglobulin A nephropathy, PSGN post-streptococcal GN, SLE lupus nephritis, CGN ESRD chronic GN not otherwise specified at end-stage renal disease, HUS hemolytic uremic syndrome

Comparisons of GN incidence in Kurdistan, Olmstead County, Minnesota, and Victoria, Australia

Table 6 compares the incidence of all GN, FSGS, IGAN, SLE, MGN, and ESRD in Kurdistan (2012–2013), Olmsted County (1994–2003), and Victoria (1995 and 1997) with the proportion of diabetics entering ESRD programs. The differences in all GN between Kurdistan, Olmsted County, and Victoria were largely due to the much higher rates of IGAN in Olmstead County and Victoria and the high rate of SLE in Victoria. The standardized rates for MGN and

Table 3 Biopsies having histologic features of end-stage kidneys

ESKD diagnosis	biopsies	Biopsies in category	% for category	% for ESKD biopsies
CGN-NOS, end-stage	24	24	NA	30.8
FSGS, end-stage	6	135	4.4	7.7
SLE class VI	3	51	5.9	3.8
IgAN Haas V	3	28	10.7	3.8
Crescentic GN, sclerotic class	7	26	26.9	9.0
Arterionephrosclerosis, end-stage	2	52	3.8	2.6
diabetes	5	5	100.0	6.4
Amyloid AA	6	19	31.2	7.7
Myeloma cast nephropathy	2	4	50	2.5
TIN, end-stage	13	46	28.3	16.7
CKG-NOS, end-stage	7	10	70	9.0
Total	78	400		100.0

Abbreviations: ESKD end-stage kidney disease, FSGS focal segmental glomerulosclerosis, SLE lupus nephritis, IGAN immunoglobulin A nephropathy, CGN-NOS chronic glomerulonephritis not otherwise specified, GN glomerulonephritis, TIN tubulointerstitial nephritis, CKD NOS chronic kidney disease, not otherwise specified

Table 4 Population of Kurdistan in 2011 from WHO Population Division estimates

Age	Female	Male	Total
0–4	325,581	345,720	671,301
5–14	624,789	619,811	1,244,600
15–24	541,195	556,405	1,097,600
25–34	413,249	409,953	823,202
35–44	185,622	186,780	372,402
45–54	128,174	156,126	284,300
55–64	84,721	86,779	171,500
65+	117,384	117,816	235,200
total	2,420,715	2,479,390	4,900,105

FSGS were somewhat similar for the three regions. Olmstead county had twice the incidence of ESRD as Victoria with 25% more diabetes.

Figure 1 demonstrates the changes in age specific incidence of all GN with increasing age in Kurdistan, Olmstead County, and Victoria. The plots show a plateau and then decline of age specific rates in Kurdistan at 40–45 years and moderately elevated rates with older age in Olmstead county that began to decline at approximately age 60. This contrasts with the marked elevation in incidence with age in Victoria with little indication of a late plateau. Although, the age standardized rates for FSGS and MGN were somewhat increased in Victoria compared to Kurdistan, the differences were largely the result of the late age of onset in Victoria and their infrequency in the elderly of Kurdistan.

Incidence of end-stage renal disease in Kurdistan compared to the kingdom of Jordan

In 2017 in Sulaimaniyah, 79 patients initiated dialysis and 124 were repeatedly dialyzed for a total of 203 patients receiving dialysis and an initiation to total dialysis ratio of 0.39. A first time renal transplant was received

Table 5 Kurdistan, Iraq. Age specific and age standardized (total rate) annual incidence per 100,000 population for FSGS, MGN, SLE, and all GN for the years 2012–2013

Age (years)	FSGS	MGN	SLE	IGAN	All GN
0–4	1.4	0.1		0.1	1.8
5–14	0.8	0.1	0.2	0.2	2.0
15–24	1.2	0.5	0.6	0.2	3.2
25–34	1.6	1.2	1.0	0.4	5.7
35–44	2.8	2.6	1.6	0.5	9.5
45–54	2.3	1.9	1.1	0.5	6.9
55–64	2.0	1.5		0.6	5.9
65+	0.6	0.9	0.2	0.2	3.4
Total rate[a]	1.6	1.2	0.7	0.4	5.1

[a]The total rate is adjusted to the 2000 US standard population

by 46 Sulaimaniyah patients, but we could not identify who had been previously dialysed, and transplant patients were not included in our calculations of ESRD rates.

The age distribution and the age specific incidence (ASpI) of ESRD per million were as follows: 0–4 years old, 0 patients, ASpI = 0.0; 5–14 years old, 1 patients, ASpI = 3.0 per million; 15–24 years old, 7 patients, ASpI = 23.9 per million; 25–34 years old, 8 patients, ASpI = 36.4 per million; 35–44 years old, 11 patients, ASpI = 110.0 per million; 45–54 years old, 16 patients, ASpI = 210.5 per million; 65–64 years old, 24 patients, ASpI = 521.7 per million; ≥ 65 years old, 12 patients, ASI = 190.5 per million. The crude ESRD incidence was an estimated 60 persons per million. ESRD was attributed to diabetes in 23% of patients, hypertension in 18%, and glomerular disease in 12% as previously reported [20]. In Jordan, the age specific ESRD incidence at 55–64 years of age as well as in younger age groups was similar to that in the Kurdish region (Fig. 2). After age 65, the Jordanian rate doubled the 522 per million seen at the 55–64 years of age while the Kurdish regional rate declined. The crude incidence of Jordanian ESRD was 99 per million with 54% of ESRD ascribed to diabetes, 26% to hypertension, and 4% to glomerular disease [19]. Figure 2 graphs the changing age specific ESRD incidence for the Northern Iraqi and Jordanian populations and adds 2011 US rates for comparison [5, 19].

Estimates of obesity in the Sulaimaniyah governate

This survey was conducted out-of-hospital within city neighborhoods. Clothed body mass index (BMI) ≥ 30 kg/m^2 was the definition for obesity. Obesity was found among 4.1% of 125 males and 14% of 160 females. For persons over 50 years old, the obesity rate was 15% for men and 36% for women. In a sample of 108 children between 5 and 15 years old, 6 (5.6%) were classified as obese.

Discussion

In 2013, Anand et el. [15] proposed using estimates of use and initiation of renal replacement therapy as a method of quantitating ESRD in developing countries. They pointed out that renal disease registries are non-existent in most of the world but emphasized the need for data on regional requirements for renal replacement therapy. Northern Iraq has 14 government dialysis centers with no conditions that exclude any person from receiving services. Daily and monthly records include name, age, blood pressures, and diabetes status. Date of entry into or exit from dialysis is rarely available, and data are not collected into a regional repository for formal estimates of incidence or prevalence.

We believe that rates of the initiation and the repeated use of dialysis when sampled at multiple dialysis centers

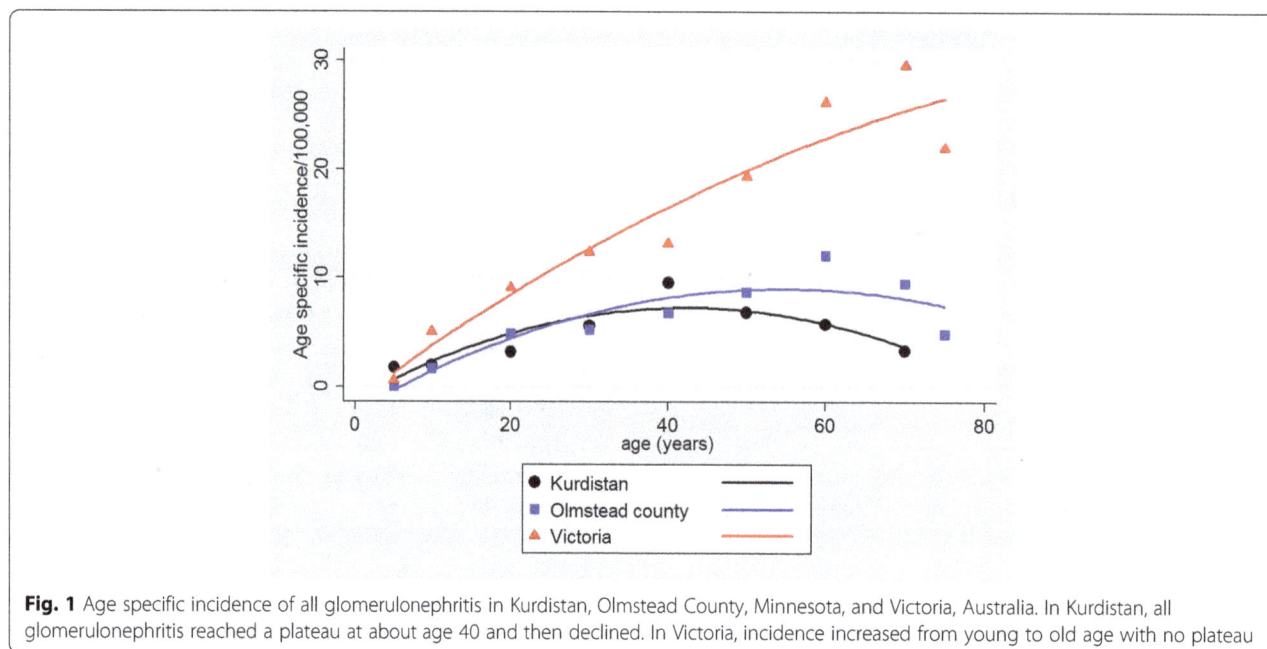

Fig. 1 Age specific incidence of all glomerulonephritis in Kurdistan, Olmstead County, Minnesota, and Victoria, Australia. In Kurdistan, all glomerulonephritis reached a plateau at about age 40 and then declined. In Victoria, incidence increased from young to old age with no plateau

can serve as surrogates for the incidence (initiation) and prevalence (total use, initiated and repeated) of ESRD. Our proportion of patients initiating dialysis in 2017 to the total number of patients using dialysis was 0.39. This is very close to the 0.34 reported by Anand et al. [15] for the Middle-East and North Africa as a whole and supports the validity of the concept as it is applied to our region. Using this approach, the annual crude incidence of ESRD for Iraqi Kurdistan was estimated at 60 per million. This is similar to an incidence of 64 per million reported in a 2014 review [21] from Iran that lies just to the East of Iraq but is considerably lower than Jordan that is on the Western Iraqi border [19].

Nevertheless, before 65 years old, age specific incidence rates for Jordan and Kurdistan were very similar to each other and to the US suggesting that before late middle age, ESRD rates in the Middle East resemble other geographic regions and that the major difference between low and high incidence regions is the accrual of CKD in aging populations. In this regard, it is important to recognize that Kurdistan and Jordan have young populations that contrast with the older population

structures of the US and Australia. When standardized to the 2000 US population, the ESRD incidence for Kurdistan was still comparatively low at 124 per million; while the age standardized rate for Jordan was 237 per million, a value close to that for Olmstead County and twice as high as Australia [13, 22].

In Northern Iraq, FSGS was the most frequently diagnosed type of GN. FSGS had an age adjusted incidence of 1.6 per 100,000 that was close to the incidence of 1.8 per 100,000 seen in Olmstead County and was not markedly lower than the incidence of 2.2 per 100,000 in Victoria [13, 14]. Nevertheless, FSGS was diagnosed at a younger age in Kurdistan than in Olmstead County or Victoria. The incidence of FSGS and all GN in Kurdistan peaked at approximately age 40 and then began to decline; whereas, in Victoria and Olmstead County there was a continued rise in later years [13, 14].

The rates of diagnosis and the age of FSGS in a population raise at least two epidemiologic issues. One concerns the variable frequency of FSGS in different populations in which there is little relationship to the population risk for ESRD. This is in part because the

Table 6 Comparison of age standardized annual incidence (per 100,000) of all glomerulonephritis, FSGS, IgAN, LN, and MGN in Olmsted County MN (USA); Victoria, Australia; and Kurdistan of Iraq. The ESRD incidence and the percent of diabetic ESRD is provided for each region

Country	All GN	FSGS	IgAN	SLE	MGN	ESRD incidence[a]	% ESRD diabetics
Olmsted Cty 1994–03	9.0	1.8	2.1	0.7	1.0	257	43
Victoria 1995–97	12.9	2.2	4.3	1.8	1.3	101	35
Kurdistan 2012–13	5.1	1.6	0.4	0.7	1.2	60	23

Age standardized annual incidence adjusted to the 2000 US standard population
[a] Incidence of ESRD per million population is unadjusted

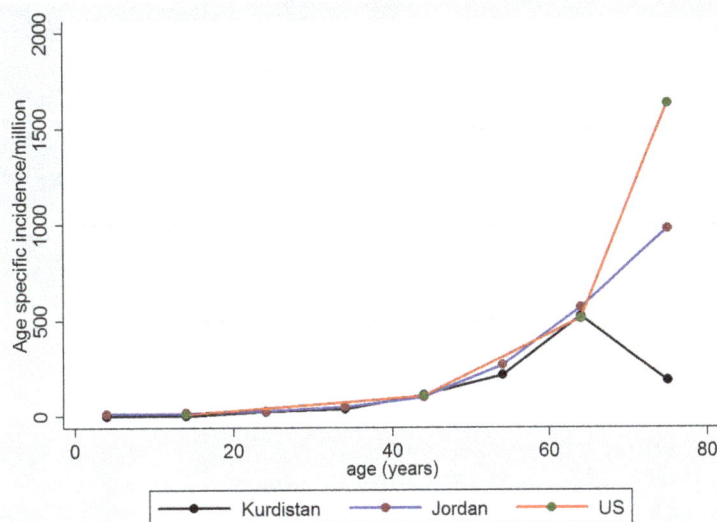

Fig. 2 Age specific incidence of end-stage renal disease (ESRD) in Kurdistan, Jordan, and the United States (US. After approximately 55 years of age, there is a marked increase in age specific ESRD incidence in Jordan and the US. This is not seen in Kurdistan and is attributed to low rates of diabetic ESRD in the elderly (assigned cause of ESRD: Kurdistan, diabetes 23%, hypertension, 18%, glomerulonephritis, 12%; Jordan, diabetes 54%, hypertension, 26%, glomerulonephritis, 4%; US, diabetes 44%, hypertension, 28%, glomerulonephritis, 6%)

major cause of ESRD in high incidence populations is diabetes. The US has the highest national incidence of ESRD in the world at a 2010 unadjusted rate of 369 per million with approximately 44% of new US ESRD patients being diabetic [4, 5]. In Australia, the rate of ESRD is considerably lower than the US at 101 per million, and just fewer than 35% of patients are diabetic [13]. IGAN is the most common form of GN in Australia, and contributes to nearly twice the frequency of GN-related ESRD as FSGS (IGAN 44% vs FSGS 23%) [13]. While these data do not indicate that FSGS or GN overall will add to a large future burden of ESRD in regions where diabetes is prevalent, the impact on lower risk regions is not known, and if FSGS in Iraq begins at an early age, a second issue is whether FSGS will increase in frequency as the young population ages.

In the US, FSGS was not always a commonly recognized disease, but it is currently the leading cause of nephrotic syndrome in both African Americans and whites [9, 23–27]. In the US, the risk of ESRD owing to FSGS is 4-times greater in African Americans, and African Americans are diagnosed with more severe disease at a peak age of 35 to 43 years old compared to 47 to 57 years old among whites [27, 28]. There is not any indication that age per se has any effect on prognosis, but FSGS has a generally poor out-come, and early versus late age of onset of any CKD results in a significantly increased loss of "kidney life" [29, 30].

FSGS appears to be increasing in many countries of the Middle-East and replacing SLE as the most common type of GN [31–33]. SLE is well known to have geographic,

racial, and ethnic variations [13, 34, 35]. Some of the geographic differences are undoubtedly due to biopsy practices. The Australian biopsy rate is > 20 per 100,000. The US rate is approximately 17 per 100,000, less than Australia but higher than the 4–8 per 100,000 practiced by nephrologists in most parts of the world and the 7.8 per 100,000 in Kurdistan [13, 36]. High biopsy rates, particularly for minor abnormalities, will certainly increase rates of IGAN and less active forms of SLE.

The validity of the reported causes of ESRD in the US and other developed countries has been questioned [37]. A patient with long-standing diabetes will be appropriately considered to have diabetic nephropathy, but hypertension is problematic, as physician biases have been shown to influence the assignment of hypertensive nephropathy to ESRD patients rather than exploring other causes [37].

With biopsies, a diagnosis of a specific cause of late stage kidney disease can often be made [38]. End-stage glomerulonephritis is characterized by solidified glomeruli that in the case of immune-complex disease frequently contain immunoglobulin deposits, and in IGAN, IgA deposits usually remain with advanced glomerulosclerosis [38]. Hypertension progresses by increasingly severe arteriosclerosis and glomerular loss that is primarily the result of ischemic glomerular obsolescence [39]. A predominance of glomerular solidification with hyalinosis lesions and IgM and C3 deposits favors primary FSGS as a cause of ESRD [39, 40]. Our analysis of causes of biopsy determined ESRD in Iraqi patients indicates that the proportional contribution of FSGS to non-diabetic ESRD could be as high as 41% and suggests that FSGS could raise ESRD rates if the disease followed the patterns in the US and Australia and became more common in older members of the population.

One hypotheses for the lowered rates of ESRD and FSGS in the elderly of Northern Iraq is that physicians stop looking for disease in older patients, or older persons become oblivious to their illnesses and do not seek medical help. We believe that these are unlikely explanations. The elderly are valued members of Iraqi and Kurdish society, and there is no age discrimination for any form of medical service.

A second hypothesis is an age cohort effect in which older members of the population have not been exposed to the factors causing the disease. This certainly could affect rates of diabetes and ESRD, as older Iraqis have been living in deprived conditions imposed by international trade restrictions since the 1980s. A current 26–30% rate of obesity is reported for Southern Iraq [41, 42], but this is excessive for Sulaimaniyah, where the all-age obesity rate was less than 10%. The obesity rate of 36% in Jordan [41] may portend changes that will be seen in the future, but we do not see a large segment of the Kurdish population currently at risk for diabetic kidney disease.

Although both Iraq and Jordan have similarly young populations, the estimated risk of ESRD in Northern Iraq was low; while the Jordanian population when adjusted for age had a risk of ESRD that more resembled the US. These differences highlight the impact of undernutrition and over nutrition on kidney health. Political instability is an unfortunate fact-of-life in many parts of the Middle-East and North Africa. Somalia and Sudan are examples where war and continuous undernutrition have lead to endemically high rates of hypertension and non-diabetic CKD possibly influenced by an intra-uterine derived nephron deficit [43, 44]. Diabetes as a disease of overnutrition and ageing will almost certainly become more common as economies improve. FSGS appears to be increasing throughout the Middle-East, and we suggest that GN and particularly FSGS are also age-dependent with effects on ESRD that are unlikely to be known for many years.

Conclusions

At an annual rate of 60 per million, the incidence of ESRD in Northern Iraq is much lower than the crude incidences of 100 and 390 per million for Jordan and the US respectively. This difference is primarily the result of low identified rates of renal disease in the Iraqi elderly and a relative infrequency of diabetes. With the exception of IGAN, that has a low incidence in the region, rates of the major types of glomerular diseases are similar to the West. FSGS is the most common primary glomerular disease in Northern Iraq. It has an age adjusted annual incidence of 1.6 cases per 100,000 population and makes an apparent major contribution to regional ESRD.

Abbreviations
ASI: Age standardized incidence; ASpI: Age specific incidence; CGN-NOS: End-stage chronic GN not otherwise specified; CKD: Chronic kidney disease; ESKD: End-stage kidney disease; ESRD: End-stage renal disease; FSGS: Focal segmental glomerulosclerosis; GN: Glomerulonephritis; HUS: Hemolytic uremic syndrome; IGAN: Immunoglobulin A nephropathy; MCD: Minimal change disease; MGN: Membranous GN; MPGN: Membranoproliferative GN; SLE: Lupus nephritis; TIN: Tubulointerstitial nephritis; US: United States

Funding
The research was supported by the Ministry of Health of the Kurdistan Regional Government. The Ministry of Health played no role in the design of the study nor in the collection, analysis, and interpretation of data or the writing of the manuscript.

Authors' contributions
Study design: AAA, DAS, MDH. Data collection and analysis: AAA, DAS, SEA, KHA, ZSMS. Wrote first draft of manuscript: AAA, MDH. MDH coordinated manuscript revisions that were read and approved by all authors.

Competing interests
The authors declare that they have no competing interests.

Author details
[1]Department of Pathology, Shorsh General Hospital, Qirga Road, Sulaimaniyah, Kurdistan, Iraq. [2]Department of Medicine, Sulaimaniyah University, Sulaimaniyah, Iraq. [3]Hawler University College of Medicine, Erbil, Iraq. [4]Dohuk University, Dohuk, Iraq.

References
1. Couser WG, Remuzzi G, Mendio S, Tonelli M. The contribution of chronic kidney disease to the global burden of major noncommunicable diseases. Kidney Int. 2001;80:1258–70.
2. Nugent RA, Fathima SF, Feifl AB, Chyung D. The burden of chronic kidney disease on developing nations: a 21st century challenge in global health. Nephron Clin Pract. 2011;118:c269–77.
3. El Nahas AM, Bello AK. Chronic kidney disease: the global challenge. Lancet. 2005;365:331–40.
4. US Renal Data Systen. USRDS 2012 Annual data report: chapter 12, international comparisons. Bethesda: National Institutes of Health. National Institutes of Diabetes and Digesive and Kidney Disease; 2012. p. 341–52.
5. US Renal Data System. USRDS 2013 Annual Data Report, Atlas of chronic kidney disease and end-stage renal disease in the U.S, Vol 2: Incidence, prevalence, patient characteristics, and treatment modalities. Bethesda: National Institutes of Health. National Institutes of Diabetes and Digesive and Kidney Disease; 2013.
6. Shaheen FAM, Sougiyyeh MZ. Kidney health in the Middle East. Clin Nephrol. 2010;74(suppl 1):S85–8.
7. Pesce F, Schena FP. Worldwide distribution of glomerular diseases: the role of renal biopsy registries. Nephrol Dial Transplant. 2010;25:334–6.
8. Ossareh S, Asgari M, Abdi E, Nejad-Gashti H, Ataipour Y, Aris S, Proushani F, Ghorbani G, Hayati F, Ghods AJ. Renal biopsy findings in Iran: case series report from a referral kidney center. Int Uro Nephrol. 2010;42:1031–40.
9. Haas M, Meechan SM, Karrison TG, Spargo BH. Changing etiologies of unexplained adult nephrotic syndrome: a comparison of renal biopsy findings from 1976–1979 and 1996–1997. Am J Kidney Dis. 1997;30:621–31.
10. Woo KT, Chan CM, Mooi CY, Choong HL, Tan HK, Foo M, Lee GS, Anantharaman V, Lim CH, Tan CC, Lee EJ, Chaing GS, Tan PH, Boon TH, Fook-Chong S, Wong KS. The changing patterns of primary glomerulonephritis in Singapore and other countries over the past 3 decades. Clin Nephrol. 2010;74:372–83.
11. Bahiense-Oliveira M, Saldana LB, Mota EL, Penna DO, Barros RT, Romao-Jumioe JE. Primary glomerular diseases in Brazil (1979-1999): is the frequency of focal and segmental glomerulosclerosis increasing. Clin Nephrol. 2004;61:90 7.

12. Das U, Dakshinamurty KV, Prayaga A. Pattern of biopsy proven renal disease in a single center of South India: 19 years experience. Indian J Nephrol. 2011;21:250–7.

13. Briganti EM, Dowling J, Finlay M, Hill PA, Jones CL, Kincaid-Smith PS, Sinclair R, McNeil JJ, Atkins RC. The incidence of biopsy-proven glomerulonephritis in Australia. Nephrol Dial Transplan. 2001;16:1364–7.

14. Swaminathan S, Leung N, Lager DJ, Melton J III, Bergstralh EJ, Rohlinger A, Fervenza FC. Changing incidence of glomerular diseases in Olmstead county, Minnesota: a 30 year renal biopsy study. Clin J Am Soc Nephrol. 2006;1:483–7.

15. Anand S, Bitton A, Gaziano T. The gap between estimated incidence of end-stage renal disease and use of therapy. PLoS One. 2013;8:e72860.

16. United Nations, Department of Economic and Social Affairs, Population Division (2017), World population prospects (2017 revision). PopulationPyramid.net. Last accessed 6/8/2018.

17. Iraqi Cancer Registry 2012. Iraqi Cancer board, Ministry of Health, Republic of Iraq. 2014,

18. United States Census 2000. US census Bureau, US Department of Commerce, Economics and Statistis Administration (www.census.gov/prod/2001pubs/c2kbr01-12.pdf), Accessed 26 Sept 2017.

19. National Registry of End-Stage Renal Disease 2013. Part four, incidence of ESRD patients. Non-communicable disease directorate: The Hashimite Kingdome of Jordan Ministry of Heath Annual Report; 2013. p. 50–3.

20. Sharif DA, Awn AH, Murad KM, Meran IMA. Demographic and characteristic distribution of end-stage renal failure in Sulaimani Governate, Kurdistan region, Iraq. Int J Med Res Prof. 2017;3:155–8.

21. Mousavi SSB, Soleiman A, Mousav MB. Epidemiology of end-stage renal disease in Iran: a review article. Saudi J Kidney Dis Transplant. 2014;25:697–702.

22. Midwest Kidney Network, Annual Report 2011, Midwest kidney network.org/about/annual report. Accessed 21 Mar 2018.

23. Haas M, Spargo BH, Coventry S. Increasing incidence of focal-segmental glomerulosclerosis among adult nephropathies: a 20 year biopsy study. Am J Kidney Dis. 1996;26:740–50.

24. Korbet SM, Genchi RM, Borok RZ, Schwartz MM. The racial prevalence of glomerular lesions in nephrotic adults. Am J Kidney Dis. 1996;27:647–51.

25. Braden GL, Mulhern JG, O'Shea MH, Nash SV, Ucci AA Jr, Germain MJ. Changing incidence of glomerular diseases in adults. Am J Kidney Dis. 2000; 35:878–83.

26. Dragovic D, Rosenstok JL, Wah SJ, Panagopoulus G, Devita MV, Michelis MF. Increasing incidence of focal segmental glomerulosclerosis and an examination of demographic patterns. Clin Nephrol. 2005;63:1–7.

27. Kitiyakara C, Eggers P, Kopp JB. Twenty-one-year trend in ESRD due to focal segmental glomerulosclerosis in the United States. Am J Kidney Dis. 2004;44: 815–25.

28. Hughson MD, Samuel T, Hoy WE, Bertram JF. Glomerular volume and clinicopathologic features related to disease severity in renal biopsies of African Americans and whites in the southeastern United States. Arch Pathol Lab Med. 2007;131:1665–72.

29. Cameron JS. Focal segmental glomerulosclerosis in adults. Nephrol Dial Transplant. 2003;18(suppl 6):vi45–51.

30. Kiberd BA, Clase CM. Cumulative risk for developing end-stage renal disease in the US population. J Am Soc Nephrol. 2002;13:1635–44.

31. Nawaz Z, Mushtaq F, Mousa D, Rehman E, Sulaiman M, Aslam N, Khawaja N. Pattern of glomerular disease in the Saudi population: a single center, five-year retrospective study. Saudi J Kidney Dis Transplant. 2013;24:1265–70.

32. Al Riyami D, Al Shaaili K, Al Bulushi Y, Al Dhahli A, Date A. The spectrum of glomerular diseases on renal biopsy: data from a single tertiary center in Oman. Oman Med J. 2013;28:213–5.

33. Karnib HH, Gharavi AG, Aftimos G, Mahfoud Z, Saad R, Gemayel E, Masri B, Assaad S, Madr KF, Ziyadeh FN. A 5-year survey of biopsy-proven kidney disease in Lebanon: significant variation in prevalence of primary glomerular diseases by age, population structure and consanguinity. Nephrol Dial Transplant. 2010;25:3962–9.

34. Feldman CH, Hiraki LT, Liu J, Fischer MA, Solomon DH, Alarcon GS, Winkelmayer WC, Costenbader KH. Epidemiology and sociodemographics of systemic lupus erythematosus and lupus nephritis among US adults with Medicaid coverage, 2000-2004. Arthritis Rheum. 2013;65:753–63.

35. Tesar V, Hruskova Z. Lupus nephritis: a different disease in European patients? Kidney Dis (Basel). 2015;1:110–8.

36. Hanko JB, Mullan RN, O'Rourke DM, McNamee PT, Maxwell AP, Courtee AE. The changing pattern of adult glomerular disease. Nephrol Dial Transplant. 2009;24:3050–4.

37. Zarif L, Covic A, Lyengar S, Sehgal AR, Sedor JR, Schelling JR. Inaccuracy of clinical phenotyping parameters for hypertensive nephrosclerosis. Nephrol Dial Transplant. 2000;15:1801–7.

38. Zhou XJ, Fenves AZ, Vaziri ND, Saxena R. Renal changes with aging and end-stage renal disease, in Heptinstall's pathology of the kidney, 7th. Jennette C, Olson JL, D' Agati VD, Silva FG. Wolters Kluwer, Philadelphia, 2015;1281–1319.

39. Hughson MD, Puelles VG, Hoy WE, Douglas-Denton RN, Mott SA, Bertram JF. Hypertension, glomerular hypertrophy and nephrosclerosis: the effect of race. Nephrol Dial Transplant. 2014;29:1399–409.

40. Hughson MD, Johnson K, Young RJ, Hoy WE, Bertram JF. Glomerular size and glomerulosclerosis: relationships to disease categories, glomerular solidification, and ischemic obsolescence. Amer J Kidney Dis. 2002;39:679–87.

41. CIA World Factbook. www.indexmundi.com. Updated Jan 1, 2018. Accessed 26 Mar 2018.

42. Monsour AA, Al-Maliky AA, Salih M. Population overweight and obesity trends over 8 years in Basrah, Iraq. Epidemiology. 2012;2:110.

43. ElHafeez SA, Bolignano D, D'Arrigo G, Dounousi E, Tripepi G, Zoccali C. Prevalence and burden of chronic kidney disease among the general population and high-risk groups in Africa: a systematic review. BMJ Open. 2018;8:e015069.

44. Hoy WE, Bertram JF, Denton RD, Zimanyi M, Samuel T, Hughson MD. Nephron number, glomerular volume, renal disease, and hypertension. Curr Opin Nephrol Hypertens. 2008;13:258–65.

3

Urinary epidermal growth factor, monocyte chemoattractant protein-1 or their ratio as predictors for rapid loss of renal function in type 2 diabetic patients with diabetic kidney disease

Bancha Satirapoj[1], Rattanawan Dispan[1], Piyanuch Radinahamed[2] and Chagriya Kitiyakara[2]* ⓘ

Abstract

Background: Increased monocyte chemoattractant protein-1 (MCP-1) and decreased epidermal growth factor (EGF) are promising biomarkers to predict progressive decline in kidney function in non-diabetic kidney diseases. We aimed to evaluate the performance of urinary EGF, MCP-1 or their ratio in predicting rapid decline of GFR in a cohort of Type 2 diabetic patients (T2DM) with diabetic kidney disease (DKD).

Methods: T2DM patients ($n = 83$) with DKD at high risk for renal progression were followed up prospectively. The baseline urine values of MCP-1 to creatinine ratio (UMCP-1), EGF to creatinine ratio (UEGF), EGF to MCP-1 ratio (UEGF/MCP-1) and albumin to creatinine ratio (UACR) were measured. The primary outcome was a decline in estimated glomerular filtration rate (GFR) of ≥25% yearly from baseline.

Results: During follow-up time of 23 months, patients with rapid decline in estimated GFR of ≥25% yearly from baseline had significantly higher baseline levels of UMCP-1, and UACR and lower UEGF and UEGF/MCP-1 ratio. All renal biomarkers predicted primary outcomes with ROC (95%CI) for UMCP-1=0.73 (0.62-0.84), UEGF=0.68 (0.57-0.80), UEGF/MCP-1=0.74 (0.63-0.85), and UACR =0.84 (0.75-0.93). By univariate analysis, blood pressure, GFR, UACR, UMCP-1, UEGF, and UEGF/MCP-1 were associated with rapid decline GFR. By multivariate analysis, UACR, systolic blood pressure, and UMCP-1 or UEGF/MCP-1 were independently associated with rapid GFR decline.

Conclusions: UMCP-1 or UEGF/MCP-1 ratio were associated with rapid renal progression independent from conventional risk factors in DKD.

Keywords: Biomarker, Diabetic nephropathy, Monocyte chemoattractant protein-1 (MCP-1), Epidermal growth factor (EGF); kidney; cytokine

* Correspondence: kitiyakc@yahoo.com; chagriya.kit@mahidol.ac.th
[2]Division of Nephrology, Department of Medicine, Faculty of Medicine Ramathibodi Hospital, Mahidol University, 270 Rama 6 Rd, Bangkok 10400, Thailand
Full list of author information is available at the end of the article

Background

Diabetic kidney disease (DKD) is a major complication of type 2 diabetes mellitus (T2DM) with up to 40% of DKD patients progressing to end stage renal disease (ESRD) [1]. Despite the improvements in the treatment for DKD, the risk of ESRD remains high. Potential new therapy must be evaluated in clinical trials, which are very costly. A successful trial must accumulate enough end-points to give adequate power for detecting a risk reduction between the placebo and the treated group. Biomarkers that can identify and target high risk patients for clinical studies or more aggressive therapy would be extremely useful. The paradigm of the natural history of DKD continues to evolve. DKD clearly does not follow the pattern of glomerular hyperfiltration progressing from microalbuminuria to increasing degrees of overt albuminuria and declining GFR in many patients [2]. Macrovascular disease rather than classical diabetic nephropathy has been increasingly recognized in the pathogenesis of GFR decline in many DKD patients [3] [4]. Although, albuminuria is an important marker to diagnose and predict the progression of DKD [2], nearly half of T2DM patients may have decreased glomerular filtration rate (GFR) before the onset of albuminuria. Conventional biomarkers cannot accurately identify T2DM patients at higher risk of rapid GFR decline and new biologic markers that can predict DKD progression are required.

DKD has been viewed traditionally as a disease of accelerated matrix deposition leading to progressive glomerular and tubulointerstitial fibrosis with the final consequence of ESRD [2]. More recently, an important role of inflammatory cells such as monocytes/macrophages has been recognized in the pathogenesis of DKD progression [5]. Monocyte chemoattractant protein-1 (MCP-1), a member of the CC chemokine family promotes macrophage accumulation both in animal models and several renal diseases [6–8]. Increased urinary MCP-1 levels have been shown to predict adverse outcomes in proliferative kidney diseases such as lupus nephritis [9]. Previous investigations have shown that the renal MCP-1 expression is also elevated in DKD. Urinary MCP-1 levels correlated with the degree of tubulointerstitial leucocyte infiltration [10, 11], but at present, its role in predicting renal prognosis in DKD remains unclear.

The balance between protective growth factors and pro-inflammatory cytokines likely determines the degree of renal tissue damage and disease progression in DKD. In contrast to MCP-1, epidermal growth factor (EGF), a peptide growth factor probably has a protective role during kidney injury. EGF expression within the kidney is decreased in several kidney diseases [12, 13]. Low urinary EGF levels have been found to be predictive of kidney function decline in non-diabetic renal diseases. Therefore, both urinary MCP-1 and EGF could serve as favorable biomarkers for kidney damage in DKD. Previously, it has been shown that urinary EGF/MCP-1 ratio was a better prognosticator of long term outcome compared to either cytokine alone in IgA nephropathy [14]. Currently, few studies have evaluated the roles of MCP-1 or EGF in predicting DKD progression across a broad spectrum of kidney function and none have evaluated the role of their ratio. This study aimed to test the hypothesis that baseline levels of urinary MCP-1 and EGF or their ratio would predict rapid decline of estimated GFR in a cohort of T2DM patients with CKD independent of conventional clinical risk factors. We also evaluated the biomarkers in subgroups with high cardiovascular risk and those low albuminuria to explore the potential value of these biomakers in subjects who may have non-classical mechanisms for DKD progression.

Methods

Study design

This prospective cohort study is comprised of T2DM subjects with DKD at risk for renal progression. The subjects were recruited in 2014 to 2016 and followed for at least 12 months at the outpatient clinic, Department of Internal Medicine, Phramongkutklao Hospital. The study was conducted according to the Declaration of Helsinki, and approved by the Ethics Committee of the Faculty of Medicine, Ramathibodi Hospital and the Royal Thai Army Medical Department. All the subjects gave written informed consent. Inclusion criteria were: age $\geq$ 18 years, T2DM with predialysis CKD stage 1 to 5 (persistent micro or macroalbuminuria or estimated GFR < 60 mL/min/1.73 m^2 not on dialysis) and a duration of diabetes of at least 5 years or uncontrolled blood pressure (BP) for 6 months (> 150/90 mmHg). Exclusion criteria included urinary tract infection, ESRD, acute kidney injury, as defined by a rapid rise in serum creatinine and/or fall in urine output according to KDIGO classification 3 months prior to inclusion or during follow-up [15], pregnancy, T1DM and patient life expectancy < 1 year.

Patient history was recorded by interview and confirmed by assessment of medical records and drug prescriptions. Demographic and anthropometric parameters were recorded. Blood pressure (BP) was measured using a standard mercury sphygmomanometer. An average of three measurement values was used. After the baseline assessments, patients were followed prospectively until the end of the observation period. To avoid loss during follow-up, patients were personally contacted if they missed any appointments and at the end of the study.

Patients were also classified according to cardiovascular risks. Patients with prior myocardial infarction, angina or stroke were classified as having a 'history of cardiovascular events'. Patients with a 'high cardiovascular disease' was defined as a 10-year cardiovascular risk ≥10% by Framingham Coronary Heart Disease Risk Score [16].

Laboratory measurements

Blood and urine samples were taken in the morning before any food intake. Common biochemical parameters including urea, creatinine, hemoglobin A1C, serum lipids and electrolytes, albumin, hemoglobin and proteinuria were measured at baseline in all patients, according to standard methods in a routine clinical laboratory. Estimated GFR (eGFR) was calculated using the Chronic Kidney Disease Epidemiology Collaboration (CKD-EPI) equation [17]. Urine albumin was measured on a nephelometric analyzer and urine creatinine was measured on a multiple analyzer (Modular P Chemistry Analyzer; Roche Diagnostics). Urine albumin and creatinine for urine samples collected from participants and albuminuria was reported as UACR.

Urine MCP-1 and EGF assay

Urine samples were collected at baseline. Thirty milliliters of fresh urine was centrifuged at 4000 rpm for 10 min, then stored at − 80 °C until assayed. Sandwich ELISA kits (Quantikine ELISA Immunoassay R&D systems, Minneapolis, USA) was used to quantitate urinary MCP-1 and EGF levels using the manufacturer's instructions. Duplicate samples were measured by a researcher who did not have information on the clinical data using TECAN Infinite M200 Pro microplate reader. The results were calculated using Magellan Tracker software (Tecan Group Ltd., Mannedorf, Switzerland). Urine MCP-1 and EGF levels were expressed as ng per mg of creatinine (UMCP-1 and UEGF). Ratio of Urine EGF and MCP-1 were also calculated. The intra- assay coefficients of variation were 3.2% for EGF and 2.6% for MCP-1.

Renal outcome

The primary outcome was *Rapid GFR decline*, defined as decreased estimated GFR decline ≥ 25% per year. This was determined for each follow-up time point by calculating the percent GFR change from baseline for time points within 1 year of urine collection or from the preceding 12 months for time-points beyond one year.

Statistical analyses

Normally distributed variables are shown as mean ± standard deviation and compared using the Pearson correlation or unpaired t-test. Variables that are Non-normally distributed are presented as median [25th, 75th percentile] and compared by the Spearman coefficients or the Mann-Whitney U test. Categorical variables are summarized as percentages and compared using the chi-square test. Receiver-operating characteristic (ROC) curves were generated and the area under the curves (AUC) were calculated to evaluate the sensitivity and specificity for UMCP-1, UEGF, UEGF/MCP-1 ratio, and UACR for *Rapid GFR decline*. The Youden index was used to determine the optimal cut-off value [18]. To evaluate the prognostic value of each biomarker to predict *Rapid GFR decline*, event-free survival times were compared between patients with high and low biomarker levels. Time to event was the period to *Rapid GFR decline*. Patients were censored if they reached November 30th, 2017 without events. Survival functions were assessed with Kaplan-Meier. Hazard ratios for outcomes associated with *Rapid GFR decline* were determined by Cox proportional hazards for each biomarker and conventional risk factors using three models separately for UMCP-1, UEGF or UEGF/MCP-1. In addition to the analysis of all subjects, we also performed subgroup analysis of subjects with high cardiovascular risk or those low albuminuria. A p value of < 0.05 was considered statistically significant.

Results

Baseline characteristics

The baseline characteristics of the study cohort ($n = 83$) are shown in Table 1. The mean age was 66.6 ± 9.8 years, and more than half were male (63.8%). Duration of T2DM was 13.9 ± 8.9 years and all patients had follow-up time of 24 [11, 19] months. Mean estimated GFR was 45.0 ± 28.4 mL/min/1.73 m², UACR was 283.69 [34.47, 762.85] mg/gCr and HbA1c was 7.4 ± 1.6%. Seventy-nine patients (96.3%) were hypertensive, and 57 (68.7%) had GFR < 60 mL/min/1.73 m². The prevalence of patients with prior cardiovascular events was 3.7% and 44.6% were considered to have high cardiovascular risk.

Comparisons between patients with rapid versus non-rapid renal progression

During the observational period, 37 patients (44.6%) had GFR decline ≥ 25% yearly and were classified as the rapid renal progression group. Mean baseline estimated GFR of subjects with rapid renal progression were significantly lower than those in the non-rapid renal progression group ($P = 0.012$). The patients with rapid renal progression had increased systolic and diastolic BP (Table 1). The prevalence of those with a history of cardiovascular event, the Framingham risk score or high cardiovascular risk were not different between rapid versus non-rapid progression.

UMCP-1 (Rapid: 3.12 [2.17, 7.97] vs. Non-rapid: 1.66 [1, 2.38] ng/mgCr ($P < 0.001$)) and UACR (Rapid: 673.4 [412.5 to 2627.6] vs. Non-rapid: 49.7 [19.9, 261.3] mg/gCr ($P < 0.001$)) were significantly higher in the rapid

Table 1 Baseline characteristics and laboratory data

Parameters	All patients (N = 83)	GFR decline < 25% per year (N = 46)	GFR decline ≥ 25% per year (N = 37)	P-value
Age (year)	66.6 ± 9.8	67.1 ± 8.9	65.9 ± 10.9	0.595
Male (%)	53 (63.9%)	29 (63.0%)	24 (64.9%)	0.864
Duration of DM (years)	13.9 ± 8.9	14.8 ± 8.3	13.2 ± 9.6	0.463
CKD staging				
CKD I	7 (8.4%)	4 (8.7%)	3 (8.1%)	0.065
CKD II	19 (22.9%)	14 (30.4%)	5 (13.5%)	
CKD III	26 (31.3%)	17 (36.9%)	9 (24.3%)	
CKD IV	16 (19.3%)	5 (10.9%)	11 (29.7%)	
CKD V	15 (18.1%)	6 (13.0%)	9 (24.3%)	
Comorbid diseases				
Hypertension (%)	79 (96.3%)	44 (95.7%)	35 (94.6%)	0.586
Dyslipidemia (%)	72 (87.8%)	43 (95.6%)	29 (78.4%)	0.037
History of cardiovascular events (%)	3 (3.7%)	2 (4.4%)	1 (2.7%)	1.000
Framingham risk score	15.63 ± 10.29	13.83 ± 8.07	17.76 ± 12.22	0.152
High cardiovascular risk[a] (%)	37 (44.6%)	21 (45.7%)	16 (43.2%)	0.605
Anemia (%)	51 (61.5%)	22 (47.8%)	29 (78.4%)	0.004
Medications				
RAAS blockers (%)	45 (54.2%)	27 (58.7%)	18 (48.7%)	0.361
Insulin (%)	29 (35.4%)	14 (31.1%)	15 (40.5%)	0.374
ASA (%)	50 (60.9%)	28 (62.2%)	22 (59.5%)	0.799
Clinical parameters				
SBP (mmHg)	143.1 ± 22.4	135.5 ± 16.3	152.4 ± 25.4	0.001
DBP (mmHg)	77.7 ± 13.9	74.8 ± 12.2	81.2 ± 15.2	0.037
BMI (kg/m^2)	27.5 ± 5.0	27.3 ± 5.2	27.73 ± 4.9	0.736
Laboratory parameters				
GFR (mL/min/1.73m^2)	45.0 ± 28.4	51.9 ± 27.6	36.4 ± 27.4	0.012
Median UACR (mg/g creatinine)	283.7 [34.5, 762.9]	49.7 [19.9, 261.3]	673.4 [412.6, 2627.6]	< 0.001
FPG (mg/dL)	150.6 ± 74.7	146.4 ± 78.9	155.8 ± 69.8	0.574
HbA1c (%)	7.4 ± 1.6	7.4 ± 1.7	7.4 ± 1.5	0.931
Hemoglobin (g/dL)	11.9 ± 3.1	12.2 ± 1.7	11.7 ± 4.2	0.517
Phosphate (mg/dL)	3.5 ± 0.9	3.7 ± 0.9	3.4 ± 0.8	0.167
Median intact-PTH (pg/mL)	120.5 [66.9, 256.6]	133.55 [63.9, 269.2]	120.5 [70.6, 214.1]	0.887

Note: Values for categorical variables are given as number (percentage); values for continuous variables, as *mean ± standard deviation or median [interquartile range]*

Abbreviations: ASA Aspirin, BMI Body Mass Index, DBP Diastolic Blood Pressure, FPG Fasting Plasma Glucose, GFR Glomerular Filtration Rate, HbA1c Hemoglobin A1 C, PTH Parathyroid hormone, RAAS Renin Angiotensin Aldosterone System, SBP Systolic Blood Pressure, UACR Urine Albumin Creatinine Ratio
[a]A high cardiovascular risk was defined a 10-year cardiovascular disease ≥ 10% by Framingham Coronary Heart Disease Risk Score

renal progression group compared to non-rapid renal progression group. In contrast, UEGF levels (Rapid: 19.5 [11.1, 36.3] vs. Non-Rapid: 42.8 [23.4, 65.1] ng/mgCr (P < 0.001)), and UEGF/MCP-1 ratios (Rapid: 5.4 [1.5, 17.5] vs. Non-rapid: 27.3 [11.5, 65.3] ng/ng (P < 0.001)), were significantly lower in the rapid renal progression group when compared with non-rapid renal progression group as shown in Fig. 1.

Urine MCP-1 and EGF correlated with other renal injury markers

UMCP-1 showed an inverse correlation with estimated GFR (R = – 0.29, P = 0.008) and a strong positive correlation with albuminuria (R = 0.79, P < 0.001) at baseline. By contrast, UEGF showed a positive correlation with estimated GFR (R = 0.39, P < 0.001), but did not correlate with albuminuria (R = – 0.19, P = 0.078). UEGF/MCP-1

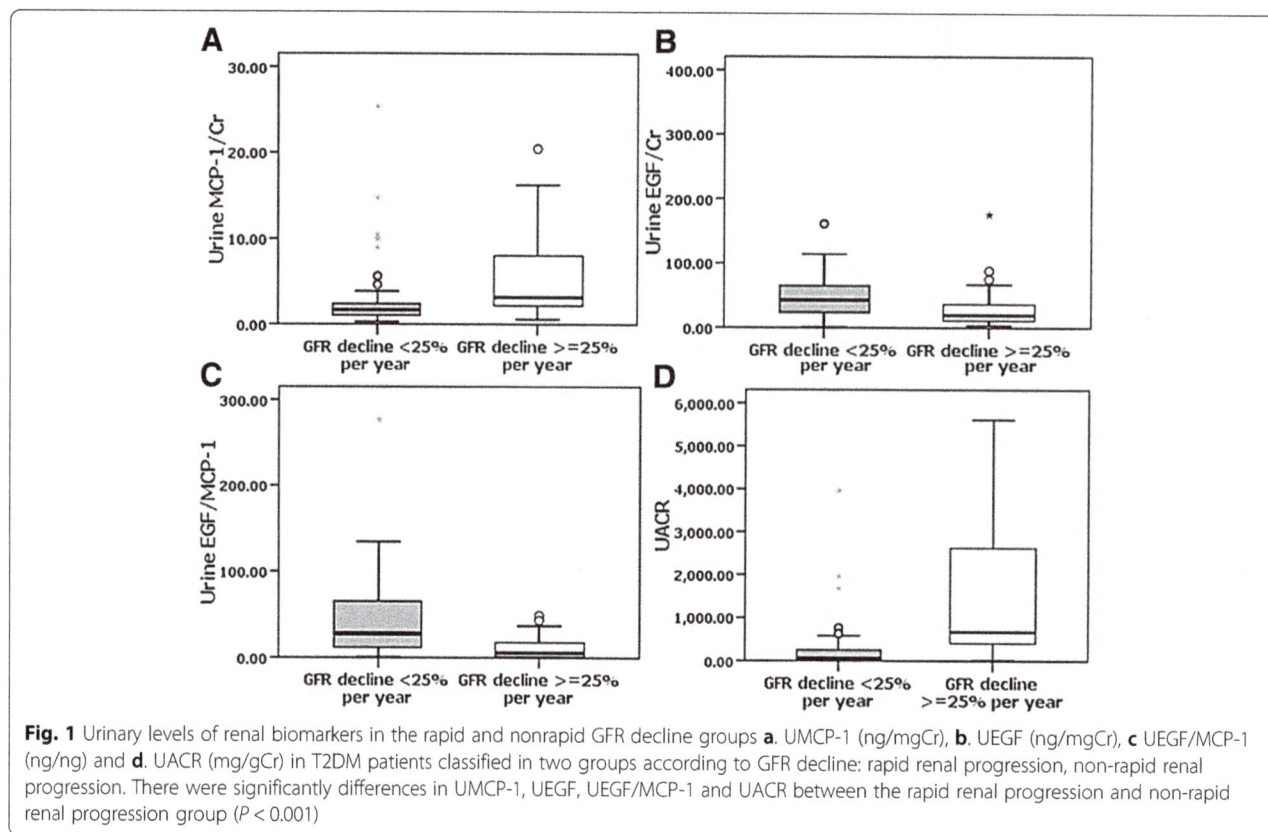

Fig. 1 Urinary levels of renal biomarkers in the rapid and nonrapid GFR decline groups **a**. UMCP-1 (ng/mgCr), **b**. UEGF (ng/mgCr), **c** UEGF/MCP-1 (ng/ng) and **d**. UACR (mg/gCr) in T2DM patients classified in two groups according to GFR decline: rapid renal progression, non-rapid renal progression. There were significantly differences in UMCP-1, UEGF, UEGF/MCP-1 and UACR between the rapid renal progression and non-rapid renal progression group ($P < 0.001$)

ratio showed a moderate correlation with estimated GFR ($R = 0.63$, $P < 0.001$) and a significant inverse correlation with albuminuria ($R = -0.34$, $P < 0.001$) (Additional file 1: Table S1).

Performance of the biomarkers to predict rapid renal progression
The ROC analysis showed an AUC (95%CI) for UMCP-1, UEGF, UEGF/MCP-1 ratio and UACR of 0.73 (0.62–0.84), 0.68 (0.57 to 0.80), 0.74 (0.63–0.85) and 0.84 (0.75–0.93), respectively as shown in Fig. 2. For UMCP-1, the best cut-off level was 2.1 ng/mgCr (sensitivity 75.7%, specificity 73.9%), UEGF was 29.9 ng/mgCr (sensitivity 70.3%, specificity 69.6%), UEGF/MCP-1 ratio was 9.2 ng/ng (sensitivity 64.9%, specificity 80.4%) and UACR was 330.9 mg/gCr (sensitivity 83.8%, specificity 84.8%). All renal biomarkers demonstrated intermediate performance to predict rapid renal progression in T2DM patients. When the levels of biomarkers were combined with UACR, The AUC (95%CI) for combined markers were: UACR+UMCP-1, 0.84 (0.75–0.93); UACR+UEGF, 0.83 (0.75–0.93); UACR +UEGF/MCP-1 0.82 (0.74–0.92). There was no improvement in the AUC compared to UACR alone.

Kaplan-Meier survival curves of *Rapid GFR decline* in patients with UMCP-1, UEGF, UEGF/MCP-1 ratio and UACR levels above and below the optimal cutoff defined

by ROC analysis are presented in Fig. 3. Subjects with high UMCP-1 or UACR UEGF and low UEGF or UEGF/MCP-1 ratio values experienced a significantly faster evolution to endpoint ($P < 0.001$). SBP.

Urine MCP-1 or EGF/MCP-1 ratio as independent predictors of rapid decline GFR
Univariate analysis of clinical and biomarkers showed that systolic blood pressure, diastolic blood pressure, GFR, UACR, UMCP-1, UEGF, and UEGF/MCP-1 ratio

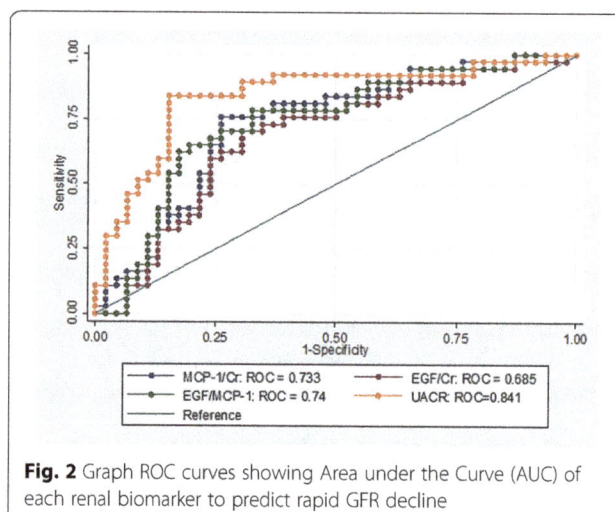

Fig. 2 Graph ROC curves showing Area under the Curve (AUC) of each renal biomarker to predict rapid GFR decline

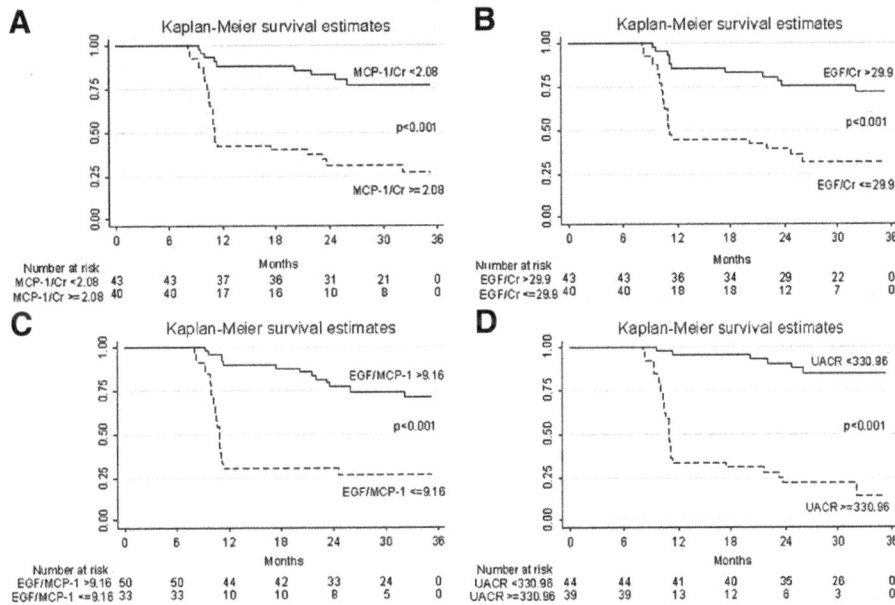

Fig. 3 Kaplan-Meier survival curves of renal endpoint in patients with UMCP-1 (ng/mgCr), UEGF (ng/mgCr), UEGF/MCP-1 (ng/ng) and UACR (mg/gCr) above and below the optimal receiver operating characteristics cutoff level of each tubular biomarkers. **a)** UMCP-1 ≥ 2.08 ng/mgCr, **b)** UEGF ≤29.9 ng/mgCr, **c)** UEGF/MCP-1 ≤ 9.16 ng/ng, **d)** UACR ≥330.96 mg/gCr showed a significantly faster progression to endpoint (p < 0.001, log-rank test). *Abbreviations: UACR* urine albumin creatinine ratio, *UEGF* urine epidermal growth factor creatinine ratio, *UEGF/MCP-1* urine epidermal growth factor and monocyte chemoattractant protein-1 ratio, *UMCP-1* urine monocyte chemoattractant protein-1 creatinine ratio

were associated with *Rapid GFR decline*. In multivariate regression analysis, systolic blood pressure, UMCP-1 in the model 1 and UEGF/MCP-1 ratio in the model 3 were independently associated with *Rapid GFR decline*, respectively (Table 2).

Subgroup analysis
Patients with high cardiovascular risk
Of all patients, 37 (44.6%) were classified as high cardiovascular risk. When patients with high cardiovascular risk were analyzed as a separate subgroup, none of the clinical or biomarker factors including UACR were significant predictors for rapid GFR decline by univariate analysis (*data not shown*).

Patients with low albuminuria
We further evaluated the sub-group of patients with low albuminuria (UACR< 330.9 mg/gCr of median UACR). Figure 4 showed that among patients with low albuminuria, patients with either high EGF or EGF/MCP-1 had

Table 2 Univariate and multivariate analysis of traditional and biomarkers for rapid GFR decline

Parameters	Univariate			Multivariate					
	HR (95% CI.)	P value		Model 1 HR (95% CI.)	P value	Model 2 HR (95% CI.)	P value	Model 3 HR (95% CI.)	P value
SBP (mmHg)	1.03 (1.02, 1.05)	< 0.001		1.03 (1.01, 1.06)	0.002	1.03 (1.01, 1.05)	0.015	1.02 (1, 1.04)	0.102
DBP (mmHg)	1.04 (1.01, 1.06)	0.006		1.02 (0.98, 1.05)	0.357	1.03 (0.99, 1.07)	0.119	1.04 (1, 1.08)	0.052
GFR (mL/min/1.73m²)	0.98 (0.97, 0.99)	0.003		0.99 (0.98, 1.01)	0.506	1 (0.98, 1.02)	0.852	1.01 (0.99, 1.03)	0.59
Age	0.99 (0.96, 1.02)	0.547		0.99 (0.96, 1.03)	0.776	1.02 (0.98, 1.06)	0.379	1.02 (0.99, 1.06)	0.211
Male	1.02 (0.52, 2.01)	0.947		1.54 (0.72, 3.31)	0.263	1.18 (0.54, 2.57)	0.677	1.07 (0.49, 2.35)	0.858
Use of RAAS blockers	0.59 (0.31, 1.14	0.115		0.64 (0.27, 1.5)	0.301	0.92 (0.4, 2.09)	0.834	0.8 (0.34, 1.9)	0.616
UACR (mg/gCr)	1.01 (1.01, 1.02)	< 0.001		1.01 (1.01, 1.02)	< 0.001	1.01 (1.01, 1.02)	< 0.001	1.01 (1.01, 1.02)	0.003
UMCP-1 (ng/mgCr)	1.03 (1.01, 1.05)	0.004		0.93 (0.89, 0.97)	0.001				
UEGF (ng/mgCr)	0.98 (0.97, 0.99)	0.011				0.99 (0.97, 1.01)	0.274		
UEGF/MCP-1 (ng/ng)	0.97 (0.95, 0.99)	0.001						0.97 (0.94, 0.99)	0.018

Abbreviations: DBP Diastolic Blood Pressure, *GFR* Glomerular Filtration Rate, *RAAS* Renin Angiotensin Aldosterone System, *SBP* Systolic Blood Pressure, *UACR* Urine Albumin Creatinine Ratio, *UMCP-1* urinary monocyte chemoattractant protein-1/creatinine, *UEGF* urinary epidermal growth factor/creatinine, *UEGF/MCP* urinary epidermal growth factor/urinary monocyte chemoattractant protein-1 ratio

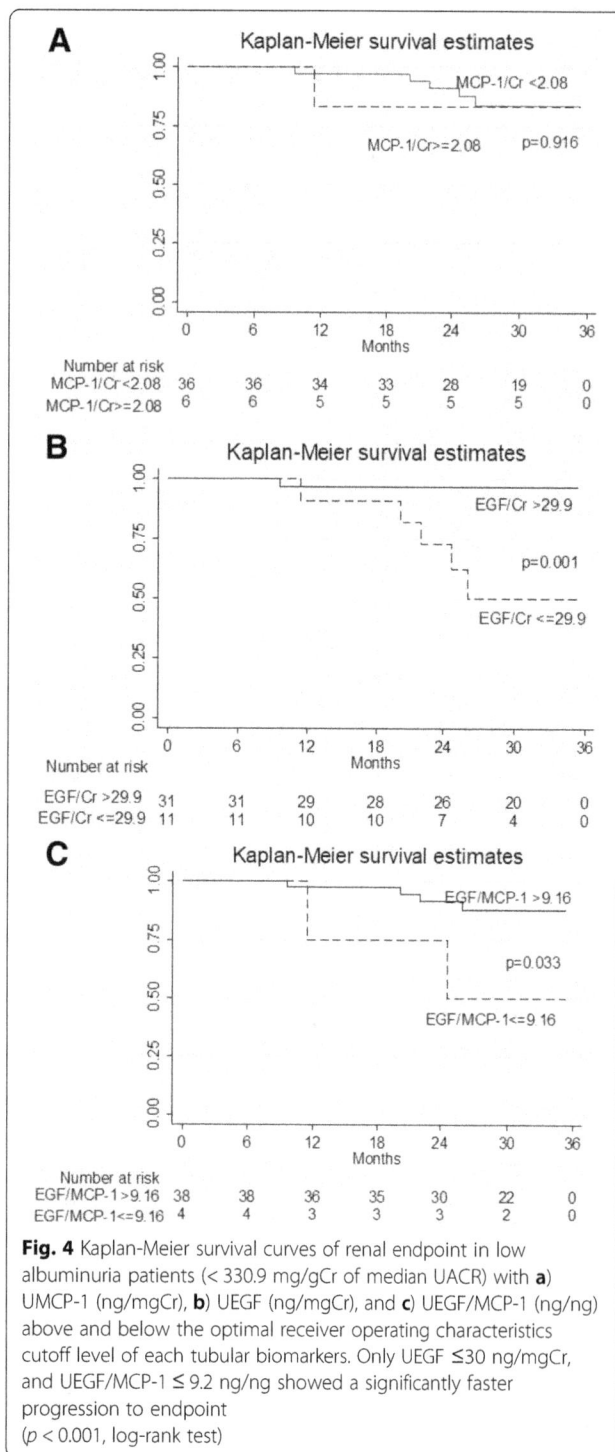

Fig. 4 Kaplan-Meier survival curves of renal endpoint in low albuminuria patients (< 330.9 mg/gCr of median UACR) with **a)** UMCP-1 (ng/mgCr), **b)** UEGF (ng/mgCr), and **c)** UEGF/MCP-1 (ng/ng) above and below the optimal receiver operating characteristics cutoff level of each tubular biomarkers. Only UEGF ≤30 ng/mgCr, and UEGF/MCP-1 ≤ 9.2 ng/ng showed a significantly faster progression to endpoint ($p < 0.001$, log-rank test)

significantly faster progression to end-point by univariate analysis.

Discussion

The ability to identify which DKD patients will develop rapid decline in kidney function is essential and currently available clinical tests cannot predict renal

outcomes accurately. The present study indicate that MCP-1, EGF, and the EGF/MCP-1 ratio represent potential biomarkers of rapid progression in DKD. UMCP-1, and UEGF/MCP-1 ratio showed significant predictive power after multivariate analysis with conventional factors (blood pressure, GFR and UACR). This might suggest that these biomarkers would not be simple surrogate indexes of baseline estimated GFR, but potential markers on their own, predicting DKD progression beyond the conventional risk factors.

The recruitment of inflammatory cells into renal tissue has a pivotal role in the progression of various renal diseases by promoting a microenvironment that amplifies tissue injury and fibrosis [20, 21]. MCP-1-mediated macrophage accumulation and activation are critical events in the development of diabetic renal injury in animal models [20, 21]. MCP-1 protein and mRNA were detected in cortical tubuli, and infiltrating mononuclear cells in the kidneys of patients with DKD [10], Urinary MCP-1 levels correlated with the severity of both the tubulointerstitial and glomerular lesions. Other studies have also shown correlations between urinary MCP-1 with baseline proteinuria and renal function in DKD [10, 22, 23]. In line with previous studies, we also found that UMCP-1 strongly correlated with the level of albuminuria. In addition, we also found that high UMCP-1 was a predictor of rapid GFR loss in DKD. The relationship between urinary MCP-1 levels and subsequent GFR decline had been observed in earlier studies. In a small study, urine MCP-1 levels was found to correlate with the rate of renal function decline in DKD patients over a 6 year period [24], but the authors did not adjust for conventional risk factors in the study. Recently, urinary MCP-1 was found to be independently associated with the rate of GFR decline in a Canadian cohort with advanced stage 3 to 4 DKD [25]. Our study extended previous observations by showing that high UMCP-1 was predictive of rapid renal function loss across a broad spectrum of kidney function that was independent of conventional factors in Asian patients with stage 1 to 5 DKD.

EGF plays important role in restoring barrier function in the healing phase of renal injury and is also a critical tubular cell survival factor [26, 27]. A role for EGF in predicting outcome in chronic kidney diseases is being increasingly recognized, but there is limited data in DKD. Urinary EGF levels have been shown to correlate with the severity of tubulointerstitial fibrosis in primary glomerulonephritis [13], and low urinary EGF has been shown to be a risk predictor of kidney progression in non-diabetic kidney diseases [28]. More recently, urine EGF was identified as a marker for DKD by urine peptidomic profiling of a diabetic rodent model [29], and reduced urinary EGF levels had been reported in patients with DKD [30, 31]. In this study, we demonstrated the predictive role of low UEGF for detecting rapid kidney decline across a broad spectrum of GFR and albuminuria including a subgroup of patients with low albuminuria (mostly in the microalbuminuria range). Previously, the predictive role of urinary EGF has been investigated in diabetic patients with preserved GFR and normoalbuminuria [29]. The investigators found that low urinary EGF was associated with rapid decline in renal function and predicted incident CKD independent of standard risk factors. DKD is associated with many alterations in the structure of glomeruli, tubulointerstitial and vascular compartments [32]. In line with previous studies, we showed that UEGF correlated with GFR, but not with albuminuria consistent with a predominant role of UEGF as a marker of renal tubulointerstitial involvement than of glomerular damage [13, 33]. However, unlike the previous study of patients with preserved GFR and normoalbuminuria [29], the utility of urine EGF to predict rapid decline in GFR was not apparent after adjustments for albuminuria in our study. Overall, this data is consistent with the hypothesis that EGF may be important in the pathogenesis of DKD and low UEGF may be a useful marker for progression especially in patients with normo- or low albuminuria. It is possible that the benefit of UEGF as a biomarker of rapid progression over traditional markers may be diminished in the context of more advanced DKD or marked proteinuria.

DKD is typically characterized by a high prevalence of cardiovascular risk factors and increased risk for cardiovascular events [2]. Macrovascular disease has been proposed as a mechanism for decreased GFR in some DKD patients [3, 4]. Biomarkers that can identify either cardiovascular or renal outcomes in patients with high cardiovascular risk would be especially useful as interventions may have the greatest benefit in this group [2]. We explored the role of the biomarkers specifically in a subgroup with high cardiovascular risk defined as > 10% probability for developing cardiovascular event at 10 years based on the Framingham risk score. Although the proportion with high risk was quite high (44.6%), only 3.7% actually had already had CV events. Thus most patients may not have extensive macrovascular disease at baseline. The proportion with high cardiovascular risk or the Framingham risk score at baseline did not differ between those who developed rapid GFR decline compared to those who did not suggesting that high CV risk might not be a major factor for GFR decline in our study population. None of the clinical parameters or biomarkers were predictive of rapid GFR decline in the high cardiovascular risk subgroup, which probably reflected the small number of patients in the subgroup. Larger studies are necessary to allow firm conclusions on the role of these biomarkers in high cardiovascular risk patients.

Albuminuria is commonly used to assess kidney disease progression among patients with DKD, but some studies have shown that this marker may have insufficient ability to predict kidney disease end points on its own [19]. On this basis, exploring novel biomarkers that can more reliably identify individuals at risk of experiencing adverse renal outcomes is warranted. Inflammatory cytokines and growth factors are logical candidates for biomarkers of progressive DKD as they have been involved in the pathogenesis of renal fibrosis and are easily measurable in the urine. In our study, albuminuria was still the strongest predictor for rapid GFR decline. The benefit of adding additional biomarkers varied depending on the statistical method used. The C-statistics test showed that UACR had a fairly good discrimination for rapid GFR decline. The addition of other biomarkers did not improve the area under the curve. However, the C-statistics test may be insensitive when adding a new predictor to a model and may occasionally produce incorrect estimates [34]. This phenomenon is particularly perceptible when the baseline model includes strong predictors especially in the context of low numbers of patients such as in our study. On the other hand, by using the multivariate model, we showed that MCP-1 or EGF/MCP-1 were independent predictors of rapid GFR decline. Together with findings from previous studies, our results suggest that urine MCP-1 could be a promising biomarker for rapid GFR decline in DKD across a broad range of GFR, but additional studies are necessary to confirm the added benefit to conventional factors including UACR. Findings of this study has several implications. Urine MCP-1 might be utilized to identify high risk patients for inclusion into clinical trials or for more aggressive intervention. The findings also provide additional support for the role of MCP-1 in the pathogenesis of human DKD progression. This is especially important as specific inhibitors of MCP-1 are now available for clinical studies with the potential to impact proteinuria [35]. It would be of interest to see if high urinary MCP-1 could identify those who would mostly likely to respond to MCP-1 blockade. To our knowledge, this is the first study to evaluate the role of EGF in addition to MCP-1 as a ratio in DKD. Earlier studies have shown that combinations of EGF with MCP-1 in the form of EGF/MCP-1 ratio was a better predictor of eGFR decline in non-diabetic kidney disease compared to either biomarker alone [14]. In this study, although high EGF/MCP-1 was an independent of rapid loss of GFR in DKD, the overall performance of the ratio was comparable to UMCP-1 alone. Therefore, our study does not support the benefit of routine EGF measurement in addition to MCP-1 given the additional costs. EGF or EGF/MCP-1 may be useful in the DKD subgroup with normo- or low grade albuminuria and decreased GFR.

This subgroup may constitute a larger proportion of DKD than previously recognized [2, 4] but larger studies are necessary to evaluate the cost-benefit of EGF measurement to predict adverse renal outcomes in this group.

This study has several limitations. This is a single center study involving small numbers of subjects with a short follow-up period of 24 months. Urine biomarkers were measured in a cohort of high risk of DKD patients who might have had a more rapid decline in renal function in a limited time of follow-up. The inclusion of higher risk patients and single-center nature of the study design may have an impact on its external validity to a broader group of T2DM patients. It remains to be seen if urinary MCP-1 and or EGF really predict future loss of kidney function in more or less stable, comparable patients or if these values are "just" independently associated with more rapid loss of kidney function. In keeping with standard clinical practice, we did not perform kidney biopsies routinely in patients with DKD in the absence of clinical features suggestive of other kidney diseases [3]. The prevalence of non-diabetic kidney diseases in patients with diabetes reported in the literature is highly variable, but about 10% of unselected patients with early DKD and albuminuria may have non-DKD as an underlying kidney disease [3]. A number of our patients had low albuminuria. However, a lack of albuminuria may not necessarily preclude structural DKD and almost all histopathologic classes of DKD may be present in such patients [36]. However, given that our inclusion criteria of poorly controlled hypertension or longer duration of diabetes, other diagnoses such as hypertensive nephropathy or other glomerular diseases could not be excluded. Finally, given the limited time, our study did not collect data of major renal outcomes such as ESRD.

Conclusions

This study suggests that urinary MCP-1, EGF and EGF/MCP-1 ratio may be promising markers of renal progression among T2DM patients. High urinary MCP-1 may be an independent predictor for rapid GFR decline after adjustments for conventional markers. Further prospective studies in larger populations with longer follow-up are warranted to fully evaluate the roles of urine MCP-1 or EGF/MCP-1 in disease management or as a guide for clinical trial entry in DKD.

Abbreviations

AUC: Area under the curves; CKD-EPI: Chronic Kidney Disease Epidemiology Collaboration; DKD: Diabetic kidney disease; EGF: Epidermal growth factor; ESRD: End stage renal disease; GFR: Glomerular filtration rate; MCP-1: Monocyte chemoattractant protein-1; ROC: Receiver operating characteristic; T2DM: Type 2 diabetes mellitus; UACR: Urine albumin creatinine ratio; UEGF: Urine epidermal growth factor creatinine ratio; UEGF/MCP-1: Urine epidermal growth factor epidermal growth factor ratio; UMCP-1: Urine monocyte chemoattractant protein-1 creatinine ratio

Acknowledgements
We would like to thank all Fellows and Staff of the Nephrology Division for assistance with patient recruitment.

Funding
This study was supported by a grant from Phramongkutklao Hospital and College of Medicine, Ramathibodi Hospital, and the National Science and Technology Development Agency (NSTDA, P-13-00505), Bangkok, Thailand).

Authors' contributions
All author contributions are in line with the ICMJE guidelines. All listed authors made substantial contributions to conception and design, or acquisition of data, or analysis and interpretation of data; been involved in drafting the manuscript or revising it critically for important intellectual content; gave final approval of the version to be published, and agreed to be accountable for all aspects of the work.

Competing interests
The authors declare that they have no competing interests.

Author details
Division of Nephrology, Department of Medicine, Phramongkutklao Hospital and College of Medicine, Bangkok, Thailand. [2]Division of Nephrology, Department of Medicine, Faculty of Medicine Ramathibodi Hospital, Mahidol University, 270 Rama 6 Rd, Bangkok 10400, Thailand.

References
1. Saran R, Li Y, Robinson B, Ayanian J, Balkrishnan R, Bragg-Gresham J, Chen JT, Cope E, Gipson D, He K, et al. US Renal Data System 2014 Annual Data Report: Epidemiology of Kidney Disease in the United States. Am J Kidney Dis. 2015;66(1 Suppl 1):Svii, S1–305.
2. Satirapoj B, Adler SG. Comprehensive approach to diabetic nephropathy. Kidney Res Clin Pract. 2014;33(3):121–31.
3. Fioretto P, Caramori ML, Mauer M. The kidney in diabetes: dynamic pathways of injury and repair. The Camillo Golgi lecture. Diabetologia 2008. 2007;51(8):1347–55.
4. Penno G, Solini A, Bonora E, Fondelli C, Orsi E, Zerbini G, Trevisan R, Vedovato M, Gruden G, Cavalot F, et al. Clinical significance of nonalbuminuric renal impairment in type 2 diabetes. J Hypertens. 2011;29(9):1802–9.
5. Furuta T, Saito T, Ootaka T, Soma J, Obara K, Abe K, Yoshinaga K. The role of macrophages in diabetic glomerulosclerosis. Am J Kidney Dis. 1993;21(5):480–5.
6. Segerer S, Nelson PJ, Schlondorff D. Chemokines, chemokine receptors, and renal disease: from basic science to pathophysiologic and therapeutic studies. J Am Soc Nephrol. 2000;11(1):152–76.
7. Grandaliano G, Gesualdo L, Ranieri E, Monno R, Montinaro V, Marra F, Schena FP. Monocyte chemotactic peptide-1 expression in acute and chronic human nephrites: a pathogenetic role in interstitial monocytes recruitment. J Am Soc Nephrol. 1996;7(6):906–13.
8. Rovin BH, Doe N, Tan LC. Monocyte chemoattractant protein-1 levels in patients with glomerular disease. Am J Kidney Dis. 1996;27(5):640–6.
9. Abujam B, Cheekatla S, Aggarwal A. Urinary CXCL-10/IP-10 and MCP-1 as markers to assess activity of lupus nephritis. Lupus. 2013;22(6):614–23.
10. Wada T, Furuichi K, Sakai N, Iwata Y, Yoshimoto K, Shimizu M, Takeda SI, Takasawa K, Yoshimura M, Kida H, et al. Up-regulation of monocyte chemoattractant protein-1 in tubulointerstitial lesions of human diabetic nephropathy. Kidney Int. 2000;58(4):1492–9.
11. Banba N, Nakamura T, Matsumura M, Kuroda H, Hattori Y, Kasai K. Possible relationship of monocyte chemoattractant protein-1 with diabetic nephropathy. Kidney Int. 2000;58(2):684–90.
12. Gesualdo L, Di Paolo S, Calabro A, Milani S, Maiorano E, Ranieri E, Pannarale G, Schena FP. Expression of epidermal growth factor and its receptor in normal and diseased human kidney: an immunohistochemical and in situ hybridization study. Kidney Int. 1996;49(3):656–65.
13. Worawichawong S, Worawichawong S, Radinahamed P, Muntham D, Sathirapongsasuti N, Nongnuch A, Assanatham M, Kitiyakara C. Urine

Urinary epidermal growth factor, monocyte chemoattractant protein-1 or their ratio as predictors for rapid loss...

29

epidermal growth factor, monocyte Chemoattractant Protein-1 or their ratio as biomarkers for interstitial fibrosis and tubular atrophy in primary glomerulonephritis. Kidney Blood Press Res. 2016;41(6):997–1007.

14. Torres DD, Rossini M, Manno C, Mattace-Raso F, D'Altri C, Ranieri E, Pontrelli P, Grandaliano G, Gesualdo L, Schena FP. The ratio of epidermal growth factor to monocyte chemotactic peptide-1 in the urine predicts renal prognosis in IgA nephropathy. Kidney Int. 2008;73(3):327–33.

15. KDIGO. 2012 clinical practice guideline for the evaluation and Management of Chronic Kidney Disease. Kidney Int Suppl. 2013;3(1):150.

16. D'Agostino RB Sr, Vasan RS, Pencina MJ, Wolf PA, Cobain M, Massaro JM, Kannel WB. General cardiovascular risk profile for use in primary care: the Framingham heart study. Circulation. 2008;117(6):743–53.

17. Levey AS, Stevens LA, Schmid CH, Zhang YL, Castro AF 3rd, Feldman HI, Kusek JW, Eggers P, Van Lente F, Greene T, et al. A new equation to estimate glomerular filtration rate. Ann Intern Med. 2009;150(9):604–12.

18. Youden WJ. Index for rating diagnostic tests. Cancer. 1950;3(1):32–5.

19. Norris KC, Smoyer KE, Rolland C, Van der Vaart J, Grubb EB. Albuminuria, serum creatinine, and estimated glomerular filtration rate as predictors of cardio-renal outcomes in patients with type 2 diabetes mellitus and kidney disease: a systematic literature review. BMC Nephrol. 2018;19(1):36.

20. Haller H, Bertram A, Nadrowitz F, Menne J. Monocyte chemoattractant protein-1 and the kidney. Curr Opin Nephrol Hypertens. 2016;25(1):42–9.

21. Kim MJ, Tam FW. Urinary monocyte chemoattractant protein-1 in renal disease. Clin Chim Acta. 2011;412(23–24):2022–30.

22. Morii T, Fujita H, Narita T, Shimotomai T, Fujishima H, Yoshioka N, Imai H, Kakei M, Ito S. Association of monocyte chemoattractant protein-1 with renal tubular damage in diabetic nephropathy. J Diabetes Complicat. 2003;17(1):11–5.

23. Tashiro K, Koyanagi I, Saitoh A, Shimizu A, Shike T, Ishiguro C, Koizumi M, Funabiki K, Horikoshi S, Shirato I, et al. Urinary levels of monocyte chemoattractant protein-1 (MCP-1) and interleukin-8 (IL-8), and renal injuries in patients with type 2 diabetic nephropathy. J Clin Lab Anal. 2002;16(1):1–4.

24. Tam FW, Riser BL, Meeran K, Rambow J, Pusey CD, Frankel AH. Urinary monocyte chemoattractant protein-1 (MCP-1) and connective tissue growth factor (CCN2) as prognostic markers for progression of diabetic nephropathy. Cytokine. 2009;47(1):37–42.

25. Verhave JC, Bouchard J, Goupil R, Pichette V, Brachemi S, Madore F, Troyanov S. Clinical value of inflammatory urinary biomarkers in overt diabetic nephropathy: a prospective study. Diabetes Res Clin Pract. 2013;101(3):333–40.

26. Lechner J, Malloth NA, Jennings P, Heckl D, Pfaller W, Seppi T. Opposing roles of EGF in IFN-alpha-induced epithelial barrier destabilization and tissue repair. Am J Physiol Cell Physiol. 2007;293(6):C1843–50.

27. Kennedy WA 2nd, Buttyan R, Garcia-Montes E, D'Agati V, Olsson CA, Sawczuk IS. Epidermal growth factor suppresses renal tubular apoptosis following ureteral obstruction. Urology. 1997;49(6):973–80.

28. Ju W, Nair V, Smith S, Zhu L, Shedden K, Song PXK, Mariani LH, Eichinger FH, Berthier CC, Randolph A, et al. Tissue transcriptome-driven identification of epidermal growth factor as a chronic kidney disease biomarker. Sci Transl Med. 2015;7(316):316ra193.

29. Betz BB, Jenks SJ, Cronshaw AD, Lamont DJ, Cairns C, Manning JR, Goddard J, Webb DJ, Mullins JJ, Hughes J, et al. Urinary peptidomics in a rodent model of diabetic nephropathy highlights epidermal growth factor as a biomarker for renal deterioration in patients with type 2 diabetes. Kidney Int. 2016;89(5):1125–35.

30. Mathiesen ER, Nexo E, Hommel E, Parving HH. Reduced urinary excretion of epidermal growth factor in incipient and overt diabetic nephropathy. Diabet Med. 1989;6(2):121–6.

31. Tsau Y, Chen C. Urinary epidermal growth factor excretion in children with chronic renal failure. Am J Nephrol. 1999;19(3):400–4.

32. Tervaert TW, Mooyaart AL, Amann K, Cohen AH, Cook HT, Drachenberg CB, Ferrario F, Fogo AB, Haas M, de Heer E, et al. Pathologic classification of diabetic nephropathy. J Am Soc Nephrol. 2010;21(4):556–63.

33. Nonclercq D, Toubeau G, Lambricht P, Heuson-Stiennon JA, Laurent G. Redistribution of epidermal growth factor immunoreactivity in renal tissue after nephrotoxin-induced tubular injury. Nephron. 1991;57(2):210–5.

34. Parikh CR, Thiessen-Philbrook H. Key concepts and limitations of statistical methods for evaluating biomarkers of kidney disease. J Am Soc Nephrol. 2014;25(8):1621–9.

35. Menne J, Eulberg D, Beyer D, Baumann M, Saudek F, Valkusz Z, Wiecek A, Haller H, Emapticap Study G. C-C motif-ligand 2 inhibition with emapticap pegol (NOX-E36) in type 2 diabetic patients with albuminuria. Nephrol Dial Transplant. 2017;32(2):307–15.

36. Klessens CQ, Woutman TD, Veraar KA, Zandbergen M, Valk EJ, Rotmans JI, Wolterbeek R, Bruijn JA, Bajema IM. An autopsy study suggests that diabetic nephropathy is underdiagnosed. Kidney Int. 2016;90(1):149–56.

4

Mineral and bone disorder management in hemodialysis patients: comparing PTH control practices in Japan with Europe and North America: the Dialysis Outcomes and Practice Patterns Study (DOPPS)

Suguru Yamamoto[1*], Angelo Karaboyas[2], Hirotaka Komaba[3], Masatomo Taniguchi[4], Takanobu Nomura[5], Brian A. Bieber[2], Patricia De Sequera[6], Anders Christensson[7], Ronald L. Pisoni[2], Bruce M. Robinson[2] and Masafumi Fukagawa[3]

Abstract

Background: High-circulating level of parathyroid hormone (PTH) is associated with elevated mortality in dialysis patients. The Japanese Society for Dialysis Therapy guideline suggests a lower PTH target than other international guidelines; thus, PTH control may differ in Japan compared with other regions, and be associated with mortality.

Methods: We analyzed data from hemodialysis patients with ≥3 measurements of PTH during the first 9 months after enrollment in the Dialysis Outcomes and Practice Patterns Study (DOPPS) phases 4–5 (2009–2015). PTH control was assessed by the mean, slope, and mean squared error (MSE) of all PTH measurements over the 9-month run-in period. Distribution of each PTH control was assessed by regions (Europe/Australia/New Zealand [Eur/ANZ], Japan and North America) and dialysis vintage. Mortality rates were compared across PTH control categories using Cox regression models.

Results: Mean PTH was lower in Japan than in other regions across dialysis vintage categories. In patients with dialysis vintage < 90 days, PTH level was more likely to decline > 5% per month in Japan (48% of patients) versus Eur/ANZ (35%) and North America (35%). In patients with dialysis vintage > 1 year, Japanese patients maintained steady PTH, while patients in Eur/ANZ and North America were more likely to experience a PTH increase. Mean PTH was associated with mortality in the overall samples (highest mortality rate for PTH > 600 pg/mL, hazard ratio, 1.35; 95% confidence interval, 1.20 to 1.52 vs PTH 200–399 pg/mL), and the association was obvious in the prevalent patients (hazard ratio, 1.44; 95% confidence interval, 1.26 to 1.65). PTH slope and MSE did not show significant association with mortality in the overall sample as well as in subjects stratified both by region and dialysis vintage.

Conclusion: PTH control in hemodialysis patients, as measured by keeping a stable PTH level over 9 months, was observed in Japan contrasted with other regions. High PTH mean, but not increased PTH slope and MSE, was associated with mortality especially in prevalent patients.

Keywords: Parathyroid hormone, Hemodialysis, Dialysis outcomes and practice patterns study, PTH slope, Japanese society for Dialysis therapy

* Correspondence: yamamots@med.niigata-u.ac.jp
[1]Division of Clinical Nephrology and Rheumatology, Niigata University Graduate School of Medical and Dental Sciences, 1-757 Asahimachi-dori, Niigata 951-8510, Japan
Full list of author information is available at the end of the article

Background

Mortality of patients with chronic kidney disease (CKD), especially undergoing maintenance hemodialysis (HD) treatment remain higher than the general population [1]. Abnormal mineral and bone metabolism induced by kidney disease accelerate cardiovascular disease, fracture, and other adverse clinical outcomes [2–4]. High serum parathyroid hormone (PTH) level is associated with higher all cause and cardiovascular mortality as well as higher incidence of fracture in patients with maintenance HD [5–10]. Lower PTH level is associated with mortality [5, 7–9] probably owing to malnutrition, and also associated with adynamic bone disease owing to skeletal resistance to PTH [11]. One of important strategies to improve survival in maintenance dialysis patients will be maintaining PTH levels lower with interventions, such as intravenous (IV) vitamin D analogs and calcimimetics [12].The target level of intact PTH was recommended from 150 pg/mL to 300 pg/mL by the National Kidney Foundation in 2003 [13]. The clinical practice guideline for CKD-mineral and bone disorder (CKD-MBD) from Kidney Disease: Improving Global Outcomes (KDIGO) in 2010 [14] suggests maintaining PTH level in the range of approximately 2 to 9 times the upper normal limit for assay, which is the same with a renewed guideline in 2017 considering better survival [15]. The international Dialysis Outcomes and Practice Patterns Study (DOPPS) reported that serum PTH levels have increased in all regions except for Japan, while prescriptions of IV vitamin D analogs and cinacalcet increased during a 15-year period [5]. On the other hand, the Japanese Society for Dialysis Therapy (JSDT) guideline suggests a low and narrow PTH target (60–240 pg/mL) [16], and the serum PTH level remained low and stable in Japanese HD patients [5]. We can find the difference of absolute level of PTH in each regions while there is little information about the practice for PTH control in Japan compared with other regions.

HD practice, such as vascular access, treatment time and dialysis adequacy, has changed globally; however, mortality in Japanese maintenance HD patients was better than in other regions [17, 18]. The management of PTH in HD patients may explain the difference of survival in Japan and other regions. To understand PTH management in each region, it should be evaluated not only with PTH level at one-point measurement, but with several PTH control during certain periods of dialysis treatment, including mean as cumulative expose with PTH, slope as trend of PTH control, or variability as trend of PTH stability. PTH control, as measured by these 3 characteristics, will be different across regions and dialysis vintage and may be associated with survival in dialysis patients. On the basis of data from the international DOPPS, we investigated measures of PTH control in HD patients in Japan compared with other countries and evaluate their association with mortality.

Methods

Patients and data collection

The DOPPS is an international prospective cohort study of patients on in-center HD who are ≥18 years of age, which is currently in phase 6. At each phase, a random sample of chronic HD facilities was selected; within each participating facility, a census of patients on prevalent in-center HD was used to select at random 20–40 patients. Study approval was obtained by a central institutional review board and local ethics committees, as required. Data on monthly laboratory values, medication prescription, and death were abstracted from patient records at baseline and every 4 months. In this study, HD patients with ≥3 measurements of PTH during the first 9 months in DOPPS phase 4 and 5 (2009–2015) were selected in Japan, North America, and Europe / Australia / New Zealand (Eur/ANZ). For the majority of the study period, intact PTH was the only assay available for clinical practice; 10% of DOPPS facilities reported using biointact PTH assays. Patients who had a parathyroidectomy prior to DOPPS enrollment were excluded.

Exposure and outcome

We first log-transformed PTH due to the skewed distribution. We then used linear regression to model log (PTH) separately for each patient over the 9-month run-in period (3 to 9 PTH measurements), with time (month) as the only covariate. Three different measures of PTH control were defined: PTH slope, PTH-mean squared error (MSE), and PTH mean. The slope of log (PTH) was estimated from the regression models, with PTH slope parameterized as % change (per month) over the 9-month run-in period. The MSE of the model, representing PTH variability along the fitted slope, was calculated as the mean of the squared residuals from the regression models. PTH mean was defined as the geometric mean, exp. (mean [log (PTH)]) of all measurements over the 9-month run-in period to lessen the influence of outlier values.

Distributions of these three measures of PTH control were assessed by regions (Eur/ANZ, North America, and Japan) and dialysis vintage at DOPPS enrollment (< 90 days, 90 days-1 year and > 1 year). We also present prescription of PTH-lowering therapies (active vitamin D and cinacalcet; any usage over the 9 month run-in period) by region and dialysis vintage.

Statistical analyses

To investigate the association between each of these three measures of PTH control with all-cause mortality, we used Cox regression using robust sandwich covariance estimators to account for facility clustering, and stratified by DOPPS phase, country, and indicators for black race and large dialysis organization (US only).

Follow-up began after the 9-month run-in period and continued until death, study phase end, or 7 days after leaving the facility due to loss to follow-up, transplantation, or modality switch (whichever occurred first). Exposures were categorized into five groups to assess the functional form of the associations. Covariate adjustment was made for age, sex, vintage, catheter use, 13 comorbidities (Table 1), and mean values of body mass index (BMI), normalized protein catabolic rate (nPCR), hemoglobin (Hgb), creatinine, and albumin over the 9-month run-in period. Other covariates that may potentially be mediators on the causal pathway between PTH control and mortality were additionally adjusted for in a sensitivity analysis, but were not included in the primary analysis: prescription of phosphate binder, cinacalcet, IV and oral vitamin D, plus the mean and slope of serum phosphorus and calcium calculated over the 9-month run-in period (as done for PTH above).

Effect heterogeneity by dialysis vintage was assessed because PTH slopes and means may differ by vintage; PTH levels among patients on dialysis for many years may reflect treatment, while PTH levels among incident dialysis patients may depend more on predialysis PTH levels. Effect heterogeneity by region was assessed because PTH targets vary greatly by region; the same PTH level (e.g., 300 pg/mL) may be in-target in one region (US), but out of target in another region (Japan), and thus likely treated differently.

To deal with missing covariate data, we used multiple imputation, assuming data were missing at random. Missing covariate values were multiply imputed using the Sequential Regression Multiple Imputation Method by IVEware [19]. Results from 20 such imputed data sets were combined for the final analysis using Rubin's formula [20]. The proportion of missing data was below 10% for all variables used for covariate adjustment, with the exception of eight comorbidities (coronary artery disease, cerebrovascular disease, other cardiovascular disease, neurologic disease, psychiatric disorder, lung disease, gastrointestinal bleeding, and recurrent cellulitis/gangrene; 40% missing) that were not collected in a subset of US facilities. All analyses were conducted using SAS software, version 9.4 (SAS institute, Cary, NC).

Results

Comparing PTH control practices in Japan with Europe and North America

Our sample included 5910 patients in Eur/ANZ, 2627 in Japan, and 18,251 in North America. Table 1 shows patient characteristics in those regions. In Japan, patients showed longer dialysis vintage, less use of catheter as vascular access, and lower BMI. The median (IQR) of patients' geometric mean PTH over 9 months was lower in Japan, as compared with Eur/ANZ and North America [Japan: 126 (77, 192) pg/mL, Eur/ANZ: 233 (140, 377) and North America: 283 (194, 425) pg/mL]. PTH slope was centered near zero (no change) in all three regions, as each region included many patients with both increasing, decreasing, and steady PTH: the median (interquartile range [IQR]) % change in PTH per month was − 1.0 (− 7.0, 4.9) in Japan, 0.6 (− 6.1, 7.1) in Eur/ANZ, and 0.5 (− 6.0, 7.1) in North America. Next, we assessed the 3 measures of PTH control, including mean of PTH, slope, and MSE by region and dialysis vintage (Fig. 1). Geometric mean of PTH over 9 months was much lower in Japan than in other regions across dialysis vintage categories (Fig. 1a). In Japan, PTH mean showed highest in patients with dialysis vintage < 90 days (median 139 pg/mL; IQR: 89–217), and was getting smaller with vintage (Fig. 1a). Among patients with baseline vintage < 90 days, the median (IQR) PTH mean was 206 (122–316) in Eur/ANZ and 249 (169–372) in North America; in contrast to Japan, PTH mean was larger at greater dialysis vintage in these regions (Fig. 1a). In patients with dialysis vintage < 90 days, PTH level was more likely to decline > 5% per month in Japan (48% of patients) versus Eur/ANZ (35%) and North America (35%) (Fig. 1b). In patients with dialysis vintage > 1 year, Japanese patients were most likely to maintain steady PTH (PTH slope within +/− 5% per month: 47% in Japan vs. 42% in Eur/ANZ and 41% in North America), and patients in Eur/ANZ and North America more likely to experience increase in PTH (Fig. 1b). When we assessed the distribution of within-patient residuals of log (PTH) in Japan, higher PTH-MSE was found in patients with dialysis vintage < 90 days, while MSE got smaller in those with dialysis vintage > 90 days, an indicator of more stable PTH control (Fig. 1c). There was no difference of residuals of log (PTH) with dialysis vintage both in Eur/ANZ and North America (Fig. 1c).

The prescription of PTH-lowering therapies (any over the 9 month run-in period) is illustrated in Fig. 2 by region and dialysis vintage. Cinacalcet use was similar across regions: about 10% during the first year of HD and 30% among patients on HD for over 1 year. Active vitamin D use also increased with dialysis vintage, and was lower in Eur/ANZ (where oral vitamin D is preferred over IV vitamin D) than in North American and Japan, consistent with a previous DOPPS report [5].

Association between PTH control practices and mortality

Median follow-up was 14.4 (IQR, 6.8–23.7) months, and associations between the 3 measures of PTH control and mortality are shown in Table 3, with Model 3 being the primary analysis. PTH slope had minimal association with mortality (Table 2, Model 3). Results further stratified by region are shown in Table 3, and results stratified by vintage category are shown in Table 4. We also observed minimal

Table 1 Patient characteristics by region

Patient characteristic	Europe	Japan	North America
N patients	5910	2627	18,251
Characteristics at study entry			
Age (years)	65.9 ± 14.7	64.3 ± 12.3	62.7 ± 14.9
Sex (% male)	62%	66%	55%
Race (% black)	2%	0%	37%
Vintage (years)	1.9 (0.4, 5.1)	3.8 (0.7, 9.2)	2.0 (0.5, 4.6)
Catheter use (%)	26%	1%	32%
Dialysate calcium (mEq/L)	2.9 ± 0.3	2.8 ± 0.2	2.5 ± 0.2
Mean over 9-month run-in period			
BMI (kg/m^2)	26.3 ± 5.5	21.5 ± 3.5	28.7 ± 7.1
Normalized PCR (g/kg/day)	1.00 ± 0.22	0.93 ± 0.18	0.95 ± 0.22
Hgb (g/dL)	11.5 ± 1.0	10.6 ± 0.9	11.0 ± 0.9
Serum creatinine (mg/dL)	7.9 ± 2.4	10.4 ± 2.8	7.9 ± 2.8
Serum albumin (g/dL)	3.73 ± 0.43	3.71 ± 0.36	3.76 ± 0.38
Serum calcium (mg/dL)	9.0 ± 0.6	8.9 ± 0.6	9.0 ± 0.6
Serum phosphorus (mg/dL)	4.9 ± 1.2	5.4 ± 1.0	5.2 ± 1.2
PTH (pg/mL)*	233 (140, 377)	126 (77, 192)	283 (194, 425)
Slope over 9-month run-in period			
Calcium (mg/dL per year)	0.1 (−0.5, 0.8)	0.1 (− 0.4, 0.7)	0.1 (− 0.5, 0.7)
Phosphorus (mg/dL per year)	−0.1 (− 1.5, 1.4)	−0.2 (− 1.5, 1.2)	0.1 (− 1.3, 1.5)
PTH (% change per month)	0.6 (− 6.1, 7.1)	−1.0 (− 7.0, 4.9)	0.5 (− 6.0, 7.1)
MSE over 9-month run-in period**			
Calcium	0.1 (0.1, 0.2)	0.1 (0.1, 0.2)	0.1 (0.1, 0.2)
Phosphorus	0.6 (0.3, 1.1)	0.5 (0.3, 1.0)	0.7 (0.4, 1.3)
Log(PTH)	0.1 (0.0, 0.2)	0.1 (0.0, 0.2)	0.1 (0.0, 0.3)
Medications over 9-month run-in period (% any prescription over 9 months)			
Phosphate binder	85%	88%	80%
Cinacalcet	23%	22%	22%
IV vitamin D	24%	45%	71%
Oral vitamin D	51%	45%	26%
Any active vitamin D	69%	81%	86%
Comorbid conditions (%)			
Coronary artery disease	37%	28%	34%
Congestive heart failure	20%	19%	30%
Cerebrovascular disease	16%	13%	11%
Peripheral vascular disease	31%	15%	15%
Other cardiovascular disease	31%	24%	19%
Hypertension	87%	81%	82%
Diabetes	38%	41%	62%
Neurologic disease	12%	7%	8%
Psychiatric disorder	18%	5%	15%
Lung disease	15%	4%	12%

Table 1 Patient characteristics by region *(Continued)*

Patient characteristic	Europe	Japan	North America
Cancer (non-skin)	16%	10%	7%
Gastrointestinal bleeding	5%	4%	3%
Recurrent cellulitis, gangrene	9%	3%	9%

Mean ± SD or median (IQR) or % shown
*Geometric mean: Exp(mean(log(PTH)))
**MSE mean squared error from fitted regression model over 9-month run-in period

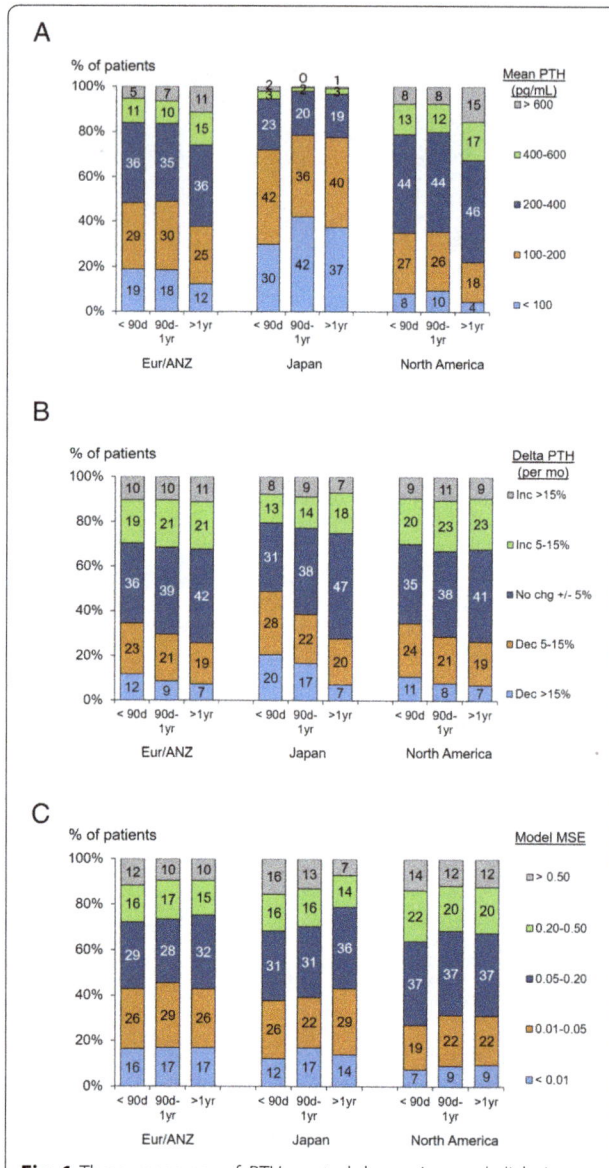

Fig. 1 Three measures of PTH control, by region and dialysis vintage. PTH control was defined as: (**a**) mean of absolute PTH (PTH mean); (**b**) slope of log (PTH) (PTH slope); and (**c**) mean squared error of PTH (PTH-MSE) over the 9 month run-in period. Each figure shows the distribution of PTH control by region [Europe/Australia/New Zealand (Eur/ANZ), North America and Japan] and dialysis vintage at DOPPS enrollment (< 90 days, 90 days-1 year and > 1 year)

association between PTH-MSE and mortality in the overall sample (Table 2, Model 3) as well as in subjects stratified both by region (Table 3) and dialysis vintage (Table 4). Regarding the geometric mean of PTH over 9 months, patients with the highest mean PTH (> 600 pg/mL) had the highest mortality rate in the adjusted model (hazard ratio [HR] = 1.35 (95% confidence interval [CI] 1.20–1.52) vs. PTH 200–399 pg/mL) (Table 2, Model 3). The association weakened after adjusting with several covariates related with calcium and phosphate control (Table 2, HR 1.19 [95% CI 1.04–1.35] in Model 3a), which may reflect an over-adjustment for factors in the causal pathway. The effect was much clearer in prevalent patients who had been on dialysis for over 1 year at study enrollment (vintage > 1 year) [HR = 1.44 (95% CI 1.26–1.65)], as compared with those with dialysis vintage < 90 days [HR = 1.13 (95% CI 0.75–1.77)] and 90 days-1 year [HR = 1.00 (95% CI 0.74–1.36)] (Table 4).

Discussion

In this study, we reported three different measures of PTH control in HD patients from three regions using worldwide DOPPS data. We compared PTH control in Japan versus other countries and evaluated the association between PTH control and mortality. In Japan, we found that PTH level decreased over the first year of dialysis (over 9 months among patients on dialysis < 90 days at DOPPS enrollment), and remained stable

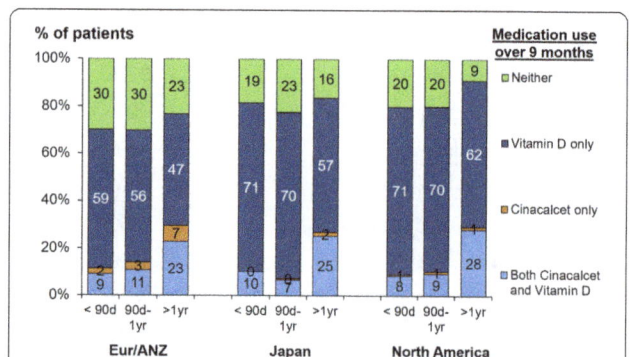

Fig. 2 Prescription of PTH-lowering therapies by region and dialysis vintage. The figure shows any prescription of active vitamin D or cinacalcet over the subsequent 9 month run-in period, by region [Europe/Australia/New Zealand (Eur/ANZ), North America and Japan] and dialysis vintage at DOPPS enrollment (< 90 days, 90 days-1 year and > 1 year)

Table 2 Association between PTH slope/residuals/mean and mortality, by level of adjustment

Exposure	N (%)	Model 1	Model 2	Model 3	Model 3a
PTH slope (% change per month)					
Decreased > 15%	2189 (8%)	1.09 (0.97–1.22)	1.08 (0.96–1.21)	1.10 (0.98–1.25)	1.13 (1.00–1.28)
Decreased 5–15%	5479 (20%)	1.12 (1.03–1.21)	1.05 (0.97–1.14)	1.06 (0.98–1.15)	1.07 (0.98–1.16)
No change ±5%	10,776 (40%)	1 (Ref.)	1 (Ref.)	1 (Ref.)	1 (Ref.)
Increased 5–15%	5750 (21%)	1.05 (0.97–1.13)	1.04 (0.97–1.13)	1.05 (0.97–1.13)	1.03 (0.96–1.12)
Increased > 15%	2594 (10%)	1.07 (0.96–1.19)	1.06 (0.95–1.18)	1.08 (0.97–1.20)	1.04 (0.93–1.16)
PTH mean squared residuals					
< 0.01	2967 (11%)	0.98 (0.89–1.09)	1.01 (0.91–1.13)	1.01 (0.90–1.12)	1.01 (0.90–1.13)
0.01–0.05	6205 (23%)	0.93 (0.86–1.01)	0.94 (0.87–1.02)	0.93 (0.86–1.01)	0.94 (0.86–1.02)
0.05–0.20	9481 (35%)	1 (Ref.)	1 (Ref.)	1 (Ref.)	1 (Ref.)
0.20–0.50	5043 (19%)	1.02 (0.94–1.11)	0.99 (0.91–1.08)	1.00 (0.92–1.09)	1.00 (0.92–1.09)
> 0.50	3092 (12%)	0.95 (0.86–1.05)	0.97 (0.88–1.08)	0.98 (0.89–1.09)	0.99 (0.89–1.11)
PTH geometric mean (pg/mL)					
< 100	2975 (11%)	1.28 (1.16–1.41)	1.01 (0.91–1.12)	1.00 (0.90–1.11)	0.99 (0.89–1.11)
100–199	6395 (24%)	1.09 (1.01–1.18)	0.93 (0.86–1.00)	0.92 (0.85–1.00)	0.94 (0.87–1.02)
200–399	10,887 (41%)	1 (Ref.)	1 (Ref.)	1 (Ref.)	1 (Ref.)
400–599	3666 (14%)	0.92 (0.83–1.01)	1.10 (1.00–1.22)	1.11 (1.01–1.22)	1.05 (0.95–1.17)
≥ 600	2865 (11%)	0.90 (0.81–1.00)	1.33 (1.18–1.50)	1.35 (1.20–1.52)	1.19 (1.04–1.35)

HR (95% CI) of all-cause mortality for each exposure displayed
Model 1: Stratified by phase, country, US-black race
Model 2: Model 1 + adjusted for age, sex, vintage, catheter use, 13 comorbidities, mean values of BMI, nPCR, Hgb, creatinine, albumin over 9-month run-in period
Model 3: Model 2 + simultaneous adjustment for all 3 exposures (PTH slope/residuals/mean)
Model 3a: Model 3 + adjusted for potential mediators: prescription of phosphate binders, cinacalcet, IV vitamin D, and oral vitamin D, P mean, (P mean)^2, P slope, Ca mean, and Ca slope over 9-month run-in period

thereafter. In contrast, PTH level tended to increase with dialysis vintage in both Eur/ANZ and North America. In the parameters of PTH control, when analyzing PTH control and mortality, the strongest association was observed for a high PTH mean (> 600 pg/mL) sustained over the 9 months, especially among prevalent (vintage > 1 year) patients.

Practice patterns for dialysis treatment are different in each country, and survival in Japan is superior to that in other regions [17, 18]. Several factors, including race, purity of dialysate, and variation in vascular access are thought to be associated with mortality [18]. Previous reports showed that high level of absolute PTH is one of risk of mortality in HD patients, and the level in Japan is smaller than that in other regions [5]. We then hypothesized that the practice pattern for PTH control is different between Japan and other regions, and that measures of PTH control are associated with mortality in HD patients.

In this study, PTH slope in Japan was lower in dialysis vintage < 90 days, kept low and stable after 1 year of dialysis duration. JSDT guideline for CKD-MBD management recommends PTH target from 60 to 240 pg/mL for better survival [16]. In the guideline, frequency of PTH measurement is recommended once every 3 months, however, monthly measurement of PTH is required until the PTH concentration is stabilized in target range with intervention [16]. JSDT guideline was recommended to manage PTH from 60 to 180 pg/mL in 2008 [21] which was the narrow target to be achieved, and revised it to PTH 60–240 pg/mL with reanalyzed JSDT data and for avoidance of very low PTH level. Furthermore, adequate PTH levels makes easy to control serum phosphorus and calcium [22]. Adopting JSDT guideline, the physicians in Japan may try to reach the target aggressively soon after initiation of dialysis treatment. Since prescription rate of PTH-lowering therapies in Japan was not high compared with other regions (Fig. 2), it is possible that effectiveness of medication may be different between Japan and other regions. Another possibility of decreasing PTH may be that initiation of dialysis treatment induces reduction of PTH due to supplementation of calcium from dialysate. In addition to aggressive intervention for PTH control after initiation of dialysis, proper PTH control at the pre-dialysis stage will be important to get better PTH control in incident dialysis patients while a European group reported insufficient CKD-MBD management in non-dialysis patients even with regular nephrology care [23]. On the other hand, Eur/ANZ and North America showed higher PTH level with dialysis vintage, contrary to the trend in Japan. One major reason for the difference

Table 3 Association between PTH slope/residuals/mean and mortality, by region

Exposure	Europe + Australia/NZ		Japan		North America	
	N (%)	Adjusted* HR (95% CI)	N (%)	Adjusted* HR (95% CI)	N (%)	Adjusted* HR (95% CI)
PTH slope (% change per month)						
Decreased > 15%	487 (8%)	1.08 (0.85–1.37)	271 (10%)	1.14 (0.72–1.80)	1431 (8%)	1.12 (0.97–1.30)
Decreased 5–15%	1166 (20%)	0.92 (0.77–1.09)	566 (22%)	1.25 (0.92–1.71)	3747 (21%)	1.10 (1.00–1.21)
No change ±5%	2375 (40%)	1 (Ref.)	1152 (44%)	1 (Ref.)	7249 (40%)	1 (Ref.)
Increased 5–15%	1244 (21%)	1.05 (0.91–1.21)	443 (17%)	0.81 (0.56–1.18)	4063 (22%)	1.07 (0.98–1.18)
Increased > 15%	638 (11%)	0.94 (0.75–1.17)	195 (7%)	1.57 (0.95–2.59)	1761 (10%)	1.11 (0.98–1.26)
PTH mean squared residuals						
< 0.01	991 (17%)	1.09 (0.92–1.30)	373 (14%)	1.13 (0.75–1.72)	1603 (9%)	0.94 (0.81–1.10)
0.01–0.05	1576 (27%)	0.95 (0.82–1.10)	728 (28%)	1.09 (0.78–1.53)	3901 (21%)	0.92 (0.83–1.02)
0.05–0.20	1833 (31%)	1 (Ref.)	901 (34%)	1 (Ref.)	6747 (37%)	1 (Ref.)
0.20–0.50	920 (16%)	0.91 (0.76–1.09)	384 (15%)	1.17 (0.74–1.88)	3739 (20%)	1.00 (0.91–1.11)
> 0.50	590 (10%)	1.04 (0.83–1.31)	241 (9%)	1.22 (0.73–2.05)	2261 (12%)	0.94 (0.83–1.06)
PTH geometric mean (pg/mL)						
< 100	862 (15%)	1.04 (0.86–1.25)	983 (37%)	1.22 (0.83–1.79)	1130 (6%)	0.97 (0.83–1.13)
100–199	1598 (27%)	0.90 (0.76–1.05)	1041 (40%)	1.35 (0.93–1.97)	3756 (21%)	0.93 (0.84–1.02)
200–399	2120 (36%)	1 (Ref.)	514 (20%)	1 (Ref.)	8253 (45%)	1 (Ref.)
400–599	774 (13%)	1.23 (1.01–1.51)	65 (2%)	–	2827 (15%)	1.04 (0.93–1.17)
≥ 600	556 (9%)	1.26 (0.97–1.62)	24 (1%)	–	2285 (13%)	1.31 (1.14–1.50)

*Adjusted as in Table 2, Model 3

Table 4 Association between PTH slope/residuals/mean and mortality, by vintage

Exposure	Vintage < 90 days		Vintage 90 days - 1 year		Vintage > 1 year	
	N (%)	Adjusted* HR (95% CI)	N (%)	Adjusted* HR (95% CI)	N (%)	Adjusted* HR (95% CI)
PTH slope (% change per month)						
Decreased > 15%	459 (12%)	1.06 (0.74–1.52)	445 (9%)	1.12 (0.83–1.52)	1189 (7%)	1.16 (1.00–1.35)
Decreased 5–15%	935 (24%)	1.06 (0.81–1.38)	1075 (21%)	0.92 (0.75–1.14)	3267 (19%)	1.13 (1.03–1.24)
No change ±5%	1373 (35%)	1 (Ref.)	1949 (38%)	1 (Ref.)	7082 (42%)	1 (Ref.)
Increased 5–15%	766 (20%)	1.20 (0.91–1.58)	1095 (22%)	0.94 (0.77–1.14)	3689 (22%)	1.06 (0.97–1.17)
Increased > 15%	374 (10%)	1.34 (0.99–1.82)	527 (10%)	0.79 (0.60–1.06)	1612 (10%)	1.15 (1.01–1.31)
PTH mean squared residuals						
< 0.01	386 (10%)	1.09 (0.79–1.51)	589 (12%)	1.23 (0.96–1.56)	1936 (12%)	0.98 (0.86–1.12)
0.01–0.05	844 (22%)	0.78 (0.59–1.03)	1214 (24%)	0.97 (0.81–1.16)	3964 (24%)	0.96 (0.87–1.06)
0.05–0.20	1358 (35%)	1 (Ref.)	1757 (35%)	1 (Ref.)	5981 (36%)	1 (Ref.)
0.20–0.50	793 (20%)	0.83 (0.64–1.08)	950 (19%)	0.91 (0.74–1.11)	3081 (18%)	1.07 (0.97–1.19)
> 0.50	526 (13%)	0.77 (0.57–1.05)	581 (11%)	0.88 (0.66–1.17)	1877 (11%)	1.05 (0.92–1.19)
PTH geometric mean (pg/mL)						
< 100	482 (12%)	1.10 (0.81–1.49)	739 (15%)	0.93 (0.75–1.16)	1658 (10%)	1.07 (0.94–1.22)
100–199	1114 (29%)	0.92 (0.74–1.15)	1421 (28%)	0.93 (0.78–1.10)	3663 (22%)	0.96 (0.87–1.05)
200–399	1581 (40%)	1 (Ref.)	2034 (40%)	1 (Ref.)	6838 (41%)	1 (Ref.)
400–599	470 (12%)	0.82 (0.56–1.20)	554 (11%)	1.15 (0.89–1.49)	2511 (15%)	1.13 (1.01–1.26)
≥ 600	260 (7%)	1.13 (0.73–1.77)	343 (7%)	1.00 (0.74–1.36)	2169 (13%)	1.44 (1.26–1.65)

*Adjusted as in Table 2, Model

of PTH level between Japan and other regions may be due to the CKD-MBD guidelines that physicians adopt. The revised KDIGO guideline in 2017 recommends target of PTH level as 2 to 9 times the upper limit of the assay [15]. Physicians in Eur/ANZ and North America who adopt the KDIGO guideline will try to control PTH level not exceeding 600 pg/mL, which is about 9 times the upper limit of the assay; however, 11% and 16% of dialysis patients in Eur/ANZ and North America, respectively, have serum PTH level over 600 pg/mL. In this study, there was not so much difference of MBD treatment between Japan and other regions [ex. Medication rate of cinacalcet: 23% vs. 22% vs. 23% and any active vitamin D: 69% vs. 81% vs. 86% in Eur/ANZ vs. Japan vs. North America, respectively, Table 1 and Fig. 2]. Then, the intervention not only in pre-dialysis stage, but in earlier dialysis vintage and/or before reaching high PTH level may be recommended to avoid excessive increase of PTH.

There are several reports about the association between absolute PTH level and mortality in dialysis patients [5–9]. In this study, we examined the relation of parameters for PTH control and survival using worldwide DOPPS data, and found that high PTH mean for 9-month periods was associated with mortality, but not high PTH slope, or a large MSE that reflects greater variation around the fitted slope. The association between mean PTH > 600 pg/mL and mortality was strong in the primary model and even remained after adjustment for potential mediators related to calcium and phosphate control (Table 2, Model 3 vs. Model 3a). PTH mean > 600 pg/mL increased mortality risk, and the effect was strongest in patients with dialysis vintage > 1 year as compared with those with dialysis vintage < 90 days and 90 days-1 year (Table 4). In incident patients, the association between PTH and mortality was not strong, potentially because PTH will be changed easily with control of calcium and phosphorus. The stronger association in prevalent patients may be owing to sustainable hyperparathyroidism with parathyroid hyperplasia which may induce vascular calcification and abnormal bone metabolism with the prolonged exposure of PTH to vascular and bone. Fibroblast growth factor 23 (FGF23) may be associated with clinical outcomes in patients with high PTH mean because high PTH is related with higher FGF23 level which is strongly associated with mortality in CKD and dialysis patients [24, 25]. In this study, data of FGF23 were not widely available, and a future study will be needed to examine FGF23 control in dialysis patients to understand better CKD-MBD management. Although increased PTH slope did not show increase of risk for mortality, a steep (> 15% per month) decrease in PTH was associated with a slightly elevated – not lower – mortality rate, which was strongest in patients with dialysis vintage more than 1 year (Table 4). The Current Management of Secondary Hyperparathyroidism, a Multi-Center Observational Study (COSMOS) study

showed the survival benefit with increase of PTH level in HD patients with baseline PTH < 168 pg/mL, but not those with decrease of PTH [8]. Another study showed that a small increase of PTH < 300 pg/mL within 12 months was associated with better survival, while decreased PTH showed the increase of mortality in prevalent HD patients whose baseline PTH was 205 (116.5, 400) pg/mL [26]. One of the reasons why decrease of PTH is associated with increase of mortality may be malnutrition [27]. In fact, our data showed that HR of mortality in patients with PTH mean < 100 pg/mL decreased when several markers associated with nutrition were added as covariates (Table 2, Model 1 vs. Model 2). Thus, to keep stable and lower PTH level will lead to better survival in prevalent HD patients. Japanese practice patterns for PTH management, such as decreased PTH levels after initiation of dialysis treatment, and keeping stable and lower PTH levels in the maintenance dialysis phase, may be better to avoid PTH > 600 pg/mL, as well as major increases or decreases of PTH in prevalent patients. To clarify the usefulness of Japanese PTH management, further studies will be needed to examine survival benefit with stable and low PTH management across countries.

The DOPPS study design allowed us to present trends in PTH control and the association with outcomes in a cohort of real-world patients, similar to what physicians may encounter when rounding in the dialysis unit. However, we must acknowledge some important limitations. Multiple assays are available for measurement of intact PTH, and large interassay variability may have contributed to misclassification of specific patients. Assuming this variation is random with respect to patient characteristics, this would tend to bias associations of PTH, with mortality to the null. As with any observational study, the reported associations do not prove causality and may be affected by unmeasured confounders. HD patients with ≥3 measurements of PTH during the first 9 months were enrolled. This would tend to bias associations that may select dialysis units to control PTH management carefully, or patients who have to measure PTH frequently. Patients on HD were enrolled in this study, and there was no information regarding CKD-MBD treatment in predialysis stage.

Conclusion

PTH control, as measured by keeping a stable PTH level over 9 months, was better in Japan versus other regions. High PTH mean, but not increased PTH slope and MSE, was associated with mortality, especially among prevalent hemodialysis patients. PTH management of treating aggressively after initiation of dialysis, and subsequently sustaining PTH within a low target range, might be preferable to avoid the potentially harmful consequences of high PTH level in HD patients.

Abbreviations

BMI: Body mass index; CI: Confidence interval; CKD: Chronic kidney disease; CKD-MBD: CKD-mineral and bone disorder; COSMOS: Current Management of Secondary Hyperparathyroidism, a Multi-Center Observational Study; DOPPS: Dialysis Outcomes and Practice Patterns Study; Eur/ANZ: Europe / Australia / New Zealand; HD: Hemodialysis; Hgb: Hemoglobin; HR: Hazard ratio; IQR: Interquartile range; IV: Intravenous; JSDT: Japanese Society for Dialysis Therapy; KDIGO: Kidney Disease: Improving Global Outcomes; MSE: Mean squared error; nPCR: Normalized protein catabolic rate; PTH: Parathyroid hormone

Acknowledgements

Heather Van Doren, MFA, senior medical editor with Arbor Research Collaborative for Health, provided editorial assistance on this manuscript.

Funding

The DOPPS Program is supported by Amgen, Kyowa Hakko Kirin, and Baxter Healthcare, Fresenius Medical Care Asia-Pacific Ltd., Fresenius Medical Care Canada Inc., Kidney Care UK, MEDICE Arzneimittel Pütter GmbH & Co KG, Otsuka America Pharmaceutical, Inc., and The Association of German Nephrology Centres (Verband Deutsche Nierenzentren e.V.). Additional support for specific projects and countries is provided by Amgen, AstraZeneca, European Renal Association-European Dialysis & Transplant Association (ERA-EDTA), German Society of Nephrology (DGfN), Janssen, Japanese Society for Peritoneal Dialysis (JSPD), Keryx, Proteon, Società Italiana di Nefrologia (SIN), and Vifor Fresenius Medical Care Renal Pharma. Public funding and support is provided for specific DOPPS projects, ancillary studies, or affiliated research projects by the Belgian Federal Public Service of Public Health in Belgium; the French National Institute of Health and Medical Research (INSERM) in France; Cancer Care Ontario (CCO) through the Ontario Renal Network (ORN) in Canada; the National Health & Medical Research Council (NHMRC) in Australia; the National Institute for Health Research (NIHR) via the Comprehensive Clinical Research Network (CCRN) in the United Kingdom; and the Thailand Research Foundation (TRF), Chulalongkorn University Matching Fund, King Chulalongkorn Memorial Hospital Matching Fund, and National Research Council of Thailand (NRCT) in Thailand. All support is provided without restrictions on publications.

Authors' contributions

SY, AK, HK, MT, TN, BB, PDS, AC, RLP, BMR, MF made substantial contributions to conception and design, or acquisition of data, or analysis and interpretation of data; SY, AK, HK, MT, TN, BB, RLP, BMR, MF have been involved in drafting the manuscript or revising it critically for important intellectual content; SY, AK, HK, MT, TN, BB, PDS, AC, RLP, BMR, MF have given final approval of the version to be published. Each author should have participated sufficiently in the work to take public responsibility for appropriate portions of the content; and all authors agreed to be accountable for all aspects of the work in ensuring that questions related to the accuracy or integrity of any part of the work are appropriately investigated and resolved. All authors read and approved the final manuscript.

Competing interests

S.Y. has received honoraria from Kyowa Hakko Kirin. H.K. has received honoraria, consulting fees, and/or grant/research support from Bayer Yakuhin and Kyowa Hakko Kirin. M.T. has received consulting fees from Kyowa Hakko Kirin. T.N. is an employee of Kyowa Hakko Kirin. M.F. has received honoraria, consulting fees, and/or grant/research support from Astellas Pharma, Bayer Yakuhin, Kyowa Hakko Kirin, Ono Pharmaceutical, and Torii Pharmaceutical. A.K., B.A.B., R.L.P., and B.M.R. are employees for the non-profit research organization Arbor Research Collaborative for Health, which has designed and carries out the Dialysis Outcomes and Practice Patterns Study (DOPPS) Program. Grants are made to Arbor Research Collaborative for Health and not to individual investigators. The remaining authors have no conflicts to report.

Author details

[1]Division of Clinical Nephrology and Rheumatology, Niigata University Graduate School of Medical and Dental Sciences, 1-757 Asahimachi-dori, Niigata 951-8510, Japan. [2]Arbor Research Collaborative for Health, Ann Arbor, MI, USA. [3]Division of Nephrology, Endocrinology and Metabolism, Tokai University School of Medicine, Isehara, Japan. [4]Fukuoka Renal Clinic, Fukuoka, Japan. [5]Medical Affairs Department, Kyowa Hakko Kirin Co. Ltd., Tokyo, Japan. [6]University Hospital Infanta Leonor, Madrid, Spain. [7]Department of Nephrology, Skåne University Hospital, Malmö-, Lund, Sweden.

References

1. Saran R, Robinson B, Abbott KC, Agodoa LYC, Bhave N, Bragg-Gresham J, Balkrishnan R, Dietrich X, Eckard A, Eggers PW, et al. US renal data system 2017 annual data report: epidemiology of kidney disease in the United States. Am J Kidney Dis. 2018;71(3S1):A7.
2. Moe S, Drueke T, Cunningham J, Goodman W, Martin K, Olgaard K, Ott S, Sprague S, Lameire N, Eknoyan G, et al. Definition, evaluation, and classification of renal osteodystrophy: a position statement from kidney disease: improving global outcomes (KDIGO). Kidney Int. 2006;69(11):1945–53.
3. Bover J, Bailone L, Lopez-Baez V, Benito S, Ciceri P, Galassi A, Cozzolino M. Osteoporosis, bone mineral density and CKD-MBD: treatment considerations. J Nephrol. 2017;30(5):677–87.
4. Torres PAU, Cohen-Solal M. Evaluation of fracture risk in chronic kidney disease. J Nephrol. 2017;30(5):653–61.
5. Tentori F, Wang M, Bieber BA, Karaboyas A, Li Y, Jacobson SH, Andreucci VE, Fukagawa M, Frimat L, Mendelssohn DC, et al. Recent changes in therapeutic approaches and association with outcomes among patients with secondary hyperparathyroidism on chronic hemodialysis: the DOPPS study. Clin J Am Soc Nephrol. 2015;10(1):98–109.
6. Tentori F, Blayney MJ, Albert JM, Gillespie BW, Kerr PG, Bommer J, Young EW, Akizawa T, Akiba T, Pisoni RL, et al. Mortality risk for dialysis patients with different levels of serum calcium, phosphorus, and PTH: the Dialysis outcomes and practice patterns study (DOPPS). Am J Kidney Dis. 2008;52(3):519–30.
7. Floege J, Kim J, Ireland E, Chazot C, Drueke T, de Francisco A, Kronenberg F, Marcelli D, Passlick-Deetjen J, Schernthaner G et al. Serum iPTH, calcium and phosphate, and the risk of mortality in a European haemodialysis population. Nephrol Dial Transplant 2011, 26(6):1948–1955.
8. Fernandez-Martin JL, Martinez-Camblor P, Dionisi MP, Floege J, Ketteler M, London G, Locatelli F, Gorriz JL, Rutkowski B, Ferreira A, et al. Improvement of mineral and bone metabolism markers is associated with better survival in haemodialysis patients: the COSMOS study. Nephrol Dial Transplant. 2015; 30(9):1542–51.
9. Taniguchi M, Fukagawa M, Fujii N, Hamano T, Shoji T, Yokoyama K, Nakai S, Shigematsu T, Iseki K, Tsubakihara Y, et al. Serum phosphate and calcium should be primarily and consistently controlled in prevalent hemodialysis patients. Ther Apher Dial. 2013;17(2):221–8.
10. Jadoul M, Albert JM, Akiba T, Akizawa T, Arab L, Bragg-Gresham JL, Mason N, Prutz KG, Young EW, Pisoni RL. Incidence and risk factors for hip or other bone fractures among hemodialysis patients in the Dialysis outcomes and practice patterns study. Kidney Int. 2006;70(7):1358–66.
11. Yamamoto S, Fukagawa M. Uremic toxicity and bone in CKD. J Nephrol. 2017;30(5):623–7.
12. Bellasi A, Cozzolino M, Russo D, Molony D, Di Iorio B: Cinacalcet but not vitamin D use modulates the survival benefit associated with sevelamer in the INDEPENDENT study. Clin Nephrol 2016, 86(9):113–124.
13. National Kidney F. K/DOQI clinical practice guidelines for bone metabolism and disease in chronic kidney disease. Am J Kidney Dis. 2003;42(4 Suppl 3):S1–201.
14. Uhlig K, Berns JS, Kestenbaum B, Kumar R, Leonard MB, Martin KJ, Sprague SM, Goldfarb S. KDOQI US commentary on the 2009 KDIGO clinical practice guideline for the diagnosis, evaluation, and treatment of CKD-mineral and bone disorder (CKD-MBD). Am J Kidney Dis. 2010;55(5):773–99.

15. Isakova T, Nickolas TL, Denburg M, Yarlagadda S, Weiner DE, Gutierrez OM, Bansal V, Rosas SE, Nigwekar S, Yee J, et al. KDOQI US commentary on the 2017 KDIGO clinical practice guideline update for the diagnosis, evaluation, prevention, and treatment of chronic kidney disease-mineral and bone disorder (CKD-MBD). Am J Kidney Dis. 2017;70(6):737–51.

16. Fukagawa M, Yokoyama K, Koiwa F, Taniguchi M, Shoji T, Kazama JJ, Komaba H, Ando R, Kakuta T, Fujii H, et al. Clinical practice guideline for the management of chronic kidney disease-mineral and bone disorder. Ther Apher Dial. 2013;17(3):247–88.

17. Goodkin DA, Bragg-Gresham JL, Koenig KG, Wolfe RA, Akiba T, Andreucci VE, Saito A, Rayner HC, Kurokawa K, Port FK, et al. Association of comorbid conditions and mortality in hemodialysis patients in Europe, Japan, and the United States: the Dialysis outcomes and practice patterns study (DOPPS). J Am Soc Nephrol. 2003;14(12):3270–7.

18. Robinson BM, Akizawa T, Jager KJ, Kerr PG, Saran R, Pisoni RL. Factors affecting outcomes in patients reaching end-stage kidney disease worldwide: differences in access to renal replacement therapy, modality use, and haemodialysis practices. Lancet. 2016;388(10041):294–306.

19. Yamamoto S, Kazama JJ, Fukagawa M. Autophagy: a two-edged sword in diabetes mellitus. Biochem J. 2013;456(3):e1–3.

20. Taylor JM, Cooper KL, Wei JT, Sarma AV, Raghunathan TE, Heeringa SG. Use of multiple imputation to correct for nonresponse bias in a survey of urologic symptoms among African-American men. Am J Epidemiol. 2002; 156(8):774–82.

21. Guideline Working Group JSfDT. Clinical practice guideline for the management of secondary hyperparathyroidism in chronic dialysis patients. Ther Apher Dial. 2008;12(6):514–25.

22. Fukagawa M, Komaba H, Onishi Y, Fukuhara S, Akizawa T, Kurokawa K, Group M-DS. Mineral metabolism management in hemodialysis patients with secondary hyperparathyroidism in Japan: baseline data from the MBD-5D. Am J Nephrol. 2011;33(5):427–37.

23. Gallieni M, De Luca N, Santoro D, Meneghel G, Formica M, Grandaliano G, Pizzarelli F, Cossu M, Segoloni G, Quintaliani G et al: Management of CKD-MBD in non-dialysis patients under regular nephrology care: a prospective multicenter study. J Nephrol 2016, 29(1):71–78.

24. Moe SM, Chertow GM, Parfrey PS, Kubo Y, Block GA, Correa-Rotter R, Drueke TB, Herzog CA, London GM, Mahaffey KW, et al. Cinacalcet, fibroblast growth Factor-23, and cardiovascular disease in hemodialysis: the evaluation of Cinacalcet HCl therapy to lower cardiovascular events (EVOLVE) trial. Circulation. 2015;132(1):27–39.

25. Gutierrez OM, Mannstadt M, Isakova T, Rauh-Hain JA, Tamez H, Shah A, Smith K, Lee H, Thadhani R, Juppner H, et al. Fibroblast growth factor 23 and mortality among patients undergoing hemodialysis. N Engl J Med. 2008;359(6):584–92.

26. Villa-Bellosta R, Rodriguez-Osorio L, Mas S, Abadi Y, Rubert M, de la Piedra C, Gracia-Iguacel C, Mahillo I, Ortiz A, Egido J et al: A decrease in intact parathyroid hormone (iPTH) levels is associated with higher mortality in prevalent hemodialysis patients. PLoS One 2017, 12(3):e0173831.

27. Drechsler C, Krane V, Grootendorst DC, Ritz E, Winkler K, Marz W, Dekker F, Wanner C, German D, Dialysis Study I. The association between parathyroid hormone and mortality in dialysis patients is modified by wasting. Nephrol Dial Transplant. 2009;24(10):3151–7.

5

Prevalence, socio-demographic characteristics, and comorbid health conditions in pre-dialysis chronic kidney disease: results from the Manitoba chronic kidney disease cohort

Mariette J Chartier[1*], Navdeep Tangri[2], Paul Komenda[2], Randy Walld[1], Ina Koseva[1], Charles Burchill[1], Kari-Lynne McGowan[1] and Allison Dart[3]

Abstract

Background: Chronic Kidney Disease (CKD) is common and its prevalence has increased steadily over several decades. Monitoring of rates and severity of CKD across populations is critical for policy development and resource planning. Administrative health data alone has insufficient sensitivity for this purpose, therefore utilizing population level laboratory data and novel methodology is required for population-based surveillance. The aims of this study include a) develop the Manitoba CKD Cohort, b) estimate CKD prevalence, c) identify individuals at high risk of progression to kidney failure and d) determine rates of comorbid health conditions.

Methods: Administrative health and laboratory data from April 1996 to March 2012 were linked from the data repository at the Manitoba Centre for Health Policy. Prevalence was estimated using three methods: a) all CKD cases in administrative and laboratory databases; b) all CKD cases captured only through the laboratory data; c) and the capture-recapture method. Patients were stratified by risk by estimated Glomerular Filtration Rate (eGFR) and albuminuria based on Kidney Disease Improving Global Outcomes (KDIGO) criteria. For comorbid health conditions, the counts were modelled using a Generalized Linear Model (GLM).

Results: The Manitoba CKD Cohort consisted of 55,876 people with CKD. Of these, 18,342 were identified using administrative health data, 27,393 with laboratory data, and 10,141 people were identified in both databases. The CKD prevalence was 5.6% using the standard definition, 10.6% using only people captured by the laboratory data and 10.6% using the capture-recapture method. Of the identified cases, 46% were at high risk of progression to end-stage kidney disease (ESKD), 41% were at low risk and 13% were not classified, due to unavailable laboratory data. High risk cases had a higher burden of comorbid conditions.

Conclusion: This study reports a novel methodology for population based CKD surveillance utilizing a combination of administrative health and laboratory data. High rates of CKD at risk of progression to ESKD have been identified with this approach. Given the high rates of comorbidity and associated healthcare costs, these data can be used to develop a targeted and comprehensive public health surveillance strategy that encompass a range of interrelated chronic diseases.

Keywords: Chronic kidney disease, Prevalence, Comorbidity, Epidemiology, Cohort, Administrative data, Surveillance

* Correspondence: Mariette_chartier@cpe.umanitoba.ca
[1]Manitoba Centre for Health Policy, Department of Community Health Sciences, University of Manitoba, Winnipeg, Canada
Full list of author information is available at the end of the article

Background

Chronic kidney disease (CKD) is a common disorder requiring a public health surveillance strategy to identify those at risk of progression and treat them with disease modifying therapies [1]. Epidemiological studies report that CKD is highly prevalent in the general population and that it has increased steadily over several decades [2–4]. Not surprisingly, parallel to these increases in CKD, increases in the prevalence of kidney failure, or End Stage Kidney Disease (ESKD), have also been reported [5, 6]. ESKD is associated with comorbid health conditions, poor quality of life, and high health care costs [7].

It is critical to develop innovative methods to estimate CKD prevalence and identify affected individuals requiring treatment. Kidney failure affects more Manitobans per capita than most other provinces in Canada, with a prevalence rate of 1530 per million population compared to the Canadian rate of 1193 per million population [5]. The under-recognition and treatment of CKD in its earlier stages and the increasing prevalence of risk factors associated with CKD are implicated in high ESKD rates [8]. Appropriate screening for, monitoring and treatment of certain types of CKD can prevent or delay progression to ESKD. Understanding the geographic variations in prevalence informs health services planning.

Unfortunately, information about the incidence and prevalence of earlier stages of CKD in the general population is limited. Estimates of CKD prevalence in Canada range from 10 to 15%, representing approximately 3 million affected adults [2]. Prevalence rates of CKD across Europe, Asia, North America and Australia range between 2.5 and 11.2% [3] and are highest among low to middle income countries [4]. ESKD represents a small fraction of the total CKD population, with early CKD affecting 50 times more individuals than ESKD [6]. Determining patients who are at greater risk of progression to ESKD is an important aspect of CKD surveillance.

In this study, we propose a novel methodologic approach by combining both laboratory and administrative health data to monitor CKD prevalence. Combining these types of data with novel methods to calculate prevalence could overcome the challenges of the low sensitivity of administrative data. The aims of this study are to: a) develop the Manitoba CKD cohort from a wide range of administrative health databases including medical claims, hospitalization records, prescriptions and laboratory data; b) estimate the CKD prevalence in the province of Manitoba using all sources of data and a capture-recapture method; c) determine the percentage of cases who are at highest risk for progression to ESKD; and d) determine rates of comorbid health conditions among people identified in the CKD cohort.

Methods

Setting and design

This study was conducted in the Canadian province of Manitoba, with a population of about 1.2 million inhabitants. The majority of the population (59%) live in the capital city of Winnipeg, 36% live in rural southern regions and 5% in the northern region located above the 52 parallel. Given the high prevalence rates of dialysis patients in the province, Manitoba Health requested a comprehensive CKD study. Researchers from the Manitoba Centre for Health Policy (MCHP) and the Manitoba Renal Program collaborated on creating the Manitoba CKD Cohort. This focus included Manitoba adults who were 18 years old and over. A separate pediatric cohort was also created and will be described in a separate paper. The study was approved by the Health Research Ethics Board (HREB) at the University of Manitoba (#H2012:297). Obtaining individual consent for use of administrative health databases has been waived by HREB.

The Manitoba CKD Cohort is based on data collected from the publically funded health care system housed at MCHP. These health services datasets include person-level health records virtually capturing the entire population (> 99%). All records within these datasets are de-identified, and personal health identifiers such as Personal Health Identification Numbers (PHINs) are scrambled [9–11]. The data are linkable across files and over time because the PHIN is scrambled in the same way for each dataset. The following datasets were used in this study: Manitoba Health Insurance Registry, Medical Claims/Medical Services, Physician Registry, Hospital Abstracts, Drug Program Information Network, Diagnostic Services Manitoba Laboratory Data, Vital Statistics and Canada Census Files. Detailed information about these data is available on the MCHP website [12].

CKD definition using administrative data

The Manitoba CKD cohort included adults living in Manitoba as of March 31, 2012 who met the definition for CKD at some point between April 1, 1996 and March 31, 2012. The CKD cohort was defined using a combination of administrative health and laboratory data. Within the administrative health data, CKD was defined as having at least two CKD-related medical claims by physician visit *or* one CKD-related hospitalization *or* one filled prescription of a medication specifically used in the treatment or management of CKD within a three-year period [13]. To ensure that acute kidney disease was not counted as CKD, ICD codes related to acute kidney disease were excluded and two abnormal blood tests at least 3 months apart were required to count as a CKD case. The medications listed are those used to treat CKD-related anemia, hyperkalemia, elevated phosphate and hyperparathyroidism. Details of the definitions are found in Table 1.

Table 1 Chronic kidney disease definitions and codes

Indicators	Definitions and Codes

Chronic kidney disease (using administrative data)	Defined as an adult with the following diagnoses from physician claims and hospital records, and drug prescriptions:
	• Two or more physician claims with diagnoses for hypertensive chronic kidney disease, hypertensive heart and chronic kidney disease, acute glomerulonephritis, nephrotic syndrome, chronic glomerulonephritis, nephritis and nephropathy not specified as acute or chronic, chronic kidney disease, renal failure (unspecified), renal sclerosis (unspecified), disorders resulting from impaired renal function, hydronephrosis, other disorders of kidney and ureter, congenital anomalies of urinary system (ICD-9-CM: 403, 404, 580, 581, 582, 583, 585, 586, 587, 588, 591, 593, 753), or
	• One or more hospital episodes with diagnoses for diabetes with renal manifestations, hypertensive chronic kidney disease, hypertensive heart and chronic kidney disease, acute glomerulonephritis, nephrotic syndrome, chronic glomerulonephritis, nephritis and nephropathy not specified as acute or chronic, chronic kidney disease, renal failure (unspecified), renal sclerosis (unspecified), disorders resulting from impaired renal function, hydronephrosis, unspecified disorder of kidney and ureter, congenital anomalies of urinary system (ICD-9-CM: 250.4, 403, 404, 580, 581, 582, 583, 585, 586, 587, 588, 591, 593.9, 753; ICD-10-CA: E10.2, E11.2, I12, I13, N18, N19, N00–16, N25, N26, N28.82, N39.1, Q60–64), or
	• One or more filled drug prescriptions used in CKD management:
	  o generic names: Epoetin Alfa, Darbepoetin Alfa, Peginesatide, Sodium Polystyrene Sulfonate, Calcium Polystyrene sulphonate, Polystyrene Sod Sulfonate 454, Sevelamer HCL, Cinacalcet HCL, Lanthanum;
	  o Anatomical Therapeutic Chemical (ATC) codes: B03XA01, B03XA02, B03XA04, V03AE01, V03AE02, H05BX01, V03AE03.

Chronic kidney disease (using laboratory data)	Defined as an adult with: 1) Two abnormal estimated Glomerular Filtration Rate (eGFR) tests at least 90 days apart using the following equation: Modification of Diet in Renal Disease (MDRD) equation [14] Men: $(175 \times (S_{cr}/88.4)^{-1.154})) \times (AGE)^{-0.203}$ Women: multiply results by 0.74). OR 2) Two abnormal tests for proteinuria (either Protein-Creatinine Ratio (PCR), Albumin-Creatinine Ratio (ACR) or dipstick protein urinalysis) at least 90 days apart. Abnormal test values were defined as: • eGFR values < 60 ml/min/1.73m^2 • PCR > =15 mg/mmol or ACR > =3 mg/mmol [14] • Dipstick Protein Urinalysis gives a categorical measurement of urine protein (0 to 4) which is less precise than a Urine Protein test*. A dipstick protein level greater than or equal to 0.3 g/L is considered abnormally high. * Note: A comparison of same-day Dipstick and Urine Protein test results showed moderate agreement (kappa = 0.48): • Dipstick Protein = 0 comparable to Urine Protein < 15 mg/mmol • Dipstick Protein = 1 comparable to Urine Protein 15–50 mg/mmol • Dipstick Protein = 2–4 comparable to Urine Protein > 50 mg/mmol

CKD definition using laboratory data

For people with laboratory results, we defined CKD by estimating the Glomerular Filtration Rate (eGFR) and level of proteinuria. We determined that an adult had CKD if he/she had at least two tests indicating eGFR < 60 ml/min/1.73m^2 at least 90 days apart as shown in Table 1. The Modification of Diet in Renal Disease (MDRD) equation was chosen to estimate the eGFR because it was being used locally by the provincial laboratories. Proteinuria was assessed by urine protein to creatinine ratio (PCR), urine albumin to creatinine ratio (ACR) or dipstick protein urinalysis. As shown in Table 1, we compared dipstick and urine protein results and oufnd a moderate agreement (kappa = 0.48). We ensured that the two tests were at least 90 days apart to address concerns of one-off testing which may lead to overestimation of CKD cases [15]. Tests with missing date of collection were excluded.

Risk of progression to ESKD

As shown in Fig. 1, we adapted a heat map, colour-coded classification, developed by the Kidney Disease Improving Global Outcomes (KDIGO) Work Group [14]. The heat map incorporated albuminuria levels, given that albuminuria is an important marker of kidney function and risk of progression to ESKD. We categorized the CKD cases by risk of progression to ESKD, using the eGFR and albuminuria levels to identify four levels of risk: a) lowest risk (green), b) moderately increased risk (yellow); c) high risk (orange) and d) the highest risk of all (red).

We adapted the KDIGO heat map by adding an additional category as shown by the light and dark purple boxes, because we wanted to use the available laboratory data to categorize as many cases as possible. Some CKD cases identified through the administrative health data had some laboratory data, but were missing either the creatinine or albuminuria. These cases could be categorized as low risk (light purple) or high risk (dark purple). CKD cases with no laboratory data were categorized as "unknown risk" given that no information about kidney function impairment was available. These classifications were then combined into a low risk (green, yellow, and light purple) and high risk (orange, red, and dark purple). This classification permitted us to examine these CDK groups: the low-risk group that includes earlier stages of CKD, the high-risk group that includes later stages of CKD, unknown CKD group, where the risk to progression to ESKD was unknown.

Sociodemographic characteristics and health conditions

We estimated the CKD prevalence by age and sex, as obtained in the health registry data files, and by income quintiles. The income quintiles were based on the

				Persistent albuminuria categories Description and range			
				A1	A2	A3	
				Normal to mildly increased	Moderately increased	Severely increased	Albuminuria unknown
				<30 mg/g <3 mg/mmol	30-300 mg/g 3-30 mg/mmol	>300 mg/g >30 mg/mmol	
eGFR categories (ml/min/1.73m²) Description and range	G1/G2	Normal or high	≥60	2,186	4,691	5,906	3,138
	G3a	Mildly to moderately decreased	45-59	3,974	2,885	4,238	3,142
	G3b	Moderately to severely decreased	30-44	2,219	2,109	3,502	1,609
	G4	Severely decreased	15-29	598	917	2,262	393
	G5	Kidney failure	<15	84	188	834	86
		eGFR unknown		638	2,076	857	7,344*

* Identified as CKD using only administrative health data with no available laboratory data

These cases are at LOW RISK of progression to ESKD
These cases are at HIGH RISK of progression to ESKD

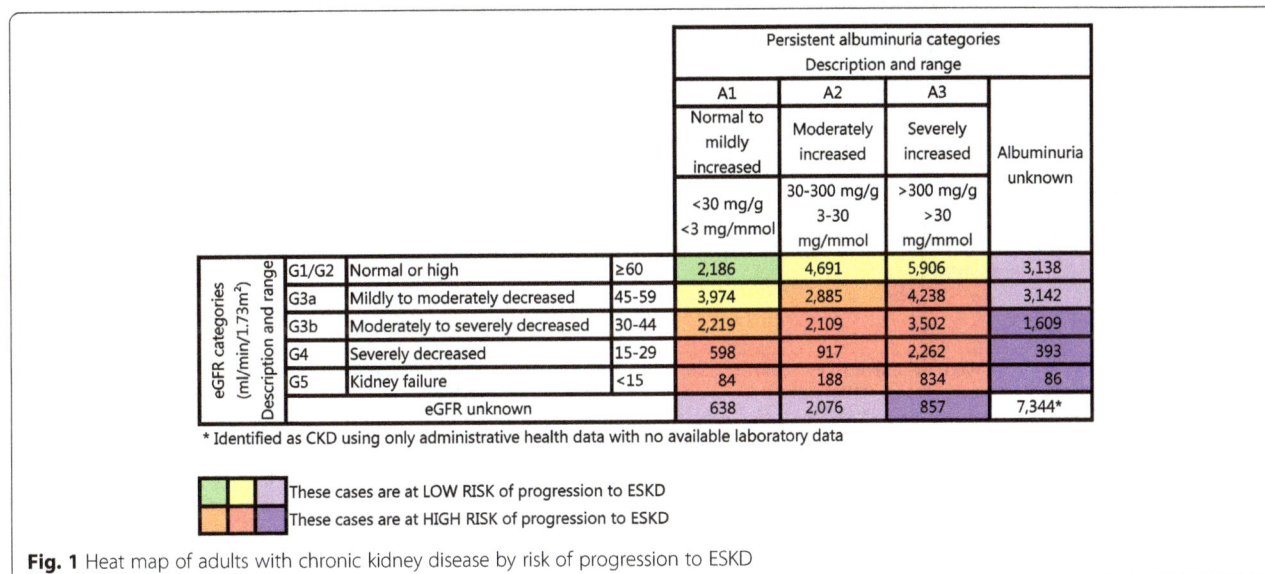

Fig. 1 Heat map of adults with chronic kidney disease by risk of progression to ESKD

average household income of small geographical areas (made up of 400 to 700 people) from the 2006 and 2011 Canadian census data, and ranking incomes in these areas from lowest to highest. Indicators for the following health conditions were defined utilizing the physician claims, hospital records and prescription data: diabetes, lower-limb amputation (among those with diabetes), hypertension, ischemic health disease, congestive heart failure, acute myocardial infarction, stroke, and atrial fibrillation. The codes for these definitions are found in the Additional file 1: Table S1 entitled, *Definitions of Comorbid Health Conditions.*

Statistical analyses

CKD prevalence was estimated using three methods. The first consisted of counting all CKD cases in administrative health and laboratory databases and dividing by the total Manitoba population. The second used exclusively laboratory data and divided CKD cases by all persons with laboratory data required to make a CKD diagnosis. For the third estimate, we used the following capture-recapture method or Chapman formula [16]:

((number of cases in administrative health data + 1) x (number of cases in laboratory data + 1) / (number of cases in both + 1)) -1.

The capture-recapture methodology is a novel approach to estimating disease prevalence, a method originally used to determine the size of animal populations [17, 18]. This method requires databases of cases from two different but potentially overlapping sources, thus taking advantage of the administrative data and the laboratory data from the Manitoba population. The idea is that disease prevalence will be higher in populations where there are fewer overlapping cases from two separate data sources. The standard practice of simply

merging several data sources will likely miss cases and underestimate the disease prevalence [19].

Generalized Linear Model (GLM) was used estimate the prevalence of comorbid health conditions in the CKD cohort as it is suitable for non–normally distributed data such as indicator counts. Depending on which fit the data best, various distributions were used for different indicators, including Poisson distribution, negative binomial distribution, or binomial distribution. Rates were age and sex adjusted. SAS® version 9.3 software was used to conduct all data management, programming and analyses on MCHP's secure server.

Results

Figure 2 illustrates how the cohort was created. The total number of Manitoba adults (18 years and older) with CKD found in all databases was 55,876. Of these, 18,342 were identified using administrative health data, 27,393 were found in the laboratory data, and 10,141 people were found in both databases. Table 2 shows the characteristics of the Manitoba CKD Cohort (n = 55, 876). We note that these characteristics differ from the total Manitoba population (n = 991,823). More women than men were captured in the CKD cohort. Over half of CKD cases were 65 years and older. When comparing the percentages of people residing in the rural health regions and the main urban health region, we note that CKD cases in some rural regions appear to be underrepresented.

CKD prevalence

The prevalence among all adults with CKD identified in both administrative and laboratory data was 5.6% (n = 55,876). Among adults in Manitoba with laboratory data, the CKD prevalence was 10.6% (n = 37,534). Prevalence based on the capture-recapture method, which uses cases defined both by

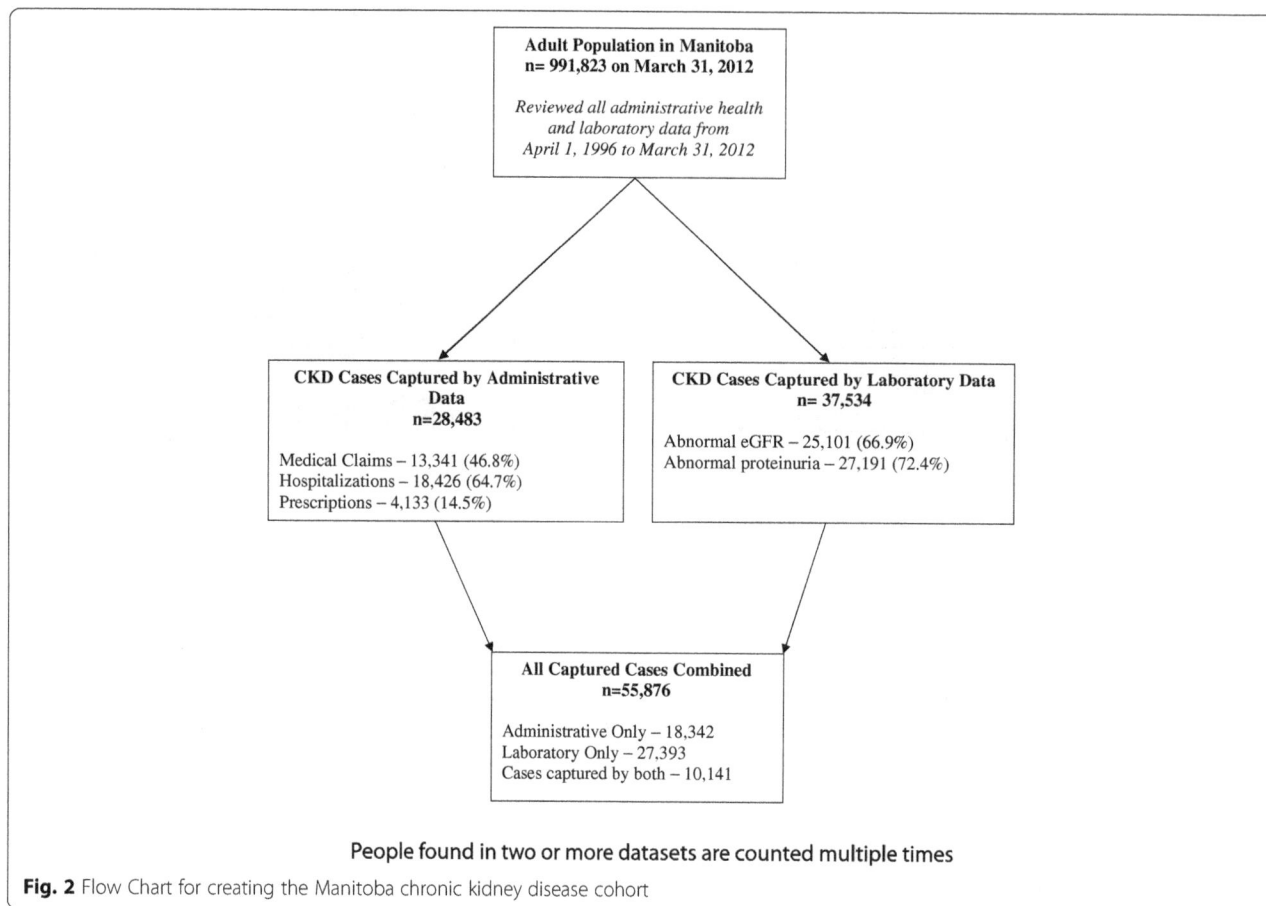

Fig. 2 Flow Chart for creating the Manitoba chronic kidney disease cohort

administrative and laboratory data, also reached 10.6% (n = 105,417). These estimates exclude ESKD cases (n = 1854) on dialysis in the Manitoba Renal Program and with kidney transplants.

Figure 1 shows the CKD cohort categorized by level of risk of progression to ESKD based on available laboratory data. Of the 55,876 people with CKD, approximately 41% (n = 23,037) were at low risk (green, yellow, and light purple). About 46% (n = 25,495) had more advanced CKD and were at higher risk of progression. The CKD stage and risk level were unknown for 13% (n = 7344) due to unavailable laboratory data.

Socio-demographic characteristics

Rates of CKD were higher in women. For women, 31.8/1000 were found to be have CKD with high risk of progression to ESKD versus 25.9/1000 for men. Higher rates of all categories of CKD were found among older compared to younger populations. Rates of high risk CKD among adults aged 65 years and older were 97.9/1000, adults aged 45 to 64 years, 20.6/1000, and adults aged 18 to 44 years, 7.9/1000 (Table 3).

In urban areas, with the exception of the group of unknown risk, there was a linear trend across income

quintiles, meaning that as income increased, a lower prevalence of CKD was found (Fig. 3). The converse was found in the rural areas, where this linear trend was found only in the group of unknown risk. The different patterns between urban and rural areas are likely due to incomplete coverage of laboratory data in rural areas.

We also noted important differences in CKD prevalence across health regions in Manitoba as shown in Fig. 4. The most northern area in the province, particularly in the remote areas (denoted by the diagonal lines), has consistently high rates. The South Eastern region of the province has the lowest CKD rates of the province.

Comorbid health conditions

The overall burden of comorbid medical conditions was considerably higher among people with CKD than among those without CKD (Table 4). For example, the prevalence of ischemic heart disease among the high risk CKD group was 24.55% compared to 4.72% in the No CKD group. Rates of comorbid medical conditions also increased with severity of CKD. For example, relative to those without CKD, rates of hypertension were higher among people classified with CKD at lower risk (RR: 2.24) and higher still among people with CKD at higher

Table 2 Chronic kidney disease cohort and total Manitoba population characteristics

Characteristics	CKD Cohort Counts (%) n = 55,876	Manitoba 2012 Population Counts (%) n = 991,823
Sex		
Men	24,947 (44.6%)	485,948 (49.0%)
Women	30,929 (55.4%)	505,875 (51.0%)
Age Groups		
18–44 years old	9681 (17.3%)	469,102 (47.3%)
45 to 64 years old	15,750 (28.2%)	338,726 (34.2%)
65 and older	30,445 (54.5%)	183,995 (49.0%)
Income Quintiles		
Rural 1 (lowest)	3614 (6.5%)	66,555 (6.7%)
Rural 2	3203 (5.7%)	74,715 (7.5%)
Rural 3	3322 (5.9%)	76,648 (7.7%)
Rural 4	3270 (5.9%)	71,984 (7.3%)
Rural 5 (highest)	2828 (5.1%)	74,853 (7.5%)
Urban 1 (lowest)	9593 (17.2%)	121,379 (12.2%)
Urban 2	8213 (14.7%)	125,383 (12.6%)
Urban 3	7213 (12.9%)	123,252 (12.4%)
Urban 4	6414 (11.5%)	123,541 (12.5%)
Urban 5 (highest)	6051 (10.8%)	124,367 (12.5%)
Health Regions		
Southern Health (rural)	4649 (8.3%)	133,549 (13.5%)
Winnipeg (urban)	38,055 (68.1%)	582,923 (58.8%)
Prairie Mountain Health (rural)	4918 (8.8%)	129,480 (13.1%)
Interlake-Eastern (rural)	5468 (9.8%)	97,375 (9.8%)
Northern (rural)	2782 (5.0%)	48,491 (4.9%)
Remote Communities*	1925 (3.4%)	18,077 (1.8%)

* These are remote northern communities that do not have permanent road access, are more than a four-hour drive from a major rural hospital or have rail or fly-in access only. These communities are found in Interlake-Eastern and Northern Health Regions, therefore the numbers in these remote communities overlap with the numbers of these health regions

Table 3 CKD prevalence by sex, age and risk of progression. Crude rates per 1000 adults as of March 31, 2012

Indicators	CKD Risk of Progression		
	Unknown	Low	High
Sex			
Males	6.9	18.6	25.9
Females*	7.9	21.4	31.8
Age (years)			
18–44	4.3	8.5	7.9
45–64*	6.4	19.6	20.6
65 and older*	17.3	50.3	97.9

* Indicates all categories of risk to progression were statistically different from the reference group (age: 18–44 or Sex: Male)

risk (RR: 3.02). Similarly, rates of diabetes and lower-limb amputation were higher among all groups of

CKD compared to those without CKD, but highest among people with high risk of progressing to ESKD. While the unknown risk group has lower rates of comorbid health conditions compared with the low-risk and high-risk groups, they have statistically higher rates of several of the conditions including diabetes, amputation, congestive heart failure, stroke and atrial fibrillation.

Risk factors associated with CKD

Table 5 shows that the highest percentages of CKD cases were found among adults older than 65 and with hypertension and diabetes. This suggests that the Manitoba CKD Cohort is capturing adults at greatest risk of developing CKD. The unknown cases were identified through the administrative health data, but no lab data was available to categorize them by low

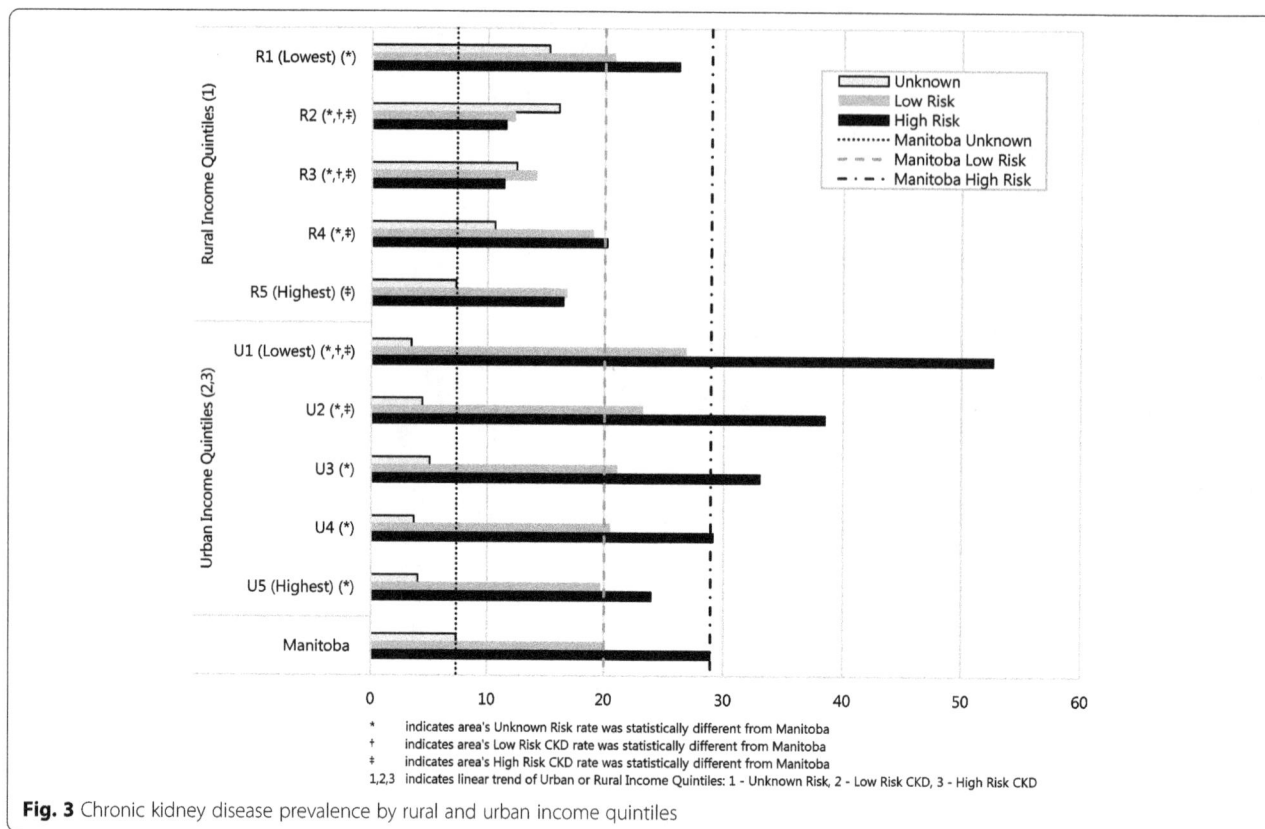

Fig. 3 Chronic kidney disease prevalence by rural and urban income quintiles

risk or high risk. It is reassuring to see that a greater percentage of lab tests were available on the groups with hypertension, diabetes and older age than the group with no risk factors.

Discussion

This study describes the development of the Manitoba CKD Cohort using a combination of administrative health and laboratory data, as well as how adult CKD prevalence was estimated. We found that the CKD prevalence was 5.6%, using the standard method and 10.6% using only people with laboratory data. Using the capture-recapture method, CKD prevalence was also estimated at 10.6% which is in line with previous studies [2]. Of the identified adult CKD cases, 46% were at high risk of progression to ESKD and 41% were at low risk. The remaining 13% did not have any laboratory data and were therefore not categorized by risk. This study also found the expected high rates of comorbid health conditions among adults with CKD, which increased from the low to the high risk cohort, supporting the methodology utilized to assess cases.

The estimated prevalence of 10.6% found in two of the methods used supports the face validity of our approach, although given that ESKD rates in Manitoba are amongst the highest in Canada, these may be underestimates. In a national study, using the Canadian Health Measures survey, Arora et al. [2] found that the

prevalence of CKD in Canadian adults ranged from 10 to 15%. Similarly, other investigators, reported CKD rates ranging between 2.5 and 11% across Europe, Asia and North America, and found CKD rates ranging from 4.7 to 33% in low- to middle-income countries. Our results suggest that CKD rates in Manitoba may be at the higher end of the range for high-income countries.

The burden of other health conditions in our CKD cohort is much higher than the provincial average for all the indicators we examined [20]. In the high-risk CKD group alone, the rate of stroke was over 14 times higher than the Manitoba average in 2011/12, and the prevalence of diabetes was over five times higher. Previous studies have found that comorbidities are common in CKD, even in the early stages of the disease and that these comorbidities are associated with increased treatment burden and poorer quality of life [21]. In addition, we found a trend of increasing comorbidity with increasing risk of progression. Previous research shows that rates of comorbid diseases at the CKD stages 3–5 are double the rates at stages 1–2 [2, 22]. Go, Chertow, Fan et al., [23] in a large epidemiologic study, found a graded association between a reduced eGFR and the risk of death and cardiovascular events. A meta-analysis reported that the risk of myocardial infarction increased with lower eGFRs [24].

Our study enabled us to capture individuals through the health care system, who may be difficult to reach in

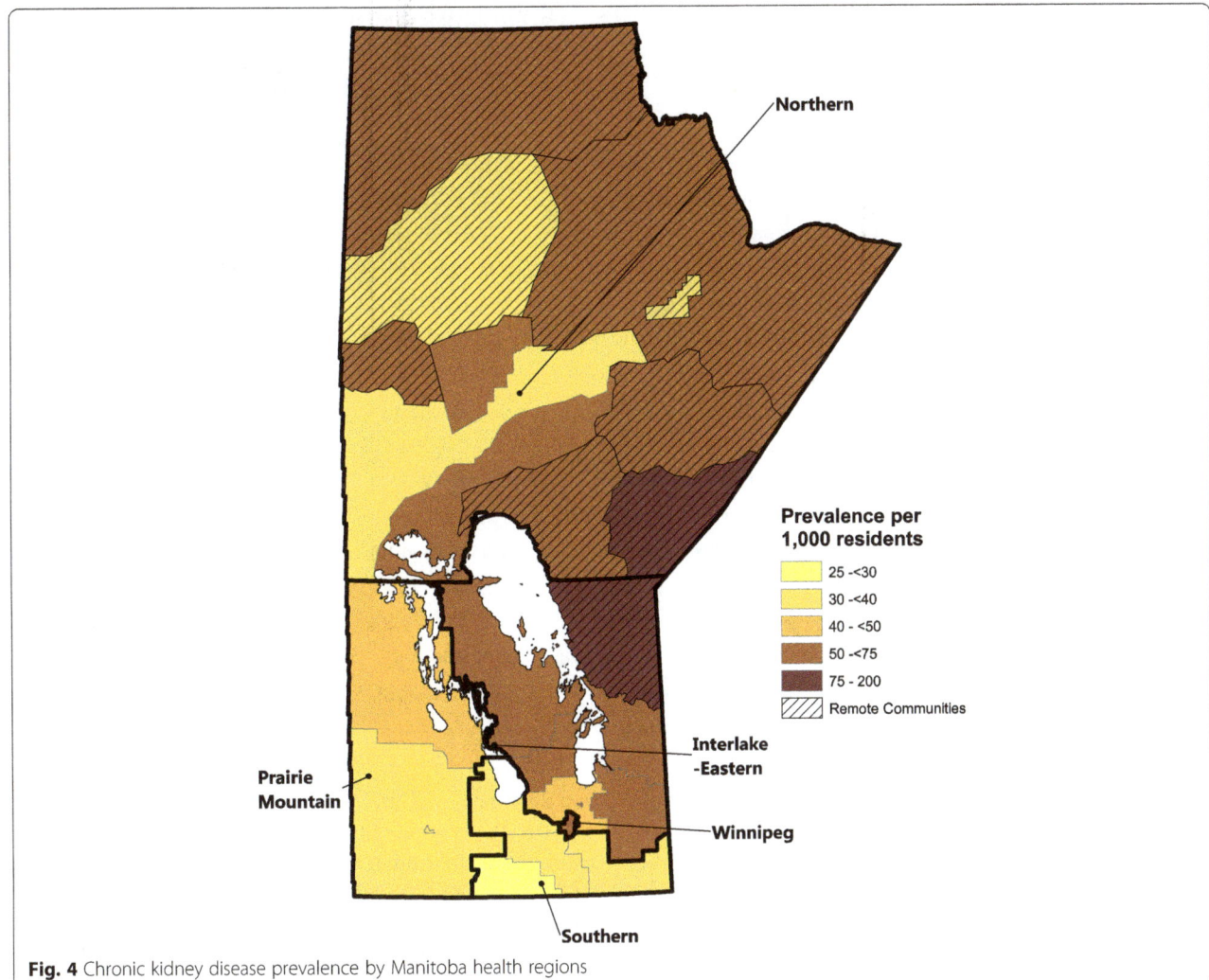

Fig. 4 Chronic kidney disease prevalence by Manitoba health regions

screening/surveillance studies. This allowed us to evaluate the geographical distribution and social factors associated with CKD. Our findings suggest that CKD is not equally distributed across geographic regions and socio-economic status. The CKD rates increase with decreases in income. We also observed that the highest rates of CKD in remote communities. These remote communities are largely populated by Indigenous peoples where living conditions are challenging due to economic conditions, poor water supply and access to affordable food, as well as limited health, social and recreational services. These findings are consistent with previous research. A recent review found that socially disadvantaged CKD patients had poorer access to health services, and higher rates of cardiovascular events and mortality than more advantaged patients [25]. Despite Canada's universal healthcare system, people living in poverty and in remote communities, face barriers to accessing early intervention strategies and treatments that are required to prevent and manage CKD. Improving living conditions

and ensuring that economic and social resources are available throughout the province would potentially decrease the development of CKD and other chronic diseases. While there are no simple solutions to reducing poverty, some existing strategies have demonstrated improved outcomes [26, 27].

Estimating CKD prevalence has proven to be challenging because the disease is typically without symptoms in the early stages, general population screening is not currently recommended and vulnerable populations at risk may not present for opportunistic screening even if it is offered. Given that survey respondents might be unaware of indicators of kidney disease, health questionnaires are problematic, and incur considerable cost and effort to collect the information. Remote and isolated regions are often not included in large surveys due to lack of infrastructure such as telephones and roads.

Epidemiological studies have relied on either laboratory testing or administrative health data to estimate population prevalence. Arora and colleagues [2] collected health

Table 4 Comorbid health conditions among adults with chronic kidney disease by risk of progression. Age and sex adjusted prevalence and relative risks, 95% confidence intervals

Indicators		No CKD N = 935,947	CKD by Risk of Progression to ESKD		
			Unknown n = 7344	Low n = 23,037	High n = 25,495
Diabetes (%) (2009/10–2011/12)	Prevalence	7.02 (6.96–7.07)	12.44 (8.64–17.92)	28.59 (19.80–41.30)	37.10 (25.62–53.73)
	Relative Risk	reference	**1.77 (1.23–2.55)**	**4.08 (2.82–5.89)**	**5.29 (3.65–7.66)**
Hypertension (%) (2011/12)	Prevalence	21.45 (21.36–21.55)	31.06 (19.91–48.45)	43.84 (28.01–68.61)	61.46 (39.06–96.72)
	Relative Risk	reference	1.45 (0.93–2.26)	**2.04 (1.31–3.20)**	**2.87 (1.82–4.51)**
Ischemic Heart Disease (%) (2007/08–2011/12)	Prevalence	4.72 (4.68–4.77)	7.30 (4.29–12.43)	12.22 (7.20–20.74)	24.55 (14.25–42.27)
	Relative Risk	reference	1.55 (0.91–2.63)	**2.59 (1.52–4.39)**	**5.20 (3.02–8.95)**
Acute Myocardial Infarction (%) (2007/08–2011/12)	Prevalence	0.99 (0.96–1.01)	1.10 (0.63–1.93)	2.29 (1.37–3.81)	5.29 (3.12–8.97)
	Relative Risk	reference	1.12 (0.64–1.96)	**2.32 (1.40–3.87)**	**5.37 (3.16–9.11)**
Congestive Heart Failure (%) (2009/10–2011/12)	Prevalence	1.38 (1.35–1.41)	4.51 (2.47–8.26)	5.19 (2.88–9.35)	25.09 (13.64–46.17)
	Relative Risk	reference	**3.27 (1.79–5.98)**	**3.76 (2.09–6.77)**	**18.17 (9.88–33.43)**
Stroke (%) (2007/08–2011/12)	Prevalence	0.41 (0.39–0.43)	0.92 (0.51–1.67)	2.01 (1.17–3.45)	5.59 (3.13–9.98)
	Relative Risk	reference	**2.26 (1.25–4.10)**	**4.94 (2.88–8.47)**	**13.72 (7.68–24.50)**
Atrial Fibrillation (%) (2009/10–2011/12)	Prevalence	1.92 (1.89–1.94)	3.09 (2.20–4.33)	5.03 (3.64–6.94)	9.72 (6.97–13.57)
	Relative Risk	reference	**1.61 (1.15–2.26)**	**2.63 (1.90–3.63)**	**5.08 (3.64–7.09)**
Lower-Limb Amputation Among Diabetics (%) (2007/08–2011/12)	Prevalence	0.33 (0.29–0.38)	0.79 (0.44–1.42)	0.77 (0.52–1.13)	2.65 (1.83–3.84)
	Relative Risk	reference	**2.37 (1.32–4.27)**	**2.30 (1.55–3.42)**	**8.00 (5.53–11.57)**

Bolded values indicate statistically significant difference from the No CKD group

information as well as laboratory tests required to identify CKD cases, from a representative sample of 3689 respondents across Canada. Laboratory tests to detect CKD including proteinuria and eGFR, can not only determine the presence of CKD, but also the risk of the disease progressing to ESKD. Specifically, by categorizing these tests, individuals can be stratified into low risk, moderately increased risk, high risk, and very high risk for progression to ESKD [14, 28–33]. Administrative databases can be an additional tool to overcome some of the challenges related to cost, time and reaching affected populations. In Alberta for example, a series of definitions for CKD using medical claims and hospitalizations based on the province's health system were compared to a gold standard [13]. Despite using a longer period, the study found that the definition

had 23% sensitivity and 96% specificity. These results indicate that using administrative data to estimate CKD prevalence tends to underreport the true rates and requires validation with population-based laboratory data or large-scale screening initiatives.

In our study, we found that many cases of CKD were not identified through the administrative health data, suggesting that these CKD cases may go undetected and undiagnosed. Given the high prevalence of CKD, it is imperative that primary care physicians conduct routine health checks for at-risk populations. The KDIGO clinical guidelines for CKD [14] and the Canadian Diabetes Association guidelines [34] include recommendations for lifestyle counselling, control of blood sugar and hypertension and avoidance of nephrotoxic substances.

Table 5 The percentage and number* of adults at risk of progression to ESKD among those with and without risk factors for ESKD, March 31, 2012

Risk of Progression ESKD	No risk factors (N = 672,495)	Hypertension (N = 232,797)	Diabetes (N = 84,405)	Over 65 (N = 183,375)
	% (n)	% (n)	% (n)	% (n)
No CKD (no risk)	98.4% (661,404)	83.5% (194,447)	75.7% (63,907)	83.4%(152,930)
CKD Unknown Risk	0.4% (2905)	1.6% (3661)	1.7% (1394)	1.7% (3188)
CKD Low Risk	1.0% (6751)	6.7% (15,629)	11.0% (9278)	5.9% (10,783)
CKD High Risk	0.2% (1435)	8.2% (19,060)	11.6% (9826)	9.0% (16,474)

*The numbers to not add up to the total population because there is overlap between the risk factors

Early identification of people at greater risk for progressing to ESKD provides the opportunity for lifestyle counselling to address risk factors and treatments to slow the progression of the disease. Clinical care pathways are available to guide primary care practitioners in the treatment of CKD patients [35]. Furthermore, there is opportunity for increased knowledge translation to ensure that all care practitioners are aware of these guidelines and have access to them in their practices. To ensure that remote communities have access to primary and renal healthcare, alternative models of care should be considered, include increasing recruitment of healthcare providers and using technology to link remote areas to specialized services in larger urban areas. It is important to develop a rigorous evaluation framework to monitor changes in the prevalence of ESKD and high-risk CKD over time in order to increase our understanding of the effectiveness of established screening, surveillance and intervention strategies and shed light on how to improve them.

This study has demonstrated the value of using of innovative methods to estimate CKD prevalence by taking advantage of the overlap between administrative and laboratory datasets. The prevalence estimated by the capture-recapture method is consistent with epidemiologic studies and with the estimate calculated using the laboratory data only. This method has previously been utilized for estimating prevalence of diseases such as acute hepatitis A, diabetes, spina bifida and infants' congenital anomaly [36]. The prevalence by the capture-recapture method may be an underestimation. Two assumptions are required when using the capture-recapture method: that the dataset includes individual identifiers and that one list does not affect the chance of being on the other list. The second assumption may not be met, because laboratory reports and physician claims are likely related.

Strengths and limitations

A strength of the Manitoba CKD Cohort is the population-based data sources on which it was created. These data sources included medical claims, hospitalization records, and prescription records that covered virtually all Manitoba residents. It also included laboratory records that covered large portions of the population. The time and costs of linking data is considerably less than collecting large-scale survey data. Previous studies found that CKD rates using administrative health data alone are underestimated, because many CKD cases are not detected by physicians and may not be coded as a diagnosis in the context of other chronic diseases. The addition of laboratory databases addresses some of these limitations by increasing the amount of cases detected. This study shows that using a combination of health and laboratory data provides a more reliable estimate of the CKD prevalence and could be utilized to monitor population-level CKD rates over time.

The availability of the laboratory data permitted us to categorize CKD cases by risk to progression to ESKD. Unfortunately, 13% were of unknown risk because we did not have laboratory data on all CKD cases. Based on the rates of comorbid health conditions in this unknown risk group, we suspect that these cases are in early stages of CKD and being followed in the community by general practitioners.

We acknowledge that relying on prescriptions to determine CKD cases will require further validation. Although, the medications were given careful consideration and are believed to be primarily used in the treatment of CKD, we cannot be certain that all individuals using these medications have CKD. Our rationale for using prescriptions for capturing CKD cases is that using only medical claims and hospitalization records would significantly underestimate the CKD prevalence as shown by Ronksley and colleagues (2012). Even when CKD has been diagnosed, physicians may be coding another co-occurring disorder on the medical claim.

We also recognize possible limitations in how GFR was estimated and challenges with our laboratory data coverage. Measuring GFR accurately requires using multiple blood and urine samples, which are costly and cumbersome [15]. It is important to keep in mind that estimating GFR may be associated with an overestimation. With regards to the laboratory data, these are collected in facilities that provide public laboratory services and diagnostic imaging. However, data from some hospitals, private laboratories and laboratories in Western Manitoba were not captured [37]. Additionally, the geographical distribution of available DSM data was unequal. Whereas 59% of the Manitoba population resides in Winnipeg, 78% of the lab data was from these residents. This resulted in an underestimation of the disease burden in some rural areas. A more accurate picture of CKD in Manitoba will emerge once additional data is added to the Repository, which will be a valuable resource for future studies.

Conclusions

Chronic kidney disease (CKD) is a health issue of increasing worldwide importance. Utilizing a combination of administrative health and laboratory data, this study found high CKD rates in Manitoba, with a large proportion at risk for progressing to ESKD. Given the high rates of comorbidity, it is important to have a comprehensive public health strategy that encompasses a range of interrelated chronic diseases. Our methodology may be well suited in the creation of passive CKD surveillance systems to target patients who may benefit from early intervention to prevent progression to more advanced forms of CKD and ESKD.

Abbreviations

ACR: Albumin-creatinine ratio; CKD: Chronic kidney disease; DSM: Diagnostic Services Manitoba; eGFR: estimated Glomerular Filtration Rate; ESKD: End stage kidney disease; KDIGO: Kidney Disease Improving Global Outcomes; MCHP: Manitoba Centre for Health Policy; MDRD: Modification of Diet in Renal Disease; PCR: Protein-creatinine ratio; PHIN: Personal Health Identification Number; RR: Relative risk; SCr: Serum creatinine

Acknowledgements

The authors wish to acknowledge the contributions of Leanne Rajotte and Susan Burchill for their assistance in preparing the manuscript. We are indebted to Manitoba Health, Seniors and Active Living, the Winnipeg Regional Health Authority and Diagnostic Services Manitoba for provision of data. We acknowledge the Manitoba Centre for Health Policy (MCHP) for use of data contained in the Manitoba Population Research Data Repository (HIPC # 2012/2013 - 21).

Funding

This study was supported through funding provided by the Department of Health of the Province of Manitoba to the University of Manitoba (HIPC 2012/2013–21). The funding body did not have a role in any aspect of this manuscript.

Authors' contributions

MJC conceived, designed and supervised the study and wrote the initial draft of the paper. AD, NT and PK were instrumental in the conception, design and interpretation of the data and assisted in writing the paper. RW and CB were instrumental in the design, conducted the analysis and reviewed the paper. IK and KLM contributed to the design and interpretation of the data and reviewed the paper. All authors have read and approved the final version.

Competing interests

The authors declare that they have no competing interests

Author details

[1]Manitoba Centre for Health Policy, Department of Community Health Sciences, University of Manitoba, Winnipeg, Canada. [2]Chronic Disease Innovation Centre, Seven Oaks General Hospital, Department of Medicine and Community Health Sciences, Max Rady College of Medicine, University of Manitoba, Winnipeg, Canada. [3]Department of Pediatrics and Child Health, Section of Nephrology, University of Manitoba, Winnipeg, Canada.

References

1. Levey AS, Coresh J. Chronic kidney disease. Lancet. 2012;379:165–80. https://doi.org/10.1016/S0140-6736(11)60178-5.
2. Arora P, Vasa P, Brenner D, Iglar K, McFarlane P, Morrison H, et al. Prevalence estimates of chronic kidney disease in Canada: results of a nationally representative survey. CMAJ. 2013;185:E417–23.
3. James MT, Hemmelgarn BR, Tonelli M. Early recognition and prevention of chronic kidney disease. Lancet. 2010;375:1296–309. https://doi.org/10.1016/S0140-6736(09)62004-3.
4. Stanifer JW, Muiru A, Jafar TH, Patel UD. Chronic kidney disease in low- and middle-income countries. Nephrol Dial Transplant. 2016;31:868–74. https://doi.org/10.1093/ndt/gfv466.
5. Canadian Institute for Health Information (CIHI). Canadian organ replacement register annual report: treatment of end-stage organ failure in Canada, 2004 to 2013. Author. 2015. https://secure.cihi.ca/free_products/2015_CORR_AnnualReport_ENweb.pdf. Accessed 31 Jul 2017.
6. Saran R, Robinson B, Abbott KC, Agodoa LYC, Albertus P, Ayanian J, et al. US renal data system 2016 annual data report: epidemiology of kidney disease in the United States. Am J Kidney Dis. 2017;69:A7–8.
7. Klarenbach SW, Tonelli M, Chui B, Manns BJ. Economic evaluation of dialysis therapies. Nat Rev Nephrol. 2014;10:644–52. https://doi.org/10.1038/nrneph.2014.145.
8. Obrador GT, Pereira BJG, Kausz AT. Chronic kidney disease in the United States: an underrecognized problem. Semin Nephrol. 2002;22:441–8.
9. Roos LL, Gupta S, Soodeen R-A, Jebamani L. Data quality in an information-rich environment: Canada as an example. Can J Aging. 2005;24(Suppl 1):153–70.
10. Roos LL, Nicol JP. A research registry: uses, development, and accuracy. J Clin Epidemiol. 1999;52:39–47.
11. Roos LL, Brownell M, Lix L, Roos NP, Walld R, MacWilliam L. From health research to social research: privacy, methods, approaches. Soc Sci Med. 2008;66:117–29. https://doi.org/10.1016/j.socscimed.2007.08.017.
12. Manitoba Centre for Health Policy. Manitoba Population Research Data Repository Data List. 2017. http://umanitoba.ca/faculties/medicine/units/community_health_sciences/departmental_units/mchp/resources/repository/datalist.html. Accessed 31 Jul 2017.
13. Ronksley PE, Tonelli M, Quan H, Manns BJ, James MT, Clement FM, et al. Validating a case definition for chronic kidney disease using administrative data. Nephrol Dial Transplant. 2012;27:1826–31. https://doi.org/10.1093/ndt/gfr598.
14. Kidney Disease Improving Global Outcomes (KDIGO). KDIGO 2012 Clinical practice guideline for the evaluation and Management of Chronic Kidney Disease. Author 2013. http://kdigo.org/clinical_practice_guidelines/pdf/CKD/KDIGO_2012_CKD_GL.pdf. Accessed 1 May 2015.
15. Glassock RJ, Warnock DG, Delanaye P. The global burden of chronic kidney disease: estimates, variability and pitfalls. Nat Rev Nephrol. 2017;13:104–14. https://doi.org/10.1038/nrneph.2016.163.
16. Chapman DG. Some properties of the hypergeometric distribution with applications to zoological sample censuses. Berkeley: University of California Press; 1951.
17. International Working Group for Disease Monitoring and Forecasting. Capture-recapture and multiple-record systems estimation I: history and theoretical development. Am J Epidemiol. 1995;142:1047–58.
18. International Working Group for Disease Monitoring and Forecasting. Capture-recapture and multiple-record systems estimation II: applications in human diseases. Am J Epidemiol. 1995;142:1059–68.
19. Hook EB, Regal RR. Accuracy of alternative approaches to capture-recapture estimates of disease frequency: internal validity analysis of data from five sources. Am J Epidemiol. 2000;152:771–9.
20. Fransoo R, Martens P, Team TN to K, Prior H, Burchill C, Koseva I, et al. The 2013 RHA indicators atlas. Manitoba Centre for health policy. 2013. http://mchp-appserv.cpe.umanitoba.ca/reference//RHA_2013_web_version.pdf. Accessed 1 Jan 2015.
21. Fraser SDS, Taal MW. Multimorbidity in people with chronic kidney disease: implications for outcomes and treatment. Curr Opin Nephrol Hypertens. 2016;25:465–72. https://doi.org/10.1097/MNH.0000000000000270.
22. Foster MC, Rawlings AM, Marrett E, Neff D, Willis K, Inker LA, et al. Cardiovascular risk factor burden, treatment, and control among adults with chronic kidney disease in the United States. Am Heart J. 2013;166:150–6. https://doi.org/10.1016/j.ahj.2013.03.016.
23. Go AS, Chertow GM, Fan D, McCulloch CE, Hsu C. Chronic kidney disease and the risks of death, cardiovascular events, and hospitalization. N Engl J Med. 2004;351:1296–305. https://doi.org/10.1056/NEJMoa041031.
24. Vashistha V, Lee M, Wu Y-L, Kaur S, Ovbiagele B. Low glomerular filtration rate and risk of myocardial infarction: a systematic review and meta-analysis. Int J Cardiol. 2016;223:401–9. https://doi.org/10.1016/j.ijcard.2016.07.175.
25. Morton RL, Schlackow I, Mihaylova B, Staplin ND, Gray A, Cass A. The impact of social disadvantage in moderate-to-severe chronic kidney disease: an equity-focused systematic review. Nephrol Dial Transplant. 2016;31:46–56. https://doi.org/10.1093/ndt/gfu394.
26. Forget EL. New questions, new data, old interventions: the health effects of a guaranteed annual income. Prev Med (Baltim). 2013;57:925–8. https://doi.org/10.1016/j.ypmed.2013.05.029.
27. The Manitoba College of Family Physicians (MCFP). It's a fact: Better income can lead to better health. Get Your Benefits. 2017. http://mcfp.mb.ca/wp-content/uploads/2014/10/1._New_PovertyTool_FINALDec04__14.pdf. 2017. Accessed 31 Jul 2017.
28. Astor BC, Matsushita K, Gansevoort RT, van der Velde M, Woodward M, Levey AS, et al. Lower estimated glomerular filtration rate and higher albuminuria are associated with mortality and end-stage renal disease. A collaborative meta-analysis of kidney disease population cohorts. Kidney Int. 2011;79:1331–40.
29. de Jong PE, Curhan GC. Screening, monitoring, and treatment of albuminuria: public health perspectives. J Am Soc Nephrol. 2006;17:2120–6. https://doi.org/10.1681/ASN.2006010097
30. Gansevoort RT, Matsushita K, van der Velde M, Astor BC, Woodward M, Levey AS, et al. Lower estimated GFR and higher albuminuria are associated with adverse kidney outcomes. A collaborative meta-analysis of general and high-risk population cohorts. Kidney Int. 2011;80:93–104. https://doi.org/10.1038/ki.2010.531

31. Hemmelgarn BR, Manns BJ, Lloyd A, James MT, Klarenbach S, Quinn RR, et al. Relation between kidney function, proteinuria, and adverse outcomes. JAMA. 2010;303:423–9. https://doi.org/10.1001/jama.2010.39.

32. Remuzzi G, Benigni A, Remuzzi A. Mechanisms of progression and regression of renal lesions of chronic nephropathies and diabetes. J Clin Invest. 2006;116:288–96. https://doi.org/10.1172/JCI27699.

33. van der Velde M, Matsushita K, Coresh J, Astor BC, Woodward M, Levey A, et al. Lower estimated glomerular filtration rate and higher albuminuria are associated with all-cause and cardiovascular mortality. A collaborative meta-analysis of high-risk population cohorts. Kidney Int. 2011;79:1341–52. https://doi.org/10.1038/ki.2010.536.

34. Canadian Diabetes Association Clinical Practice Guidelines Expert Committee. Canadian Diabetes Association 2013 clinical practice guidelines for the prevention and management of diabetes in Canada. Can J Diabetes. 2013;37(Suppl 1):S1–212.

35. Manitoba Renal Program. Kidney disease referral pathways. Author. 2017. http://www.kidneyhealth.ca/wp/wp-content/uploads/pdfs/MRP-CKD-pathway.pdf. Accessed 31 Jul 2017.

36. Chao A, Tsay PK, Lin SH, Shau WY, Chao DY. The applications of capture-recapture models to epidemiological data. Stat Med. 2001;20:3123–57 http://www.ncbi.nlm.nih.gov/pubmed/11590637.

37. Diagnostic Services Manitoba. Annual report to the Ministry of Health, 2015/16. Author. 2016. http://dsmanitoba.ca/wp-content/uploads/2016/09/DSM_2015-16AR_Final.pdf. Accessed 31 Jul 2017.

6

Design and methodology of the screening for CKD among older patients across Europe (SCOPE) study: a multicenter cohort observational study

Andrea Corsonello[1], Lisanne Tap[2], Regina Roller-Wirnsberger[3*] [iD], Gerhard Wirnsberger[3], Carmine Zoccali[4], Tomasz Kostka[5], Agnieszka Guligowska[5], Francesco Mattace-Raso[2], Pedro Gil[6], Lara Guardado Fuentes[6], Itshak Meltzer[7], Ilan Yehoshua[8], Francesc Formiga-Perez[9], Rafael Moreno-González[9], Christian Weingart[10], Ellen Freiberger[10], Johan Ärnlöv[11,12,13], Axel C. Carlsson[11,13], Silvia Bustacchini[1], Fabrizia Lattanzio[1] on behalf of SCOPE investigators

Abstract

Background: Decline of renal function is common in older persons and the prevalence of chronic kidney disease (CKD) is rising with ageing. CKD affects different outcomes relevant to older persons, additionally to morbidity and mortality which makes CKD a relevant health burden in this population. Still, accurate laboratory measurement of kidney function is under debate, since current creatinine-based equations have a certain degree of inaccuracy when used in the older population. The aims of the study are as follows: to assess kidney function in a cohort of 75+ older persons using existing methodologies for CKD screening; to investigate existing and innovative biomarkers of CKD in this cohort, and to align laboratory and biomarker results with medical and functional data obtained from this cohort. The study was registered at ClinicalTrials.gov, identifier NCT02691546, February 25th 2016.

Methods/design: An observational, multinational, multicenter, prospective cohort study in community dwelling persons aged 75 years and over, visiting the outpatient clinics of participating institutions. The study will enroll 2450 participants and is carried out in Austria, Germany, Israel, Italy, the Netherlands, Poland and Spain. Participants will undergo clinical and laboratory evaluations at baseline and after 12 and 24 months- follow-up. Clinical evaluation also includes a comprehensive geriatric assessment (CGA). Local laboratory will be used for 'basic' parameters (including serum creatinine and albumin-to-creatinine ratio), whereas biomarker assessment will be conducted centrally. An intermediate telephone follow-up will be carried out at 6 and 18 months.

Discussion: Combining the use of CGA and the investigation of novel and existing independent biomarkers within the SCOPE study will help to provide evidence in the development of European guidelines and recommendations in the screening and management of CKD in older people.

Keywords: Chronic kidney disease, Older people, Disability, Frailty, Ageing

* Correspondence: Regina.Roller-Wirnsberger@medunigraz.at
[3]Department of Internal Medicine, Medical University of Graz,
Auenbruggerplatz 15, 8036, Graz, Austria
Full list of author information is available at the end of the article

Background

Evidence from epidemiological and clinical literature suggests that ageing contributes to the incidence of reduced renal filtration capacity [1]. In the presence of risk factors during ageing, such as diabetes, hypertension and others, filtration capacity further declines. This concept is underlined by many epidemiological studies showing a decline of measured estimated glomerular filtration rate (eGFR) with advancing age [2]. Kidney function is usually assessed by creatinine-based estimated glomerular filtration rate (eGFR) equations. However, those formulae have a certain degree of inaccuracy when used in older people due to changes in anthropometry and renal physiology during ageing [3]. Alternative filtration markers yielded different eGFR values for different cohorts of people tested [4]. This inaccuracy of laboratory measurements of kidney function suggests a risk of underdetection or overdetection of CKD, especially with advancing age [5]. Indeed, the eGFR threshold at which the risk of negative outcomes increases among older patients is hotly debated [6], and current evidence suggests that such a threshold may be lower among older people compared to adult ones [7–9]. Additionally, the eGFR cut-offs at which the risk of death starts to increase may change as a function of the equation used among older people [10]. Thus, improving accuracy of CKD screening measures for older populations would be of help in reducing the risk of underdiagnosis to maximize prevention of CKD and its consequences while minimising the risks and cost of overdiagnosis [6].

Diminished kidney function has become a relevant public health burden for all age groups, as CKD frequently results in an increased risk of end stage renal disease (ESRD), morbidity and mortality [11]. Besides "traditional" endpoints, CKD has been shown to impact nutritional status, inflammatory processes and anemia [12], thereby affecting different outcomes especially relevant to older people. These include impaired physical function, frailty and disability [13–16], cognitive impairment and dementia [17–19], depression [20–22], sensory impairment [23], undernutrition and sarcopenia [24–26], and adverse drug reactions (ADRs) [27, 28]. Therefore, early and sensitive detection of diminished renal function is essential to individually address care needs of older people with CKD and to address one of the major health burden in public health for the incoming decades [29].

Incorporating scoring risk models for care planning of older people at risk for CKD has come into focus recently [30]. Risk prediction models are generally based on equations designed on the basis of prognostic factors and clinical outcomes, available at the time the prediction is made, and collected in specific and representative cohorts of individuals followed up for a given period of time [31]. Built on evidence of such models, screening

programmes for CKD can take into account the characteristics of the target population in addition to simple laboratory measures, biomarkers and disease-based investigations. Multi- and co-morbidity, polypharmacy, frailty, functional and cognitive impairment and disability should be considered as part of a patient centered approach in CKD management especially in older adults [15, 23–26, 32–35].

So far, no CKD screening program has included all those variables also including data from comprehensive geriatric assessment (CGA), the only assessment technology able to capture the numerous domains of health status and their complex interactions in older people. Accordingly, the need for laboratory measurements able to identify accurately older people with CKD is a demand to address the public health challenges arising from the current demographic shifts. Indeed, this view is widely shared by the geriatric and nephrology communities, both in EU and USA [36, 37].

The aims of this multicenter study in Europe are to assess existing methodologies for CKD screening and investigate existing and innovative biomarkers of CKD in older persons. Furthermore, the Screening for CKD among Older People across Europe (SCOPE) study will provide evidence for including physical and functional health parameters of older people across Europe and help design a tailored risk prediction model for CKD in old age.

Methods

Study design

The SCOPE study is designed as an observational, multinational, multicenter, prospective cohort study in persons older than 75 years across Europe. This study is carried out in seven countries, including Austria, Germany, Israel, Italy, the Netherlands, Poland and Spain. Participants will undergo clinical and laboratory evaluations at the baseline (recruitment), and will be followed up at face to face visits at months 12 and 24 following enrollment. An intermediate telephone follow-up will be carried out at 6 and 18 months following recruitment. Figure 1 shows the schematic flow of the observational clinical study.

The study design complies with the Declaration of Helsinki and Good Clinical Practice Guidelines. The enrollment has started in August 2016 and is ongoing.

Ethical approval/ monitoring

The study protocol was approved by ethics committees at all participating institutions. Patients are requested to sign a written informed consent before entering the study. Patients are also asked to sign a separate informed consent to the collection of DNA samples to be used for genetic testing, while those not giving their consent will be retained in the main cohort study.

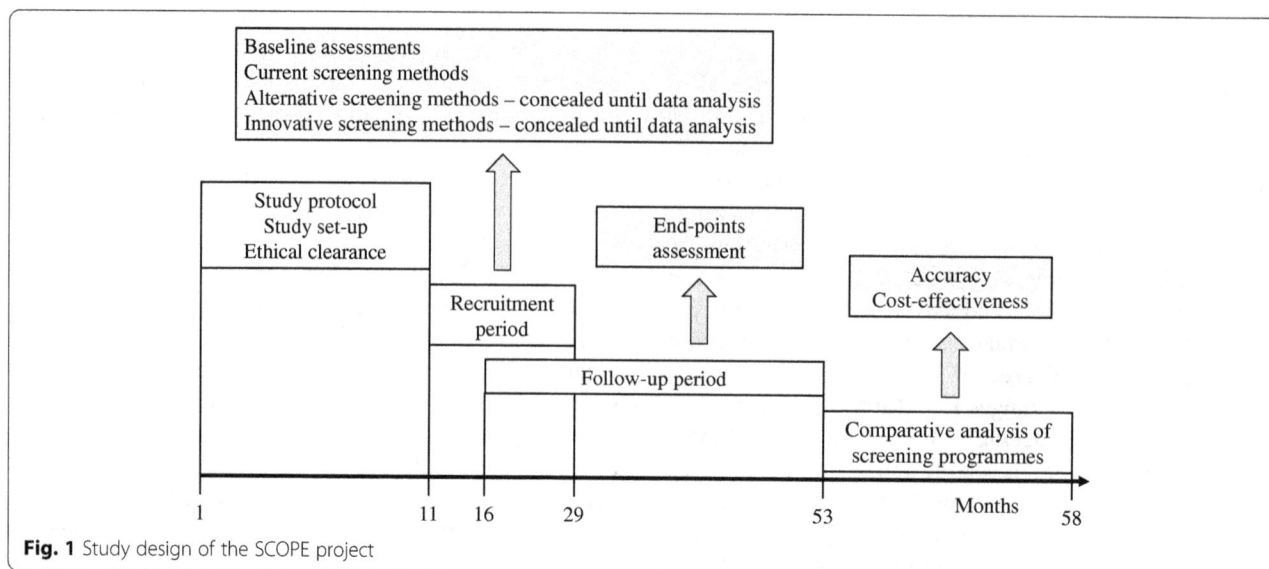

Fig. 1 Study design of the SCOPE project

In order to ensure high ethical and scientific standards of the project and to monitor the progress of the clinical study a Scientific Advisory Board (SAB) and a Data and Ethics Management Board (DEMB) was implemented within the Governance Structure. The SAB ensures a high standard of research, monitors the progress of the project by taking part in the project meetings, and provides final approval to any required study amendments. The DEMB supports the preparation of the relevant end-points for ethical review, advises on local research Ethical Committee applications, and reviews the relevant safety, morbidity and mortality end-points during the course of the study. The DEMB maintains an overview of the work throughout the whole course of the project and helps to foresee possible problems that might arise and how they can be addressed.

Study population

Persons aged 75 years and older, visiting the outpatient clinics of participating institutions are eligible for inclusion. The study design aims at minimizing self-selection bias and enrolling real-world patients without stringent inclusion/exclusion criteria. The few exclusion criteria are outlined in Table 1. Therefore, no other inclusion criteria will be considered. The SCOPE study aims to finally enroll 2450 participants.

Study visits

Following enrollment, participants will be seen by the study teams at 12 and 24 months at a face to face meeting. Demographic data and socioeconomic status (occupation before retiring, economic status, formal and informal care) will be documented and followed up at each visit. Physical examination will be performed by medical doctors due to standardized procedure given in

the visit protocol. Medical history and use of medication and adverse drug reactions classified according to the World Health Organization (WHO) definition [38] will be collected during follow-up visits. During all face to face visits a comprehensive geriatric assessment (CGA) will be performed. Table 2 shows all domains checked during study visits [39–51] [52].

Healthcare resource consumption will be evaluated using a resource use questionnaire within a 6-month recall time-frame [50]. Following information will be retrieved: previous physician visits (GPs, specialists, or physician at the Emergency Room), use of diagnostic tests and specialist clinic procedures, use of care services (e.g. Nurse home visit, Physiotherapy, Home help, Social transport, Day care center) and hospital admissions (number and duration of hospitalization, type of reimbursement).

Furthermore, caregiver burden will be measured using the Zarit Burden Interview (ZBI) [53].

Table 1 Exclusion criteria for participants enrollment into the SCOPE project

- Age < 75 years
- End stage renal disease (< 15 mL/min/1.73 m2) or dialysis at time of enrollment
- History of solid organ or bone marrow transplantation
- Active malignancy within 24 months prior to screening or metastatic cancer
- Life expectancy less than 6 months
- Severe cognitive impairment (Mini Mental State Examination < 10)
- Any medical or other reason (e.g. known or suspected inability of the patient to comply with the protocol procedure) in the judgement of the investigators, that the patient is unsuitable for the study
- Unwilling to provide consent and those who cannot be followed-up

Table 2 Comprehensive Geriatric Assessment domains tested during the SCOPE project

- Basic (ADL) and Instrumental Activities of Daily Living (IADL)/self-reported disability [39, 40]
- Mini Mental State Examination (MMSE)/cognitive status [41]
- 15-items Geriatric Depression Scale (GDS)/mood [42]
- Cumulative Illness Rating Scale (CIRS)/overall comorbidity [43]
- History of falls and incident falls
- Vision and hearing impairment will be coded on a scale from 0 (adequate) to 4 (no vision/hearing present) [44].
- Lower urinary tract symptoms (LUTS): The presence of LUTS will be ascertained by asking the patient to rate on a 5-point (0–4) Likert scale how big a problem, if any, has each of the following items been during the last 4 weeks: 1. Dripping or leaking urine, 2. Pain or burning in urination, 3. Bleeding with urination, 4. Weak urine stream or incomplete emptying, 5. Waking up to urinate, 6. Need to urinate frequently during the day [45].
- Nutritional status: anthropometric parameters (calf circumference, arm circumference, Body mass index (kg/m2), waist-hip ratio, waist-to-height ratio), Mini Nutritional Assessment (MNA) [46] and 24-h dietary recall[a] [47].
- Short Physical Performance Battery (SPPB) [48].
- Grip strength [49] measured by using JAMAR hydraulic dynamometer.
- Bioelectrical impedance analysis (BIA)[b] [50] Muscle mass will be calculated using the Janssen et al. equation [51], using the instrument Akern BIA101.
- Health related quality of life will be rated by the Euro-QoL 5D.

[a]Data obtained from the 24-h dietary recall will be analyzed using nutritional databases suitable for the patient's country. Following the analysis, a detailed report (containing levels of consumption of various nutrients and energy) will be available. This level will be compared with recommended levels of intake
[b]BIA will not be performed in patients with pacemaker or implantable cardioverter defibrillator

During enrollment and at the two face to face follow up visits blood and urine samples will be collected and analysed for serum creatinine, urinary albumin and albumin-to-creatinine ratio.

Telephone follow-up

At 6- and 18-month participants and/or caregivers will be interviewed by phone to collect information on vital and functional status and healthcare resource consumption. Changes in medical history and adverse drug reactions will also be collected.

Laboratory parameters and biomarkers

Serum creatinine measurement will be standardised to Isotope-Dilution Mass Spectrometry at local level, when the method is available. Creatinine-based eGFR will be calculated using the Berlin Initiative Study 1 (BIS1) equation, which is the only method specifically developed in a population older than 70 years [54]. ESRD will be defined as GFR < 15 mL/min/1.73 m2 or dialysis [55]. In case of unavailability of standardized creatinine methodology at local level, this measurement will be made by

INRCA laboratories afterwards. The panel of laboratory parameters to be measured at baseline, 12-month and 24 months by local laboratories will also include: complete blood cells count, lipids profile, electrolytes, nutritional status, and urine analysis.

The project will also include the collection of blood and urine samples to investigate existing and innovative biomarkers of kidney function. Existing biomarkers of CKD like Cystatin C (CysC) [56], β-Trace protein (BTP), also known as lipocalin prostaglandin D2 synthase [57, 58] Beta2-microglobulin [59] will be measured using published and established methods. Potential and new biomarkers will be also evaluated. Furthermore, the evaluation of experimental kidney damage biomarkers as well as untargeted analysis of metabolomics in serum and urine is currently be performed in ULSAM [60] and PIVUS [61] studies, in order to identify additional kidney damage biomarkers that may be validated in the SCOPE project. Table 3 shows an overview on current, alternative and innovative biomarkers for CKD whose applicability in old age will be investigated within the SCOPE project.

The assessment of selected genetic and epigenetic parameters involved in hallmarks of aging will be also carried out to investigate their relationship with kidney function. This latter assessment will be limited to participants who signed a separate informed consent (patients not giving informed consent for genetic and epigenetic analysis will be retained in the main cohort study), and will include: DNA methylation, polymorphisms of mitochondrial DNA, polymorphisms of genes coding for pro- and anti-inflammatory cytokines (IL-6, IL-1, TNF-alpha,

Table 3 Biomarkers research in the SCOPE project

Current screening methods[a]	Alternative screening methods[b]	Innovative screening methods[b]
Serum creatinine	Serum cystatin C	Serum fibroblast growth factor 23
Creatinine-based eGFR	Serum β-trace protein	Serum and urinary soluble TNF receptor 1
Urinary albumin	Serum β2-microglobulin	Seerum and urinary soluble TNF receptor 2
Albumin-to-creatinine ratio		Serum and urinary osteopontin
		Serum penthraxin 3
		Serum and urinary endostatin
		Serum and urinary TIM-1 (KIM-1)
		Serum TRAIL R2
		Serum and urinary endostatin

[a]current screening measures will be assessed at local laboratories and are immediately available after enrollment and follow-up visits;
[b]alternative and innovative screening measures will be centrally assessed and will be concealed until data analysis

IL-10, IL-2, IL-17, IL-8) and chemokines (MCP-1 and RANTES), polymorphisms associated with molecules involved in the pathogenesis of metabolic and neurodegenerative diseases such as insulin and IGF-1 signaling pathway and APOE, Klotho, mTOR, and whole genome analysis by Affymetrix Chip Array 6.0.

Measured glomerular filtration rate

The assessment of measured glomerular filtration rate (mGFR) will be performed by single-dose inulin clearance [62, 63]. Participants will be asked to sign a separate informed consent to participate in this sub-study, while those not giving their consent will be retained in the main cohort study. The objective of this sub-study will be the derivation of new eGFR equation(s) based on already known and/or novel biomarkers. The accuracy of new equation(s) in predicting mGFR will represent the primary study endpoint. Accuracy will be assessed by P30 (percentage of estimates within 30% of the mGFR). A sample of 400 participants will enable us to detect a difference of 2% in P30 between the new equations (based on the innovative and novel biomarkers) and the BIS equations, with significance level 0.05 and power 0.8 (considering a 1-sample and 1-sided test). In addition, we have evaluated that the sample will be sufficient to detect a statistically significant difference in 4,3 points in the Area under the ROC curve using the new equation(s) for discriminating participants below the critical threshold of 60 ml/min/1.73 m². Finally, the availability of mGFR in a subgroup of participants enrolled in the study will be used to investigate the relationship between innovative biomarkers and objectively measured kidney function.

Study endpoints

The primary study endpoints will be the rate of eGFR decline and the incidence of ESRD.

The secondary endpoints will include measures of conventional and geriatric outcome measures, such as: rate of CKD complications (anemia, hyperphosphatemia, acidosis, hypoalbuminemia, hyperparathyroidism, hyperkaliemia); rate of major comorbidities (e.g. hypertension and CV diseases) [43]; overall and CV mortality; adverse drug reactions (ADRs); self-reported disability and objectively measured physical performance decline [39, 40, 48]; cognitive impairment [41]; depression [42]; malnutrition/undernutrition [46, 47]; health-related quality of life [52]; healthcare resource consumption, including the estimation of caregiver burden [53].

Informations on vital status during follow-up will be obtained by interviewing the patients and/or their formal and/or informal caregivers. For mortality during the follow-up period, date, place and cause of death will be retrieved by certificates of death exhibited by relatives or caregivers.

Data management and statistics

The SCOPE project will enroll a total of 2450 participants. On the basis of the primary end-points, a sample of 1900 patients will be able to differentiate between two equally sized subgroups according to a standardized difference in yearly rate of GFR decline of 0.13 mL/min/1.73m² with a power of 80%. The same sample size allows to detect a hazard ratio of 1.2 in time-to-event analyses with 80% power for incidence of ESRD. Thus, even a 20% drop out rate will not affect statistical power of the study.

Every effort will be made to collect all data at the specified time points. In the case of missing (and not recoverable) data on primary endpoints, we will make the assumption that data are missing completely at random. Analyses will be carried out applying the list-wise deletion of cases with missing values in order to obtain unbiased estimations. Multiple imputation of missing data will be applied only for secondary endpoints and co-variates when found appropriate.

For continuous outcomes, generalized mixed models will be used while for dichotomous outcomes, random effect logistic or Cox regression will be applied. Effect modification by age and gender will be investigated using multiplicative interaction analyses.

Relevant exposure and co-variates will be selected based on plausible underlying hypothesis. Directed acyclic graphs may be used in order to create parsimonious multivariable models with minimized confounding. If appropriate, repeated measurements of exposure and co-variates will be included in the models.

Economic monitoring

The economic analysis of the SCOPE project will include: i) cost of screening/diagnosis; ii) cost of follow-up (e.g. pharmacological treatment, specialist visits, laboratory visits over the 2-year follow-up); iii) cost of CKD complications (e.g. emergency room access, hospital admission, haemodialysis, etc.); iv) other health-related costs (e.g. hospital out-patient care referrals, nursing home placements, use of home care services). With this analysis, it will be possible to determine main predictors of costs in CKD using multivariate regression and to establish cost-effective ratio of the intervention (overall healthcare costs, divided by efficacy, expressed as survival or quality-adjusted survival).

In order to assess the cost-benefit profile of the screening program on a longer time horizon, clinical and economic results of the SCOPE project will be used to run a projection (10–15 years) using Markov modelling. The analysis consists in evaluating a hypothetical cohort of CKD patients, whose healthcare status is categorized into different initial Markov states, based on CKD biomarkers. Patients can move from one state to another, according to certain probabilities that will be derived from the SCOPE project, and can develop complications, such as cardiovascular morbidity, renal failure and need of dialysis, CKD related and non-related death.

Discussion

The SCOPE study is one of the largest prospective observational cohort studies aimed at screening for CKD among older persons across Europe. The current paper outlines the study protocol including statistical analysis of data, risk prediction modeling and economic evaluation of costs arising from CKD during the advanced ageing process.

The strength of the protocol outlined in this paper is the real life setting for recruitment of participants. All persons with age ≥ 75 years attending the outpatient services at participating institutions will be requested to participate in the study. No other inclusion criteria will be considered. This seems the primary strength of the SCOPE study. The collection of real life data in a longitudinal fashion over a two- years period of time will allow insight on the impact of renal function on the management and advanced care planning of older subjects prone to renal impairment.

It is expected that many of the participants enrolled will be affected by multimorbidity [64]. The impact of disease clusters and management strategies from experts in the field of nephrology and geriatrics will open access to comparative effectiveness analysis of data and interventions [65]. People older than 75 years or people with impaired renal function have so far been rarely included into clinical trials. Aging population heralds a new geriatric "reality", namely an increase in older adults with CKD. Conversely, many older adults are living healthy and active, even with several chronic conditions. In this context longitudinal epidemiological studies are extremely valuable tools in observational research and have many uses and strengths [66].

Multimorbidity, and in this context CKD have been shown to impact functional status, especially of older patients [66]. The systematic use of a CGA makes possible the investigation of multiple domains of health status in older persons. CGA is part of clinical practice of Geriatric Medicine [67] and is also useful in research investigating consequences of CKD [68, 69] since it has been shown to affect different kind of outcomes relevant to older people. The inclusion of functional domains, as recently postulated by the World Health Organization (WHO) [70] in the design of screening models for CKD in older persons aligns the SCOPE projects with future demands for all Health Care systems around the globe [71, 72]. Health care is currently provided and funded on a disease-centered approach in many health care systems. The inclusion of CGA in the longitudinal evaluation of study participants of the SCOPE project will allow a more patient-centered and individualized approach for screening and advanced care planning for older subjects prone to kidney function decline [31, 69]. Furthermore, the search for biomarkers which are less influenced by muscle mass and more accurate in predicting outcomes compared to circulating creatinine is of special interest and will be further investigated. Thus, combining the use of CGA and the investigation of novel and existing independent biomarkers in within the SCOPE project, could help in building new evidence in the development of recommendations and guidelines for a patient-centered approach in the screening and management of older people at risk for CKD.

The alignment of an economic evaluation of care pathways and histories of study participants during the study period will give new input for care providers and planners in different health care and funding systems. Inclusion of costs of screening to achieve accurate diagnosis of CKD and related follow-up costs (e.g. pharmacological treatment, specialist visits, laboratory visits over the 2-year follow-up) will answer current call for actions coming from different bodies [73]. The focus on CKD related consumption of healthcare resources (e.g. emergency room access, hospital admission, hospital out-patient care referrals, nursing home placements, use of home care services and others) using Markov modelling will provide key information for developments in public health.

Major drawback or limitation of the project is the lack of standardized management and care plans for older people currently available for all participating centres. Centres enrolling participants in the SCOPE projects are highly experienced in the management of older multimorbidity subjects at risk for renal impairment and related clinical complications, including changes in functional status. Guidelines on CKD management are mainly disease-centred and put a focus on morbidities and mortality. It is to be foreseen that the care pathways for participants will therefore still be tailored individually and according to needs, driven by expertise of staff in the participating centres. However, important information may be expected though, as the implementation of the CGA per se into care pathways has already been proven effective [67]. It seems noteworthy that the individualized care approach during complex care management of older subjects is part of daily routine in geriatric medicine. Alignment of care processes along CGA results seems feasible in the context of current scientific evidence.

In conclusion, the SCOPE project will close essential gaps in the care of older people with declining kidney function. Due to the extremely comprehensive study setting and data analysis it is to be expected that evidence arising from the SCOPE project will impact the management of older people suffering from CKD, as well as the quality of care delivered for older subjects at risk for CKD in daily routine. The high quality of data retrieved will however, also open doors for new research and innovation in the field of nephrology and geriatrics. Building on solid evidence arising from the current project, SCOPE will support the development of European recommendations and guidelines, as well as a European education program in the field of screening and management of CKD in older adults across Europe.

Abbreviations
ADL: Activities of Daily Living; ADRs: Adverse drug reactions; APOE: Apolipoprotein E; BIA: Bio-impedance analysis; BIS: Berlin Initiative Study; BTP: Beta-trace proetin; CGA: Comprehensive geriatric assessment; CKD: Chronic kidney disease; CysC: Cystatin C; DEMB: Data and Ethics Management Board; eGFR: Estimated glomerular filtration rate; ESRD: End-stage renal disease; GDS: Geriatric Depression Scale; IADL: Instrumental Activities of Daily Living; IL: Interleukin; LUTS: lower urinary tract symproms; MCP-1: Monocyte Chemoattractant Protein-1; MMSE: Mini Mental State Exam; MNA: Mini Nutritional Assessment; mTOR: Mammalian target of rapamycin; PIVUS: Prospective Investigation of Vasculature in Uppsala Seniors; RANTES: Regulated on Activation, Normal T Cell Expressed and Secreted; SAB: Scientific Advisory Board; SCOPE: Screening for CKD among Older People across Europe; SPPB: Short Physical Performance Battery; TNF: Tumor Necrosis Factor; ULSAM: Uppsala Longitudinal Study of Adult Men; WHO: World Health Organization; ZBI: Zarit Burden Interview

Funding
The work reported in this publication was granted by the European Union Horizon 2020 program, under the Grant Agreement n° 634869, following a peer review process.

SCOPE study investigators
Coordinating center.
Fabrizia Lattanzio, Italian National Research Center on Aging (INRCA), Ancona, Italy – Principal Investigator.
Andrea Corsonello, Silvia Bustacchini, Silvia Bolognini, Paola D'Ascoli, Raffaella Moresi, Giuseppina Di Stefano, Laura Cassetta, Anna Rita Bonfigli, Roberta Galeazzi, Federica Lenci, Stefano Della Bella, Enrico Bordoni, Mauro Provinciali, Robertina Giacconi, Cinzia Giuli, Demetrio Postacchini, Sabrina Garasto, Annalisa Cozza - Italian National Research Center on Aging (INRCA), Ancona, Fermo and Cosenza, Italy – Coordinating staff.
Romano Firmani, Moreno Nacciariti, Mirko Di Rosa, Paolo Fabbietti – Technical and statistical support.
Participating centers

- Department of Internal Medicine, Medical University of Graz, Austria: Gerhard Hubert Wirnsberger, Regina Elisabeth Roller-Wirnsberger.
- Section of Geriatric Medicine, Department of Internal Medicine, Erasmus University Medical Center Rotterdam, The Netherlands: Francesco Mattace-Raso, Lisanne Tap.
- Department of Geriatrics, Healthy Ageing Research Centre, Medical University of Lodz, Poland: Tomasz Kostka, Agnieszka Guligowska, Łukasz Kroc, Bartłomiej K Sołtysik, Katarzyna Smyj, Elizaveta Fife, Joanna Kostka, Małgorzata Pigłowska.
- The Recanati School for Community Health Professions at the faculty of Health Sciences at Ben-Gurion University of the Negev, Israel: Rada Artzi-Medvedik, Yehudit Melzer, Mark Clarfield, Itshak Melzer; and Maccabi Healthcare services southern region, Israel: Rada Artzi-Medvedik, Ilan Yehoshua, Yehudit Melzer.
- Geriatric Unit, Internal Medicine Department and Nephrology Department, Bellvitge University Hospital – IDIBELL - L'Hospitalet de Llobregat, Barcelona, Spain: Francesc Formiga-Perez, Rafael Moreno-González, Josep Maria Cruzado.
- Department of Geriatric Medicine, Hospital Clínico San Carlos, Madrid: Pedro Gil Gregorio, Jose A. Herrero Calvo, Fernando Tornero Molina, Lara Guardado Fuentes, Pamela Carrillo García, María Mombiedro Pérez.

- Department of General Internal Medicine and Geriatrics, Krankenhaus Barmherzige Brüder Regensburg and Institute for Biomedicine of Aging, Friedrich-Alexander-Universität Erlangen-Nürnberg, Germany: Christian Weingart, Ellen Freiberger, Cornel Sieber
- Department of Medical Sciences, Uppsala University, Sweden: Johan Ärnlöv, Axel Carlsson, Tobias Feldreich.

Scientific advisory board (SAB).
Roberto Bernabei, Catholic University of Sacred Heart, Rome, Italy.
Christophe Bula, University of Lausanne, Switzerland.
Hermann Haller, Hannover Medical School, Hannover, Germany.
Carmine Zoccali, CNR-IBIM Clinical Epidemiology and Pathophysiology of Renal Diseases and Hypertension, Reggio Calabria, Italy.
Data and Ethics Management Board (DEMB).
Dr. Kitty Jager, University of Amsterdam, The Netherlands.
Dr. Wim Van Biesen, University Hospital of Ghent, Belgium.
Paul E. Stevens, East Kent Hospitals University NHS Foundation Trust, Canterbury, United Kingdom.

Authors' contributions
AC and FL conceived the study, coordinated study protocol and data collection, participated in manuscript drafting and revising. LT participated in study protocol design, data collection, manuscript drafting and revising. RRW participated in study protocol design, data collection, writing of the manuscript and taking responsibility for the publication process. GW, TK, AG, FMR, PG, LGF, IM, IY, FFP, RMG, CW, EF, SB participated in study protocol design, data collection, and manuscript revision and approval. JA, ACC participated in study protocol design and biomarkers identification and assessment. CZ reviewed the manuscript for important intellectual content. All authors read and approved the final manuscript.

Ethics approval and consent to participate
Ethics approvals have been obtained by Ethics Committees in participating institutions as follows:

- Italian National Research Center on Aging (INRCA), Italy, #2015 0522 IN, January 27, 2016.
- University of Lodz, Poland, #RNN/314/15/KE, November 17, 2015.
- Medizinische Universität Graz, Austria, #28–314 ex 15/16, August 5, 2016
- Erasmus Medical Center Rotterdam, The Netherland, #MEC-2016-036 - #NL56039.078.15, v.4, March 7, 2016.
- Hospital Clínico San Carlos, Madrid, Spain, # 15/532-E_BC, September 16, 2016
- Bellvitge University Hospital Barcellona, Spain, #PR204/15, January 29, 2016.
- Friedrich-Alexander University Erlangen-Nürnberg, Germany, #340_15B, January 21, 2016.
- Helsinki committee in Maccabi Healthcare services, Bait Ba-lev, Bat Yam, Israel, #45/2016, July 24, 2016.

All patients must give their written informed consent before entering the study.

Competing interests
The authors declare that they have no competing interests.

Author details
[1]Italian National Research Center on Aging (INRCA), Ancona, Fermo and Cosenza, Italy. [2]Section of Geriatric Medicine, Department of Internal Medicine, Erasmus University Medical Center Rotterdam, Rotterdam, The Netherlands. [3]Department of Internal Medicine, Medical University of Graz, Auenbruggerplatz 15, 8036, Graz, Austria. [4]CNR-IFC, Clinical Epidemiology and Pathophysiology of Hypertension and Renal Diseases, Ospedali Riuniti,

Reggio Calabria, Italy. [5]Department of Geriatrics, Healthy Ageing Research Centre, Medical University of Lodz, Lodz, Poland. [6]Department of Geriatric Medicine, Hospital Clinico San Carlos, Madrid, Spain. [7]The Recanati School for Community Health Professions at the faculty of Health Sciences, Ben-Gurion University of the Negev, Beersheba, Israel. [8]Maccabi Healthcare Services Southern Region, Tel Aviv, Israel. [9]Geriatric Unit, Internal Medicine Department and Nephrology Department, Bellvitge University Hospital – IDIBELL – L'Hospitalet de Llobregat, Barcelona, Spain. [10]Department of General Internal Medicine and Geriatrics, Krankenhaus Barmherzige Brüder Regensburg and Institute for Biomedicine of Aging, Friedrich-Alexander-Universität Erlangen-Nürnberg, Erlangen, Germany. [11]Department of Medical Sciences, Uppsala University, Uppsala, Sweden. [12]School of Health and Social Studies, Dalarna University, Falun, Sweden. [13]Division of Family Medicine, Department of Neurobiology, Care Sciences and Society, Karolinska Institutet, Stockholm, Sweden.

References

1. Schmitt R, Melk A. Molecular mechanisms of renal aging. Kidney Int. 2017; 92(3):569–79.
2. Davies DF, Shock NW. Age changes in glomerular filtration rate, effective renal plasma flow, and tubular excretory capacity in adult males. J Clin Invest. 1950;29(5):496–507.
3. Farrington K, Covic A, Aucella F, Clyne N, de Vos L, Findlay A, Fouque D, Grodzicki T, Iyasere O, Jager KJ et al: Clinical Practice Guideline on management of older patients with chronic kidney disease stage 3b or higher (eGFR <45 mL/min/1.73 m2). Nephrol Dial Transplant 2016, 31(suppl 2):ii1-ii66.
4. Christensson A, Elmstahl S. Estimation of the age-dependent decline of glomerular filtration rate from formulas based on creatinine and cystatin C in the general elderly population. Nephron Clinical practice. 2011;117(1):c40–50.
5. Glassock RJ, Winearls C. Ageing and the glomerular filtration rate: truths and consequences. Trans Am Clin Climatol Assoc. 2009;120:419–28.
6. Moynihan R, Heneghan C, Godlee F. Too much medicine: from evidence to action. BMJ. 2013;347:f7141.
7. Shastri S, Katz R, Rifkin DE, Fried LF, Odden MC, Peralta CA, Chonchol M, Siscovick D, Shlipak MG, Newman AB, et al. Kidney function and mortality in octogenarians: cardiovascular health study all stars. J Am Geriatr Soc. 2012; 60(7):1201–7.
8. Esposito C, Torreggiani M, Arazzi M, Serpieri N, Scaramuzzi ML, Manini A, Grosjean F, Esposito V, Catucci D, La Porta E, et al. Loss of renal function in the elderly Italians: a physiologic or pathologic process? J Gerontol A Biol Sci Med Sci. 2012;67(12):1387–93.
9. Lattanzio F, Corsonello A, Montesanto A, Abbatecola AM, Lofaro D, Passarino G, Fusco S, Corica F, Pedone C, Maggio M, et al. Disentangling the impact of chronic kidney disease, Anemia, and mobility limitation on mortality in older patients discharged from hospital. The journals of gerontology Series A, Biological sciences and medical. sciences. 2015;70(9):1120–7.
10. Corsonello A, Pedone C, Bandinelli S, Ferrucci L, Antonelli Incalzi R. Predicting survival of older community-dwelling individuals according to five estimated glomerular filtration rate equations: the InChianti study. Geriatr Gerontol Int. 2018;
11. Astor BC, Matsushita K, Gansevoort RT, van der Velde M, Woodward M, Levey AS, Jong PE, Coresh J, de Jong PE, El-Nahas M, et al. Lower estimated glomerular filtration rate and higher albuminuria are associated with mortality and end-stage renal disease. A collaborative meta-analysis of kidney disease population cohorts. Kidney Int. 2011;79(12):1331–40.
12. Pecoits-Filho R, Lindholm B, Stenvinkel P. The malnutrition, inflammation, and atherosclerosis (MIA) syndrome -- the heart of the matter. Nephrology, dialysis, transplantation : official publication of the European Dialysis and Transplant Association - European Renal Association. 2002;17(Suppl 11):28–31.
13. Lattanzio FCA, Abbatecola AM, Volpato S, Pedone C, Pranno L, Laino I, Garasto S, Corica F, Passarino G, Antonelli Incalzi R. Relationship between renal function and physical performance in elderly hospitalized patients. Rejuvenation Res. 2012;15(6):545–52.
14. Shlipak MG, Stehman-Breen C, Fried LF, Song X, Siscovick D, Fried LP, Psaty BM, Newman AB. The presence of frailty in elderly persons with chronic

15. Pedone C, Corsonello A, Bandinelli S, Pizzarelli F, Ferrucci L, Incalzi RA. Relationship between renal function and functional decline: role of the estimating equation. J Am Med Dir Assoc. 2012;13(1):84–e11–84.
16. Walker SR, Gill K, Macdonald K, Komenda P, Rigatto C, Sood MM, Bohm CJ, Storsley LJ, Tangri N. Association of frailty and physical function in patients with non-dialysis CKD: a systematic review. BMC Nephrol. 2013;14(1):228.
17. Yaffe K, Ackerson L, Kurella Tamura M, Le Blanc P, Kusek JW, Sehgal AR, Cohen D, Anderson C, Appel L, Desalvo K, et al. Chronic kidney disease and cognitive function in older adults: findings from the chronic renal insufficiency cohort cognitive study. J Am Geriatr Soc. 2010;58(2):338–45.
18. Seliger SL, Siscovick DS, Stehman-Breen CO, Gillen DL, Fitzpatrick A, Bleyer A, Kuller LH. Moderate renal impairment and risk of dementia among older adults: the cardiovascular health cognition study. Journal of the American Society of Nephrology : JASN. 2004;15(7):1904–11.
19. Madero M, Gul A, Sarnak MJ. Cognitive function in chronic kidney disease. Semin Dial. 2008;21(1):29–37.
20. Reckert A, Hinrichs J, Pavenstadt H, Frye B, Heuft G. Prevalence and correlates of anxiety and depression in patients with end-stage renal disease (ESRD). Z Psychosom Med Psychother. 2013;59(2):170–88.
21. Tsai YC, Chiu YW, Hung CC, Hwang SJ, Tsai JC, Wang SL, Lin MY, Chen HC. Association of symptoms of depression with progression of CKD. American journal of kidney diseases : the official journal of the National Kidney Foundation. 2012;60(1):54–61.
22. Balogun RA, Abdel-Rahman EM, Balogun SA, Lott EH, Lu JL, Malakauskas SM, Ma JZ, Kalantar-Zadeh K, Kovesdy CP. Association of depression and antidepressant use with mortality in a large cohort of patients with nondialysis-dependent CKD. Clin J Am Soc Nephrol. 2012;7(11):1793–800.
23. Deva R, Alias MA, Colville D, Tow FK, Ooi QL, Chew S, Mohamad N, Hutchinson A, Koukouras I, Power DA, et al. Vision-threatening retinal abnormalities in chronic kidney disease stages 3 to 5. Clin J Am Soc Nephrol. 2011;6(8):1866–71.
24. Duenhas MR, Draibe SA, Avesani CM, Sesso R, Cuppari L. Influence of renal function on spontaneous dietary intake and on nutritional status of chronic renal insufficiency patients. Eur J Clin Nutr. 2003;57(11):1473–8.
25. Morley JE, Abbatecola AM, Argiles JM, Baracos V, Bauer J, Bhasin S, Cederholm T, Coats AJ, Cummings SR, Evans WJ, et al. Sarcopenia with limited mobility: an international consensus. J Am Med Dir Assoc. 2011; 12(6):403–9.
26. Foley RN, Wang C, Ishani A, Collins AJ, Murray AM. Kidney function and sarcopenia in the United States general population: NHANES III. Am J Nephrol. 2007;27(3):279–86.
27. Doogue MP, Polasek TM. Drug dosing in renal disease. Clin Biochem Rev. 2011;32(2):69–73.
28. Corsonello A, Pedone C, Corica F, Mazzei B, Di Iorio A, Carbonin P, Incalzi RA. Concealed renal failure and adverse drug reactions in older patients with type 2 diabetes mellitus. J Gerontol A Biol Sci Med Sci. 2005;60(9):1147–51.
29. Burch JB, Augustine AD, Frieden LA, Hadley E, Howcroft TK, Johnson R, Khalsa PS, Kohanski RA, Li XL, Macchiarini F, et al. Advances in geroscience: impact on healthspan and chronic disease. J Gerontol A Biol Sci Med Sci. 2014;69(Suppl 1):S1–3.
30. Santos J, Fonseca I. Incorporating scoring risk models for care planning of the elderly with chronic kidney disease. Current Gerontology and Geriatrics Research. 2017;2017
31. Steyerberg EW, Vickers AJ, Cook NR, Gerds T, Gonen M, Obuchowski N, Pencina MJ, Kattan MW. Assessing the performance of prediction models: a framework for traditional and novel measures. Epidemiology (Cambridge, Mass). 2010;21(1):128–38.
32. Lattanzio F, Corsonello A, Abbatecola AM, Volpato S, Pedone C, Pranno L, Laino I, Garasto S, Corica F, Passarino G, et al. Relationship between renal function and physical performance in elderly hospitalized patients. Rejuvenation Res. 2012;15(6):545–52.
33. Roshanravan B, Khatri M, Robinson-Cohen C, Levin G, Patel KV, de Boer IH, Seliger S, Ruzinski J, Himmelfarb J, Kestenbaum B. A prospective study of frailty in nephrology-referred patients with CKD. Am J Kidney Dis. 2012; 60(6):912–21.
34. Fried LF, Lee JS, Shlipak M, Chertow GM, Green C, Ding J, Harris T, Newman AB. Chronic kidney disease and functional limitation in older people: health,

aging and body composition study. Journal of the American Geriatrics Society. 2006;54(5):750–6.

35. Kurella M, Chertow GM, Fried LF, Cummings SR, Harris T, Simonsick E, Satterfield S, Ayonayon H, Yaffe K. Chronic kidney disease and cognitive impairment in the elderly: the health, aging, and body composition study. Journal of the American Society of Nephrology : JASN. 2005;16(7):2127–33.

36. Levey AS, Inker LA, Coresh J. GFR estimation: from physiology to public health. Am J Kidney Dis. 2014;63(5):820–34.

37. Stevens PE, Lamb EJ, Levin A, Integrating Guidelines CKD. Multimorbidity, and Older Adults. Am J Kidney Dis. 2014;

38. Adverse Drug Reactions Monitoring [http://www.who.int/medicines/areas/quality_safety/safety_efficacy/advdrugreactions/en/].

39. Katz S, Ford AB, Moskowitz RW, Jackson BA, Jaffe MW. Studies of illness in the aged. The index of Adl: a standardized measure of biological and psychosocial function. JAMA. 1963;185:914–9.

40. Lawton MP, Brody EM. Assessment of older people: self-maintaining and instrumental activities of daily living. Gerontologist. 1969;9(3):179–86.

41. Folstein MF, Folstein SE, McHugh PR. "Mini-mental state". A practical method for grading the cognitive state of patients for the clinician. J Psychiatr Res. 1975;12(3):189–98.

42. Lesher EL, Berryhill JS. Validation of the geriatric depression scale--short form among inpatients. J Clin Psychol. 1994;50(2):256–60.

43. Conwell Y, Forbes NT, Cox C, Caine ED. Validation of a measure of physical illness burden at autopsy: the cumulative illness rating scale. J Am Geriatr Soc. 1993;41(1):38–41.

44. Yamada Y, Vlachova M, Richter T, Finne-Soveri H, Gindin J, van der Roest H, Denkinger MD, Bernabei R, Onder G, Topinkova E. Prevalence and correlates of hearing and visual impairments in European nursing homes: results from the SHELTER study. J Am Med Dir Assoc. 2014;15(10):738–43.

45. Rosenberg MT, Staskin DR, Kaplan SA, MacDiarmid SA, Newman DK, Ohl DA. A practical guide to the evaluation and treatment of male lower urinary tract symptoms in the primary care setting. Int J Clin Pract. 2007;61(9):1535–46.

46. Vellas B, Balardy L, Gillette-Guyonnet S, Abellan Van Kan G, Ghisolfi-Marque A, Subra J, Bismuth S, Oustric S, Cesari M. Looking for frailty in community-dwelling older persons: the Gerontopole frailty screening tool (GFST). J Nutr Health Aging. 2013;17(7):629–31.

47. Aglago EK, Landais E, Nicolas G, Margetts B, Leclercq C, Allemand P, Aderibigbe O, Agueh VD, Amuna P, Annor GA, et al. Evaluation of the international standardized 24-h dietary recall methodology (GloboDiet) for potential application in research and surveillance within African settings. Glob Health. 2017;13(1):35.

48. Guralnik JM, Fried LP, Salive ME. Disability as a public health outcome in the aging population. Annu Rev Public Health. 1996;17(1):25–46.

49. Cooper C, Fielding R, Visser M, van Loon LJ, Rolland Y, Orwoll E, Reid K, Boonen S, Dere W, Epstein S, et al. Tools in the assessment of sarcopenia. Calcif Tissue Int. 2013;93(3):201–10.

50. Shim JS, Oh K, Kim HC. Dietary assessment methods in epidemiologic studies. Epidemiology and health. 2014;36:e2014009.

51. Janssen I, Heymsfield SB, Baumgartner RN, Ross R. Estimation of skeletal muscle mass by bioelectrical impedance analysis. J Appl Physiol (1985). 2000;89(2):465–71.

52. The EuroQol Group. http:\\www.euroqol.org

53. Zarit SH, Reever KE, Bach-Peterson J. Relatives of the impaired elderly: correlates of feelings of burden. Gerontologist. 1980;20(6):649–55.

54. Schaeffner ES, Ebert N, Delanaye P, Frei U, Gaedeke J, Jakob O, Kuhlmann MK, Schuchardt M, Tolle M, Ziebig R, et al. Two novel equations to estimate kidney function in persons aged 70 years or older. Ann Intern Med. 2012;157(7):471–81.

55. Chapter 1. Definition and classification of CKD. Kidney Int Suppl (2011). 2013;3(1):19–62.

56. Onopiuk A, Tokarzewicz A, Gorodkiewicz E: Chapter two - cystatin C: a kidney function biomarker. In: Advances in Clinical Chemistry. Edited by Gregory SM, vol. Volume 68: Elsevier; 2015: 57–69.

57. White CA, Ghazan-Shahi S, Adams MA. Beta-trace protein: a marker of GFR and other biological pathways. Am J Kidney Dis. 2015;65(1):131–46.

58. Donadio C, Bozzoli L. Urinary β-trace protein: a unique biomarker to screen early glomerular filtration rate impairment. Medicine. 2016;95(49):e5553.

59. Astor BC, Shaikh S, Chaudhry M. Associations of endogenous markers of kidney function with outcomes: more and less than glomerular filtration rate. Curr Opin Nephrol Hypertens. 2013;22(3):331–5.

60. Lind L, Fors N, Hall J, Marttala K, Stenborg A. A comparison of three different methods to evaluate endothelium-dependent vasodilation in the elderly: the prospective investigation of the vasculature in Uppsala seniors (PIVUS) study. Arterioscler Thromb Vasc Biol. 2005;25(11):2368–75.

61. Helmersson J, Vessby B, Larsson A, Basu S. Association of type 2 diabetes with cyclooxygenase-mediated inflammation and oxidative stress in an elderly population. Circulation. 2004;109(14):1729–34.

62. Zitta S, Schrabmair W, Reibnegger G, Meinitzer A, Wagner D, Estelberger W, Rosenkranz AR. Glomerular filtration rate (GFR) determination via individual kinetics of the inulin-like polyfructosan sinistrin versus creatinine-based population-derived regression formulae. BMC Nephrol. 2013;14:159.

63. Zitta S, Stoschitzky K, Zweiker R, Lang T, Holzer H, Mayer F, Reibnegger G, Estelberer W. Determination of renal reserve capacity by identification of kinetic systems. Math Comput Model Dyn Syst. 2000;6(2):190–207.

64. Barnett K, Mercer SW, Norbury M, Watt G, Wyke S, Guthrie B. Epidemiology of multimorbidity and implications for health care, research, and medical education: a cross-sectional study. Lancet (London, England). 2012;380(9836):37–43.

65. Tinetti ME, Studenski SA. Comparative effectiveness research and patients with multiple chronic conditions. N Engl J Med. 2011;364(26):2478–81.

66. Guralnik JM, Kritchevsky SB. Translating research to promote healthy aging: the complementary role of longitudinal studies and clinical trials. J Am Geriatr Soc. 2010;58(Suppl 2):S337–42.

67. Ellis G, Whitehead MA, O'Neill D, Langhorne P, Robinson D. Comprehensive geriatric assessment for older adults admitted to hospital. Cochrane Database Syst Rev. 2011;(7):CD006211. https://doi.org/10.1002/14651858.CD006211.pub2.

68. Hall RK, Haines C, Gorbatkin SM, Schlanger L, Shaban H, Schell JO, Gurley SB, Colon-Emeric CS, Bowling CB. Incorporating geriatric assessment into a nephrology clinic: preliminary data from two models of care. J Am Geriatr Soc. 2016;64(10):2154–8.

69. Pilotto A, Sancarlo D, Franceschi M, Aucella F, D'Ambrosio P, Scarcelli C, Ferrucci L. A multidimensional approach to the geriatric patient with chronic kidney disease. J Nephrol. 2010;23(Suppl 15):S5–10.

70. World Health Organization: World report on ageing and health. 2015.

71. Framework on integrated, people-centred health services, Report on the Secretariat [http://apps.who.int/gb/ebwha/pdf_files/WHA69/A69_39-en.pdf?ua=1&ua=1].

72. Sandier SP, Poltomn D V. Health care systems in transition: France. Copenhagen: WHO Regional Office for Europe on behalf of the European Observatory on Health Systems and Policies; 2004.

73. Kerr M, Bray B, Medcalf J, O'Donoghue DJ, Matthews B. Estimating the financial cost of chronic kidney disease to the NHS in England. Nephrol Dial Transplant. 2012;27(Suppl 3):iii73–80.

7

Pediatric continuous renal replacement therapy: have practice changes changed outcomes? A large single-center ten-year retrospective evaluation

Alyssa A. Riley[1,3], Mary Watson[2], Carolyn Smith[2], Danielle Guffey[4], Charles G. Minard[4], Helen Currier[2] and Ayse Akcan Arikan[1*] [iD]

Abstract

Background: To evaluate changes in population characteristics and outcomes in a large single-center pediatric patient cohort treated with continuous renal replacement therapy (CRRT) over a 10 year course, coincident with multiple institutional practice changes in CRRT delivery.

Methods: A retrospective cohort study with comparative analysis of all patients treated from 2004 to 2013 with CRRT in the neonatal, pediatric, and cardiovascular intensive care units within a free-standing pediatric tertiary care hospital.

Results: Three hundred eleven total patients were identified, 38 of whom received concurrent treatment with extracorporeal membrane oxygenation. 273 patients received CRRT only and were compared in two study eras (2004–2008 $n = 129$; 2009–2013 $n = 144$). Across eras, mean patient age decreased (9.2 vs 7.7 years, $p = 0.08$), and the most common principal diagnosis changed from cardiac to liver disease. There was an increase in patients treated with continuous renal replacement therapy between cohorts for acute kidney injury of multi factorial etiology (44% vs 56%) and a decrease in treated patients with sepsis (21% vs 11%, $p = 0.04$). There was no significant difference in survival to hospital discharge between eras (47% vs 49%). Improvement in outpatient follow-up after discharge amongst survivors was seen between study eras (33% vs 54%).

Conclusions: Despite multiple institutional practice changes in provision of CRRT, few changes were seen regarding patient demographics, diseases treated, indications for therapy, and survival over 10 years at a single tertiary care. Recognition of need for follow-up nephrology care following CRRT is improving. Ongoing assessment of the patient population in a changing landscape of care for critically ill pediatric patients remains important.

Keywords: Acute kidney injury, Children, Pediatric, Continuous renal replacement therapy, Renal replacement therapy acute, Pediatric CRRT

* Correspondence: aaarikan@texaschildrens.org
[1]Department of Pediatrics, Renal Section, Baylor College of Medicine, Houston, TX, USA
Full list of author information is available at the end of the article

Background

Continuous renal replacement therapy (CRRT) has been established as the gold standard for management of critically ill pediatric patients with acute kidney injury (AKI) in resource replete settings. Provision of CRRT to pediatric patients was initially guided by extrapolation of adult data, as far more critically ill adult than pediatric patients require CRRT, allowing for larger cohort studies. Available pediatric data largely stem from the Prospective Pediatric CRRT (ppCRRT) Registry, a North American multi-center registry enrolling patients between 2001 through 2005. ppCRRT has been instrumental in describing demographics, outcomes, and practice patterns [1–11] for pediatric CRRT and has established CRRT as a safe and effective therapy in pediatric AKI. However, this registry predates the standardization of pediatric AKI definition, new generation of scale based machines and other improvements in the care of critically ill children such as lung protective ventilation strategies, sepsis care bundles, improvement in mechanical support device technology. In fact, pediatric critical illness mortality has decreased from 4.6% in the 1990s to a current rate of 2.4% [12, 13]. In addition, more recent awareness of an association between fluid overload and adverse outcomes, as well as the possibility that earlier CRRT starts portend a better prognosis may have resulted in a practice drift where CRRT is being started earlier at a lower cumulative fluid overload [14].

We hypothesized that with improvements and changes in delivery of critical care and parallel longitudinal improvements in delivery of CRRT, the demographics of CRRT patient population would change over time, not unlike changes previously reported in the epidemiology of pediatric AKI [15–19]. Additionally, we hypothesized that with the improved recognition of AKI and advances in critical care practice and CRRT technology, we would see a survival benefit over time. Our objectives were to determine if there were measurable changes in patient characteristics and outcomes over a 10-year course in a large single-center pediatric CRRT cohort, and to provide insight as to whether those changes, if any, could be related to institutional CRRT practice patterns.

Methods

Retrospective chart review

All patients who received CRRT, including neonatal, pediatric, and young adults, treated with CRRT at Texas Children's Hospital from 2004 to 2013 were identified from an administrative database and included in the study. Study period was divided into two cohorts, from 2004 to 2008 and from 2009 to 2013, roughly paralleling several institutional practice changes to evaluate for difference in outcomes (Table 1). For patients having multiple CRRT courses, each unique hospitalization was

Table 1 Institutional changes affecting changes in the delivery process for pediatric continuous renal replacement therapy

- Equipment change from Prisma to Prismaflex
- Standard prescription changed from CVVHD to CVVHDF
- Standard anticoagulation changed from systemic heparin to regional citrate
- Filter change from mostly AN69 to HF2000 membranes
- Adoption of 24 h in-house dialysis nursing staff
- Introduction of emergency department sepsis protocol[a]
- Establishment of a dedicated Renal ICU physician team
- Institutional CRRT Policies & Procedures manual written
- Creation of an institutional CRRT prospective database
- Creation of a prospective CRRT Quality Improvement Team

CVVHD: continuous venovenous hemodialysis; CVVHDF: continuous venovenous hemodialfiltration
[a] Akcan Arikan A, Williams EA, Graf JM, et al. Resuscitation Bundle in Pediatric Shock Decreases Acute Kidney Injury and Improves Outcomes. *J Pediatr.* Dec 2015;167(6):1301–1305

considered as a separate patient case. The study was approved by the Baylor College of Medicine Institutional Review Board and informed consent was waived.

Medical records were reviewed to determine principal diagnosis, cause of AKI, indication for CRRT, and other clinical information. Additional data obtained based on hospital charges included sex, age at start of CRRT, total days and number of courses of CRRT, ventilation days, intensive care unit (ICU) and hospital length of stay (LOS), and discharge disposition. Patients were grouped by principal diagnosis categories, including renal disease with end stage renal disease, hematology/oncology diagnoses (excluding bone marrow transplantation), bone marrow transplant (BMT) recipients, cardiac disease (including heart transplant recipients), liver disease (including liver transplant recipients), pulmonary disease (including lung transplant recipients), primary sepsis without a pre-existing known underlying organ system disease, inborn errors of metabolism, neonatal, and other primary system involvement.

A primary etiology for kidney injury was determined based on review of nephrology and intensive care unit (ICU) physician documentation. Indications for CRRT were identified from nephrologists' notes. Additional information recorded included patient's ICU admission weight, concurrent provision of extracorporeal mechanical oxygenation (ECMO) or use of cardiac assist device, and failure of renal recovery at hospital discharge defined as ongoing need for dialysis. Percentage fluid overload prior to initiation of CRRT was determined as previously reported: [(fluid in) - (fluid out)/(ICU admission weight)] * 100 [20]. All CRRT treatments were performed using Prisma or the Prismaflex control unit (Gambro, Sweden and Baxter, USA),), with a standard initial prescription of 2000 ml/min/m2 divided equally between dialysate and replacement. Outpatient nephrology follow-up was defined as an outpatient visit within 12 months of hospital discharge with a Texas Children's Hospital nephrologist in survivors.

Statistical analysis

Summary statistics of patient characteristics are described using mean and standard deviation, median and 25th and 75th percentiles (IQR), or frequency and percentage. Summary statistics are stratified by era (2004–2008, 2009–2013) and compared using t-test, Wilcoxon rank-sum test, chi-square, or Fisher's exact test. Variables related to time and fluid overload are stratified by era and discharge disposition and eras are compared among survivors and non-survivors separately. Survival was compared between and within era by principal diagnosis, weight, CCRT indication, and immune status using Fisher's exact test. All analyses were performed using Stata version 12.1 (Stata Corp, College Station, TX).

Results

A total of 311 patients were treated with CRRT during the study period, 38 of whom were concurrently treated on ECMO. Patient characteristics of the 10-year cohort are shown in Table 2, showing inclusion and exclusion of ECMO patients. From 2004 to 2008, 129 individual patients, and from 2009 to 2013, 144 individual patients were treated with CRRT (Table 3). The institutional volume of CRRT increased 12% (15 patients) between the two eras. Three patients in the 2004–2008 cohort and 4 patients in the 2009–2013 cohort each had two separate hospitalizations during which they received CRRT, however for statistical analysis, each patient was only considered once in their respective cohorts, with the first observation of CRRT retained in statistical analysis. Although not statistically significant, patients in the latter cohort were younger than in the early cohort (7.7 vs. 9.2 years, $p = 0.08$). There was also a shift toward lower weight patients, including 12 more patients in the 0–10 kg group treated with CRRT from 2009 to 2013 ($n = 38$) than in 2004–2008 ($n = 26$), as well as 10 additional patients in the 10–20 kg treated from 2009 to 2013 ($n = 39$) compared with 29 in the 2004–2008 group. There was a modest reduction in percent fluid overload at initiation of CRRT (17% vs. 14%, $p = 0.19$). Survival to ICU discharge, 28-day survival, 60-day survival, survival to hospital discharge was comparable between groups. Follow-up with a nephrologist after hospital discharge was significantly improved over time ($p < 0.05$), with 54% of 60 surviving patients treated between 2009 and 2013 being seen in the outpatient nephrology clinic within one year of discharge. Four of the surviving patients were followed with nephrology due to reaching end-stage renal disease after critical illnesses, which were autoimmune hepatitis with

Table 2 Patient characteristics over the 10 year study period with and without ECMO patients

Characteristic, n (%)	All patients including ECMO	All patients excluding ECMO
Patients (n)	311	273
Age (n)		
0 to 1 yr.	73 (23%)	56 (21%)
1 to 3 yr	37 (12%)	34 (12%)
3 to 5 yr	23 (7%)	23 (8%)
5 to 10 yr	41 (13%)	38 (14%)
10 to 15 yr	63 (20%)	57 (21%)
15 to 21 yr	64 (21%)	55 (20%)
> 21 yr	10 (3%)	10 (4%)
Mean (SD)	8.2 (7.0)	8.4 (7.0)
Weight (n)		
0 to 10 kg	82 (26%)	64 (23%)
10 to 20 kg	71 (23%)	68 (25%)
20 to 50 kg	80 (26%)	68 (25%)
> 50 kg	78 (25%)	73 (27%)
Mean (SD)	33 (28.1)	33.5 (27.2)
Pre-existing end-stage renal disease	13 (4%)	13 (5%)
Sepsis on admission	36 (13%)	34 (14%)
Immunocompromised		
Solid organ transplant	67 (22%)	58 (21%)
BMT	33 (11%)	31 (11%)
Other immunocompromised	54 (17%)	51 (19%)
Not immunocompromised	156 (50%)	132 (49%)
% Fluid overload at CRRT Start [a]	15 (7, 26)	15 (8, 26)
Hospital Unit of CRRT Start		
Pediatric Intensive Care Unit	257 (83%)	241 (89%)
Neonatal Intensive Care Unit	22 (7%)	14 (5%)
Cardiovascular Intensive Care Unit	29 (9%)	15 (6%)
Bone Marrow Transplant Unit	1 (0.3%)	1 (0.4%)
ICU survival	154 (50%)	145 (53%)
28 day survival	176 (57%)	165 (60%)
60 day survival	156 (50%)	146 (53%)
Survival to discharge	139 (45%)	131 (48%)
Outpatient Renal Follow-up [b]	62 (45%)	58 (44%)

[a]Median with (interquartile range)
[b]Patients who received CRRT for non-renal indications were excluded from this cohort (inborn errors of metabolism, ingestion)

fulminant hepatic failure, biliary atresia requiring liver transplant, Streptococcal pneumoniae sepsis with underlying sickle cell disease, and severe combined immunodeficiency syndrome. Table 3 also displays the principal diagnosis, causes of AKI, and indications for patients treated with CRRT in the two cohort groups. The

Table 3 Comparing patient characteristics, principal diagnoses, causes of acute kidney injury, and indications for CRRT between study eras (excluding ECMO patients)

Characteristic, n (%)	2004–2008	2009–2013	p-value
Patients (n)	129	144	
Age (n)			
0 to 1 yr.	24 (19%)	32 (22%)	
1 to 3 yr	15 (12%)	19 (13%)	
3 to 5 yr	7 (5%)	16 (11%)	
5 to 10 yr	19 (15%)	19 (13%)	
10 to 15 yr	28 (22%)	29 (20%)	
15 to 21 yr	29 (22%)	26 (18%)	
> 21 yr	7 (5%)	3 (2%)	
Mean (SD)	9.2 (7.2)	7.7 (6.8)	0.08
Weight (n)			
0 to 10 kg	26 (20%)	38 (26%)	
10 to 20 kg	29 (22%)	39 (27%)	
20 to 50 kg	35 (27%)	33 (23%)	
> 50 kg	39 (30%)	34 (24%)	
Mean (SD)	36.0 (28.6)	31.3 (25.7)	0.15
Pre-existing end-stage renal disease	8 (6%)	5 (3%)	0.40
Sepsis on admission [a]	21 (20%)	13 (9%)	0.02
Immunocompromised			0.74
Solid organ transplant	25 (20%)	33 (23%)	
BMT	17 (13%)	14 (10%)	
Not immunocompromised	61 (48%)	71 (49%)	
Other immunocompromised	25 (20%)	26 (18%)	
% Fluid overload at CRRT Start [b]	17 (10, 26)	14 (6, 26)	0.19
Hospital Unit at CRRT Start			0.85
Pediatric Intensive Care Unit	115 (91%)	126 (88%)	
Neonatal Intensive Care Unit	6 (5%)	8 (6%)	
Cardiovascular Intensive Care Unit	6 (5%)	9 (6%)	
Bone Marrow Transplant Unit	0	1 (1%)	
ICU survival	68 (53%)	77 (53%)	0.90
28 day survival	79 (61%)	86 (60%)	0.81
60 day survival	68 (53%)	78 (54%)	0.90
Survival to discharge	60 (47%)	71 (49%)	0.72
Outpatient Renal Follow-up [c]	20 (33%)	38 (54%)	0.02
Diagnosis, n (%)			0.06
Cardiac	13 (10%)	11 (8%)	
Renal	9 (7%)	19 (13%)	
Liver	19 (15%)	37 (26%)	
Hematology/Oncology	18 (14%)	17 (12%)	
Post-Bone Marrow Transplant	18 (14%)	15 (10%)	
Pulmonary	11 (9%)	4 (3%)	
Inborn error of metabolism	5 (4%)	10 (7%)	

Table 3 Comparing patient characteristics, principal diagnoses, causes of acute kidney injury, and indications for CRRT between study eras (excluding ECMO patients) *(Continued)*

Characteristic, n (%)	2004–2008	2009–2013	p-value
Sepsis	10 (8%)	5 (4%)	
Neonates	10 (8%)	13 (9%)	
Other [d]	16 (12%)	13 (9%)	
Cause of acute kidney injury [a, e]	(n = 113)	(n = 124)	0.04
Multifactorial	50 (44%)	69 (56%)	
Septic shock	24 (21%)	14 (11%)	
Renal	10 (9%)	7 (6%)	
Poor cardiac function	5 (5%)	6 (5%)	
Hepatorenal syndrome	5 (4%)	8 (6%)	
Nephrotoxic drugs	4 (3%)	5 (4%)	
Abdominal compartment syndrome	1 (1%)	8 (6%)	
Other [f]	16 (13%)	7 (6%)	
Indication for CRRT	(n = 129)	(n = 144)	0.41
Fluid overload	74 (57%)	71 (49%)	
Electrolyte management	7 (5%)	9 (6%)	
Fluid overload and electrolyte management	28 (22%)	42 (29%)	
Prevent fluid overload/provide nutrition	6 (5%)	3 (2%)	
Other	14 (11%)	19 (13%)	
Hemodynamic instability	3 (21%)	4 (21%)	
Hyperammonemia	6 (43%)	12 (63%)	
Ingestion	3 (21%)	3 (16%)	
End-stage renal disease	2 (14%)	0	

[a] $p < 0.05$ comparing 2004–2008 with 2009–2013
[b] Median with (interquartile range)
[c] Patients who received CRRT for non-renal indications were excluded from this cohort (inborn errors of metabolism, ingestion)
[d] Includes rheumatology, gastroenterology, multiple organ, neurology, ingestions, hemorrhage, rhabdomyolysis, and non-accidental trauma
[e] Patients with end-stage renal disease and non-acute kidney injury indications for CRRT (i.e. inborn error of metabolism) are excluded
[f] Includes vasculitis, microangiopathy, rhabdomyolysis, tumor lysis, obstruction, cardiac arrest, and unknown

constellation of principal diagnoses was similar between the two cohorts ($p = 0.06$), however some small shifts were seen in diagnoses treated, including more renal and liver patients, and fewer pulmonary and sepsis patients. The identified causes of AKI were different ($p = 0.04$) with a greater percentage of patients in the latter era having multifactorial AKI, and fewer patients considered having AKI caused solely by septic shock. Fluid overload was the most common indication for initiation of CRRT in both eras.

Outcomes on CRRT were evaluated by measurements of days to start CRRT from hospital and ICU admission, total CRRT days, ventilation days, and ICU and hospital length of stay (LOS) (Table 4). Non-survivors had a longer time to CRRT start from hospital admission (survivors 4

Table 4 Comparison of survival on CRRT by median time from hospital admission to CRRT start, time from intensive care unit (ICU) admission to CRRT start, CRRT duration, total ventilation days, ICU days, and hospital length of stay (LOS) (median (inter-quartile range)) within and between study eras, as well as over the 10-year study period

Time Variable (days)	2004–2008			2009–2013			2004–2013		
	All Patients	Survivors	Non-survivors	All Patients	Survivors	Non-survivors	All Patients	Survivors	Non-survivors
Time from Hospital Admit to CRRT Start	8 (2, 22)	4 (2, 9)	18 ^{a} (4, 36)	7 (3, 22)	4 (1, 11)	14 ^{a} (4, 32)	8 (2, 22)	4 (1, 10)	16 ^{a} (4, 35)
Time from ICU Admit to CRRT Start	4 (1, 10)	3 (1, 6)	9 ^{a} (2, 19)	5 (2, 12)	2 (1, 5)	4.5 ^{a} (3, 14)	3 (1, 10)	3 (1, 6)	7 ^{a} (2, 16)
Total CRRT time	8 (4, 16)	7 (4, 13)	8 (4, 19)	8 (4, 18)	8 (4, 17)	8 (4, 18)	8 (4, 17)	7 (4, 15)	8 (4, 18)
Ventilation time	21 (9, 35)	19 (6, 31)	21 (11, 37)	12 (5, 29)	11 (4, 25)	13 ^{b} (7, 30)	16 (7, 31)	13 (4, 28)	18 ^{a} (8, 33)
ICU LOS	22 (13, 36)	21 (13, 34)	22 (13, 38)	19 (11, 33)	20 (11, 33)	19 (10, 33)	21 (12, 34)	21 (12, 34)	21 (11, 36)
Hospital LOS	39 (24, 63)	43 (31, 77)	36 ^{a} (19, 59)	35 (23, 60)	41 (26, 71)	31 ^{a} (20, 51)	38 (23, 61)	42 (28, 71)	32 ^{a} (19, 54)

^{a} $p < 0.05$ comparing survivors with non-survivors within the respective period cohort

^{b} $p < 0.05$ comparing non-survivors from 2004 to 2008 with non-survivors from 2009 to 2013

(1, 10) vs non-survivors 16 (4, 35) days, $p < 0.001$) and from ICU admission (survivors 3 (1, 6) vs 7 (2, 16) days, p < 0.001) than survivors. Hospital LOS was longer in survivors (survivors 42 (28, 71) vs. 32 (19, 54) days, $p = 0.003$), as expected, ICU LOS was not different. Non-survivors had more ventilation days compared to survivors across the entire 10-year study period (survivors 13 (4, 28) vs non-survivors 18 (8, 33) days, $p = 0.02$), except for the 2009–2013 period when non-survivors had fewer ventilation days than the non-survivors in the 2004–2008 period ($p = 0.01$). The total days on CRRT were not different between survivors and non-survivors or between eras. Patient hospital survival was also examined accounting for primary diagnosis, ICU admission weight, indication for CRRT, and immune status (Table 5). Patients with a hematologic/oncologic primary diagnosis (excluding patients who had undergone BMT) in the 2004–2008 cohort had fewer deaths ($p = 0.04$). Survival was not different when compared by patient weight at CRRT start, indication for CRRT, time on CRRT, and immune status.

Table 6 shows a comparison of percent fluid overload at initiation of CRRT between eras based on principal diagnoses overall and survival. BMT patients were significantly less fluid overloaded upon initiation of CRRT (2004–2008 16% (10, 20) vs 2009–2013 10% (7, 12), $p = 0.047$), however there was no difference in survival. When the entire 10-year cohort was evaluated, sepsis survivors had lower percent fluid overload at initiation of CRRT (8% (12, 21)) compared with non-survivors (27% (19, 34)) ($p = 0.05$), however this was not demonstrated between the two eras. Neonatal survivors in the 2009–2013 cohort group also had lower percentage of fluid overload (17% (12, 22)) versus non-survivors (26% (14, 37)) ($p = 0.043$). No other differences were seen in the patient survival based on fluid overload and principal diagnosis.

Discussion

This cohort study of 311 patients treated with CRRT over a 10-year period is the largest single center pediatric report published to date. To our surprise, we found only a 12% increase in treatment volume over time and very similar patient characteristics in the two eras. There was a shift towards treatment of younger patients by 2.5 years, as well a nearly 5 kg shift towards smaller patients. Overall, the mean weight and age of this patient population were similar to those of the ppCRRT registry studies (33.5 kg vs 34.3 kg (ppCRRT) and 8.4 yr. vs 8.5 yr. (ppCRRT), with similar interval subcategorizations (Table 7) [3, 6]. It is worth noting that there may be a small measure of overlap in the ppCRRT registry data with our patients, as patients from our institution in years 2004 and 2005 were enrolled in that registry. We were unable to identify which patients were enrolled, and ppCRRT

Table 5 Comparison of survival on CRRT by principal diagnosis, weight, CRRT indication, and immune status between study eras and shown over the 10 year study period

	2004–2008	2009–2013	2004–2013
	Survivor n (%)	Survivor n (%)	Survivor n (%)
Principal Diagnosis Category			
Cardiac	7 (54%)	3 (27%)	10 (42%)
Renal	4 (44%)	14 (74%)	18 (64%)
Liver	6 (32%)	17 (46%)	23 (41%)
Hematology/Oncology [a]	10 (56%)	3 (18%)	13 (37%)
Bone marrow transplant	3 (17%)	5 (33%)	8 (24%)
Pulmonary	4 (36%)	2 (50%)	6 (40%)
Inborn error of metabolism	5 (100%)	7 (70%)	12 (80%)
Sepsis	3 (30%)	2 (40%)	5 (33%)
Neonates	8 (80%)	8 (62%)	16 (70%)
Other [b]	10 (63%)	10 (77%)	20 (69%)
Weight			
0-10 kg	9 (35%)	19 (50%)	28 (44%)
10-25 kg	13 (45%)	22 (56%)	35 (51%)
25-50 kg	17 (49%)	13 (39%)	30 (44%)
> 50 kg	21 (54%)	17 (50%)	38 (52%)
Indications for CRRT			
Fluid overload	31 (42%)	35 (49%)	66 (46%)
Fluid overload & electrolyte management	12 (43%)	17 (41%)	29 (41%)
Prevent fluid overload/provide nutrition	3 (50%)	2 (67%)	5 (56%)
Electrolyte management	4 (57%)	4 (44%)	8 (50%)
Other [c]	10 (71%)	13 (68%)	23 (70%)
Days on CRRT			
1 day	8 (47%)	5 (55%)	12 (50%)
2–7 days	24 (42%)	34 (45%)	58 (44%)
8–14 days	18 (50%)	12 (36%)	30 (43%)
15–21 days	10 (53%)	11 (48%)	21 (50%)
22–28 days	1 (17%)	7 (50%)	8 (40%)
> 28 days	3 (25%)	7 (50%)	10 (38%)
Immune Status			
Solid organ transplant	11 (44%)	17 (52%)	28 (48%)
Bone marrow transplant	5 (29%)	5 (36%)	10 (32%)
Other immunocompromised	12 (48%)	11 (42%)	23 (45%)
Not immunocompromised	32 (52%)	38 (54%)	70 (53%)

[a]$p < 0.05$ comparing 2004–2008 survivors with 2009–2013 survivors
[b]Includes rheumatologic, gastroenterologic, multiple organ, neurologic, ingestions, hemorrhage, rhabdomyolysis, and non-accidental trauma
[c]Includes hemodynamic instability, hyperammonemia, ingestion, and end-stage renal disease

Table 6 Comparison of median percent fluid overload upon initiation of CRRT in all patients, survivors, and non-survivors between eras (median (inter-quartile range)), as well as over the 10-year study period

Principal Diagnosis	2004–2008			2009–2013			2004–2013		
	All Patients	Survivors	Non-survivors	All Patients	Survivors	Non-survivors	All Patients	Survivors	Non-survivors
Cardiac	19 (2, 26)	5 (2, 22)	20 (19, 33)	4 (3, 11)	12 (3,29)	4 (0, 7)	7 (2, 22)	9 (3, 24)	7 (0, 20)
Renal	10 (6, 30)	10 (6, 30)	–	23 (13, 30)	17 (13, 30)	28 (28,28)	20 (12, 30)	17 (11, 30)	28 (28, 28)
Liver	20 (15, 31)	37 (17, 42)	18 (14, 24)	20 (12, 30)	19 (12, 30)	20 (12, 30)	20 (12, 30)	20 (12, 35)	19 (13, 27)
Hematology/ Oncology	15 (8, 22)	20 (12, 22)	12 (8, 15)	17 (5, 29)	14 (0, 29)	21 (5, 29)	17 (8, 28)	17 (8, 22)	16 (8, 29)
Bone marrow transplant	16 (10, 20)	15 (9,20)	16 (10, 20)	10 [a] (7, 12)	9 (7, 11)	10 (7, 13)	11 (9, 18)	10 (8, 12)	11 (10, 19)
Pulmonary	15 (9, 18)	20 (5, 26)	15 (11, 15)	13 (4, 22)	13 (8, 18)	13 (0, 25)	15 (7, 19)	18 (8, 20)	15 (7, 16)
Inborn Error of Metabolism	0 (0, 0)	0 (0, 0)	–	0 (0, 16)	0 (0, 0)	17 (0, 35)	0 (0, 16)	0 (0, 0)	17 (0, 35)
Sepsis	20 (9, 28)	8 (0, 21)	25 (13, 30)	22 (20, 38)	17 (12, 22)	38 (20, 46)	21 (12, 30)	12 (8, 21)	27 [b] (19, 34)
Neonates	20 (9, 32)	21 (8, 39)	20 (20, 20)	14 (0, 26)	6 (0, 14)	26 [b] (14, 37)	14 (6, 29)	10 (0, 15)	23 (14, 37)
Other [c]	21 (13, 40)	21 (13, 28)	28 (12, 48)	11 (4, 21)	17 (5, 21)	4 (0, 12)	17 (8, 30)	17 (10, 28)	12 (4, 36)

[a] $p < 0.05$ comparing all patient median percent fluid overload between the 2004–2008 and 2009–2013 cohorts

[b] $p \leq 0.05$ comparing median percent fluid overload between survivors and non-survivors within the respective cohort period

[c] Includes rheumatologic, gastroenterologic, multiple organ, neurologic, ingestions, hemorrhage, rhabdomyolysis, and non-accidental trauma

Table 7 Comparative outcomes of present study with previously published pediatric CRRT studies; FO, fluid overload, EM electrolyte management

	Our Study	ppCRRT Registry [a, b]	Spain [c, d]	Birmingham [e]	Alberta (CRRT only) [f]
N	273	344	174	76	49
Weight					
Mean/Median Wt (kg)	33.5	34.3		19.5(2.5–150)	19.5 (5.5–45)
Less than 10 kg (%)	23	24	43		
10 to 20 kg (%)	25	20			
20 to 50 kg (%)	25	29			
> 50 kg (%)	27	27			
Age					
Mean / Median Age (yr)	8.4	8.5	4.3 (±5.3)	5.8 (0–17.8)	5.4 (0.3–13.8)
0 to 1 yr. (%)	21	20	43.7		
1 to 3 yr. (%)	12	13			
3 to 5 yr. (%)	8	8			
5 to 10 yr. (%)	14	17			
10 to 15 yr. (%)	21	19			
15 to 21 yr. (%)	20	20			
> 21 yr. (%)	4	3			
Survival to discharge (%)	48	58	64	55	67
Principle diagnosis (%)					
Sepsis	5	24	20	12	
BMT	12	16		16	
Cardiac	9	12	56	9	
Renal	10	9	10	20	
Liver	21	8		6	
Malignancy	13	8		8	
Ischemia/shock		6			
Inborn error of metabolism	5	4	7		
Drug intoxication		4	2		
Tumor lysis syndrome		3	3	14	
Pulmonary	5	3			
Other	11	2	05	14	
Survival on CRRT by Weight (N (%))					
< 10 kg	28 (43%)	36 (43%)	57%		
> 10 kg	105 (49%)	165 (63%)	73%		
ICU days before CRRT	4 (1,10)	2			2 (1–5)
Days on CRRT	8 (4,16)				7 (3–18)
% FO	15 (8, 26)			12.9 (0–66.4)	20.1 (5.4–32.5)
Indication for CRRT & survival (%)					
FO and EM	29 (41%)	15	32[g]		
FO	67 (45%)	18			
EM	8(50%)	20	42[h]		
Prevent FO /provide nutrition	5(56%)	20			
Other	24 (55%)	21			

a. Symons JM, Chua AN, Somers MJ, et al. Demographic characteristics of pediatric continuous renal replacement therapy: a report of the prospective pediatric continuous renal replacement therapy registry. *Clin J Am Soc Nephrol.* July 2007;2(4):732–738

b. Sutherland SM, Zappitelli M, Alexander SR, et al. Fluid overload and mortality in children receiving continuous renal replacement therapy: the prospective pediatric continuous renal replacement therapy registry. *Am J Kidney Dis.* Feb 2010;55(2):316–25

c. Lopez-Herc J, Santiago MJ, Solana MJ et al. Clinical course of children requiring prolonged continuous renal replacement therapy. *Pediatr Nephrol.* Dec 2010; 25:523–528

d. Santiago MJ, Lopez-Herce J, Urbando J, et al. Clinical course and mortality risk factors in critically ill children requiring continuous renal replacement therapy. *Intensive Care Med.* May 2010;36(5):843–9

e. Hayes LW, Oster RA, Tofil NM, et al. Outcomes of critically ill children requiring continuous renal replacement therapy. *J Crit Care.* Sep 2009;24(3):394–400

f. Boschee E, Cave D, Garros D, et al. Indications and outcomes in children receiving renal replacement therapy in pediatric intensive care. *J Crit Care.* Feb 2014;29(1):37–42

g. Patients with diagnosis of AKI and hypervolemia

h. Patients with diagnosis of AKI

was a voluntary registry for which only those patients who were consented were included, thus it is extremely unlikely that every patient from those years was also in ppCRRT. In the modern era of CRRT, nearly half (46%) the patients treated were younger than 5 years old. Additionally, 53% of our patients were less than 20 kg and more than a quarter were less than 10 kg. This may be due to improving recognition of AKI in younger patients, and increasing comfort with providing CRRT for neonatal patients. The shift towards smaller, younger patients also falls in line with more recently published single-center cohort studies, as shown in Table 7 [21–24].

The shift towards younger, smaller patients continues to speak loudly to the need for equipment specially designed for treating the smallest patients, especially as our CRRT equipment is not United States Food and Drug Administration approved for use in patients weighing less than 20 kg. Following the ppCRRT evaluation, CRRT equipment evolved with the introduction of a new generation of machines now in use with better safeguards in place for delivery of CRRT to smaller patients [25]. A specialized pediatric CRRT circuit, the PrismaFlex HF20, with an extracorpeal volume of 60 ml [26] is currently being tested for FDA approval at pediatric centers throughout the USA. CARPEDIEM is RRT equipment with a 27 ml extracorpeal circuit volume and capability to handle blood flow rates 5–50 ml/hr., that once approved should dramatically improve the mechanics of treating the smallest patients [27, 28]. Additionally, the Newcastle infant dialysis and ultrafiltration system (NIDUS) is hemodialysis equipment designed for use in infants 800 g to 8 kg, without need for blood priming as well as using only single lumen vascular access, and successful use has been published on 9 babies weighing 1.8 kg to 5.9 kg in the United Kingdom [29]. There is additional work on pediatric equipment occurring, including the Aquadex™ continuous venovenous hemofiltration system [30], the KIDS-CRRT Device machine for pediatric fluid management [31], and a volumetric-based scale system for pediatric patients [32].

While not notably different, we did see shifts in the primary diagnoses of patients treated with CRRT in our institution over just 10 years. Across eras, there were double the number of patients treated with primary liver disease (19 vs 37) and nearly doubling of patients treated for inborn errors of metabolism (5 vs 10). This most likely reflects an institutional increase in tertiary referrals, where more patients with liver disease and inborn errors of metabolism are transported to our facility from around the region. Our institution does have an Extracorporeal Liver Support program; however, the cohort presented here predates the launch of that program so is unlikely to explain the increased numbers of liver failure patients placed on CRRT. Rather, this might be a reflection in the shift towards offering more CRRT to liver transplant candidates for AKI with or without hepatorenal syndrome, with the

more recent reports of renal recovery after liver transplantation in pediatric and adult patients [33, 34]. Almost 3-fold fewer patients with pulmonary disease were treated with CRRT in the modern era (11 vs 4), which likely reflects the referral patients our center receives for its busy lung transplant program. A comparison of the primary diagnostic categories of published pediatric CRRT cohorts shown in Table 4 demonstrates the heterogeneity of the populations likely reflecting unique program strengths and referral regions. In our institution, cardiac population largely received acute peritoneal dialysis as the RRT of choice when possible. With the introduction of rasburicase, CRRT treatment for tumor lysis syndrome has become increasingly rare.

An important difference to note across the two eras was a significant decline in the number of patients treated with CRRT for an initial presentation of sepsis. We suspect this is largely due to the introduction of a septic shock protocol in early 2010, an early resuscitation bundle initiated upon patient presentation to the emergency department when meeting abnormal vital sign criteria within an electronic triage system to provide earlier recognition and treatment interventions [35]. The protocol has been shown to reduce AKI, the need for renal replacement therapy, hospital LOS, and patient mortality [36]. When evaluated alongside the ppCRRT registry and other single center studies, our center clearly has the smallest percentage of CRRT patients presenting with sepsis (Table 7). It is worth noting that the patient population with a primary diagnosis of sepsis was the only group to show a difference in percentage fluid overload between survivors and non-survivors when looking at the entire cohort over 10 years. An obvious predilection in either direction was not demonstrable for any other principal diagnoses. In many studies, the percentage of fluid overload at initiation of CRRT has repeatedly shown to be an independent risk factor for increased morbidity and mortality [3, 9, 20, 21, 37, 38], although conflicting reports also exist [39]. Awareness of the association between fluid overload and adverse outcomes has certainly increased, with pediatric data paving the way. In the initial report by Goldstein in 2001 [20], non-survivors of CRRT had almost 35% fluid overload at CRRT start. The lack of a clear schism in the percentage fluid overload between survivors and non-survivors in the current report originating from the same institution as the 2001 paper might reflect a drift in practice where CRRT is started earlier, thus avoiding a higher initial degree of fluid overload. Our patients had an average of 15% fluid overload at CRRT start, with a shift between eras from 17 to 14%, although not statistically significant. The time to CRRT initiation seemed shorter in the modern era, although this difference was not statistically significant. The difference in percentage fluid overload might at least in part reflect a more careful attention to fluid balance by the general healthcare team.

Our results confirm that patients requiring treatment with CRRT are rarely patients with primary renal disease; rather they are patients who secondarily suffer from kidney injury in the context of their primary disease condition and comorbidities. In fact, half of the patients treated across both eras were immunocompromised, including cancer, organ transplantation, and autoimmune conditions. Patients who have undergone stem cell transplants and received renal replacement therapy have been studied, but little has been studied to date surrounding the immune status of patients requiring CRRT [5, 40, 41]. While the difference in survival did not achieve statistical significance, we observed a trend towards decreased survival rates amongst patients who were immunocompromised. There is very limited pharmacokinetic data in pediatric CRRT, potentially impacting optimal treatment of CRRT patients particularly with antimicrobials, as pediatric CRRT patients are reported to have increased infections [42]. Further study is warranted to determine if higher infection susceptibility translates to increased morbidity from suboptimal treatment.

Our patient population showed no difference in survival based on the total time spent on CRRT, examined both as total median days on CRRT and when categorized incrementally. This is consistent with reporting from the ppCRRT registry, as well as a much smaller study of 39 patients, for whom there was no significant difference in survival rates based on duration of CRRT for greater than or less than 4 weeks [6, 43]. Across all groupings in our study, survivors consistently demonstrated shorter times from both hospital and ICU admissions to initiation of CRRT compared to non-survivors, but an overall shorter hospital length of stay. In pediatrics, Hayes et al. showed no difference in the number of hospital days prior to starting CRRT, however Modem et al. did find a significantly longer time to CRRT initiation amongst non-survivors [14, 21]. Adult CRRT investigations have evaluated the benefits of early versus late start CRRT, defined by timing to initiate CRRT in the setting of AKI severity, without any clearly demonstrable benefit [44–46]. We suspect differential survival outcomes with respect to time to initiation of CRRT may be more indicative of severe, progressive multi-organ illness with eventual AKI development rather than a beneficial impact of earlier CRRT initiation on outcomes. While percentage of fluid overload at initiation of CRRT has been linked to longer ventilation times [21], ventilation time alone in pediatric patients treated with CRRT has not been previously evaluated for survival, and suggests increased severity of illness associated with patient mortality.

For those patients who survive their hospital course that includes CRRT, we found that overall only 44% of patients were subsequently seen for dedicated outpatient nephrology care, however between eras, that number improved from 33 to 54%. Only one-third of pediatric and adult patients follow up with a nephrologist after an episode of AKI [47, 48]. While the exact time course for developing chronic kidney disease (CKD) is unknown, a progressively higher rate of CKD is observed over time amongst AKI survivors [47, 49]. In pediatric patients with CKD, increasing proteinuria is associated with decreased renal function, and excellent blood pressure control has been correlated with slowed progression of renal disease [50, 51]. Thus, early intervention is critical in slowing the relentless progression of CKD, and patients whose course of critical illness has included AKI may benefit from dedicated longitudinal follow-up with a nephrologist for monitoring of blood pressure, urinary protein, and kidney function. More importantly, this finding underscores the need to educate fellow physicians, patients, and parents on the importance of monitoring kidney function and maintaining nephrology follow-up over the patient's lifetime.

Our study has several limitations. The retrospective nature of the study did not allow us to determine certain important patient characteristics, such as severity of illness indices, which would have been helpful in refining the definition of the cohorts and to examine if indeed sicker patients were being treated with CRRT in the latter era, perhaps accounting for the lack of improvement in survival, at least partially. We were also only able to determine outpatient follow-up in patients who came to our nephrology clinic, and may have missed some patients who were followed at other centers. Lack of an AKI/CRRT survivors' clinic or a formal outreach program where these patients are being followed in conjunction with primary care physician is partially responsible for the incomplete follow-up.

The largest and most comprehensive evaluation of pediatric AKI was recently published, demonstrating an AKI rate of 26.9% in pediatric ICU around the world [52]. Studies have shown that AKI, regardless of the criterion scoring used and with or without provision of CRRT, portend the greatest risk for mortality [18, 53, 54]. Since the ppCRRT registry was concluded more than ten years ago, the pediatric nephrology and critical care communities gained a wealth of information, including data on the demographics, epidemiologic, and technical aspects of pediatric CRRT [25]. The field of AKI clinical research has exploded in the last decade, improving our understanding of the impact of AKI on survival as well as other morbidity such as new disability [55]. While feasibility of pediatric CRRT was still being questioned in the early 2000s, it has now become the standard of care. Our study provides evidence for a need to continue performing interval assessments of this patient population, especially with advances across critical care medicine, not limited to renal replacement devices.

It is especially disheartening to see that mortality rate has not decreased at all despite technological advances and accumulating clinical experience. The reasons underlying this observation require further exploration. While it is certainly possible that we are treating sicker patients with CRRT, in the absence of severity of illness indicators, we cannot conclude this to be the only reason. Lack of specialized renal replacement equipment for pediatric patients, uncertainty about optimal antibiotic dosing on CRRT, and under nutrition likely all play roles in little improvement seen in survival among patients treated with CRRT during their hospital course. While we benefit from good patient volume numbers, this is still a single-center study, reflecting the unique aspects of CRRT prescription and delivery at one location. Multi-center assessments to amass collaborative patient evaluations will continue to help further assess multi-layered aspects of patient care, including a clarification of who is most affected by fluid overload, changing demographics of the population and their needs, and how duration of CRRT correlates with patient outcomes. Additionally, longitudinal care of these patients who survive with AKI is for maintaining maximal health in the face of progressive chronic kidney disease.

Conclusions

Over the last decade, the demographics of our pediatric CRRT population have shifted slightly to younger and smaller patients, but overall diagnostic categories and outcomes have not changed. Although nephrology outpatient follow-up in AKI survivors has improved over time, it remains poor at around 50%. Further studies focusing on pediatric CRRT patients to examine areas of limited data such as pharmacokinetics, dose delivery, quality indicators, and renal recovery will enhance our practice of CRRT and might improve outcomes.

Acknowledgements
The authors wish to acknowledge Dr. Michael C. Braun, Chief of the Pediatric Renal Section, Baylor College of Medicine, for his support of this study.

Funding
This study was performed without additional financial support.

Authors' contributions
Dr. AAR – study conceptualization & design, data collection, data analysis, data interpretation, drafting the manuscript, revising and editing the final article. Ms. MW – data collection, revising and editing the final article. Ms. CS – data collection, revising and editing the final article. Ms. DG – data analysis and interpretation, revising and editing the final article. Dr. CGM – data analysis and interpretation, revising and editing the final article. Ms. HC – study conceptualization & design, revising and editing the final article. Dr. AAA – study conceptualization & design, data collection, data analysis, data interpretation, revising and editing the final article. All authors read and approved the final manuscript.

Competing interests
Baylor College of Medicine received payments in 2013 totaling $8587.68 from Amgen, Inc. under Dr. Alyssa Riley's name while she was the site PI for two of their sponsored pediatric cinacalcet studies.

Author details
[1]Department of Pediatrics, Renal Section, Baylor College of Medicine, Houston, TX, USA. [2]Texas Children's Hospital, Houston, TX, USA. [3]Department of Pediatrics, Dell Medical School, The University of Texas at Austin, Austin, TX, USA. [4]Dan L. Duncan Institute for Clinical and Translational Research, Baylor College of Medicine, Houston, TX, USA.

References
1. Askenazi DJ, Goldstein SL, Koralkar R, et al. Continuous renal replacement therapy for children ≤10 kg: a report from the prospective pediatric continuous renal replacement therapy registry. J Pediatr. 2013;162(3):587–92.
2. Fleming GM, Walters S, Goldstein SL. Nonrenal indications for continuous renal replacement therapy: A report from the Prospective Pediatric Continuous Renal Replacement Therapy Registry Group. Pediatr Crit Care Med. 2012;13(5):e299–304.
3. Sutherland SM, Zappitelli M, Alexander SR, et al. Fluid overload and mortality in children receiving continuous renal replacement therapy: the prospective pediatric continuous renal replacement therapy registry. Am J Kidney Dis. 2010;55(2):316–25.
4. Zappitell M, Goldstein SL, Symons JM, et al. Protein and calorie prescription for children and young adults receiving continuous renal replacement therapy: a report from the Prospective Pediatric Continuous Renal Replacement Therapy Registry Group. Crit Care Med. 2008;36(12):3239–45.
5. Flores FX, Brophy PD, Symons JM, et al. Continuous renal replacement therapy (CRRT) after stem cell transplantation. A report from the prospective pediatric CRRT Registry Group. Pediatr Nephrol. 2008;23(4):625–30.
6. Symons JM, Chua AN, Somers MJ, et al. Demographic characteristics of pediatric continuous renal replacement therapy: a report of the prospective pediatric continuous renal replacement therapy registry. Clin J Am Soc Nephrol. 2007;2(4):732–8.
7. Goldstein SL, Somers MJ, Brophy PD, et al. The Prospective Pediatric Continuous Renal Replacement Therapy (ppCRRT) Registry: design, development and data assessed. Int J Artif Organs. 2004;27(1):9–14.
8. Brophy PD, Somers MJ, Baum MA, et al. Multi-centre evaluation of anticoagulation in patients receiving continuous renal replacement therapy (CRRT). Nephrol Dial Transplant. 2005;20(7):1416–21.
9. Goldstein SL, Somers MJ, Baum MA, et al. Pediatric patients with multi-organ dysfunction syndrome receiving continuous renal replacement therapy. Kindey Int. 2005;67(2):653–8.
10. Goldstein SL, Hackbarth R, Bunchman TE, et al. Evaluation of the PRISMA M10 circuit in critically ill infants with acute kidney injury: A report from the Prospective Pediatric CRRT Registry Group. Int J Artif Organs. 2006;29(12):1105–8.
11. Hackbarth R, Bunchman TE, Chua AN. al e. The effect of vascular access location and size on circuit survival in pediatric continuous renal replacement therapy: a report from the PPCRRT registry. Int J Artif Organs. 2007;30(12):1116–21.
12. Fiser D, Tilford J, Roberson P. Relationship of illness severity and length of stay to functional outcomes in the pediatric intensive care unit: a multi-institutional study. Crit Care Med. 2000;28(4):1173–9.
13. Pollack M, Holubkov R, Funai T, Clark A, et al. Pediatric intensive care outcomes: development of new morbidities during pediatric critical care. Pediatr Crit Care Med. 2014;15(9):821–7.
14. Modem V, Thompson M, Gollhofer D, et al. Timing of continuous renal replacement therapy and mortality in critcally ill children. Crit Care Med. 2014;42(4):943–53.
15. Hui-Stickle S, Brewer ED, Goldstein SL. Pediatric ARF epidemiology at a tertiary care center from 1999 to 2001. Am J Kidney Dis. 2005;45(1):96–101.
16. Bailey D, Phan V, Litalien C, et al. Risk factors of acute renal failure in critically ill children: a prospective decriptive epidemiological study. Pediatr Crit Care Med. 2007;8(1):29–35.
17. McGregor TL, Jones DP, Wang L, et al. Acute kidney injury incidence in noncritically ill hospitalized children, adolescents, and young adults: a retrospective observational study. Am J Kidney Dis. 2016;67(3):384–90.

18. Schneider K, Khemani R, Grushkin C, Bart R. Serum creatinine as stratified in the RIFLE score for acute kidney injury is associated with mortality and length of stay for children in the pediatric intensive care unit. Crit Care Med. 2010;38(3):933–9.

19. Sutherland SM, Ji J, Sheikhi FH, et al. AKI in hospitalized children: epidemiology and clinical associations in a national cohort. Clin J Am Soc Nephrol. 2013;8(10):1661–9.

20. Goldstein SL, Currier H, Graf C, et al. Outcome in children receiving continuous venovenous hemofiltration. Pediatics. 2001;107(6):1309–12.

21. Hayes LW, Oster RA, Tofil NM, et al. Outcomes of critically ill children requiring continuous renal replacement therapy. J Crit Care. 2009; 24(3):394–400.

22. Boschee E, Cave D, Garros D, et al. Indications and outcomes in children receiving renal replacement therapy in pediatric intensive care. J Crit Care. 2014;29(1):37–42.

23. Santiago M, Lopez-Herce J, Urbano J, et al. Clinical course and mortality risk factors in critically ill children requiring continuous renal replacement therapy. Intensive Care Med. 2010;36(5):843–9.

24. Lopez-Herce J, Santiago M, Solana M, et al. Clinical course of children requiring prolonged continuous renal replacement therapy. Pediatr Nephrol. 2010;25:523–8.

25. Sutherland SM, Goldstein SL, Alexander SL. The Prospective Pediatric Continuous Renal Replacement Therapy (ppCRRT) Registry: a critical appraisal. Pediatr Nephrol. 2014;29(11):2069–76.

26. Liu ID, Ng KH, Lau PY, et al. Use of HF20 membrane in critically ill unstable low-body-weight infants on inotropic support. Pediatr Nephrol. 2013;28(5):819–22.

27. Ronco C, Garzotto F, Brendolan A, et al. Continuous renal replacement therapy in neonates and small infants: development and first-in-human use of a miniaturised machine (CARPEDIEM). Lancet. 2014;383(9931):1807–13.

28. Peruzzi L, Bonaudo R, Amore A, et al. Neonatal sepsis with multi-organ failure and treated with a new dialysis device specifically designed for newborns. Case Rep Nephrol Urol. 2014;4(2):113–9.

29. Askenazi D, Ingram D, White S, et al. Smaller circuits for smaller patients: improving renal support therapy with AquadexTM. Pediatr Nephrol. 2016; 31(5):853–60.

30. Coulthard MG, Crosier J, Griffiths C, et al. Haemodialysing babies weighing < 8 kg with the Newcastle infant dialysis and ultrafiltration system (Nidus): comparison with peritoneal and conventional haemodialysis. Pediatr Nephrol. 2014;29(10):1873–81.

31. Santhanakrishnan A, Nestle TT, Moore BL, et al. Development of an accurate fluid management system for a pediatric continuous renal replacement therapy device. ASAIO J. 2013;59(3):294–301.

32. Hanudel MR, Salusky IB, Zaritsky JJ. The accuracy of a continuous volumetric balancing system in pediatric continuous renal replacement therapy. Int J Artif Organs. 2014;37(3):215–21.

33. Deep A, Stewart C, Dhawan A, Douiri A. Effect of continuous renal replacement therapy on outcome in pediatric acute liver failure. Crit Care Med. 2016;44(10):1910–9.

34. Rana A, Kueht M, Desai M, et al. No child left behind: Liver transplantion in critically ill children. J Am Coll Surg. 2017;224(4):671–7.

35. Cruz AT, Perry AM, Williams EA, et al. Implementation of goal-directed therapy for children with suspected sepsis in the emergency department. Pediatrics. 2011;127(3):e758–66.

36. Akcan Arikan A, Williams EA, Graf JM, et al. Resuscitation Bundle in Pediatric Shock Decreases Acute Kidney Injury and Improves Outcomes. J Pediatr. 2015;167(6):1301–5.

37. Foland JA, Fortenberry JD, Warshaw BL. Fluid overload before continuous hemofiltration and survival in critically ill children: A retrospective analysis. Crit Care Med. 2004;32(8):1771–6.

38. Gillespie RS, Seidel K, Symons JM. Effect of fluid overload and dose of replacement fluid on survival in hemofiltration. Pediatr Nephrol. 2004;19(12):1394–9.

39. de Galasso L, Emma F, Picca S, et al. Continuous renal replacement therapy in children: fluid overload does not always predict mortality. Pediatr Nephrol. 2016;31(4):651–9.

40. Elbahlawan L, West NK, Avent Y, et al. Impact of continuous renal replacement therapy on oxygenation in children with acute lung injury after allogeneic hematopoietic stem cell transplantation. Pediatr Blood Cancer. 2010;55(3):540–5.

41. Rajesekaran S, Jones DP, Avent Y, et al. Outcomes of hematopoietic stem cell transplant patients who received continuous renal replacement therapy in a pediatric oncology intensive care unit. Pediatr Crit Care Med. 2010;11(6):699–706.

42. Santiago M, Lopez-Herce J, Vierge E, et al. Infection in critically ill pediatric patients on continuous renal replacement therapy. Int J Artif Organs. 2017;40(5):224–9.

43. Baird JS, Wald EL. Long-duration (> 4 weeks) continuous renal replacement therapy in critical illness. Int J Artif Organs. 2010;33(10):716–20.

44. Wierstra B, Kadri S, Alomar S, et al. The impact of "early" versus "late" initiation of renal replacement therapy in critical care patients with acute kidney injury: a systematic review and evidence synthesis. Crit Care. 2016;20:122.

45. Zarbock A, Kellum J, Schmidt C, et al. Effect of early vs delayed initiation of renal replacement therapy on mortality in critically ill patients with acute kidney injury: The ELAIN randomized clinica trial. JAMA. 2016;315(20):2190–9.

46. Gaudry S, Hajage D, Schortgen F, et al. Initiation strategies for renal-replacement therapy in the intensive care unit. N Engl J Med. 2016;375(2):122–33.

47. Askenazi DJ, Feig DI, Graham NM, et al. 3–5 year longitudinal follow-up of pediatric patients after acute renal failure. Kidney Int. 2006;69(1):184–9.

48. Ali T, Tachibana A, Khan I, et al. The changing pattern of referral in acute kidney injury. QJM. 2011;104(6):497–503.

49. Mammen C, Al Abbas A, Skippen P, et al. Long-term risk of CKD in children surviving episodes of acute kidney injury in the intensive care unit: a prospective cohort study. Am J Kidney Dis. 2012;59(4):523–30.

50. Wong CS, Pierce CB, Cole SR, et al. Association of proteinuria with race, cause of chronic kidney disease, and glomerular filtration rate in the chronic kidney disease in children study. Clin J Am Soc Nephrol. 2009;4(4):812–9.

51. ESCAPE Trial Group, Wuhl E, Trivelli A, et al. Strict blood-pressure control and progression of renal failure in children. N Engl J Med. 2009;361(17):1639–50.

52. Kaddourah A, Basu RK, Bagshaw SM, Goldstein SL. AWARE Investigators. Epidemiology of Acute Kidney Injury in Critically Ill Children and Young Adults. N Engl J Med. 2017;376(1):11–20.

53. Sutherland SM, Byrnes JJ, Kothari M, et al. AKI in hospitalized children: comparing the pRIFLE, AKIN, and KDIGO definitions. Clin J Am Soc Nephrol. 2015;10(4):554–61.

54. Sanchez-Pinto LN, Goldstein SL, Schneider JB, Khemani RG. Association Between Progression and Improvement of Acute Kidney Injury and Mortality in Critically Ill Children. Pediatr Crit Care Med. 2015;16(8):703–10.

55. Fitzgerald JC, Basu RK, Akcan-Arikan A, et al. Acute Kidney Injury in Pediatric Severe Sepsis: An Independent Risk Factor for Death and New Disability. Crit Care Med. 2016;44(12):2241–50.

8

Rituximab, plasma exchange and immunoglobulins: an ineffective treatment for chronic active antibody-mediated rejection

Gastón J Piñeiro[1,2], Erika De Sousa-Amorim[1], Manel Solé[3], José Ríos[4,5], Miguel Lozano[6], Frederic Cofán[1], Pedro Ventura-Aguiar[1,2], David Cucchiari[1,2], Ignacio Revuelta[1,2,7], Joan Cid[6], Eduard Palou[8], Josep M Campistol[1,7], Federico Oppenheimer[1], Jordi Rovira[2,7*†] [ID] and Fritz Diekmann[1,2,7*†]

Abstract

Background: Chronic active antibody-mediated rejection (c-aABMR) is an important cause of allograft failure and graft loss in long-term kidney transplants.

Methods: To determine the efficacy and safety of combined therapy with rituximab, plasma exchange (PE) and intravenous immunoglobulins (IVIG), a cohort of patients with transplant glomerulopathy (TG) that met criteria of active cABMR, according to BANFF'17 classification, was identified.

Results: We identified 62 patients with active c-aABMR and TG (cg ≥ 1). Twenty-three patients were treated with the combination therapy and, 39 patients did not receive treatment and were considered the control group. There were no significant differences in the graft survival between the two groups. The number of graft losses at 12 and 24 months and the decline of eGFR were not different and independent of the treatment. A decrease of eGFR≥13 ml/min between 6 months before and c-aABMR diagnosis, was an independent risk factor for graft loss at 24 months (OR = 5; $P = 0.01$). Infections that required hospitalization during the first year after c-aABMR diagnosis were significantly more frequent in treated patients (OR = 4.22; $P = 0.013$), with a ratio infection/patient-year of 0.65 and 0.20 respectively.

Conclusions: Treatment with rituximab, PE, and IVIG in kidney transplants with c-aABMR did not improve graft survival and was associated with a significant increase in severe infectious complications.

Keywords: Kidney transplantation, Transplant glomerulopathy, Chronic active antibody-mediated rejection, Rituximab, Infections

Background

Chronic active antibody-mediated rejection (c-aABMR) is a major cause of renal allograft failure in kidney transplants [1, 2]. Transplant glomerulopathy (TG), one of the histological features of c-aABMR, results from continuous endothelial injury and repair processes, leading to pathological multi-layering of the glomerular basement membrane [3]. The prevalence of TG increases over time after transplantation and has been associated with reduced allograft outcomes, with a mean allograft survival of 2 years after diagnosis [2, 4–6].

Despite its clinical significance the available evidence on treatment of c-aABMR with TG is scarce. Similar to the treatment of active antibody-mediated rejection, many centers use combinations of plasma exchange (PE), immunoglobulin (IVIG) and rituximab (RTX)

* Correspondence: jrovira1@clinic.cat; fdiekman@clinic.cat
†Jordi Rovira and Fritz Diekmann contributed equally to this work.
[2]Laboratori Experimental de Nefrologia i Trasplantament (LENIT), IDIBAPS, Barcelona, Spain
[1]Department of Nephrology and Renal Transplantation, ICNU, Hospital Clinic, Barcelona, Spain
Full list of author information is available at the end of the article

therapy for c-aABMR. Small and retrospective series of cases reported a slight improvement in patients with c-aABMR under IVIG and rituximab treatment [7–10]. In contrast, in two recent patients series, improvements of graft survival were not observed when comparing untreated with treated patients, whereas treated patients suffered a higher incidence of complications and adverse effects [11, 12]. However, untreated groups were small in both studies.

Recently in a randomized trial, the efficacy of rituximab and IVIG vs. placebo was tested in 24 patients with TG and DSA. There was no difference in eGFR decline. Unfortunately the study was underpowered, because the recruitment was stopped early due to low inclusion rate [13].

In the present study, we retrospectively reviewed 62 patients with c-aABMR and TG to determine the efficacy and safety of the combined therapy of RTX, PE, and IVIG.

Methods
Study population
We retrospectively reviewed our pathology database between 2006 and 2015, identified all patients with TG (cg ≥ 1 in the Banff histopathological classification) and re-evaluated them according to Banff 2017 classification criteria [3].

The inclusion criteria were the coexistence of c-aABMR TG with microvascular injury (MVI) ≥2 (g + ptc ≥ 2), with positive or negative C4d staining in peritubular capillaries and positive donor-specific antibodies (DSA). The patients with compatible histology, but negative DSA were included in the analysis as suspicious of c-aABMR. Also, TG plus positive C4d or TG with MVI =1 plus positive DSA were included. The presence of concomitant cellular rejection required at least g of 1.

The decisions to perform a renal biopsy and patient treatment were based on the clinical judgment at c-aABMR diagnosis.

Every patient who received treatment with RTX, IVIG, and PE after diagnosis of c-aABMR was included in the treatment group. Patients who did not receive RTX, IVIG neither PE, alone or in combination, were included in the control group.

PE was performed in Cobe Spectra or Spectra Optia separators (Terumo BCT, Lakewood, CO, USA) using 5% albumin (Albutein® 5%, Grífols, Spain) as a replacement solution. One plasma volume was exchanged in each session as previously reported [14].

The primary endpoint was graft survival. Secondary endpoints were the evolution of glomerular filtration rate and complications related to treatment.

The Institutional Ethics Committee approved the study. The registration number was 14,566/RG 24161

(Agencia Española del Medicamento y Producto Sanitario, AEMPS).

Clinical data
The clinical characteristics, immunosuppression, and treatment were analyzed at the time of c-aABMR diagnosis and in the follow-up period. We assessed Charlson comorbidity index (CCI) at diagnosis of c-aABMR [15]. In accordance with other groups, CCI was unadjusted for age, and the minimum score of our patients was 0 (2 points for renal insufficiency were not added) [16–19].

We assessed renal function and proteinuria at c-aABMR diagnosis, 6 months before and 6, 12, 24 months after diagnosis and at the end of follow-up. Renal function was determined by serum creatinine and by estimated glomerular filtration rate (eGFR) using the Modification of Diet in Renal Disease (MDRD) formula [20]. Proteinuria was evaluated using the proteinuria/creatinine index [21].

Serum samples obtained at the moment of transplantation and rejection were screened for HLA class I and II antibodies using the Lifecodes LifeScreen Deluxe flow bead assay (Immucor, Stamford, CT, USA). Antibody specificities were determined using the Lifecodes Single Antigen bead assay (Immucor, Stamford, CT, USA) in patients with positive HLA antibodies.

Infections that required hospitalization at least 48 h during the first year after c-aABMR diagnosis were analyzed. All immediate adverse events (AE), after IVIG, PE and RTX infusion were registered.

Statistical analysis
Data were described as mean with standard deviation (SD) or standard error of the mean (SEM), in case of graphical presentation for quantitative variables and as absolute and relative (%) frequencies for qualitative variables. Group comparisons between patients with or without the intake of rituximab were made by Fisher's exact, t-test or Mann Whitney U test for independent groups. Kaplan-Meier and comparison between both groups were made using Log-Rank test, considering non-related death as censure. We performed a crude estimation of the effect of treatment on the evolution of eGFR by generalized estimating equation (GEE) model using an AR(1) matrix to estimate the intra-subject correlation. These models included treatment effect, time of follow-up and their interaction with treatment. GEE models of treatment effect were adjusted for confounding factors including infectious disease. As a useful clinical evaluation of prediction values of change of eGFR (Δ of change) from 6 months before to rejection, we proposed a cut-off using the Likelihood Ratio (LR$^+$) defined as ratio

sensitivity/(1-specificity) from a ROC curve [22]. Estimation of risk of graft loss at 24 months due to treatment or a high delta of change of eGFR was performed calculating odds ratios (OR) and their confidence intervals at 95% (CI 95%) from logistic regression models. All statistical analyses were performed using IBM SPSS statistics V20.0 software (IBM Corp, Armonk, NY, USA). Two-sided P-values < 0.05 were used to indicate statistical significance.

Results

Sixty-two patients with TG (cg ≥ 1) and diagnosis of active c-aABMR according to Banff 2017 classification, were retrospectively identified and included in the study. Twenty-three received treatment with RTX, IVIG, and PE, whereas 39 did not receive additional treatment and were considered the control group. The median length of follow-up was 27 months.

In all patients but one, the indication of graft biopsy was in the context of deterioration of renal function or proteinuria (> 1 g/day). In the remaining patient, the biopsy was performed as follow-up biopsy after borderline rejection.

Table 1 summarized the demographic and clinical characteristics at the time of c-aABMR diagnosis. At the time of c-aABMR diagnosis, treated patients were significantly younger than those not treated 43.6 ± 13.2 vs. 53.6 ± 16.1 years ($P = 0.008$). However, CCI was not different between groups. In the two groups, the immunosuppressive regimens were similar (Table 1).

Type of donor and prior kidney transplants were not statistically different between both groups (Table 1). Mean donor age was lower in the treated group 43.05 ± 15.69 vs. 50.89 ± 11.99 years ($P = 0.035$).

Treatment

In all treated patients RTX was initiated between one and 3 weeks after c-aABMR diagnosis. 82.6% of patients treated with RTX received two doses with a mean cumulative dose of 1008 ± 342 mg.

The mean number of PE sessions was 5.8 ± 0.38, and mean total processed volume was 24.2 ± 5.4 L. The dose of IVIG was 200 mg/kg, after every second PE.

In the control group, six patients presented concomitant acute cellular rejection and were treated with corticoids.

Graft survival censoring death was not different between both groups (Fig. 1), Log Rank $P = 0.92$. The proportion of graft loss at 12 and 24 months after c-aABMR diagnosis in treated and control groups was not statistically significant, 7 patients (30%) vs. 8 patients (34.7%) and 8 (34.7%) vs.13 (33.3%) respectively.

Patient survival

Four patients died in the treated group, two of sepsis (10 and 45 months after the initiation of treatment) and two of sudden death at home (3 and 64 months after c-aABMR treatment). None of the patients in the control group died.

Kidney function, proteinuria, and presence of DSA

The mean eGFR at diagnosis of c-aABMR and 6 months before was not different between groups (Table 1 and Fig. 2a). Also, proteinuria at diagnosis was similar in both groups (Table 1).

The mean eGFR at 6, 12 and 24 months in treated and control patients was not different (Fig. 2a). Even if we split according to graft outcome eGFR follow-up was similar between treated and control patient. (Figs 2b and Additional file 1: Figure S1).

An elevated ΔeGFR (eGFR 6 months before diagnosis – eGFR at diagnosis of cABMR) was related to graft loss during the first 24 months after diagnosis. A proposed cut of 13 ml/min in ΔeGFR was obtained from ROC analysis with LR$^+$ = 3.34. A decrease of eGRF of 13 ml/min or more was an independent indicator of graft loss in the first 24 months with OR = 5 (95% CI = 1.5–16.9; $P = 0.01$). The impact of ΔeGFR was influenced neither in magnitude or statistical significance in a multivariate approach, adjusted by treatment (Table 2). Also proteinuria higher than 2.5 g/day (LR$^+$ = 3.6), adjusted for treatment, was associated with loss of graft at 24 months in both groups (OR = 3; 95% CI = 1.22–7.37; $P = 0.016$).

We have evaluated the impact of treatment on the deterioration of renal function in a longitudinal model analysis (Fig. 3), showing that the impairment of eGFR is independent of the treatment in a crude estimation model. Also, we evaluated the impact of treatment adjusted by possible confounding factors such as age, Charlson's index, graft loss, IFTA, microvascular inflammation (MVI), transplant glomerulopathy (TG), glomerulitis and peritubular capillaritis scores, proteinuria or presence of infections. However, the decrease in eGFR remains independent of the treatment (Fig. 3).

Proteinuria was not different in both groups at 6 and 12 months, mean 1.8 ± 1.2 vs. 1.7 ± 1.5 and 1.7 ± 1 vs. 1.8 ± 1.8 g/g ($P = 0.9$) creatinine respectively.

Anti-HLA antibodies were more prevalent in the treated patients, but no difference was observed in de novo DSA prevalence ($P = 0.03$ and 0.17 respectively). Regarding the DSA class, 22% were class II, 33,3% class I and, 44,4% class I and II.

The positivity of DSA and anti-HLA antibodies were not associated with worse graft survival at 24 months in our series ($P = 0.06$ and 0.65 respectively).

Table 1 Demographic and clinical characteristics

	Treatment (N = 23)	Control (N = 39)	P value
Dialysis vintage (months)	32.6 ± 24.2	41.3 ± 38.7	0.37
Donor Age	43.05 ± 15.69	50.89 ± 11.99	0.008
Donor type (Living donor)	9 (39.1%)	12 (30.7%)	0.5
First kidney transplant	13 (56.5%)	27 (69.2%)	0.31
HLA mismatch (A, B, DR)	3.27 ± 1.1	3.8 ± 1.5	0.12
Desensitization (PE + RTX)	1 (4.34%)	1 (2.56%)	0.7
Induction (Yes)	16 (69.56%)	30 (76.92%)	0.52
Thymoglobulin / ATG	10 (43.48%)	15 (38.46%)	0.7
Basiliximab	3 (13.04%)	13 (33.3%)	0.8
Other	3 (13.04%)	2 (5.12%)	0.3
IS at time of transplantation n (%)			
Tacrolimus + MMF/MPA + PDN	12 (52.2%)	24 (58.9%)	
Cyclosporine + MMF/MPA + PDN	3 (13.04%)	5 (12.82%)	
Cyclosporine + PDN	5 (21.74%)	3 (7.69%)	
mTORi + MMF/MPA + PDN	1 (4.35%)	5 (12.82%)	
Tacrolimus + mTORi + PDN	1 (4.35%)	1 (2.56%)	
Cyclosporine + mTORi + PDN		1 (2.56%)	
Cyclosporine + Azathioprine + PDN	1 (4.35%)		
Previous treated rejections of this allograft			
Cellular rejection	6 (26.1%)	10 (25%)	0.97
Humoral rejection	7 (30.4%)	6 (15.38%)	0.26
At the time of c-aABMR diagnosis			
Sex (Female/Male)	8/15	14/25	0.92
Age (years)	43.59 ± 13.2	53.6 ± 16.1	0.013
Charlson comorbidity index (CCI)	0.83 ± 1.1	0.97 ± 1.27	0.7
Time KT to active c-aABMR (months)	92.2 ± 75	93.3 ± 55.1	0.67
eGFR (mL/min) at c-aABMR diagnosis	30.9 ± 13.5	33.4 ± 11.6	0.45
eGFR (mL/min) 6 months before cABMR	40 ± 11	42.9 ± 10.2	0.3
Proteinuria (mg/g) at c-aABMR diagnosis	2286 ± 2248	1763 ± 1427	0.31
DSA (+)	6 /9	3 / 11	0.17
Anti-HLA Antibodies (+)	13 / 16	19 / 37	0.041
IS at time of c-aABMR diagnosis n (%)			
PDN + other IS	17 (73.9%)	22 (55%)	
Tacrolimus + MMF/MPA ± PDN	9 (39.1%)	17 (42.5%)	
mTORi + MMF/MPA ± PDN	2 (8.69%)	7 (17.5%)	
Cyclosporine + MMF/MPA ± PDN	4 (17.39%)	6 (15%)	
Tacrolimus + PDN	3 (13.04%)	4 (10%)	
MMF/MPA + PDN	1 (4.34%)	3 (7.5%)	
Cyclosporine ± PDN	2 (8.69%)	2 (5%)	
Tacrolimus + mTORi ± PDN	1 (4.34%)	1 (2.5%)	
Cyclosporine + mTORi	1 (4.34%)		

Results are shown as mean ± SD or absolute frequencies (%) for quantitative and qualitative variables respectively. *GFR* glomerular filtrate rate, *KT* kidney transplant, *IS* immunossupression, *mTORi* mammalian target of rapamycin inhibitor, *MMF/MPA* mycophenolate mofetil or mycophenolic acid, *cABMR* chronic antibody-mediated rejection; PDN, prednisone, *RTX* Rituximab

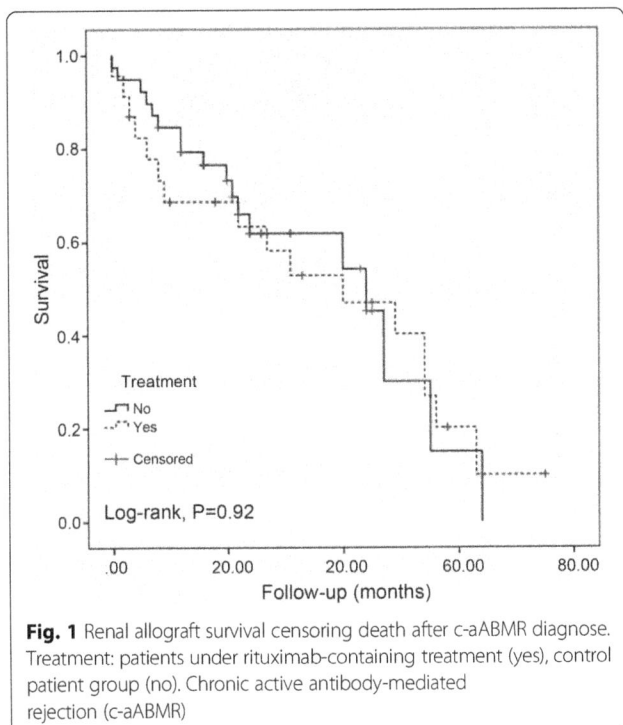

Fig. 1 Renal allograft survival censoring death after c-aABMR diagnose. Treatment: patients under rituximab-containing treatment (yes), control patient group (no). Chronic active antibody-mediated rejection (c-aABMR)

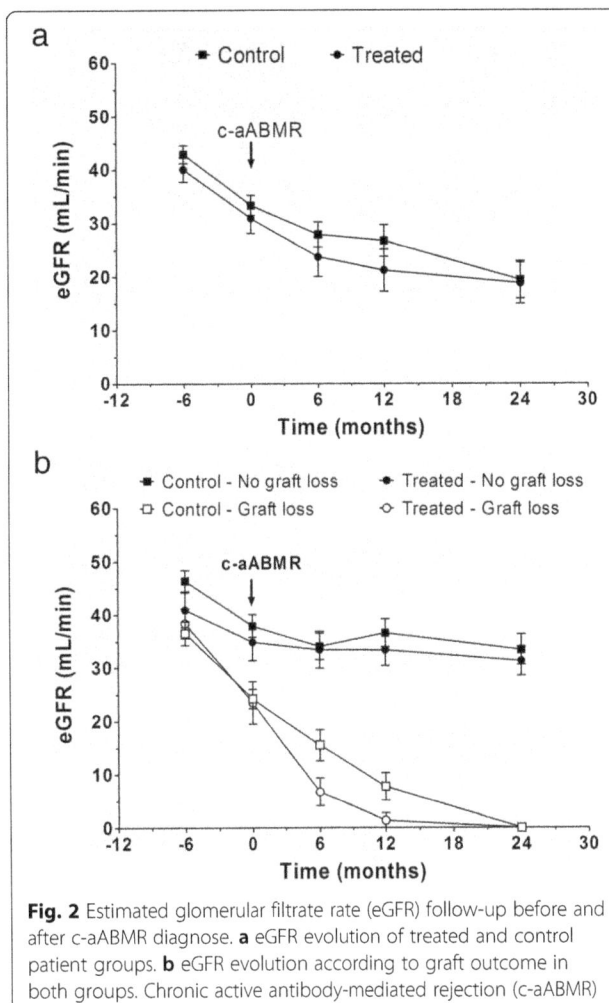

Fig. 2 Estimated glomerular filtrate rate (eGFR) follow-up before and after c-aABMR diagnose. **a** eGFR evolution of treated and control patient groups. **b** eGFR evolution according to graft outcome in both groups. Chronic active antibody-mediated rejection (c-aABMR)

Histological features

The time between renal transplantation and graft biopsy was similar in treated and control patients, 92.2 ± 75 and 93.3 ± 55 months respectively ($P = 0.94$).

At diagnosis, histologically acute inflammatory and chronic lesions related to c-aABMR and TG were similar in both groups (Table 3). Transplant glomerulopathy and IFTA were similar in treated and control patients, 1.74 ± 0.83 vs. 1.83 ± 0.77 ($P = 0.54$) and 1.61 ± 0.78 vs. 1.83 ± 0.84 ($P = 0.27$) respectively. The presence of IFTA $\geq$ two was associated with graft loss at 24 months, (OR = 4.7; 1.19–18.5; $P = 0.02$).

C4d deposition was more frequent in treated patients 19 (82.6%) vs. 17 (43.6%) ($P = 0.001$). The positivity of C4d, the severity of MVI (g + ptc) and TG degree were not associated with graft loss or worse survival.

Ten of the 23 treated patients had post-treatment follow-up biopsies within the first year after treatment with persisting active c-aABMR in all ten biopsies.

Adverse events

Infections that required hospitalization at least 48 h were more common in treated than non-treated patients during the first year after c-aABMR diagnosis, 15 vs. 8 (OR = 4.22; 95% CI = 1.37–13.1; $P = 0.012$), this reflects a ratio of infection/patient per year of 0.65 and 0.25 in treated and control patients respectively.

Infections were respiratory (8), urinary tract (6), cutaneous and mucosal (3), abdominal (4), disseminated zoster (1), and sepsis (1). The microbiological isolation was

negative in 12 cases, 3 *Pseudomonas aeruginosa*, 2 *Cytomegalovirus*, 1 *Klebsiella pneumoniae*, 1 *Escherichia coli*, 1 *Enterococcus faecalis*, 1 *Campylobacter jejuni* and 1 *Herpes Zoster* virus.

A CCI of 3 was associated with more infectious complications in the control group (OR = 8.7; 95% CI = 1.15–65.9; $P = 0.036$), but not in the treated patients ($P = 0.16$). Related to adverse reactions in PE sessions or RTX infusion, only one patient developed tetany related to hypocalcemia.

Table 2 Risk of graft loss at 24 months according to ΔeGFR and treatment

	OR & (95% CI)	P value	Model
Change in ΔeGFR > 13 ml/min	5 (1.5 – 16.9)	0.006	Univariate
Treatment	1.2 (0.4 - 3.5)	0.736	Univariate
Change in ΔeGFR > 13 ml/min	5 (1.5 – 16.9)	0.006	Multivariate
Treatment	1.1 (0.3 - 3.4)	0.897	

ΔeGFR eGFR six months before diagnosis - eGFR at diagnosis of c-aABMR

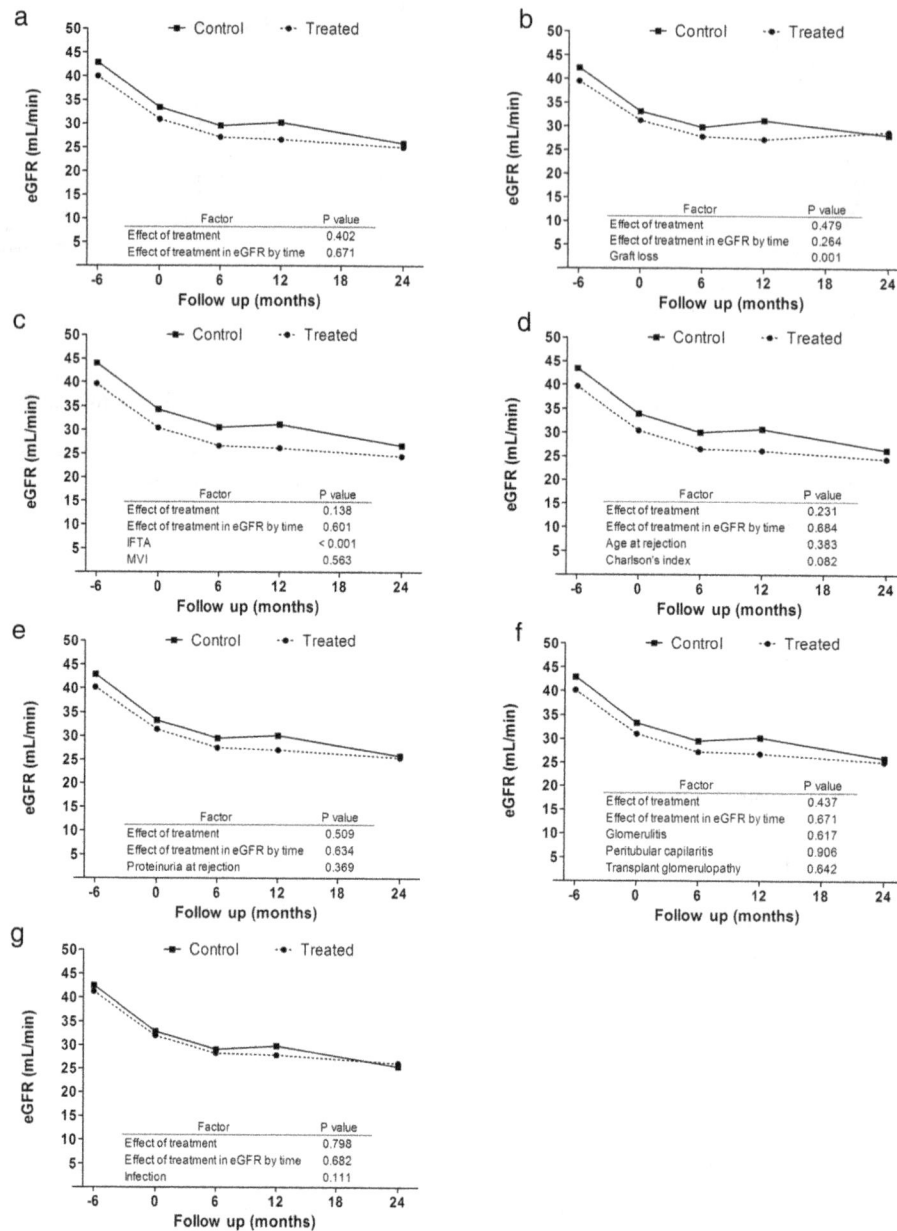

Fig. 3 Crude and adjusted estimation of eGFR according to GEE longitudinal models. Crude model (**a**); adjusted by graft loss (**b**); adjusted by IFTA (interstitial fibrosis and tubular atrophy) and MVI (microvascular inflammation) (**c**); adjusted by age and Charlson comorbidity index (**d**); adjusted by proteinuria (**e**); adjusted by glomerulitis, capillaritis and transplant glomerulopathy (**f**); adjusted by infection disease complications in the follow-up (**g**). Estimated glomerular filtrate rate (eGFR)

Discussion

In this study, treatment with rituximab + IVIG and PE was not associated with improved graft survival when compared with the control group. On the other hand, the incidence of infections requiring hospitalization within 1 year after treatment was more than doubled in the treated group.

Chronic antibody-mediated damage is the main limitation for long-term graft survival, but currently, only scarce data are available about the treatment of active c-aABMR with TG. In small retrospective series of cases, the partial effectiveness of RTX and IVIG has been reported [7–10]. Rostaing et al. reported 14 patients with TG treated with RTX and steroids showing stabilization or improvement of renal function in seven patients. Four patients (28.5%) presented severe infections in the first year after treatment [23].

A prospective study in 20 pediatric patients with c-aABMR treated with one dose of RTX and a high dose of IVIG reported good response in all the patients

Table 3 Banff histopathological features at diagnosis of cABMR

	Treatment (N=23)	Control (N=39)	P value
MVI (g+tc)	2.78 ± 1.35	2.87 ± 1.36	0.67
i	0.6 ± 0.78	0.56 ± 0.65	0.95
t	0.17 ± 0.49	0.25 ± 0.69	0.97
g	1.52 ± 0.94	1.4± 0.94	0.63
ptc	1.26 ± 0.86	1.4 ± 0.79	0.4
ah	1.43 ± 1.04	1.38 ± 1.1	0.91
cg	1.74 ± 0.83	1.83 ± 0.77	0.54
ci	1.52 ± 0.79	1.83 ± 0.88	0.17
ct	1.56 ± 0.73	1.67 ± 0.89	0.62
IFTA	1.61 ± 0.78	1.83 ± 0.84	0.27
cv	1.17 ± 0.83	1.39 ± 0.87	0.46
C4d deposition	19 (82.6%)	17 (43.6%)	0.01
acute cellular rejection	0	6	0.05

Results are shown as mean ± SD or absolute frequencies (%) for quantitative and qualitative variables respectively. *i* interstitial inflammation, *t* tubulitis, *g* glomerulitis, *ptc* peritubular capillaritis, *ah* arterial hyalinosis, *cg* transplant glomerulopathy, *ci* interstitial fibrosis, *ct* tubular atrophy, *IFTA* interstitial fibrosis + tubular atrophy, *cv* vascular fibrous intimal thickening

without TG, but only in 45% of the patients with TG [10]. The response was defined as a reduction in the decline of GFR of 30%.

In another retrospective series of 31 patients with c-aABMR and TG treated with RTX (*n* = 14) vs. no treatment (*n* = 17), only eight patients responded to treatment [24]. The response was defined as a decline or stabilization of serum creatinine for at least 1 year.

These studies highlight the importance of TG as a marker of chronic damage and a poor prognosis. On the other hand, efficacy was based on graft function stabilization, which is difficult to distinguish from the natural history of the disease in the absence of an untreated control group. Indeed, in our control group, some patients stabilized their renal function. As in other reported series, the evolution of these patients is heterogeneous in both groups, which highlights the importance of having a control group in future studies.

Other recent studies reported that RTX treatment did not improve graft survival compared to an untreated group. Moreover, a higher incidence of adverse effects was detected in the treatment groups [11, 12]. However, the untreated groups were small in both studies, and they did not evaluate the combination of RTX, PE, and IVIG.

We performed the analysis using two comparable cohorts. Also, c-aABMR treatment was homogeneous.

The decision to treat was based on individual clinical judgment and seems to be influenced by the perception of a better performance status of the patient, younger age, younger donor and less risk of infections. However, even with this potential positive selection bias, severe infections were more frequent in treated patients than in the older control group. In fact, the CCI was similar in both groups but was only associated with more infections in the control patients.

On the contrary with results presented in other studies [10], the severity of transplant glomerulopathy, (cg) score, was not associated with worse survival or loss of the graft at 24 months. Probably TG indicates a late non-reversible manifestation of antibody-mediated processes. Ten patients had a control biopsy after treatment, none presented improvement of TG.

In contrast with our data Kahwaji et al. suggest that patients with a high ptc and MVI scores may benefit from treatment with IVIG and RTX. But this was a trend that was not statistically significant [12]. Similar to our findings the authors did not find C4d positivity to be associated with worse graft outcomes, which is in contrast to the previous reports [5, 25–29].

A low eGFR at diagnosis is associated with graft loss at 24 months [11, 12]. We postulate that ΔeGFR, between 6 months before rejection and the time of diagnosis of rejection, ≥13 ml/min is more helpful to identify the patients with worse graft survival at 24 months.

In an observational study, 114 consecutive kidney transplant patients with c-ABMR were treated with steroids and IVIG. Three-fourths of patients lost their kidney grafts with a median survival of 1.9 years. The addition of rituximab or thymoglobulin in 40% of patients did not improve graft survival [30].

Recently a Spanish multicenter randomized trial has been performed in order to analyze the efficacy of rituximab and IVIG vs. placebo in 24 patients with TG and DSA positivity (12 placeboes vs. 12 treatments) [13]. The primary outcome was the difference in the decline of eGFR at 12 months. In concordance with our study, there was no difference in eGFR decline. Unfortunately, the study was stopped, after recruiting only 50% of the minimal sample calculated, due to low inclusion rate, and was underpowered, thus, highlighting the difficulty for prospective studies in this area.

Another strategy includes the use of bortezomib, a proteasome inhibitor. Recently a randomized trial has been presented comparing bortezomib treatment vs. placebo in late ABMR, which included 28 patients with cABMR. Bortezomib treatment failed to induce a reversal in decline of eGFR, DSA changes or morphologic and molecular features of disease activity in follow-up biopsies. In this trial, treatment was associated with substantial toxicity [31].

Given the poor results and the higher incidence of infectious complications, the unmet need is to improve diagnosis and enhance treatment options. Use of electron microscopy to detect early forms of TG (cg = 1a) or increased expression of gene transcripts indicative of endothelial injury might be helpful to improve graft survival.

New therapeutic options with more potent and less toxic immunosuppressive drugs or alternative immunological interventions are required. In this regard, two small prospective studies evaluated the complement system blockade at different levels in the treatment and prevention of c-aABMR and TG, without changes in long-term outcomes [32, 33].

In another recent report, Tocilizumab (Anti-IL6 receptor monoclonal antibody) showed promising results with stabilization of renal function in a small series of patients with c-aABMR and TG [34].

A significant cause of DSA and c-aABMR development is non-adherence to immunosuppression therapy. In this context, it seems to be more efficient and less dangerous to focus on promoting immunosuppressant therapy adherence rather than treating c-aABMR with TG aggressively.

This study presents a large group of patients with uniform pathology and treatment. However, the retrospective nature of the study is a limitation. DSA, and anti-HLA description is incomplete, hypogammaglobulinemia was not recorded and the dose of IVIG was low. In spite of the impossibility to assess the presence of DSA in all patients, the failure to demonstrate DSA does not rule out its existence [35]. The Banff´17 classification recognizes the fact that current DSA testing methods do not detect all antibodies that are potentially injurious to the allograft, and recommends the use of alternative markers that are not available in our center [3]. Recently, Sablik et al. analyzed whether cases suspicious for c-aABMR (DSA negative, $n = 24$) differ from cases of c-aABMR (DSA positive, $n = 17$) with respect to renal histology, allograft function and long-term graft survival [36]. There were no statistically significant differences on the decline of allograft function and renal allograft survival in cases with or without DSAs.

On the other hand, a strength of this study is that it shows a realistic incidence of serious infectious complications after treatment that should be taken into account in the therapeutic decision.

Conclusions

In summary, the rapid decline in GFR between 6 months before rejection diagnosis and the time of diagnosis is associated with poor prognosis. Treatment with RTX, PE, and IVIG in patients with active c-aABMR with TG was not associated with better graft survival, but a significant increase in serious infectious complications was observed.

Abbreviations

c-aABMR: Chronic active antibody-mediated rejection; CCI: Charlson comorbidity index; DSA: Donor specific antibodies; eGFR: Estimated glomerular filtrated rate; IFTA: Interstitial fibrosis and tubular atrophy; IVIG: Intravenous immunoglobulin; MMF/MPA: Mycophenolate mofetil or mycophenolic acid; MVI: Microvascular inflammation; PDN: Prednisone; PE: Plasma exchange; RTX: Rituximab; TG: Transplant glomerulopathy

Funding

This study has been funded by "Premio fin de residencia Emili Letang 2016" by Hospital Clínic de Barcelona and REDINREN (RD12/0021/0028 and RD16/0009/0023) by ISCIII-Subdirección General de Evaluación.

Authors' contributions

GJP participated in research design, performance of research, data analysis and writing of the paper. EDS-A, MS, JRíos, IR, ML, PV-A, DC, JC, FC and EP participated in data analysis, performance of research. JMC and FO participated in research design and performed critical revision of the manuscript for important intellectual content. JRovira and FD participated in research design, performance of research, data analysis and writing of the paper. All authors read and approved the final manuscript.

Competing interests

The authors declare that they have no competing interests.

Author details

Department of Nephrology and Renal Transplantation, ICNU, Hospital Clinic, Barcelona, Spain. ²Laboratori Experimental de Nefrologia i Trasplantament (LENIT), IDIBAPS, Barcelona, Spain. ³Department of Pathology, Hospital Clinic, Barcelona, Spain. ⁴Medical Statistics Core Facility, IDIBAPS, Hospital Clinic, Barcelona, Spain. ⁵Biostatistics Unit, Faculty of Medicine, Autonomous University of Barcelona, Barcelona, Spain. ⁶Apheresis Unit, Department of Hemotherapy and Hemostasis, IDIBAPS, Hospital Clinic, Barcelona, Spain. ⁷Red de Investigación Renal (REDinREN), Madrid, Spain. ⁸Department of Immunology, Hospital Clinic, Barcelona, Spain.

References

1. El-Zoghby ZM, Stegall MD, Lager DJ, Kremers WK, Amer H, Gloor JM, Cosio FG. Identifying specific causes of kidney allograft loss. Am J Transplant. 2009;9(3):527–35.
2. Naesens M, Kuypers DR, De Vusser K, Evenepoel P, Claes K, Bammens B, Meijers B, Sprangers B, Pirenne J, Monbaliu D et al: The histology of kidney transplant failure: a long-term follow-up study. Transplantation 2014, 98(4): 427–435.
3. Haas M, Loupy A, Lefaucheur C, Roufosse C, Glotz D, Seron D, Nankivell BJ, Halloran PF, Colvin RB, Akalin E, et al. The Banff 2017 kidney meeting report: revised diagnostic criteria for chronic active T cell-mediated rejection, antibody-mediated rejection, and prospects for integrative endpoints for next-generation clinical trials. Am J Transplant. 2018;18(2):293–307.
4. Remport A, Ivanyi B, Mathe Z, Tinckam K, Mucsi I, Molnar MZ. Better understanding of transplant glomerulopathy secondary to chronic antibody-mediated rejection. Nephrol Dial Transplant. 2015;30(11):1825–33.
5. John R, Konvalinka A, Tobar A, Kim SJ, Reich HN, Herzenberg AM. Determinants of long-term graft outcome in transplant glomerulopathy. Transplantation. 2010;90(7):757–64.
6. Lopez Jimenez V, Fuentes L, Jimenez T, Leon M, Garcia I, Sola E, Cabello M, Gutierrez C, Burgos D, Ruiz P, et al. Transplant glomerulopathy: clinical course and factors relating to graft survival. Transplant Proc. 2012;44(9): 2599–600.
7. Billing H, Rieger S, Ovens J, Susal C, Melk A, Waldherr R, Opelz G, Tonshoff B. Successful treatment of chronic antibody-mediated rejection with IVIG and rituximab in pediatric renal transplant recipients. Transplantation. 2008;86(9): 1214–21.
8. Fehr T, Rusi B, Fischer A, Hopfer H, Wuthrich RP, Gaspert A. Rituximab and intravenous immunoglobulin treatment of chronic antibody-mediated kidney allograft rejection. Transplantation. 2009;87(12):1837–41.

9. Hong YA, Kim HG, Choi SR, Sun IO, Park HS, Chung BH, Choi BS, Park CW, Kim YS, Yang CW. Effectiveness of rituximab and intravenous immunoglobulin therapy in renal transplant recipients with chronic active antibody-mediated rejection. Transplant Proc. 2012;44(1):182–4.

10. Billing H, Rieger S, Susal C, Waldherr R, Opelz G, Wuhl E, Tonshoff B. IVIG and rituximab for treatment of chronic antibody-mediated rejection: a prospective study in paediatric renal transplantation with a 2-year follow-up. Transpl Int. 2012;25(11):1165–73.

11. Bachelet T, Nodimar C, Taupin JL, Lepreux S, Moreau K, Morel D, Guidicelli G, Couzi L, Merville P. Intravenous immunoglobulins and rituximab therapy for severe transplant glomerulopathy in chronic antibody-mediated rejection: a pilot study. Clin Transpl. 2015;29(5):439–46.

12. Kahwaji J, Najjar R, Kancherla D, Villicana R, Peng A, Jordan S, Vo A, Haas M. Histopathologic features of transplant glomerulopathy associated with response to therapy with intravenous immune globulin and rituximab. Clin Transpl. 2014;28(5):546–53.

13. Moreso F, Crespo M, Ruiz JC, Torres A, Gutierrez-Dalmau A, Osuna A, Perello M, Pascual J, Torres IB, Redondo-Pachon D, et al. Treatment of chronic antibody mediated rejection with intravenous immunoglobulins and rituximab: a multicenter, prospective, randomized, double-blind clinical trial. Am J Transplant. 2018;18(4):927–35.

14. Cid J, Carbasse G, Andreu B, Baltanas A, Garcia-Carulla A, Lozano M. Efficacy and safety of plasma exchange: ann 11-year single-center experience of 2730 procedures in 317 patients. Transfus Apher Sci. 2014;51(2):209–14.

15. Charlson ME, Pompei P, Ales KL, MacKenzie CR. A new method of classifying prognostic comorbidity in longitudinal studies: development and validation. J Chronic Dis. 1987;40(5):373–83.

16. Hemmelgarn BR, Manns BJ, Quan H, Ghali WA. Adapting the Charlson comorbidity index for use in patients with ESRD. Am J Kidney Dis. 2003;42(1):125–32.

17. Miskulin DC, Martin AA, Brown R, Fink NE, Coresh J, Powe NR, Zager PG, Meyer KB, Levey AS. Predicting 1 year mortality in an outpatient haemodialysis population: a comparison of comorbidity instruments. Nephrol Dial Transplant. 2004;19(2):413–20.

18. van Manen JG, Korevaar JC, Dekker FW, Boeschoten EW, Bossuyt PM, Krediet RT: How to adjust for comorbidity in survival studies in ESRD patients: a comparison of different indices. Am J Kidney Dis 2002, 40(1):82–89.

19. Laging M, Kal-van Gestel JA, van de Wetering J, JN IJ, Betjes MG, Weimar W, Roodnat JI. A high comorbidity score should not be a contraindication for kidney transplantation. Transplantation. 2016;100(2):400–6.

20. Levey AS, Bosch JP, Lewis JB, Greene T, Rogers N, Roth D. A more accurate method to estimate glomerular filtration rate from serum creatinine: a new prediction equation. Modification of diet in renal disease study group. Ann Intern Med. 1999;130(6):461–70.

21. Torng S, Rigatto C, Rush DN, Nickerson P, Jeffery JR. The urine protein to creatinine ratio (P/C) as a predictor of 24-hour urine protein excretion in renal transplant patients. Transplantation. 2001;72(8):1453–6.

22. Deeks JJ, Altman DG. Diagnostic tests 4: likelihood ratios. Bmj. 2004;329(7458):168–9.

23. Rostaing L, Guilbeau-Frugier C, Fort M, Mekhlati L, Kamar N. Treatment of symptomatic transplant glomerulopathy with rituximab. Transpl Int. 2009;22(9):906–13.

24. Smith RN, Malik F, Goes N, Farris AB, Zorn E, Saidman S, Tolkoff-Rubin N, Puri S, Wong W. Partial therapeutic response to rituximab for the treatment of chronic alloantibody mediated rejection of kidney allografts. Transpl Immunol. 2012;27(2 3):107 13.

25. Sellares J, de Freitas DG, Mengel M, Reeve J, Einecke G, Sis B, Hidalgo LG, Famulski K, Matas A, Halloran PF. Understanding the causes of kidney transplant failure: the dominant role of antibody-mediated rejection and nonadherence. Am J Transplant. 2012;12(2):388–99.

26. Einecke G, Sis B, Reeve J, Mengel M, Campbell PM, Hidalgo LG, Kaplan B, Halloran PF. Antibody-mediated microcirculation injury is the major cause of late kidney transplant failure. Am J Transplant. 2009;9(11):2520–31.

27. Gaston RS, Cecka JM, Kasiske BL, Fieberg AM, Leduc R, Cosio FC, Gourishankar S, Grande J, Halloran P, Hunsicker L, et al. Evidence for antibody-mediated injury as a major determinant of late kidney allograft failure. Transplantation. 2010;90(1):68–74.

28. Kedainis RL, Koch MJ, Brennan DC, Liapis H. Focal C4d+ in renal allografts is associated with the presence of donor-specific antibodies and decreased allograft survival. Am J Transplant. 2009;9(4):812–9.

29. Kieran N, Wang X, Perkins J, Davis C, Kendrick E, Bakthavatsalam R, Dunbar N, Warner P, Nelson K, Smith KD, et al. Combination of peritubular c4d and transplant glomerulopathy predicts late renal allograft failure. J Am Soc Nephrol. 2009;20(10):2260–8.

30. Redfield RR, Ellis TM, Zhong W, Scalea JR, Zens TJ, Mandelbrot D, Muth BL, Panzer S, Samaniego M, Kaufman DB, et al. Current outcomes of chronic active antibody mediated rejection - a large single center retrospective review using the updated BANFF 2013 criteria. Hum Immunol. 2016;77(4):346–52.

31. Eskandary F, Regele H, Baumann L, Bond G, Kozakowski N, Wahrmann M, Hidalgo LG, Haslacher H, Kaltenecker CC, Aretin MB, et al. A randomized trial of Bortezomib in late antibody-mediated kidney transplant rejection. J Am Soc Nephrol. 2018;29(2):591–605.

32. Viglietti D, Gosset C, Loupy A, Deville L, Verine J, Zeevi A, Glotz D, Lefaucheur C. C1 inhibitor in acute antibody-mediated rejection nonresponsive to conventional therapy in kidney transplant recipients: a pilot study. Am J Transplant. 2016;16(5):1596–603.

33. Cornell LD, Schinstock CA, Gandhi MJ, Kremers WK, Stegall MD. Positive Crossmatch kidney transplant recipients treated with Eculizumab: outcomes beyond 1 year. Am J Transplant. 2015;15:1293.

34. Choi J, Aubert O, Vo A, Loupy A, Haas M, Puliyanda D, Kim I, Louie S, Kang A, Peng A, et al. Assessment of Tocilizumab (anti-Interleukin-6 receptor monoclonal) as a potential treatment for chronic antibody-mediated rejection and transplant Glomerulopathy in HLA-sensitized renal allograft recipients. Am J Transplant. 2017;17(9):2381–9.

35. Martin L, Guignier F, Bocrie O, D'Athis P, Rageot D, Rifle G, Justrabo E, Mousson C. Detection of anti-HLA antibodies with flow cytometry in needle core biopsies of renal transplants recipients with chronic allograft nephropathy. Transplantation. 2005;79(10):1459–61.

36. Sablik KA, Clahsen-van Groningen MC, Looman CWN, Damman J, Roelen DL, van Agteren M, MGH B. Chronic-active antibody-mediated rejection with or without donor-specific antibodies has similar histomorphology and clinical outcome - a retrospective study. Transpl Int. 2018;31:900–8.

9

Low birth weight associates with glomerular area in young male IgA nephropathy patients

Paschal Ruggajo[1,2*], Sabine Leh[2,4], Einar Svarstad[2,3], Hans-Peter Marti[2,3] and Bjørn Egil Vikse[2,5]

Abstract

Background: In a recent study we demonstrated that low birth weight (LBW) was associated with increased risk of progressive IgA nephropathy (IgAN). In the present study we investigate whether this could be explained by differences in glomerular morphological parameters.

Methods: The Medical Birth Registry of Norway has registered all births since 1967 and the Norwegian Kidney Biopsy Registry has registered all kidney biopsies since 1988. Patients diagnosed with IgAN, registered birth weight and estimated glomerular filtration rate above 60 ml/min/1.73m^2 at time of diagnosis were eligible for inclusion. Patients were included in a case-control manner based on whether or not they had LBW or were small for gestational age (SGA). Glomerular area, volume and density were measured using high resolution digital images and differences were compared between groups.

Results: We included 51 IgAN patients with a mean age of 23.6 years, 47.1% male. Compared to IgAN patients without LBW or SGA, IgAN patients with LBW and/or SGA had larger glomerular area (16,235 ± 3744 vs 14,036 ± 3502 μm^2, p-value 0.04). This was significant for total cohort and male but not female. On separate analysis by gender, glomerular area was significantly larger only in males (17,636 ± 3285 vs 13,346 ± 2835 μm^2, p-value 0.004). Glomerular density was not different between groups. In adjusted linear regression analysis, glomerular area was negatively associated with birth weight.

Conclusion: Among young adult IgAN patients, low birth weight is associated with having larger glomerular area, especially in males. Larger glomeruli may be a sign of congenital nephron deficit that may explain the increased risk of progressive IgAN.

Background

Brenner and co-workers suggested that adverse intrauterine environment, for example due to placental insufficiency or maternal undernutrition, was associated with impaired nephron development and increased risk of hypertension and progressive kidney disease in adult life [1]. Birthweight related parameters such as low birth weight (LBW) and small for gestational age (SGA) are strong surrogate markers for adverse intrauterine environment [2, 3]. LBW has been associated with increased risk of hypertension [4], albuminuria [5, 6] and progressive

chronic kidney disease [7, 8]. Fewer studies have investigated effects of SGA, but in a previous study from Norway we showed that SGA was a stronger risk marker than LBW for development of ESRD in adult age [9].

IgA nephropathy (IgAN) is the most frequent primary idiopathic glomerulonephritis worldwide [10–12] and has a variable clinical course [13–15]. In a previous study we showed that LBW and SGA were risk factors for progression to ESRD in IgAN patients [16].

Several previous autopsy-based stereological and histomorphometric studies have reported strong correlations between LBW and reduced glomerular numbers as well as increased glomerular volume [17–19]. A previous study has also shown that IgAN patients born SGA had increased risk for glomerulosclerosis and arterial hypertension [20]. To our knowledge, the association between

* Correspondence: prugajo@yahoo.com
[1]Department of Internal Medicine, Muhimbili University of Health and Allied Sciences (MUHAS), P.O.Box 65001, Dar es Salaam, Tanzania
[2]Department of Clinical Medicine, University of Bergen, Bergen, Norway
Full list of author information is available at the end of the article

birth weight and glomerular histomorphometric changes among IgAN patients has not been investigated before.

In the present study we aimed to investigate how LBW and SGA in IgAN patients associate with specific glomerular morphological changes compared to IgAN without LBW and SGA. We hypothesized that LBW and SGA would be associated with fewer and larger glomeruli in line with the Brenner hypothesis but that the effects of LBW and SGA could be different. In our previous study cited above, associations were stronger in males, so gender differences were also investigated in the present study.

Methods
Description of registries
Since 1967, the Medical Birth Registry of Norway has registered extensive medical data on all births in Norway (total population of 5.1 million) [21]. The Norwegian Kidney Biopsy Registry has registered clinical and histopathological data (including diagnosis) for all patients who have had a kidney biopsy performed in Norway since 1988. Since 1980, the Norwegian Renal Registry has registered data on all patients in Norway who developed ESRD (defined as starting maintenance dialysis treatment or undergoing renal transplantation). The data from all registries were available until December 2013 and data were linked using the unique 11-digit national identification number.

The regional ethics committee of Western Norway gave clearance for the study (2013/553), participants were asked for consent by mail.

Variables from the medical birth registry and Norwegian kidney biopsy registry
LBW was defined as birth weight less than the 10th percentile for gender (2930 g for male, 2690 g for female) in the study population of our previous study [16]. From 1967 through 1998, gestational age was based on the last menstrual period and from 1999 onwards on routine ultrasonographic examination in gestational weeks 17 through 20. Based on national data on birth weight, gestational week, gender and plurality, a z-score denoting numbers of standard deviations from mean of birth weight for each week of gestational age was calculated for all cases and controls based on data from the Medical Birth Registry [22, 23]. Small for gestational age (SGA) was defined as birth weight less than the 10th percentile for gestational week in the study population of our previous study [16] (defined by z-score less than − 1.2900 for male and − 1.5280 for female gender). Preterm birth was defined as a gestational age less than 37 weeks [22, 23].

Maternal pregestational disease was defined as maternal rheumatic disease, renal disease, diabetes mellitus or hypertension diagnosed before pregnancy and reported at birth to the Medical Birth Registry [24]. Maternal pre-eclampsia was defined based on the 1972 recommendations of the American College of Obstetricians and Gynecologists, i.e. hypertension and proteinuria after week 20 of gestation [25].

The following clinical variables at the time of kidney biopsy were used in the present study; estimated glomerular filtration rate (eGFR), calculated using the IDMS-traceable CKD-EPI equation [26]. All patients were assumed to be of Caucasian race. For patients who had a kidney biopsy performed before year 2005, their serum creatinine levels were reduced by 5% to standardize them to IDMS-traceable levels [27]. To avoid spurious eGFR distribution in patients with very low values of serum creatinine, all eGFR values exceeding 150 ml/min/1.73m^2 were set to 150 ml/min/1.73m^2. Proteinuria (grams/24 h), systolic and diastolic blood pressure measurements (mmHg) at time of biopsy were all used as continuous variables.

Selection of cases and controls
We selected cases and controls from patients registered in the described registries (Additional file 1: Figure S1). Eligible patients had registered birth weight, eGFR > 60 ml/min/1.73m^2 at time of biopsy and did not develop ESRD during follow-up (as registered in the Norwegian Renal Registry). The last two criteria were chosen to ensure that during selection, our study population comprised of patients with lowest risk of progressive IgAN population at the time of biopsy (in addition, only 1 eligible patient had developed ESRD). Power calculations were based on extrapolations from two human studies which had published measurements of glomerular size in relation to birth weight [17, 18]. From these eligible patients, we selected 5 groups of patients:(1) 20 patients randomly selected out of the 230 eligible patients registered in the Kidney Biopsy Registry with a diagnosis of IgAN and being neither LBW nor SGA, (2) all 13 patients with LBW but not SGA, (3) all 15 patients with SGA but not LBW and (4) all 14 patients with both LBW and SGA. As some of the selected patients did not have available kidney biopsy tissue, we were able to include 18, 11, 10 and 12 case patients in these respective groups. In addition, (5) we selected 20 patients who were neither LBW nor SGA, had normal findings on kidney biopsy (indicated for proteinuria or haematuria) and had eGFR > 60 ml/min/1.73m^2 as normal controls; this control group was age-and-sex matched with the group of IgAN cases without LBW or SGA; 19 patients in this control group had available tissue and were included.

Histopathological and histomorphometric variables
Representative periodic acid Schiff stained 3 μm thick sections from paraffin embedded formalin fixed tissue

were used. Morphological evaluation was done on digital slides scanned at 40x resulting in a resolution of 0.25 μm per pixel (Aperio ScanScope™ XT System, 1360 Park Center Drive Vista, CA 92081, USA). The digital images were viewed in Imagescope (version 12, Leica/ Aperio). We recorded the total number of glomeruli, the number of glomeruli with mesangial hypercellularity, endocapillary hypercellularity, global sclerosis, segmental sclerosis and tubular atrophy as defined by the Oxford classification for IgAN and a MEST score was calculated [28]. The annotation pen tool was used to measure glomerular tuft areas and cortical area of each profile. We determined the glomerular density as a ratio of number of glomeruli per cortical area, and this was calculated for all glomeruli (reported as total glomerular density), for sclerosed glomeruli and for non-sclerosed glomeruli. We used total glomerular density during analysis. The glomerular tuft area was defined as an area bound by outer capillary loops of the glomerular tuft and the mean glomerular area was obtained by averaging the area of all eligible glomeruli in the profile. Glomerular diameter (d) was calculated from the formula d = square root of $(4A/\pi)$, where A = glomerular area and $\pi = 3.142$, assuming the glomerular tuft to be circular in shape.

For estimating glomerular volume we used the Weibel-Gomez formula expressed as $GV = (GA)^{3/2} x \ \beta/d$; where GV = glomerular volume, GA = glomerular tuft area, β = 1.38 (assuming the glomerulus is spherical in shape) and d is a size distribution coefficient that is used to adjust for the variation in glomerular size; we used d = 1.01 as adopted from other studies [29–31]. The microscopic and morphometric evaluations for all kidney biopsies in this study were performed by the first author after thorough training by an experienced nephropathologist (second author) who also verified all measurements. These evaluations were blinded for information on LBW / SGA.

Statistical analysis

Birth weight related parameters were used as exposure variables whereas histopathological and histomorphometric parameters were used as outcome variables. In the primary analyses, outcome variables were compared between the four sub-groups with IgAN described above; in further analyses all groups with LBW and/or SGA were combined. Also, IgAN patients without LBW or SGA were compared to control patients. Continuous variables were tested for normal distribution (confirmed by P-P plots for all glomerular size parameters) and compared using student t-tests while categorical variables were compared using Chi-square tests. Linear regression statistics were used to determine the association between glomerular area and birthweight-related variables and clinical variables. In the primary analysis (model 1) we adjusted for diagnostic group (IgA nephropathy vs control) as the study sample

consisted of these two separate groups. In the secondary analysis (model 2) we further adjusted for gender and age at biopsy. If not otherwise stated, values are reported as mean ± standard deviation; $P < 0.05$ was considered statistically significant, and all tests were 2 tailed. Analyses were performed using the SPSS version 21 (SPSS, Chicago, IL).

Results

A total of 51 patients with IgAN were included in the present study, of these 24 (47.1%) were males. Mean age at biopsy was 23.6 years and mean eGFR was 95.3 ml/ min/1.73m². At the time of kidney biopsy, patients without LBW or SGA had comparable clinical characteristics to patients with LBW and/or SGA (Table 1). As expected, birth weight characteristics varied between groups.

Birth weight related variables and glomerular morphological changes

As shown in Table 2, glomerular measurements and other morphological variables were similar between groups with LBW and/or SGA (explored with t-tests between groups), these groups were therefore combined in the main analysis. Glomerular morphology, as investigated with markers of glomerular damage and the Oxford classification, were similar between groups. In glomerular histomorphometric analysis, compared to IgAN patients without LBW or SGA, IgAN patients with LBW and/or SGA had larger glomerular area (16,235 ± 3744 vs 14,036 ± 3502 μm², p-value 0.004). Further analyses stratified by gender showed that glomerular area was significantly larger only in males (17,636 ± 3285 vs 13,346 ± 2835 μm², p-value 0.004) but not in females (14,588 ± 4018 vs 14,918 ± 3758 μm², p-value 0.8). Glomerular density was not different between groups. In a sensitivity analysis, we tested whether including only patients with 9 glomeruli or more [32] would change the results for glomerular area, in these analyses the differences in glomerular area were comparable, but due to a lower N it did not reach statistical significance. In an analysis in which the two groups with LBW (excluding the group with only SGA) were compared to the group without LBW and SGA, glomerular area was statistically significantly different (14,036 vs 16,383 μm², p-value 0.04).

Comparison between patients with normal biopsy and IgAN

To investigate whether development of IgAN altered glomerular area, we compared results for patients with IgAN who did not have LBW or SGA (N = 18) to a matched group of control patients with normal biopsies (N = 19). As shown in Table 3, clinical characteristics were comparable between these two groups except for proteinuria which was significantly higher among the IgAN controls (1.8 ± 1.7 vs 0.32 ± 0.28 g/d, p-value 0.002). There were no significant differences between

Table 1 Cohort characteristics among Cases and Controls in Norway, 1988–2013

	IgAN controls	IgAN cases			IgAN cases combined
	Neither LBW nor SGA	LBW but not SGA	SGA but not LBW	Both LBW and SGA	LBW and/or SGA
N	18	11	10	12	33
N (%) male	8 (44.4)	5 (45.5)	5 (50.0)	6 (50.0)	16 (48.5)
Age at Biopsy (years)	22.8 ± 9.0	21.1 ± 8.6	22.3 ± 7.1	28.3 ± 8.9	24.1 ± 8.7
Weight at Biopsy (Kg)	76.8 ± 22.6	56.8 ± 27.9	68.3 ± 18.6	75.2 ± 14.3	66.1 ± 21.8
Systolic BP (mmHg)	124.4 ± 22.9	118.8 ± 16.2	131.3 ± 9.8	126.1 ± 17.5	124.8 ± 15.6
Diastolic BP (mmHg)	76.6 ± 13.2	72.6 ± 14.9	77.8 ± 10.1	72.7 ± 11.1	74.0 ± 12.2
eGFR (ml/min/1.73m^2)	94.8.0 ± 27.3	99.4 ± 32.9	95.5 ± 23.5	92.1 ± 18.6	95.5 ± 25.0
Urinary Protein (g/d)	1.8 ± 1.7	1.7 ± 1.5	1.0 ± 1.3	2.4 ± 2.6	1.7 ± 1.9
Birth Weight (kg)	3.6 ± 0.53	1.9 ± 0.75[b]	2.9 ± 0.17[a]	2.4 ± 0.42[b]	2.4 ± 0.65[b]
Gestational age (week)	40.3 ± 1.1	32.6 ± 4.5[b]	40.40 ± 0.70	38.7 ± 1.2[b]	37.2 ± 4.3[b]
Birthweight for Gestational Age (Z-score)	−0.18 ± 1.04	− 0.28 ± 0.73	−1.56 ± 0.24[b]	−2.19 ± 0.54[b]	− 1.36 ± 0.98[b]
Maternal Pre-eclampsia	0 (0.0)	0 (0.0)	2 (20.0)	2 (16.7)	4 (12.1)
Maternal pregestational disease[b]	0 (0.0)	0 (0.0)	0 (0.0)	1 (8.3)	1 (3.0)

[a]pvalue< 0.01,[b]p-value< 0.001 as compared to IgAN controls
[b]Maternal pregestational disease was defined as maternal rheumatic disease, renal disease, diabetes mellitus or hypertension

birth weight-related and glomerular histomorphometric characteristics observed between the two groups but there was a non-significant trend towards larger glomeruli in IgAN patients.

Glomerular area against birth weight-related and clinical characteristics

In order to further analyse the associations we conducted linear regression statistics to investigate associations between glomerular area and birth-weight and clinical variables. In these analyses we included both patients with IgAN and normal controls. Glomerular area was significantly higher in those with low birth weight in the adjusted model 2 analysis (a decrease of 1357 μm^2 in glomerular area for every 1 kg increase in birthweight, p-value =0.01) but not in the primary model 1 analysis. Furthermore, maternal pre-eclampsia, gender and age at biopsy were significantly associated with glomerular area

Table 2 Glomerular histopathological and histomorphometric variables stratified by LBW and/or SGA, Norway (1988–2013)

	IgAN Controls Without	IgAN Cases			IgAN cases combined
	LBW or SGA	LBW but not SGA	SGA but not LBW	Both LBW and SGA	LBW and/or SGA
N	18	11	10	12	33
N (%) with M-score of 1	10 (55.6)	8 (72.7)	5 (50.0)	4 (33.3)	17 (51.5)
N (%) with E-score of 1	3 (16.7)	2 (18.2)	0 (0.0)	1 (8.3)	3 (9.1)
N (%) with S-score of 1	1 (5.6)	3 (27.3)	2 (20.0)	1 (8.3)	6 (18.2)
N (%) with T-score of 1	0 (0.0)	0 (0.0)	0 (0.0)	0 (0.0)	0 (0.0)
% of glomeruli with mesangial hypercellularity	49.6 ± 27.4	49.1 ± 35.6	39.8 ± 21.7	35.0 ± 29.7	41.2 ± 29.4
% of glomeruli with endocapillary hypercellularity	0.93 ± 2.7	7.3 ± 20.1	0.00 ± 0.00	2.0 ± 6.8	3.2 ± 12.3
% of glomeruli with global sclerosis	3.3 ± 6.9	12.8 ± 29.6	3.3 ± 6.2	2.5 ± 5.9	5.9 ± 17.8
% of glomeruli with segmental sclerosis	0.69 ± 2.9	2.5 ± 5.2	1.6 ± 3.3	0.25 ± 0.85	1.5 ± 3.6
Histomorphometric variables					
Number of glomeruli (N)	14.1 ± 7.8	16.0 ± 7.5	16.2 ± 6.4	14.7 ± 11.4	15.6 ± 8.6
Glomerular tuft volume (μm^{3}x10^6) [c]	2.37 ± 0.82	2.90 ± 0.97	2.81 ± 1.13	2.93 ± 0.89	2.89 ± 0.96
Glomerular tuft area (μm^2)	14,036 ± 3502	16,311 ± 3805	15,899 ± 4335	16,447 ± 3478	16,235 ± 3744[a]
Glomerular tuft diameter (μm) [c]	132.7.4 ± 16.8	143.1. ± 17.5	141.1 ± 19.5	143.9 ± 15.9	142.8 ± 17.0[a]
Glomerular density (N per 10^6 μm^2)	2.95 ± 0.85	3.54 ± 1.30	3.36 ± 0.93	2.66 ± 1.47	3.17 ± 1.30

[a]p-value< 0.01,[b]p-value< 0.001 as compared to IgAN controls
[c] Glomerular tuft volume and glomerular tuft diameter was calculated based on the measured glomerular tuft area (as described in detail in the methods section)

Table 3 Comparison of clinical, birth-related and glomerular histomorphometric characteristics between normal controls and IgAN controls

| | Normal controls | IgAN controls | |
	Not LBW or SGA	Not LBW or SGA	p-value
N	19	18	
N (%) Male	10 (52.6)	8 (44.4)	1.0
Age at Biopsy (years)	21.8 ± 8.6	22.8 ± 9.0	0.7
Systolic BP (mmHg)	114.7 ± 15.6	124.4 ± 22.9	0.1
Diastolic BP (mmHg)	71.3 ± 13.8	76.6 ± 13.2	0.2
eGFR (ml/min/1.73m^2)	92.5 ± 28.4	94.8 ± 27.3	0.8
Urinary protein (g/d)	0.32 ± 0.28	1.8 ± 1.7[a]	0.002
Birth Weight (kg)	3.7 ± 0.5	3.6 ± 0.5	0.4
Gestational age (week)	39.9 ± 1.4	40.3 ± 1.1	0.3
Birth weight for gestational age (Z-score)	0.25 ± 0.99	−0.18 ± 1.04	0.2
Glomerular tuft volume (μm^3 ×10^6) [c]	1.97 ± 0.77	2.37 ± 0.82	0.1
Glomerular tuft area (μm^2)	12,522 ± 3410	14,036 ± 3502	0.1
Glomerular tuft diameter (μm) [c]	125.0 ± 18.2	132.7 ± 16.8	0.2
Glomerular Density (N per 10^6 μm^2)	3.29 ± 1.40	2.96 ± 0.85	0.4

[a] Glomerular tuft volume and glomerular tuft diameter was calculated based on the measured glomerular tuft area (as described in detail in the methods section)

in both model 1 and 2 analyses, whereas body weight, BMI and eGFR at biopsy associated with glomerular area only in model 1 analysis (Table 4).

In Fig. 1 we show the inverse relationships between glomerular area and birthweight and z-score of birthweight for gestational age. In Fig. 2 we show the inverse relationships between glomerular area and glomerular density and eGFR.

Discussion

The present study shows that young IgAN patients who were born with LBW and/or SGA had larger glomerular area at time of diagnosis than IgAN patients born with normal birth weight. The association was statistically significant in total cohort and in males. We consider larger glomerular area to be a marker of lower number of total glomeruli and the study thus suggests that larger glomeruli may at least in part, explain the higher risk of progressive renal disease in young IgAN patients with LBW and/or SGA in Norway [16]. Furthermore, considering that our cohort comprised young adults with preserved renal function (low-risk group), our findings may indeed underestimate the importance of this association. LBW and/or SGA may thus represent a basic vulnerability (first hit) among IgAN patients upon which other insults (immunology, hypertension etc. as second hits) may accelerate progressive nephropathy.

As described, LBW and/or SGA were associated with larger glomeruli at time of diagnosis of IgAN. Importantly, this association showed a dose-response correlation between birthweight and glomerular area. Larger glomeruli were also associated with lower eGFR. Previous studies have shown that glomerular size is a sensitive measure of total kidney glomerular number [18] and is proposed to be among the adaptive compensatory glomerular changes for congenital nephron deficit [17, 18, 33]. LBW has also been associated with low nephron number [34] and higher blood pressure [35] as well as microalbuminuria and low glomerular filtration rate in those born very premature and after intrauterine growth

Table 4 Linear associations between glomerular area and birth related and clinical characteristics, Norway (1988–2013)

	Model 1 β-coefficient[a]	p-value	Model 2 β-coefficient[b]	p-value
Birthweight (Kg)	−1143	0.06	−1357	0.01
Gestational age (Weeks)	−141	0.3	−198	0.1
Birth weight for gestational age (Z-score)	−711	0.08	−521	0.2
Maternal preeclampsia (Yes/No)	4305	0.02	3577	0.046
Gender (male vs female)	1736	0.05	1849	0.03
Age at biopsy (10 years)[c]	1368	0.007	1418	0.04
Body weight at biopsy (10 kg)[c]	668	0.004	491	0.1
Body mass index at biopsy (kg/m^2)	238	0.02	141	0.6
eGFR (10 ml/min/1.73m^2)[c]	−530	0.01	−297	0.1
Systolic BP (10 mmHg)[c]	159	0.5	−164	0.54
Urinary Protein (g/d)	132	0.7	154	0.6

[a] Model 1 adjusted for IgA nephropathy diagnosis at biopsy
[b] Model 2 adjusted for IgA nephropathy diagnosis at biopsy, gender and age at biopsy
[c] Body weight at time of biopsy, eGFR and systolic BP are given per 10 unit increase to give meaningful coefficients, otherwise one unit was used for other variables

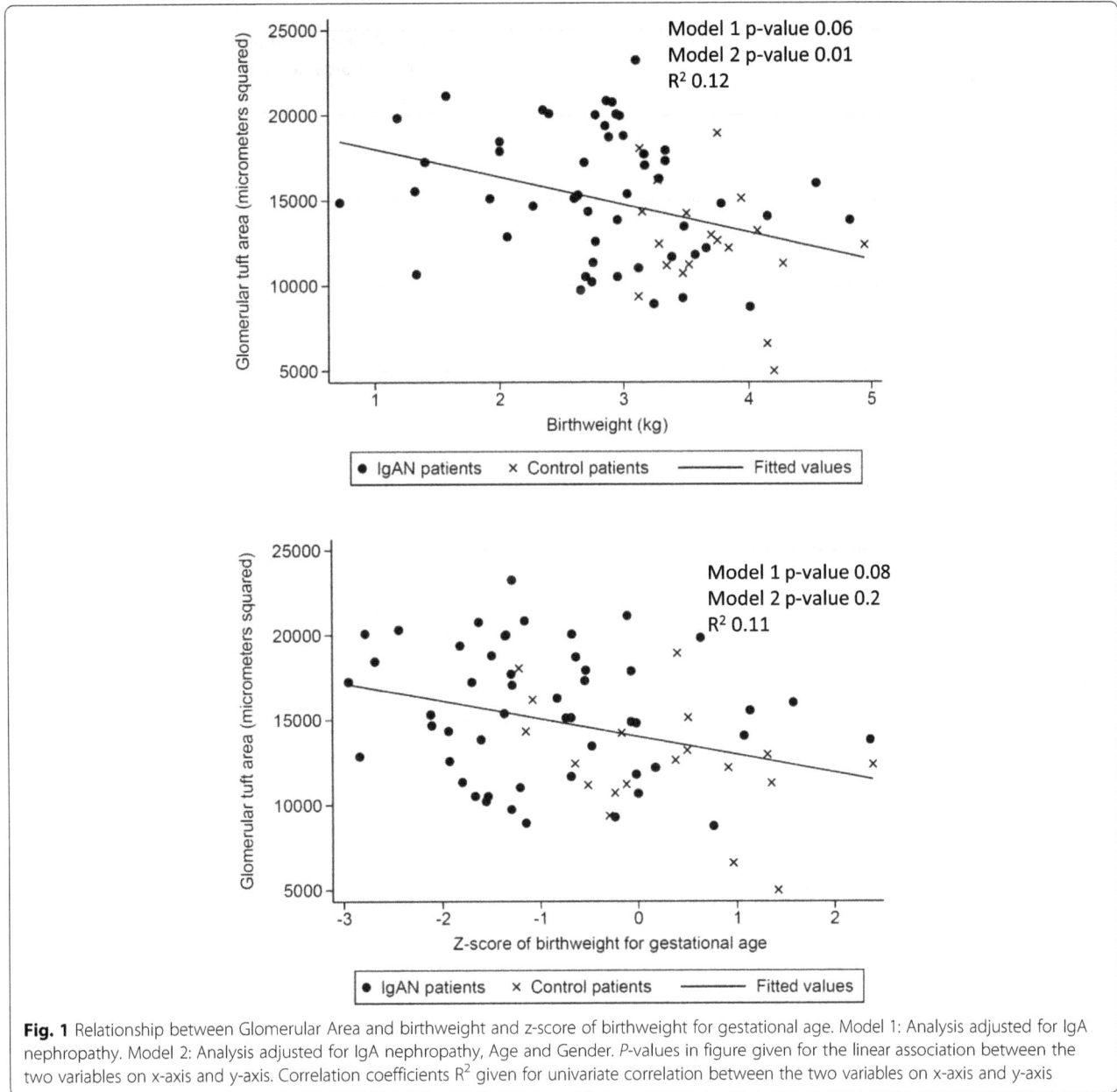

Fig. 1 Relationship between Glomerular Area and birthweight and z-score of birthweight for gestational age. Model 1: Analysis adjusted for IgA nephropathy. Model 2: Analysis adjusted for IgA nephropathy, Age and Gender. *P*-values in figure given for the linear association between the two variables on x-axis and y-axis. Correlation coefficients R² given for univariate correlation between the two variables on x-axis and y-axis

retardation [36]. In relation to IgAN in particular, a previous study has shown that progressive IgAN is associated with reduced glomerular density and increased glomerular volume [37]. The present study thus links these findings and suggests that LBW and/or SGA increase risk of progressive IgAN, mechanisms might involve lower glomerular number or higher blood pressure [1, 38]. These mechanisms might be important also in other kidney diseases as we previously have shown that LBW was associated with higher risk of ESRD in general, and also of ESRD due to glomerular disease [7, 39]. In the present study, LBW was defined by the 10th percentile in our previous study and corresponded to 2.93 kg for men and 2.69 kg for women [16]. As we

observed a dose-response relationship between birth weight and glomerular size, we hypothesize that differences might have been larger if we had used a lower cut-off (WHO definition of LBW is < 2.5 kg). Neither LBW alone nor SGA alone were however significantly associated with larger glomeruli in Table 1 and we therefore decided to combine these groups in the remaining analyses. SGA and LBW may however partly be explained by different pathophysiological mechanisms and it is uncertain which is most strongly associated with later development of kidney disease [16]. As differences between groups with LBW and/or SGA in Table 1 were negligible we believe that this is the best approach. It is interesting to note that the group with SGA but not

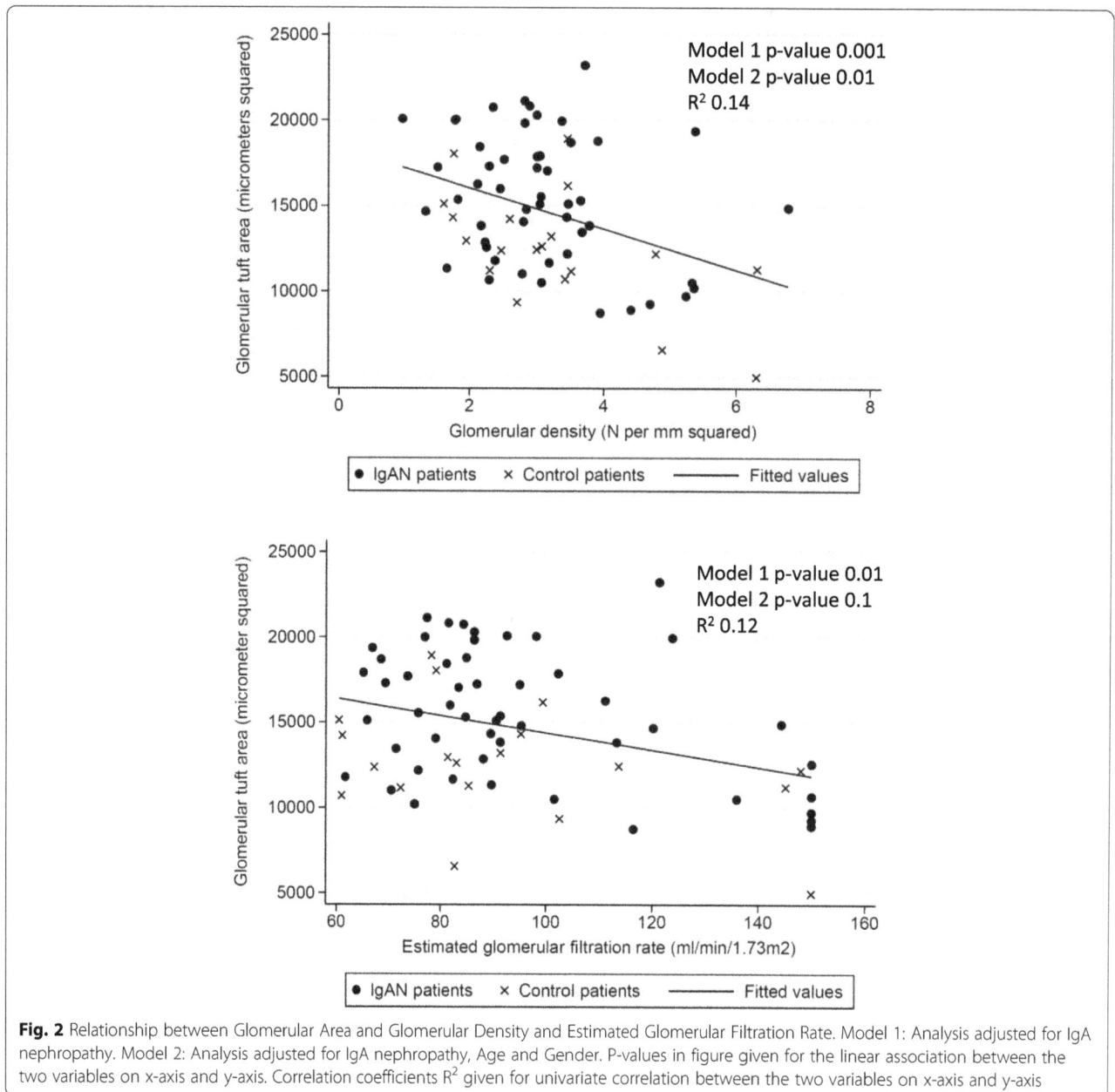

Fig. 2 Relationship between Glomerular Area and Glomerular Density and Estimated Glomerular Filtration Rate. Model 1: Analysis adjusted for IgA nephropathy. Model 2: Analysis adjusted for IgA nephropathy, Age and Gender. P-values in figure given for the linear association between the two variables on x-axis and y-axis. Correlation coefficients R^2 given for univariate correlation between the two variables on x-axis and y-axis

LBW (mean birth weight of 2.9 kg) had nearly the same glomerular area as the groups with LBW (mean birth weights of 1.9 and 2.4 kg). It should however be noted that in the comparison of only IgAN patients with vs without LBW (excluding the group with SGA and without LBW), glomerular area was statistically significantly different. Whether birthweight or birthweight for gestational age represents the most powerful predictor of later kidney disease and morphology must be analysed further in future studies.

Brenner postulated that congenital nephron deficit would lead to large glomeruli with glomerular hyperfiltration that would progressively increase risk of glomerular

damage. A previous study has reported higher mean percentage of sclerotic glomeruli among IgAN patients who had suffered intra-uterine growth retardation [20]. Further, Ikezumi et al. reported association between LBW and development of focal segmental glomerulosclerosis in children and proposed that this was probably related to glomerular prematurity and podocytopenia [38]. In fact, podocytopenia has been associated with increased disease severity in IgAN [40] and in turn, compensatory podocyte hypertrophy has been associated with progressive glomerulosclerosis [41]. In our paper, there were non-significant trends towards more glomerular sclerosis in those with low birth weight but the degree of glomerular sclerosis was mild in our study as we selected patients with pre-served kidney function. In our opinion, our study supports the Brenner hypothesis that large glomeruli with hyperfil-tration is a link between low birth weight (as a marker of congenital nephron deficit) and progressive kidney disease.

As mentioned above, the association between LBW and larger glomeruli was significant in males but not females. In our previous paper [16] on IgAN, we reported that the association between LBW and ESRD was strong and sig-nificant in males but not females. The present study in-cluded a slightly higher proportion of female IgAN patients (53%) as compared to a previous study from the same registry (26%) [42]. These findings of a possible gender dif-ference are interesting and warrant further investigation to supplement previous human and experimental studies that also have suggested that females might be protected against both progressive nephropathy [43–45] and intrauterine im-paired nephron endowment or effects thereof [46].

In adjusted analysis, maternal preeclampsia was associ-ated with a significantly larger glomerular area. Previous studies have shown that pre-eclampsia is associated with placental insufficiency and increases risk of LBW and SGA offspring [17, 47]. The present study suggests that the as-sociated placental insufficiency might have especially im-portant effects on kidney development. This finding is however limited by the small number of observations in this study (only four patients had a mother with pre-eclampsia) and should thus be interpreted with caution.

In this study, we report on glomerular morphology from kidney tissue specimens obtained from patients using per-cutaneous kidney biopsy needle as part of the routine clin-ical care. This method yields only a limited sample of glomeruli as compared to stereological methods using the physical dissector/fractionator method which is consid-ered as the gold standard. Such stereological methods e.g. Cavalieri, Weibel-Gomez, Maximal Planar Area or Dis-sector Principle yield accurate estimation for glomerular size and density but are laborious, time consuming, costly and require the whole kidney tissue and are therefore of limited accessibility for routine studies [48, 49]. A previous study has illustrated that reliable mean estimates of glom-erular size can be obtained by measuring 9 or more glom-eruli; in white patients, measuring fewer than 6 glomeruli reduced the precision [32]. In the present study, even though some patients had fewer than 6 glomeruli, and fewer glomeruli would tend to lower precision of the mean, the glomerular size estimates were statistically sig-nificant between groups. Also, results for glomerular area were comparable in a sensitivity analysis where only pa-tients with 9 glomeruli or more were included, although it did not reach statistical significance due to lower N. We would thus argue that estimates of glomerular area could be obtained also by measuring fewer glomeruli in studies with limited number of available patients and tissue.

Conclusion
In the present study we have shown that among young IgAN patients with preserved renal function, impaired intrauterine growth was associated with larger glomerular area as a sign of congenital nephron deficit. This could in part explain the increased risk of progressive kidney dis-ease in individuals born with LBW or SGA. Further larger studies should investigate why this effect seems to be more important in males than females and in population with higher frequency of offspring birthweight < 2.5 kg. However, the non-significant trend towards larger glom-eruli may mean other plausible theories such as pre-diag-nosis loss of glomeruli with compensatory hypertrophy may not be ruled out as additional/alternative explana-tions to what we observe in this study. There seems to be sufficient evidence to argue that consideration of birth weight is an important part of the clinical history of patients with chronic kidney disease.

Strengths
The strength of this study is that we directly test whether the Brenner hypothesis could explain the in-creased risk of progressive IgAN that was seen in our previous study [16] and that we test this in IgAN pa-tients with preserved kidney function at an early stage of the disease.

Limitations
The study is however limited by the fact that percutaneous kidney biopsy method samples only procures a limited number of glomeruli from a small portion of the kidney that may not adequately represent the entire kidney tissue, especially when we consider the fact that glomerular size varies within different kidney regions [50].

Abbreviations
BMI: Body Mass Index; EGFR: Estimated Glomerular Filtration Rate; ESRD: End Stage Renal Disease; GA: Glomerular Tuft Area; GD: Glomerular Density; GV: Glomerular Volume; IDMS: Isotope Dilution Mass Spectrophotometer; IgAN: IgA Nephropathy; LBW: Low Birth Weight; MEST: Mesangial hypercellularity, Endocapillary proliferation, Segmental sclerosis, Tubular atrophy; SGA: Small for Gestational Age; SPSS: Statistical Package for Social Sciences

Acknowledgements
We express our sincere gratitude to our study participants. Further, we thank the Department of Pathology at Haukeland University Hospital in Bergen, Norway.

Authors' contributions
PR, BEV and SL conceived the study. PR and SL did data collection and quality check. PR, BEV and SL analysed and interpreted the data and wrote the first draft. ES, HPM and SL reviewed and quality checked the submitted manuscript. All authors read and approved the final manuscript.

Competing interests

The authors declare that they have no competing interests.

Author details

[1]Department of Internal Medicine, Muhimbili University of Health and Allied Sciences (MUHAS), P.O.Box 65001, Dar es Salaam, Tanzania. [2]Department of Clinical Medicine, University of Bergen, Bergen, Norway. [3]Department of Medicine, Haukeland University Hospital, Bergen, Norway. [4]Department of Pathology, Haukeland University Hospital, Bergen, Norway. [5]Department of Medicine, Haugesund Hospital, Haugesund, Norway.

References

1. Brenner BM, Garcia DL, Anderson S. Glomeruli and blood pressure less of one, more the other? Am J Hypertens. 1988;1(4 1):335–47.
2. Luyckx VA, Brenner BM. Birth weight, malnutrition and kidney-associated outcomes [mdash] a global concern. Nat Rev Nephrol. 2015;11(3):135–49.
3. Lee AC, et al. National and regional estimates of term and preterm babies born small for gestational age in 138 low-income and middle-income countries in 2010. Lancet Glob Health. 2013;1(1):e26–36.
4. Mu M, et al. Birth weight and subsequent blood pressure: a meta-analysis. Arch Cardiovasc Dis. 2012;105(2):99–113.
5. Hoy WE, et al. A new dimension to the barker hypothesis: low birthweight and susceptibility to renal disease. Kidney Int. 1999;56(3):1072–7.
6. White SL, et al. Is low birth weight an antecedent of CKD in later life? A systematic review of observational studies. Am J Kidney Dis. 2009;54(2):248–61.
7. Vikse BE, et al. Low birth weight increases risk for end-stage renal disease. J Am Soc Nephrol. 2008;19(1):151–7.
8. Luyckx VA, et al. A developmental approach to the prevention of hypertension and kidney disease: a report from the low birth weight and nephron number working group. Lancet. 2017;390(10092):424–8.
9. Ruggajo P, et al. Familial factors, low birth weight, and development of ESRD: a nationwide registry study. Am J Kidney Dis. 2016;67(4):601–8.
10. D'amico G. The commonest glomerulonephritis in the world: IgA nephropathy. Qj Med. 1987;64(245):709–27.
11. Floege J, Feehally J. IgA nephropathy: recent developments. J Am Soc Nephrol. 2000;11(12):2395–403.
12. Levy M, Berger J. Worldwide perspective of IgA nephropathy. Am J Kidney Dis. 1988;12(5):340–7.
13. Barbour SJ, Reich HN. Risk stratification of patients with IgA nephropathy. Am J Kidney Dis. 2012;59(6):865–73.
14. Canetta PA, Kiryluk K, Appel GB. Glomerular diseases: emerging tests and therapies for IgA nephropathy. Clin J Am Soc Nephrol. 2014;9(3):617–25.
15. Wyatt RJ, Julian BA. IgA nephropathy. N Engl J Med. 2013;368(25):2402–14.
16. Ruggajo P, et al. Low birth weight and risk of progression to end stage renal disease in IgA nephropathy—a retrospective registry-based cohort study. PLoS One. 2016;11(4):e0153819.
17. Manalich R, et al. Relationship between weight at birth and the number and size of renal glomeruli in humans: a histomorphometric study. Kidney Int. 2000;58(2):770–3.
18. Hughson M, et al. Glomerular number and size in autopsy kidneys: the relationship to birth weight. Kidney Int. 2003;63(6):2113–22.
19. Hinchliffe S, et al. The effect of intrauterine growth retardation on the development of renal nephrons. BJOG Int J Obstet Gynaecol. 1992;99(4):296–301.
20. Zidar N, et al. Effect of intrauterine growth retardation on the clinical course and prognosis of IgA glomerulonephritis in children. Nephron. 1998;79(1):28–32.
21. Irgens LM. The medical birth registry of Norway. Epidemiological research and surveillance throughout 30 years. Acta Obstet Gynecol Scand. 2000;79(6):435–9.
22. Skjaerven R, GJESSING HK, BAKKETEIG LS. Birthweight by gestational age in Norway. Acta Obstet Gynecol Scand. 2000;79(6):440–9.
23. Glinianaia SV, Skjærven R, Magnus P. Birthweight percentiles by gestational age in multiple births: a population-based study of Norwegian twins and triplets. Acta Obstet Gynecol Scand. 2000;79(6):450–8.
24. Vikse BE, et al. Preeclampsia and the risk of end-stage renal disease. N Engl J Med. 2008;359(8):800–9.
25. Group, N.H.B.P.E.P.W. Report on high blood pressure in pregnancy (consensus report). Am J Obstet Gynecol. 1990;163:1691–712.
26. Matsushita K, et al. Comparison of risk prediction using the CKD-EPI equation and the MDRD study equation for estimated glomerular filtration rate. Jama. 2012;307(18):1941–51.
27. Stevens L, Levey A. Frequently asked questions about GFR estimates. New York: National Kidney Foundation; 2004.
28. of the International, A.W.G., et al. The Oxford classification of IgA nephropathy: pathology definitions, correlations, and reproducibility. Kidney Int. 2009;76(5):546–56.
29. Tsuboi N, et al. Glomerular density in renal biopsy specimens predicts the long-term prognosis of IgA nephropathy. Clin J Am Soc Nephrol. 2010;5(1):39–44.
30. Fulladosa X, et al. Estimation of total glomerular number in stable renal transplants. J Am Soc Nephrol. 2003;14(10):2662–8.
31. Hughson MD, Samuel T, Hoy WE. Glomerular volume and clinicopathologic features related to disease severity in renal biopsies of African Americans and whites in the southeastern United States. Arch Pathol Lab Med. 2007; 131(11):1665.
32. Puelles VG, et al. Estimating individual glomerular volume in the human kidney: clinical perspectives. Nephrol Dial Transplant. 2012;27:1880–8.
33. Merlet-Bénichou C, et al. Intrauterine growth retardation leads to a permanent nephron deficit in the rat. Pediatr Nephrol. 1994;8(2):175–80.
34. Hughson M, et al. Hypertension, glomerular number, and birth weight in African Americans and white subjects in the southeastern United States. Kidney Int. 2006;69(4):671–8.
35. Keller G, et al. Nephron number in patients with primary hypertension. N Engl J Med. 2003;348(2):101–8.
36. Keijzer-Veen MG, et al. Microalbuminuria and lower glomerular filtration rate at young adult age in subjects born very premature and after intrauterine growth retardation. J Am Soc Nephrol. 2005;16(9):2762–8.
37. Tsuboi N, et al. Changes in the glomerular density and size in serial renal biopsies during the progression of IgA nephropathy. Nephrol Dial Transplant. 2009;24(3):892–9.
38. Ikezumi Y, et al. Low birthweight and premature birth are risk factors for podocytopenia and focal segmental glomerulosclerosis. Am J Nephrol. 2013;38(2):149–57.
39. Ruggajo P, et al. Familial factors, low birth weight, and development of ESRD: a Nationwide registry study. Am J Kidney Dis. 2016;67(4):601–8.
40. Lemley KV, et al. Podocytopenia and disease severity in IgA nephropathy. Kidney Int. 2002;61(4):1475–85.
41. Wiggins R-C. The spectrum of podocytopathies: a unifying view of glomerular diseases. Kidney Int. 2007;71(12):1205–14.
42. Knoop T, et al. Mortality in patients with IgA nephropathy. Am J Kidney Dis. 2013;62(5):883–90.
43. Hannedouche T, et al. Factors affecting progression in advanced chronic renal failure. Clin Nephrol. 1993;39(6):312–20.
44. Ji H, et al. Female protection in progressive renal disease is associated with estradiol attenuation of superoxide production. Gender Med. 2007;4(1):56–71.
45. Silbiger SR, Neugarten J. The impact of gender on the progression of chronic renal disease. Am J Kidney Dis. 1995;25(4):515–33.
46. Woods LL, Ingelfinger JR, Rasch R. Modest maternal protein restriction fails to program adult hypertension in female rats. Am J Phys Regul Integr Comp Phys. 2005;289(4):R1131–6.
47. Xiao R, et al. Influence of pre-eclampsia on fetal growth. J Matern Fetal Neonatal Med. 2003;13(3):157–62.
48. Lane PH, Steffes MW, Mauer SM. Estimation of glomerular volume: a comparison of four methods. Kidney Int. 1992;41(4):1085–9.
49. Basgen JM, et al. Comparison of methods for counting cells in the mouse glomerulus. Nephron Exp Nephrol. 2006;103(4):e139–48.
50. Samuel T, et al. Determinants of glomerular volume in different cortical zones of the human kidney. J Am Soc Nephrol. 2005;16(10):3102–9.

10

Diagnosis and management of non-dialysis chronic kidney disease in ambulatory care: a systematic review of clinical practice guidelines

Gesine F C Weckmann[1,5]* (iD), Sylvia Stracke[2], Annekathrin Haase[1], Jacob Spallek[3], Fabian Ludwig[1], Aniela Angelow[1], Jetske M Emmelkamp[4], Maria Mahner[1] and Jean-François Chenot[1]

Abstract

Background: Chronic kidney disease (CKD) is age-dependent and has a high prevalence in the general population. Most patients are managed in ambulatory care. This systematic review provides an updated overview of quality and content of international clinical practice guidelines for diagnosis and management of non-dialysis CKD relevant to patients in ambulatory care.

Methods: We identified guidelines published from 2012-to March 2018 in guideline portals, databases and by manual search. Methodological quality was assessed with the Appraisal of Guidelines for Research and Evaluation II instrument. Recommendations were extracted and evaluated.

Results: Eight hundred fifty-two publications were identified, 9 of which were eligible guidelines. Methodological quality ranged from 34 to 77%, with domains "scope and purpose" and "clarity of presentation" attaining highest and "applicability" lowest scores. Guidelines were similar in recommendations on CKD definition, screening of patients with diabetes and hypertension, blood pressure targets and referral of patients with progressive or stage G4 CKD. Definition of high risk groups and recommended tests in newly diagnosed CKD varied.

Conclusions: Guidelines quality ranged from moderate to high. Guidelines generally agreed on management of patients with high risk or advanced CKD, but varied in regarding the range of recommended measurements, the need for referrals to nephrology, monitoring intervals and comprehensiveness. More research is needed on efficient management of patients with low risk of CKD progression to end stage renal disease.

Keywords: Chronic kidney disease, Management, Clinical practice guideline, Systematic review

Background

Chronic kidney disease (CKD) has a high prevalence in the general population and is defined as kidney damage or glomerular filtration rate (GFR) < 60 mL/min/1.73 m^2 for 3 months or more, irrespective of cause [1, 2]. In the general adult population, CKD stages 3–5 have a prevalence of up to 10%. Because kidney function declines with age, the prevalence of CKD is higher in the elderly population, with ca. 40–50% in the age group of over 85 years old meeting the criteria for CKD [3–6].

Most important risk factors for CKD are diabetes and hypertension [7]. CKD is associated with an increased risk of cardiovascular disease and can progress to end-stage renal disease [8]. However, only a small minority of patients with CKD will progress to end stage renal disease (ESRD) during their lifetime [9]. Medical care of non-dialysis patients is mostly provided by primary care providers.

Observational studies on management of chronic kidney disease in primary and ambulatory care, have concluded that management of patients with CKD could

* Correspondence: allgemeinmedizin@uni-greifswald.de
[1]Department of General Practice, Institute for Community Medicine, University Medicine Greifswald, Fleischmannstr. 6, 17475 Greifswald, Germany
[5]Faculty of Applied Health Sciences, European University of Applied Sciences, Rostock, Germany
Full list of author information is available at the end of the article

benefit from the implementation of clinical practice guidelines [3, 10–18]. Fundamental to the development of clinical practice guidelines is the review of existing evidence based guidelines.

The aim of this review is to compare quality, scope, consistency and methodological rigor of clinical practice guidelines on diagnosis and management of non-dialysis CKD.

Methods

This is a systematic review of clinical practice guidelines on diagnosis and management of CKD in adult patients in ambulatory care.

This systematic review was prospectively registered as CRD42016016939 in the PROSPERO registry.

Search strategy

A systematic search was performed to identify all relevant contemporary guidelines. The search strategy was confined to guidelines on diagnosis and management of adult non-pregnant ambulatory patients with chronic, non-dialysis CKD (GFR $\geq$30 ml/min/1.73m^2) that had been issued or updated between January 1, 2012 and March 20 2018. The search was limited to clinical practice guidelines in the languages English, French, Dutch/Flemish and German. Only guidelines issued in industrialized countries were considered eligible to ensure comparability.

Guideline portals

We performed a search using the following guideline portals:

- Guidelines-International-Network (G-I-N) [www.g-i-n.net].
- NHS Centre for Reviews and Dissemination (CRD) [19]
- National guideline Clearinghouse [10]
- Haute Autorité de Santé (HAS) [20]
- Ärztliches Zentrum für Qualität in der Medizin (AEZQ) [21]
- Arbeitsgemeinschaft der Wissenschaftlichen Medizinischen Fachgesellschaften (common working group of scientific medical Specialty Associations, AWMF) [www.awmf.org]

These guideline portals were searched with the terms:
"chronic kidney disease"
for the English language portals and
"chronische Niereninsuffizienz"
for the German language portals

Database

A search of the database Pubmed was performed with the algorithm (last update March 20 2018):

(((((((((("2012/01/01"[Date - Completion]: "3000"[Date - Completion])) AND ((((((clinical practice guideline) OR clinical practice guidelines) OR guideline) OR guidelines[MeSH Terms])) AND (((chronic kidney disease) OR CKD) OR chronic kidney insufficiency[-MeSH Terms]))))) NOT (child OR children or adolescents or infants)) NOT (dialysis OR intensive care))))) NOT (tumor OR malignancy)

Sciencedirect was searched with **"guideline"** AND **"chronic kidney disease"** for the years 2012–2018, article type: "practice guidelines".

Google search

A targeted search for eligible clinical practice guidelines was performed for the following European countries: Belgium, Denmark, Finland, France, Iceland, Ireland, the Netherlands, Norway, Sweden Switzerland and the United Kingdom. From the non-European countries a search was performed for Australia, Canada, Israel, New Zealand, South Africa and the United States of America. We used the following mesh terms in English and in the language of the country in question:

"<country>" AND "kidney" AND "guideline".

to search the World Wide Web with the Google browser and scanned the first 5 pages for eligible guidelines. If no guidelines were found, the nephrological society in this country was identified and its website was searched for information concerning national guidelines. If no such information was listed on the website, a request for information was sent to the organization.

Manual search

We conducted a manual search for additional guidelines in the reference lists of identified guidelines.

Selection of guidelines

For the selection of eligible guidelines we used predefined in- and exclusion criteria.

Inclusion criteria (Table 1).

A prior systematic guideline review had identified and evaluated guidelines on early CKD up to 2011 [8]. For this reason and to ascertain compliance of the guidelines with current state of research, we limited the search to guidelines that had been issued or updated since 2012. When guideline updates had been issued, we included the most recent update. Supplementary information was considered when the guideline referred to this information.

Quality assessment

All eligible guidelines were assessed by 2 authors independently, using the AGREE-II instrument for guideline quality assessment [22]. The AGREE instrument measures methodological rigor in guideline development [22]. The AGREE-II instrument consists of 6 domains,

Table 1 Inclusion and exclusion criteria for clinical guidelines on chronic kidney disease

Inclusion criteria	Excluson criteria:
guideline issued in an industrialized country	relevance limited to subspecialty or subtheme
guideline is relevant to management of patients with CKD	relevance is limited to acute renal insufficiency
guideline is targeted to adult patients	target group of children
guideline is available in one of the following languages: Dutch/Flemish, English, French, German	relevance is limited to pregnancy or childbirth
guideline is relevant to ambulatory patients	relevance is limited to KDIGO stage 4 and above
	relevance is limited to patients on dialysis
	relevance is limited to kidney transplant patients
	relevance is limited to inpatients

CKD Chronic Kidney Disease

consisting of 23 items and one overall assessment [22]. The content of the different domains of this instrument are listed in Additional file 1. Guidelines were rated by 2 independent researchers (AA, JFC, JME, FL, SS, GW). Scores indicate the extent to which a predefined quality dimension has been fulfilled and vary on an ordinal scale from 1 "strongly disagree" to 7 "strongly agree".

Individual AGREE-II-items were discussed in a consensus meeting between the first 2 reviewers, when a difference of 3 or more points was detected in individual item ratings, to allow for correction of false allocation of the ratings. A third reviewer would be appointed when 3 of the domains had an average item score standard deviation of ≥1,5 or if one of the domains had a standard deviation of > 2 [22].

Scaled domain scores were automatically calculated by an integrated program in the online version of the AGREE-II instrument: (Obtained score – Minimum possible score) / (Maximum possible score – Minimum possible score) [22]. Overall guideline scores were calculated as weighted mean of the domain scores.

Data extraction
A synthesis of recommendations of the selected guidelines regarding content, consistency and strengths of recommendations, as well as level of evidence, was compiled by extracting recommendations, strength or recommendation and level of evidence in a predefined form. Recommendations were inserted into the form by AH, CK, FL and GW and grouped by domain, to enable the identification of discrepancies and similarities. Domains were: prevention and screening, diagnostic tests in newly diagnosed CKD, monitoring, referral criteria, blood pressure and anemia management, and a group of miscellaneous recommendations.

Results

Selection of guidelines
We identified 1274 potentially relevant records. We excluded 1187 after title and/or abstract review. Eighty-seven

potentially relevant guidelines were included in full text review (Fig. 1). Of these, 76 guidelines did not meet eligibility criteria, one was a duplicate and 1 a preliminary version of an unpublished guideline. After full text review, we retained 9 guidelines and one USPSTF statement (Table 2) [23, 24].

Quality assessment
The quality of the guidelines was assessed with the Appraisal of Guidelines for Research and Evaluation instrument (AGREE-II) [22]. Interrater variability was low for all guidelines. Domains with high average scores were "scope and purpose" with 58–100% and "clarity of presentation" 53–100%. Lowest average score was found for "applicability" with 4–60% average score whereas editorial independence had a highly variable score with 0–96%. Guidelines achieving ratings of > 70% over all domains were the NICE guideline and the KDIGO guideline, with weighted mean domain scores of 75% and 73% respectively. KHA-CARI, BCMA and HAS guidelines received the lowest scores (Table 3). No correlation was found between year of publication and domain score, but total score correlated with rigor of development (data not shown).

Scope and purpose
Missing items included incomplete description of health questions and imprecise objectives. KDIGO was the only guideline scoring 100% for this domain, whereas VA-DoD and ACP scored 89% and 81% respectively.

Stakeholder and patient involvement
Several guidelines incompletely described the target user group. Guideline development groups were not always defined and often did not include methodologists, primary care physicians and health care workers other than physicians.

Rigor of development
Systematic evidence search and selection were incompletely described in several guidelines. Strengths and

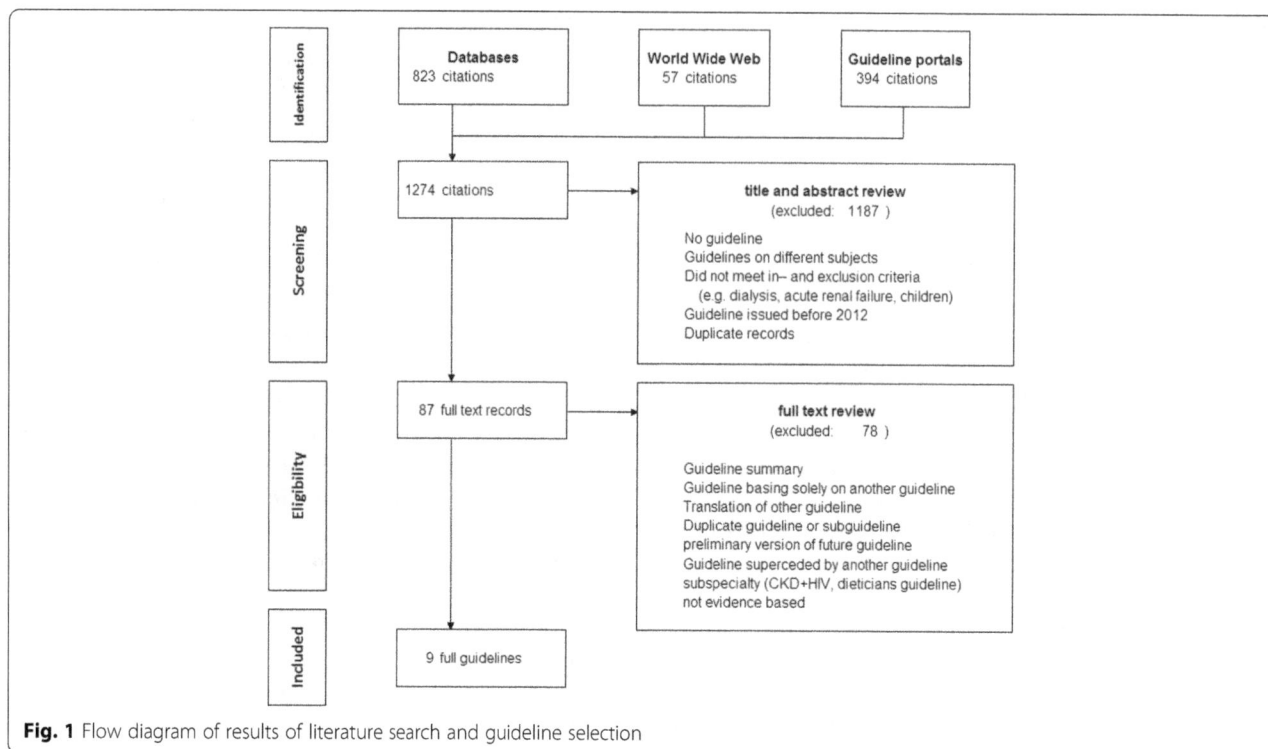

Fig. 1 Flow diagram of results of literature search and guideline selection

limitations of the evidence were not rigorously discussed by several guidelines. Health benefits and side effects were inconsistently considered in formulating recommendations. Only NICE described a structured strategy for formulating recommendations. External reviews were incompletely reported by most guidelines. Several guidelines incompletely described an updating procedure.

Clarity of presentation

Wording of recommendations was mostly unambiguous, but treatment alternatives where inconsistently addressed. The option abstaining form therapy was only mentioned by NICE.

Applicability

Facilitators and barriers and implementation strategies were incompletely addressed in most guidelines. No guideline described formal tools for barrier analysis. Only NICE consistently considered resource implications of recommendations and auditing and monitoring criteria. KDIGO provided no recommendations for implementation since it is intended to be a template for national adaptations.

Editorial Independence

Independence of the funding body was incompletely reported in several guidelines and two guidelines did not report conflicts of interest (Additional file 1).

Recommendations

Definition

The definition of CKD in the included guidelines was congruent with the KDIGO definition of CKD as abnormalities of kidney structure or function with albuminuria or GFR < 60 ml/min/1.73m^2 for > 3 months [25].

CEBAM and USPSTF restricted the definition to decreased kidney function persisting for more than 3 months. None of the guidelines provided a description of relevant structural kidney abnormalities.

Prevention

General lifestyle recommendations like weight management and sodium restriction for CKD prevention were mentioned only by KHA-CARI with medium grades of recommendation and low levels of evidence (Table 4) [26]. Other guidelines' lifestyle recommendations were aimed solely at persons with established CKD [26].

Screening

None of the guidelines recommended screening for CKD in asymptomatic persons without risk factors and NICE, ACP and USPTF guidelines explicitly advised against it (Table 4). Most guidelines recommended screening in persons with risk factors like diabetes, cardiovascular risk, or positive family history for ESRD. Notably, the UMHS guideline considered age a risk factor and recommended screening persons over 55 [23].

Table 2 Characteristics of included guidelines and one statement

	country	Issuing organization	name of guideline	initial release	revisions	target patients	target users/setting	evidence base	grading of evidence LoE	grading of evidence GoR
CEBAM	Belgium	Belgian Centre for Evidence Based Medici, Cochrane Belgium	Chronische Niereninsufficiëntie	2012		adult patients (over 18 years of age) with chronically diminished kidney function	general practitioners	systematic guideline review, additional systematic searches	GRADE	
ACP	USA	American College of Physicians	Screening, Monitoring, and Treatment of Stage 1 to 3 Chronic Kidney Disease: A Clinical Practice Guideline From the American College of Physicians	2013		target patient population for screening is adults, and the target population for treatment it is adults with stage 1 to 3 CKD	clinicians	systematic review	American College of Physicians grading system, adapted from GRADE	
HAS	France	Haute Autorité de Santé	Guide de parcours de soins Maladie Rénale Chronique de l'adulte	2012		Adult patients with chronic kidney disease. Excluded: patients with end stage renal disease, dialysis or transplantation, inpatients.	General practitioners, dieticians, nurses, pharmacists, etc., and may also concern other health professionals (Nephrologists, cardiologists, diabetologists, physiotherapists, psychologists)	unclear, existing recommendations, expert opinion	no formal grading of evidence or level of recommendation	
KDIGO	USA	Kidney Disease Improving Global Outcomes	KDIGO 2012 Clinical Practice Guideline for the Evaluation and Management of Chronic Kidney Disease	2012		individuals at risk for or with CKD	Providers: Nephrologists (adult and pediatric), dialysis providers(including nurses), Internists, and pediatricians,patients: Adult and pediatric individuals at risk for or with CKD. Policy Makers: Those in related health fields.	systematic review	GRADE	
KHA-CARI	Australia, New Zealand	Kidney Health Australia, Caring for Australasians with Renal Impairment	Early Chronic Kidney Disease	2013		patients with kidney disease in Australia & New Zealand, patients with early chronic kidney disease	clinicians and health care workers	systematic review	GRADE	
BCMA	Canada	British Columbia Medical Association	Chronic Kidney Disease - Identification, Evaluation and	2014		adults aged ≥19 years at risk of or with known chronic kidney disease	The primary audience for BC Guidelines is British Columbia physicians, nurse	not described	no formal grading of evidence or level of recommendation	

Table 2 Characteristics of included guidelines and one statement *(Continued)*

country	Issueing organization	name of guideline	initial release	revisions	target patients	target users/setting	evidence base	grading of evidence	
								LoE	GoR
		Management of Adult Patients				practitioners, and medical students. However, other audiences such as health educators, health authorities, allied health organizations, pharmacists, and nurses may also find them to be a useful resource			
UMHS USA	University of Michigan Health System	Management of Chronic Kidney Disease	2005	Interim/minor revision: March, 2014 June, 2016	adults with chronic kidney disease	clinicians, primary care providers	systematic review	GRADE, not formally stated	
VA-DoD USA	Department of Veterans Affairs, Department of Defense	VA/DoD Clinical Practice Guideline for the Management of Chronic Kidney Disease in Primary Care	2014	–	adults 18 years or older with CKD 1–4 without kidney transplant	primary care providers	systematic review	GRADE	
NICE UK	National Institute of Health and Care Excellence	Early identification and management of chronic kidney disease in adults in primary and secondary care	2014	Update 2015	Adults 18+ with or at risk of developing chronic kidney disease	Healthcare professionals Commissioners and providers People with chronic kidney disease and their families and carers	systematic review	NICE	
USPSTF USA	United States Preventive Services Task Force	Final Recommendation statement, Chronic Kidney Disease: Screening	2012		asymptomatic adults without diagnosed CKD	clinicians	probably systematic review "The USPSTF reviewed evidence on screening for CKD, including evidence on screening, accuracy of screening, early treatment, and harms of screening and early treatment."	one recommendation, not graded	

GoR grade of recommendation, *LoE* level of evidence

Table 3 Results of guideline assessment with AGREE

	CEBAM	HAS	ACP	KDIGO	KHA-CARI	BCMA	NICE	UMHS	VA-DoD	mean	range	
Scope and Purpose	72%	75%	81%	100%	61%	58%	75%	67%	89%	75%	58%	100%
Stakeholder Involvement	53%	75%	8%	89%	25%	31%	67%	39%	61%	50%	8%	89%
Rigour of Development	55%	19%	53%	70%	29%	17%	77%	40%	59%	47%	17%	77%
Clarity of Presentation	72%	53%	69%	100%	61%	78%	81%	69%	67%	72%	53%	100%
Applicability	50%	15%	4%	29%	13%	27%	60%	25%	10%	26%	4%	60%
Editorial Independence	96%	0%	88%	79%	67%	25%	88%	71%	29%	60%	0%	96%
weighted mean	61%	38%	42%	73%	34%	36%	75%	45%	54%	51%	34%	75%

Selected general clinical practice guidelines were rated with the AGREE-II instrument [22]. Scaled domain scores were calculated as percentage of the difference between the minimum possible score and the maximum possible score for a particular domain. Belgisch Centrum voor Evidence Based Medicine (CEBAM), Haute Autorité de Santé (HAS), American College of Physicians (ACP), Kidney Disease Improving Global Outcomes (KDIGO), Caring for Australians with Renal Insufficiency (KHA-CARI), British Colombia Medical Association (BCMA), National Institute of Health and Care Excellence (NICE), University of Michigan Health System (UMHS), Department of Veteran's Affairs (VA-DoD)

Table 4 Recommendation summary – Prevention and screening

	CEBAM	USPTF	ACP	HAS	KHA-CARI	BCMA	UMHS	VA-DoD	NICE
	2012	2012	2013	2013	2013	2014	2014	2014	2015
Prevention and Screening									
Prevention									
weight management					•				
sodium restriction					•				
protein restriction					−				
smoking abstinence					•				
reducing excessive alcohol intake					•				
physical exercise					•				
Screening									
asymptomatic		−	−						−
diabetes	•			•	•	•	•	•	•
hypertension				•	•	•		•	•
cardiovascular disease	•			•	•	•		•	•
acute kidney injury				•				+	•
structural renal tract disease, renal calculi, prostate hypertrophia				•					•
systemic illness (e.g. SLE, HIV)				•					•
positive family history					•	•		•	•
hematuria	•								•
nephrotoxic drugs				•					•*
smoking					•				
age							> 55		−
gender									−
ethnicity					•	•		•	−
obesity				•	•				−
occupational hazards				•				•	
socioeconomic disadvantage					•				

• recommendation, − negative recommendation, * including NSAID
American College of Physicians (ACP), Belgisch Centrum voor Evidence Based Medicine (CEBAM), British Columbia Medical Association (BCMA), Department of Veteran's Affairs (VA-DoD), Haute Autorité de Santé (HAS), Kidney Disease Improving Global Outcomes (KDIGO), Kidney Health Australia - Caring for Australasians with Renal Impairment (KHA-CARI), National Institute of Health and Care Excellence (NICE), University of Michigan Health System (UMHS)

Table 5 Recommendation summary - diagnostic tests in newly diagnosed CKD

	CEBAM 2012	ACP 2013	HAS 2013	KDIGO 2013	KHA-CARI 2013	BCMA 2014	UMHS 2014	VA-DoD 2014	NICE 2015
Diagnostic Tests in newly diagnosed CKD									
clinical blood tests									
blood pressure					▪				
serum creatinine			▪	▪	▪				
(e)GFR (creatinine)	*		▪		▪	▪	▪	▪	▪
blood count			▪		▪				
serum urea			i		▪				
serum uric acid			▪						
serum albumin			i		▪				
serum electrolytes			▪		▪				
serum glucose			▪		▪				
lipids			▪		▪				
serum cystatin C				i					
eGFR (cystatin C)									i
clearance				i					
HbA1c									
serum calcium			▪		i				
serum phosphate					i				
serum phosphorus			i						
serum PTH			▪		i				
serum 25-hydroxy-Vitamin D			▪		i				
iron					i				
serum electrophoresis			i		i				
ANA			i		i				
anti-ENA					i				
complement			i		i				
Hepatitis-B serology					i				
Hepatitis-C serology					i				
HIV-serology					i				
anti-GBM			i		i				
ANCA			i		i				
inulin									i
^{51}Cr-EDTA									i
^{125}I-iothalamate									i
iohexol									i
urine tests									
albuminuria			▪	▪	i	▪	▪		–
proteinuria - reagent strips									– ***
urine albumin-creatinin-ratio (ACR)	▪**				i	▪			n
urine protein-creatinin ratio (PCR)	▪**				i				i
urine leucocytes			▪						
hematuria			▪	(▪) ****					unclear*****
urine microscopy					▪				(–)

Table 5 Recommendation summary - diagnostic tests in newly diagnosed CKD *(Continued)*

	CEBAM 2012	ACP 2013	HAS 2013	KDIGO 2013	KHA-CARI 2013	BCMA 2014	UMHS 2014	VA-DoD 2014	NICE 2015
24 h urine			i						
urine electophoresis					i				
imaging									
renal ultrasound	i		▪		▪		i	▪	i
bladder ultrasound			i						
MRI									
CT									
Angiography									
renal artery doppler			i				i		
invasive									
kidney biopsy			i						

▪ recommendation, − negative recommendation, i: when indicated, *implicitly mentioned, **ACR or PCR, ***unless able to detect microalbuminuria, ****no explicitly formulated recommendation, but mentioned in background and a flow diagram, *****opportunistic detection
ANA anti-nuclear antibodies, anti-ENA anti extractable nuclear antibodies, ANCA anti-neutrophil cytoplasmic antibodies, anti-GBM anti-glomerular basement membrane antibodies, eGFR estimated glomerular filtration rate, PTH parathyroid hormone
American College of Physicians (ACP), Belgisch Centrum voor Evidence Based Medicine (CEBAM), British Columbia Medical Association (BCMA), Department of Veteran's Affairs (VA-DoD), Haute Autorité de Santé (HAS), Kidney Disease Improving Global Outcomes (KDIGO), Kidney Health Australia - Caring for Australasians with Renal Impairment (KHA-CARI), National Institute of Health and Care Excellence (NICE), University of Michigan Health System (UMHS)

Diagnostic tests in newly diagnosed CKD

Serum creatinine, eGFR and proteinuria testing were recommended most often (Table 5). HAS and KHA-CARI issued detailed recommendations for more extensive testing. HAS stated that some of the tests should only be ordered if recommend by a nephrologist.

Monitoring

Several guidelines issued recommendations on monitoring. Monitoring intervals were mostly congruent with KDIGO recommendations, but NICE recommended less frequent monitoring in early CKD (Table 6). Monitoring recommendations included eGFR and proteinuria, but several guidelines recommended monitoring other parameters such as weight, cardiovascular risk (BCMA, HAS), smoking status and psychosocial health (BCMA). Only HAS and BCMA and ACP explicitly recommended monitoring blood pressure and only BCMA and ACP recommended reviewing medication. BCMA recommended more extensive blood testing.

Referral criteria

Most guidelines recommend referring patients to a nephrologist if GFR falls below 30 ml/min/1.73m^2 (Table 7). HAS recommends a higher cut-off value of 45 ml/min/1.73m^2. Guidelines generally agreed in recommending referral in case of proteinuria. Only few guidelines differentiated between low-threshold consultation (NICE, KHA-CARI) or co-management versus long-term referral for management of (advanced) CKD. Multidisciplinary or co-management was mentioned by several guidelines. Only CEBAM explicitly described the role of general

practitioners (GP) and recommended GP to be responsible for detecting and monitoring CKD, detecting complications and treating cardiovascular risk.

Blood pressure

All guidelines recommended blood pressure targets of < 140/90 mmHg, with lower targets of 130/80 mmHg for patients with diabetes or albuminuria. As first line treatment, guidelines consistently recommended renin-angiotensin system antagonists, whereas diuretics, betablockers and calcium antagonists were mentioned as second line options by KHA-CARI and BCMA. Combining angiotensin converting enzyme inhibitors with angiotensin receptor blockers was explicitly not recommended by several guidelines (Table 8).

Anemia

Several guidelines issued recommendations on diagnosis, monitoring or treatment of anemia. Therapeutic targets for serum hemoglobin (6.8 moll/l; Hb, 11 g/dl) were lower than the normal values (7,5–8.1 moll/l;12-13 g/dl) (Table 9). Except for HAS and to a lesser extent CEBAM, guidelines did not contain details on the treatment of renal anemia and instead referred to specific guidelines on this topic [27–29]. Only HAS explicitly recommended avoiding blood transfusion in patients who may need kidney transplant.

Other subjects

Some guidelines issued recommendations on CKD-mineral bone disorder, patient education, and various issues

Table 6 Recommendation summary – Monitoring recommendations for patients with established CKD

	CEBAM 2012	ACP 2013	HAS 2013	KDIGO 2013	KHA-CARI 2013	BCMA 2014	UMHS 2014	VA-DoD 2014	NICE 2015
Monitoring patients with known CKD frequency (times /year)									
G1/A1	1			1		1	1		≤1
G1/A2	1			1		1	1		1
G1/A3	1			2		2	2		≥1
G2/A1	1			1		1	1		≤1
G2/A2	1			1		1	1		1
G2/A3	2			2		2	2		≥1
G3a/A1	2			1		1	1		1
G3a/A2	2			2		2	2		1
G3a/A3	2			3		3	3		2
G3b/A1	2			2		2	2		≤2
G3b/A2	2			3		3	3		2
G3b/A3	≥4			3		3	3		≥2
G4/A1	≥4			3		3	4**		2
G4/A2	≥4			3		3	3		2
G4/A3	≥4			≥4		≥4	≥4		3
G5/A1	≥4			≥4		≥4	≥4		4
G5/A2	≥4			≥4		≥4	≥4		≥4
G5/A3	≥4			≥4		≥4	≥4		≥4
parameter									
blood pressure	*	▪	▪	*		▪	*		*
weight						▪			
(e)GFR	▪	▪	▪	▪		▪	▪		▪
albuminuria/proteinuria/ACR	▪	▪	▪	▪		▪	▪		▪
complete blood count						▪			
iron saturation						▪			
HbA1c						▪			
serum calcium						▪			
serum phosphorus						▪			
serum potassium						i	i		
serum albumin						▪			
complications	▪								
inulin									i
51Cr-EDTA									i
125I-iothalamate									i
iohexol									i
cardiovascular risk			▪			▪≻			
smoking status						▪			

Table 6 Recommendation summary – Monitoring recommendations for patients with established CKD *(Continued)*

	CEBAM 2012	ACP 2013	HAS 2013	KDIGO 2013	KHA-CARI 2013	BCMA 2014	UMHS 2014	VA-DoD 2014	NICE 2015
medication		•					•		
psychosocial health							•		

▪ recommendation, − negative recommendation, i: when indicated, *not specifically mentioned, but obvious from the context (e.g. blood pressure targets), **probably transcription error, ≫ refers to British Columbian guideline "Cardiovascular disease - primary prevention"
Stages of CKD: G1, glomerular filtration rate of ≥90 ml/min/1.73m^2; G2, 60–89 ml/min/1.73m^2; G3a, 45–59 ml/min/1.73m^2; G3b, 30–44 ml/min/1.73m^2; G4, 15–29 ml/min/1.73m^2; G5, < 15 ml/min/1.73m^2
Albuminuria stages of CKD: A1, albumine-creatinine-ratio < 3 mg/mmol; A2, 3–30 mg/mmol; A3, > 30 mg/mmol
ACR albumin-creatinine-ratio, *eGFR* estimated glomerular filtration rate, *HbA1c* glycated hemoglobin, *51Cr-EDTA* chromium-51-ethylenediaminetetraacetic acid
American College of Physicians (ACP), Belgisch Centrum voor Evidence Based Medicine (CEBAM), British Columbia Medical Association (BCMA), Department of Veteran's Affairs (VA-DoD), Haute Autorité de Santé (HAS), Kidney Disease Improving Global Outcomes (KDIGO), Kidney Health Australia - Caring for Australasiansians with Renal Impairment (KHA-CARI), National Institute of Health and Care Excellence (NICE), University of Michigan Health System (UMHS)

pertaining to early or advanced CKD (Table 10). ACP and UMHS issued the general recommendation to avoid nephrotoxic medication, whereas NICE recommended using NSAID with caution. Further subjects were treatment objectives for diabetes and congestive heart failure, low protein diet, statin use, hyperuricemia, oral bicarbonate and antiplatelets and anticoagulants.

Discussion

Summary of the main results

We identified 9 clinical practice guidelines and one recommendation statement on diagnosis and management of non-dialysis CKD in adults, issued between 2012 and March 2018. Methodological quality of the guidelines ranged between 34 and 77%. All guidelines used the KDIGO definition of CKD. Recommendations for CKD screening were restricted to higher risk groups, but risk factors considered relevant for diagnostic evaluation varied. There was considerable variation of recommended tests in newly diagnosed CKD. Five guidelines published monitoring intervals for established CKD, mostly reflecting the intervals proposed by KDIGO. Monitoring tests were specified by three guidelines. Referral was usually recommended at GFR < 30 ml/min/1.73m^2 or when indicated by various other risk factors.

Quality of guidelines

A previous systematic review of clinical practice guidelines, published in 2013, analyzed 15 clinical practice guidelines issued up to 2011 for prevention, detection and management of early CKD [8]. They reported coverage and recommendations, methodological quality varying from 24 to 95%, as measured by the AGREE-II instrument. AGREE-II measures methodological rigor by rating several different aspects of guideline development, but does not appraise the content of recommendations. Low scores imply that important aspects have been omitted. Some guideline developers did not involve primary care physicians, who care for the majority of CKD patients and were target users. Most guidelines did not include the views of health care professionals other than physicians, like nurses or dieticians. Additionally, many guidelines did not describe external review procedures. External review can help to identify potential barriers related to guideline content, organization of health service provision, availability of health services, billing issues and implementation. Few guidelines explicitly discussed barriers and facilitators of guideline implementation. Identifying implementation barriers early can be valuable in resolving potential problems during the guideline development [30].

Most guidelines based recommendations on evidence from systematic literature searches. Limitations of the evidence were not consistently discussed. Only NICE described the formal procedure for formulating recommendations based on the evidence. Providing this information would help to discern recommendations based on clinical trials from those based on consensus [31]. HAS acknowledged the limited evidence and need for consensus on many topics. To reflect scientific development, clinical practice guidelines should be updated periodically, but several guidelines did not provide an expiration date or a procedure for updating.

AGREE assesses whether all treatment options are discussed and trade-offs between benefits and harms are addressed. Only NICE mentioned the option of abstaining from therapy. Potential harms of overdiagnosis and overtreatment should be more consistently incorporated in guidelines [32]. Consideration of individual patient related factors were mentioned in several guidelines. These considerations are especially important for the mostly elderly population affected by CKD. Life expectancy, comorbidities and health priorities are important factors in decisions on testing, therapy and referral for these patients [32]. KDIGO consciously excluded information on resource implications and implementation, considering itself a template for local adaptations. However, although guideline recommendations can have major impact on healthcare cost and health service utilization given the high prevalence of CKD, only few guidelines consistently addressed resource implications. Auditing and monitoring criteria to measure quality of care were only proposed by NICE.

Table 7 Recommendation summary - referral criteria

		CEBAM 2012	ACP 2013	HAS 2013	KDIGO 2013	KHA-CARI 2013	BCMA 2014	UMHS 2014	VA-DoD 2014	NICE 2015
Referral Criteria										
general	consider individual preferences					•				•
	consider individual comorbidities			•						•
	cooperation or multidisciplinary care	•			i	•			•	•
	routine follow-up after referral by patient's GP					•				•
nephrologist	GFR < 60 ml/min/1,73m^2									
	GFR < 45 ml/min/1,73m^2	i		•						
	GFR < 30 ml/min/1,73m^2	•		•		•	•	•	•	•
	ACR > 30 mg/mmol	•*		•			•			+ hematuria
	ACR ≥70 mg/mmol				•					i#
	proteinuria > 3500 mg/day								•	
	hematuria			i		•*				
	urinary cell casts						•			
	constitutional symptoms						•			
	CKD progression	•		•	•	•	•			•
	poorly controlled hypertension				•	•	•			•
	electrolyte disturbance			i	•		•		•	
	anemia			i				•		
	metabolic complications			i					•	
	complications			i				i		
	nephrolythiasis				•				•	
	suspected renal artery stenosis	•								•
	genetic etiology of CKD				•		•			•
	rare etiology of CKD									•
	etiology requiring specialist care								•	
	unclear etiology					i		i	•	
	1-year ESRD-risk of ≥10%				•					
	indication for dialysis or transplant				•		•			•
urologist	renal outflow obstruction	•								•
diabetologist	diabetic nephropathy						•			•
dietician	eGFR< 60 ml/min/1,73m^2				•	i				i
inpatient treatment	complications									•
	hypertensive crisis									•
	unknown etiology									•

• recommendation, i: when indicated *in combination with KDIGO stage A3, # unless caused by diabetes and properly treated
ACR albumin-creatinine-ratio, *CKD* chronic kidney disease, *ERSD* end stage renal disease, *GFR* glomerular filtration rate, *GP* general practitioner, *HbA1c* glycated hemoglobin
American College of Physicians (ACP), Belgisch Centrum voor Evidence Based Medicine (CEBAM), British Columbia Medical Association (BCMA), Department of Veteran's Affairs (VA-DoD), Haute Autorité de Santé (HAS), Kidney Disease Improving Global Outcomes (KDIGO), Kidney Health Australia - Caring for Australasiansians with Renal Impairment (KHA-CARI), National Institute of Health and Care Excellence (NICE), University of Michigan Health System (UMHS)

Content of guidelines
Definition and screening
There was no disagreement on the definition of CKD by laboratory tests, but all guidelines fail to precise which structural abnormalities qualify for CKD. NICE and ACP guidelines as well as the USPSTF recommended explicitly against screening of asymptomatic individuals without known risk factors. Screening was recommended for high risk groups in most guidelines, but KHA-CARI used broad definitions for at risk populations like smoking, obesity, socioeconomic disadvantage or age. This can lead to screening situations where

Table 8 Recommendation summary - blood pressure management

		CEBAM 2012	ACP 2013	HAS 2013	KDIGO 2013	KHA-CARI 2013	BCMA 2014	UMHS 2014	VA-DoD 2014	NICE 2015
Blood pressure management										
BP monitoring intervals						•				
individualized BP targets					•		•			•
BP target	< 140/90	•		•	•	•	•	•	•	•
BP target in diabetics	< 140/90							GP		
	< 140/80									
	< 130/80					•				•
BP target in ≥ microalbuminuria	< 140/90							•		
	< 130/80				•	•			i	•
medication	renin-angiotensin system antagonist						i ≻			i
	ACEI	i	i		i	i	i	•	i	
	ARB		i		i	i	i	•	i	
	combination of ACEI + ARB				−	−			−	−
	combination of ACEI/ARB + direct renin inhibitor					−			−	−
	diuretics					i	i			
	β-blocker					i	i			
	calcium channel blocker					i	i			
	side effects	•								

• recommendation, − negative recommendation, i: when indicated, ≻ recommendations in KDIGO BP guideline, *ACEI* angiotensin converting enzyme inhibitor, *ARB* angiotensin receptor blocker, *BP* blood pressure, *DM* diabetes mellitus, *ev* insufficient evidence for recommendation, GP: identical blood pressure targets as general population, n.a.: not applicable
American College of Physicians (ACP), Belgisch Centrum voor Evidence Based Medicine (CEBAM), British Columbia Medical Association (BCMA), Department of Veteran's Affairs (VA-DoD), Haute Autorité de Santé (HAS), Kidney Disease Improving Global Outcomes (KDIGO), Kidney Health Australia - Caring for Australasiansians with Renal Impairment (KHA-CARI), National Institute of Health and Care Excellence (NICE), University of Michigan Health System (UMHS)

health benefits and therapeutic consequences of CKD diagnosis are lacking.

Diagnostic tests in newly diagnosed CKD
Main purpose of the initial diagnostic work-up is to establish CKD and rule out emergencies or specifically treatable kidney disorders, e.g. glomerulonephritis. Most guidelines agree on assessing kidney function by eGFR-creatinine and proteinuria. Primarily KHA-CARI and HAS, recommend extensive additional diagnostic work-up, mainly to identify possible complications or comorbidities reflecting the epidemiology in specialized nephrology services but not in primary care. As the risk of developing complications like electrolyte disturbances, anemia or CKD-MBD is largely dependent on kidney function, a more differentiated approach according to CKD stage, could lower health service utilization and cost while maintaining quality of care. HAS explicitly stated that testing was aimed to obtain baseline values in some instances. It is debatable whether this set point information has therapeutic consequence.

Assessment of hematuria was inconsistently addressed. While NICE recommended against using urine microscopy,

KHA-CARI recommended it. Most primary care providers do not have the skills and equipment to perform urine microscopy. However NICE and KDIGO did not specify when dipstick testing for hematuria is warranted, while most guideline did not address checking for hematuria at all.

Monitoring
Guidelines recommending monitoring intervals, generally adopted these from the KDIGO recommendations, although NICE recommended less frequent monitoring for early stage CKD. Monitoring intervals are mainly based on clinical experience and consensus, given a lack of clinical studies evaluating the effect of different monitoring intervals on health outcomes. Guidelines were not always clear which parameters should be monitored continuously. Therefore, individual patients' preferences, comorbidities and progression risk, should be incorporated in decisions on monitoring frequency. Monitoring eGFR and proteinuria was recommended by all guidelines, but the latter might not be necessary if proteinuria has been ruled out.

Other parameters mentioned, were prognostic and etiological factors like diabetes, or laboratory values

Table 9 Recommendation summary - anemia management

		CEBAM 2012	ACP 2013	HAS 2013	KDIGO 2013	KHA-CARI 2013	BCMA 2014	UMHS 2014	VA-DoD 2014	NICE 2015
Management of anemia										
diagnosis	definition	•			•			•		•
	lower limit in g/dl	11			M: 13, F: 12			M: 13, F: 12		11
monitoring	monitor for anemia	•		•	•		i	•		
	tests	•			•			•		
	frequency (per year)	individual			1–4					
initial evaluation								•		
treatment options	iron	•		i					•	
	erythropoetin	•		i						
	nutritional supplements			i						
	androgens									
	blood transfusion			–/i*						
treatment	indications			•						
	target values			•						
	monitoring			•						
	erythropoietine resistance			•						
	referral			•						

• recommendation, – negative recommendation, F: female, M: male, i: when indicated, *Transfusions should be avoided (risk of allo-immunization). The only indications are symptomatic anemia in patients with an associated risk factor; acute worsening of anemia by blood loss (hemorrhage, surgery), hemolysis or resistance to erythropoietin. A search for anti-HLA antibodies should be performed before and after any transfusion in patients waiting for kidney transplant
American College of Physicians (ACP), Belgisch Centrum voor Evidence Based Medicine (CEBAM), British Columbia Medical Association (BCMA), Department of Veteran's Affairs (VA-DoD), Haute Autorité de Santé (HAS), Kidney Disease Improving Global Outcomes (KDIGO), Kidney Health Australia - Caring for Australasiansians with Renal Impairment (KHA-CARI), National Institute of Health and Care Excellence (NICE), University of Michigan Health System (UMHS)

indicative of complications like CKD-MBD or anemia, that have different monitoring intervals, which is potentially confusing. Some guidelines recommended testing for electrolyte disturbances, which usually develop in later CKD stages, so that it seems sensible to focus more extensive laboratory testing on patients with moderate or severe CKD. Although nephrotoxic medication can be an important risk factor for CKD progression, only BCMA and ACP recommended regular medication reviews. Blood pressure monitoring was not formally recommended by most guidelines except for HAS and BCMA, although almost all guidelines recommended specific blood pressure targets.

Referral criteria

Referral criteria often reflected the structure of the healthcare system and availability of resources and services. Early referral to specialist nephrology services has been linked to reduced hospitalization and mortality and increased quality of life, but was defined as more than 6 months before dialysis [33]. Because of the protracted course of CKD and low probability of most patients with CKD to progress to ESRD, only few patients with specific underlying conditions will benefit from referral to

nephrologist specialty care in early CKD [34]. No longitudinal prospective studies have been conducted in the large population of patients with early CKD to assess if referral can slow CKD progression or prevent the occurrence of complications and comorbidities in this group.

Some guidelines described interdisciplinary care, but generally, no distinction was made between referral for evaluation of CKD diagnosis and ruling out kidney specific disease like glomerulonephritis, versus continuous interdisciplinary care. Main referral criteria across guidelines were refractory hypertension and progressive or advanced CKD (G4,5). Referral intervals or criteria for determining these are not proposed.

Several guidelines state that patient preferences and comorbidities should be considered when referring patients. Formal criteria for non-referral are proposed by none of the guidelines. An important unaddressed issue in all guidelines is the definition of specific referral criteria for elderly patients (80+) or nursing home residents who are unlikely to benefit from referral although CKD prevalence is high in this population. Indiscriminate application of referral criteria in this population, could lead to substantial capacity problems with respect to the nephrology workforce and may not be feasible or desirable from a public health perspective [35, 36].

Table 10 Recommendation summary - other subjects

other subjects		CEBAM 2012	ACP 2013	HAS 2013	KDIGO 2013	KHA-CARI 2013	BCMA 2014	UMHS 2014	VA-DoD 2014	NICE 2015
patient education		•				•			•	•
diet	protein intake (in g/kg/day)				0.8	0.75–1.0			0.6–0.8	
	no low protein diet < 0.6 g/kg/day					•				•
complications	CKD-mineral bone disorder	•			•		•	•		•
diabetes	HbA1c target values (in %)				7.0				< 7.0	
	metformin	with caution					avoid/ reduce			
	cardiovascular risk					•				
hyperlipidemia					≻					≻
	statins for cardiovascular risk				i			i		
	statins for CKD progression								–	
	ezetimibe							i		
congestive heart failure		•			•					
antigoagulants and antiplatelets		•			•	•				•
nephrotoxic Medication	geneneral				–			–		
	NSAID									–
vaccinations									•	
metabolism	hyperuricemia				•					•
	oral bicarbonate				•				•	•
nephrotoxic medication		•							•	•

• recommendation, – negative recommendation, i: when indicated, ≻ referral to KDIGO and NICE guidelines on lipid management, *CKD* chronic kidney disease, *HbA1c* glycated Hemoglobin, *NSAID* nonsteroidal anti-inflammatory drugs
American College of Physicians (ACP), Belgisch Centrum voor Evidence Based Medicine (CEBAM), British Columbia Medical Association (BCMA), Department of Veteran's Affairs (VA-DoD), Haute Autorité de Santé (HAS), Kidney Disease Improving Global Outcomes (KDIGO), Kidney Health Australia - Caring for Australasiansians with Renal Impairment (KHA-CARI), National Institute of Health and Care Excellence (NICE), University of Michigan Health System (UMHS)

Blood pressure

Hypertension control is important to prevent progression of CKD and all guidelines recommended blood pressure below 140/90 mmHg, with lower reference values of 130/80 for patients with diabetes or albuminuria. Although it was obvious from the context that blood pressure monitoring was expected in all guidelines, only HAS, ACP and BMCA explicitly mentioned blood pressure measurements in their monitoring recommendations.

Anemia

Anemia is a complication of CKD that becomes more prevalent with CKD progression. NICE recommends using a lower cut-off value of < 6,8 moll/l (11 g/dl) for diagnosing anemia, corresponding with the WHO-definition of moderate anemia, whereas KDIGO's higher cut-off corresponds to WHO mild anemia [25, 28, 37]. Recommended monitoring frequency is somewhat lower than for GFR.

Other subjects

Most patients with CKD are multimorbid and the presence of CKD has implications for management of comorbid conditions. Therefore the most common associated problems should be addressed in the guideline. However, recommendations of management of comorbid conditions varied widely between the guidelines. This is a barrier for integrated management of patients with CKD.

Strengths and limitations

Although we believe that we have not missed an important guideline on the topic and have searched in several languages, we cannot exclude language bias. We have excluded guidelines for CKD and diabetes and guidelines addressing specific issues to ensure readability and conciseness.

The AGREE-II instrument is a valuable tool to assess the methodological quality of clinical practice guidelines, but does not address content-related quality considerations such as quality of the evidence base, or applicability and acceptability of the recommendations for clinicians and patients.

Therefore, some guidelines are user-friendly for clinicians, but do not attain high scores on many of the AGREE-II items. Examples are BCMA and UMHS

Table 11 Recommendations for future guidelines on CKD

1	Recommendations should specify how to consider age, multimorbidity, risk of progression, life expectancy, health goals and quality of life.
2	Recommendations on referral should distinguish between interdisciplinary or co-treatment and one-time consultations for specific problems or to rule out specific kidney diseases.
3	Guidelines should be comprehensive and include management recommendations for common CKD-related problems usually solved in primary care.
4	All relevant options including the option of abstaining from diagnosis or therapy should be incorporated in the guideline.
5	Increase involvement of stakeholders and target users, particularly non-nephrologists in the development process.
6	Implications for cost and resources in the healthcare system should be considered when formulating recommendations.
7	Facilitators and barriers to implementation and adoption of the guideline in clinical practice should be identified and analyzed and the results should be incorporated during the guideline development process.
8	A procedure and timeframe for updating the guideline should be specified.

CKD chronic kidney disease

guidelines which provide summary tables and comprehensive overviews of management options at a glance.

Directions for future research and guideline development

Currently, a research gap exists regarding the natural history of CKD in the general population, particularly in the elderly, and regarding the effectiveness and benefits of monitoring and treatment recommendations on preventing relatively rare but clinically important outcomes like ESRD. Research mostly addresses patients with advanced CKD or in secondary and tertiary care. Findings in these selected subgroups cannot be indiscriminately applied to the CKD population in primary care. This population, consisting mostly of elderly patients with slightly or moderately diminished kidney function, many of whom remain undiagnosed or are multimorbid with limited life expectancy and are therefore not likely to benefit from more intensive treatment or monitoring [32, 36]. These considerations are especially important regarding decisions about information, monitoring, treatment intensity and referral. CKD-stage or GFR may not always be the most appropriate criteria for decision making. A summary of recommendations for future guideline updates is provided in Table 11.

Conclusions

Clinical Practice Guidelines are increasingly issued by various stakeholders to promote quality of care. The KDIGO guideline on diagnosis and management of CKD has been adapted in many countries and served as model for most guidelines included in this review. There was substantial variation in the quality of the guideline development process.

Although there is good agreement on most core recommendations, the scope of recommendations issued by the guidelines varied significantly. Many recommendations for management of CKD rely on primarily on consensus. The care for CKD in multimorbid patients might require more individualization based on patient preferences and circumstances than can be reflected by

guideline recommendations based primarily on measurement of kidney function. Since subtle differences can have a significant impact on health resource utilization and increase burden of disease in affected patients, careful implementation and evaluation of benefits and harms in every health care system is warranted.

Additional file

Additional file 1: Compliance of different guidelines with AGREE-II. Description of how the included guidelines conform to AGREE-II items [22]. ACP: American College of Physicians, BMCA: British Columbia Medical Association, CEBAM: Belgian Centre for Evidence Based Medicine Cochrane Belgium, HAS: Haute Autorité de Santé, KDIGO: Kidney Disease Improving Global Outcomes, KHA-CARI: Kidney Health Australia – Caring for Australasians with Renal Insufficiency, NICE: National Institute of Health and Care Excellence, UMHS: University of Michigan Health System, VA-DoD: Veterans Affairs, Department of Defence. (DOCX 19 kb)

Abbreviations
(e)GFR: (estimated) glomerular filtration rate; ACP: American College of Physicians; AEZQ: Ärztliches Zentrum für Qualität in der Medizin [*German Agency for Quality in Medicine*]; AGREE: Appraisal of Guidelines for Research and Evaluation; AWMF: Arbeitsgemeinschaft der Wissenschaftlichen Medizinischen Fachgesellschaften [*common working group of scientific medical Specialty Associations*]; BCMA: British Columbia Medical Association; CEBAM: Belgian Centre for Evidence Based Medicine; CKD: chronic kidney disease; CKD-MBD: chronic kidney disease – mineral and bone disorder; CRD: Centre for Reviews and Dissemination; ERSD: End stage renal disease; G-I-N: Guidelines International Network; HAS: Haute Autorité de Santé; KDIGO: Kidney Disease Improving Global Outcomes; KHA-CARI: Caring for Australasians with Renal Insufficiency; MeSH: Medical Subject Headings; NHS: National Health Service (United Kingdom); NICE: National Institute of Health and Care Excellence; UMHS: University of Michigan Health System; USPSTF: United States Preventive Services Task Force; VA-DoD: United States Department of Veteran's Affairs – United States Department of Defence

Acknowledgements
The authors wish to thank Christine Klötzer und Maria Richter for assistance in preparing tables for the manuscript and Cornelie Jol for English language editing.

Funding
This systematic review was conducted as part of the REnal Function in Ambulatory CarE (REFACE) study, which was funded by the German foundations "KfH Stiftung Präventivmedizin" and "Damp Stiftung". The authors declare that the funding bodies had no role or any influence in the design of the study, in collection, analysis, and interpretation of data and in writing the manuscript.

Authors' contributions
JFC and GW designed, GW and AA performed the systematic review and GW, JS, FL evaluated citations according to the in- and exclusion criteria. GW, FL, JFC, SS, JME and MM appraised the included guidelines with the AGREE-II instrument. AH, FL, JFC and GW extracted and evaluated recommendations. GW, JS and JFC analyzed and interpreted the data. All authors discussed the results and implications and commented on the manuscript at all stages.

Competing interests
The authors declare that they have no competing interests.

Author details
[1]Department of General Practice, Institute for Community Medicine, University Medicine Greifswald, Fleischmannstr. 6, 17475 Greifswald, Germany. [2]Department of Internal Medicine A, Nephrology Dialysis and Hypertension, University Medicine Greifswald, Greifswald, Germany. [3]Department of Public Health, Brandenburg University of Technology Cottbus-Senftenberg, Senftenberg, Germany. [4]Department II – Cardiology, Clinic for Internal Medicine, Pulmonology and General Internal Medicine, DRK-Krankenhaus Teterow, Teterow, Germany. [5]Faculty of Applied Health Sciences, European University of Applied Sciences, Rostock, Germany.

References
1. KDOQI. Clinical practice guideline for diabetes and CKD: 2012 update. Am J Kidney Dis. 2012;60:850–86. https://doi.org/10.1053/j.ajkd.2012.07.005.
2. Levey AS, Eckardt K-U, Tsukamoto Y, Levin A, Coresh J, Rossert J, et al. Definition and classification of chronic kidney disease: A position statement from Kidney Disease: Improving Global Outcomes (KDIGO). 2005;67:2089–100. https://doi.org/10.1111/j.1523-1755.2005.00365.x.
3. Morgan T. Chronic kidney disease (stages 3–5) prevalence estimates using data from the Neoerica study (2007). England: Association of Public Health Observatories; 2009.
4. Kearns B. Chronic kidney disease prevalence modelling briefing document. 2009.
5. Stevens PE, O'Donoghue DJ, de LS, van Vlymen J, Klebe B, Middleton R, et al. Chronic kidney disease management in the United Kingdom: NEOERICA project results. Kidney Int. 2007;72:92–9. https://doi.org/10.1038/sj.ki.5002273.
6. Bolignano D, Mattace-Raso F, Sijbrands EJG, Zoccali C. The aging kidney revisited: a systematic review. Ageing Res Rev. 2014;14:65–80. https://doi.org/10.1016/j.arr.2014.02.003.
7. Levey AS, Jong d, Paul E, Coresh J, El Nahas M, Astor BC, Matsushita K, et al. The definition, classification, and prognosis of chronic kidney disease: a KDIGO controversies conference report. Kidney Int. 2011;80:17–28. https://doi.org/10.1038/ki.2010.483.
8. Lopez-Vargas PA, Tong A, Sureshkumar P, Johnson DW, Craig JC. Prevention, detection and management of early chronic kidney disease: a systematic review of clinical practice guidelines. Nephrology (Carlton). 2013;18:592–604. https://doi.org/10.1111/nep.12119.
9. KDIGO. Clinical practice guideline for lipid management in chronic kidney disease. New York, NY: Nature Publ. Group; 2013.
10. McIntyre NJ, Fluck R, McIntyre C, Taal M. Treatment needs and diagnosis awareness in primary care patients with chronic kidney disease. Br J Gen Pract. 2012;62:32.
11. Zhang Q-L, Rothenbacher D. Prevalence of chronic kidney disease in population-based studies: systematic review. BMC Public Health. 2008;8: 117. https://doi.org/10.1186/1471-2458-8-117.
12. Diamantidis CJ, Powe NR, Jaar BG, Greer RC, Troll MU, Boulware LE. Primary care-specialist collaboration in the care of patients with chronic kidney disease. Clin J Am Soc Nephrol. 2011;6:334–43. https://doi.org/10.2215/CJN.06240710.
13. Minutolo R, de NL, Mazzaglia G, Postorino M, Cricelli C, Mantovani LG, et al. Detection and awareness of moderate to advanced CKD by primary care practitioners: a cross-sectional study from Italy. Am J Kidney Dis. 2008;52: 444–53. https://doi.org/10.1053/j.ajkd.2008.03.002.
14. Allen AS, Forman JP, Orav EJ, Bates DW, Denker BM, Sequist TD. Primary care management of chronic kidney disease. J Gen Intern Med. 2011;26: 386–92. https://doi.org/10.1007/s11606-010-1523-6.
15. Boulware LE, Troll MU, Jaar BG, Myers DI, Powe NR. Identification and referral of patients with progressive CKD: a national study. Am J Kidney Dis. 2006;48:192–204. https://doi.org/10.1053/j.ajkd.2006.04.073.
16. Navaneethan SD, Kandula P, Jeevanantham V, Nally JV, Liebman SE. Referral patterns of primary care physicians for chronic kidney disease in general population and geriatric patients. Clin Nephrol. 2010;73:260–7.
17. Curtis BM, Barrett BJ, Djurdjev O, Singer J, Levin A. Evaluation and treatment of CKD patients before and at their first nephrologist encounter in Canada. Am J Kidney Dis. 2007;50:733–42. https://doi.org/10.1053/j.ajkd.2007.08.004.
18. Smart NA, Titus TT. Outcomes of early versus late nephrology referral in chronic kidney disease: a systematic review. Am J Med. 2011;124:1073. https://doi.org/10.1016/j.amjmed.2011.04.026.
19. CRD. www.crd.york.ac.uk.
20. Haute Autorité de Santé: Guide parcours de soins maladie rénale chronique de l'adulte; 2012. Accessed 20 Mar 2018.
21. AEZQ. www.aezq.de.
22. Brouwers MC, Kho ME, Browman GP, Burgers JS, Cluzeau F, Feder G, et al. AGREE II: advancing guideline development, reporting, and evaluation in health care. Prev Med. 2010;51:421–4. https://doi.org/10.1016/j.ypmed.2010.08.005. Accessed 20 Mar 2018.
23. Moyer VA. Screening for chronic kidney disease: U.S. preventive services task force recommendation statement. Ann Intern Med. 2012;157:567–70. https://doi.org/10.7326/0003-4819-157-8-201210160-00533.
24. Chi C, Moore M, Murphy TV, Patel PR, Pilishvili T, Strikas RA. Guidelines for vaccinating dialysis patients and patients with chronic kidney disease: Summarized from recommendations of the Advisory Committee on Immunization Practices (ACIP). Atlanta, GA: U.S. Dept. of Health & Human Services, Centers for Disease Control and Prevention (CDC); 2012.
25. Andrassy KM. KDIGO 2012 clinical practice guideline for the evaluation and Management of Chronic Kidney Disease. Kidney Int. 2013;84:622–3.
26. Johnson DW, Atai E, Chan M, Phoon RK, Scott C, Toussaint ND, et al. KHA-CARI guideline: early chronic kidney disease: detection, prevention and management. Nephrology (Carlton). 2013;18:340–50. https://doi.org/10.1111/nep.12052.
27. KDIGO. Clinical practice guideline for anemia in chronic kidney disease. New York, NY: Nature Publishing Group; 2012.
28. National Institute for Health and Clinical Excellence (Great Britain). Chronic kidney disease: Early identification and management of chronic kidney disease in adults in primary and secondary care. London: NICE; 2015.
29. NICE - National Institute of Health and Care Excellence. Chronic kidney disease: managing anaemia: NICE guideline; 2015.
30. Gagliardi AR, Brouwers MC. Do guidelines offer implementation advice to target users? A systematic review of guideline applicability. BMJ Open. 2015; 5:e007047. https://doi.org/10.1136/bmjopen-2014-007047.
31. Schoenmaker NJ, Tromp WF, van der Lee, Johanna H, Offringa M, Craig JC, Groothoff JW. Quality and consistency of clinical practice guidelines for the management of children on chronic dialysis. Nephrol Dial Transplant. 2013; 28:3052–61. https://doi.org/10.1093/ndt/gft303.
32. Moynihan R, Glassock R, Doust J. Chronic kidney disease controversy: how expanding definitions are unnecessarily labelling many people as diseased. BMJ. 2013;347:f4298. https://doi.org/10.1136/bmj.f4298.
33. Smart NA, Dieberg G, Ladhani M, Titus T. Early referral to specialist nephrology services for preventing the progression to end-stage kidney disease. Cochrane Database Syst Rev. 2014:CD007333. https://doi.org/10.1002/14651858.CD007333.pub2.
34. Black C, Sharma P, Scotland G, McCullough K, McGurn D, Robertson L, et al. Early referral strategies for management of people with markers of renal disease: a systematic review of the evidence of clinical effectiveness, cost-effectiveness and economic analysis. Health Technol Assess. 2010;14:1–184. https://doi.org/10.3310/hta14210.
35. Singh K, Waikar SS, Samal L. Evaluating the feasibility of the KDIGO CKD referral recommendations. BMC Nephrol. 2017;18:223. https://doi.org/10.1186/s12882-017-0646-y.
36. McClure M, Jorna T, Wilkinson L, Taylor J. Elderly patients with chronic kidney disease: do they really need referral to the nephrology clinic? Clin Kidney J. 2017;10:698–702. https://doi.org/10.1093/ckj/sfx034.
37. World Health Organization. Haemoglobin Concentrations for the Diagnosis of Anaemia and Assessment of Severity. 2011.

11

Relation of multi-marker panel to incident chronic kidney disease and rapid kidney function decline in African Americans: the Jackson Heart Study

Stanford E. Mwasongwe[1]* (iD), Bessie Young[2,3], Aurelian Bidulescu[5], Mario Sims[4], Adolfo Correa[4] and Solomon K. Musani[4]

Abstract

Background: Few investigations have evaluated the incremental usefulness of multiple biomarkers representing varying physiological pathways for predicting risk of renal outcomes in African Americans.

Design, setting, participants, and measurements: We related a multi-marker panel to incident chronic kidney disease (CKD) and rapid kidney function decline (RKFD) in 2813 Jackson Heart Study participants without prevalent CKD at exam 1 (2000–2004) and with complete assays at exam 1 for 9 biomarkers: adiponectin, aldosterone, B-natriuretic peptide [BNP], cortisol, high sensitivity C-reactive protein (hsCRP), endothelin, homocysteine, plasma renin activity and mass. Incident CKD was defined as estimated glomerular filtration rate (eGFR) < 60 mL/min/1.73 m^2 at exam 3 while RKFD was defined as eGFR ≥30% loss between exams 1 and 3 (8.2 median years). We employed multiple logistic regression model to describe association between the panel and incident CKD and RKFD and used backward elimination strategy to estimate the most parsimonious biomarker model while controlling for conventional risk factors.

Results: The multi-marker panel predicted the risk for both incident CKD (odds ratios [OR], 2.72; 95% confidence intervals [CI], 1.63, 4.56; $P = 0.001$) and RKFD (2.61; 95% CI, 1.67, 4.08; $P < 0.001$). Per standard deviation increase in log biomarker concentrations were significantly (multivariable adjusted odds ratios, [95% confidence interval], p-value) associated with incident CKD: plasma adiponectin (1.24 [1.07, 1.44], $p = 0.005$) and leptin (1.3 [1.06, 1.61], $p = 0.011$), and with RKFD: plasma adiponectin (1.22 [1.06, 1.40], $p = 0.006$); hsCRP (1.17 [1.01, 1.36], $p = 0.031$) and aldosterone (0.85 [0.74, 0.96], $p = 0.012$). Moderate levels (3rd quartile) of aldosterone were inversely associated with incident CKD (0.54 [0.35, 0.82], $p = 0.004$) while leptin was associated with RKFD (1.64 [1.10, 2.44], $p = 0.015$). Biomarkers improved CKD risk prediction ($P = 0.003$) but not RKFD risk prediction ($P = 0.10$).

Conclusion: In this community-based sample of African Americans, a multi-marker panel added only moderate predictive improvement compared to conventional risk factors.

Keywords: Biomarker, Chronic kidney disease, Rapid kidney function decline, Estimated glomerular filtration rate, African Americans

* Correspondence: smwasongwe@umc.edu; smwasogwe@umc.edu
[1]Jackson Heart Study, Jackson State University, 350 W. Woodrow Wilson Ave., Suite 701, Jackson, MS 39213, USA
Full list of author information is available at the end of the article

Background

Chronic kidney disease (CKD) is a significant health problem which is associated with increased morbidity and mortality, making its prevention a public health priority. Thirteen percent of the adult population of the United States have reduced kidney function or albuminuria [1]. Early identification of persons at greater risk of developing CKD is critical in prevention and management strategies. Traditionally, hypertension and diabetes are the most commonly known key risk factors for CKD. Others include advanced age, low high-density lipoprotein cholesterol (HDL) and metabolic syndrome [2]. Previous studies have shown that traditional factors alone are inadequate to explain CKD risks and improve risk stratification for CKD or progression of CKD [3–5]. Established CKD risk factors explain only 34% of renal disease progression among whites and 44% for African Americans after adjusting for sociodemographic, lifestyle and clinical factors [3, 6]. In clinical settings, CKD prognosis largely depends on traditional markers such as estimated glomerular filtration rate (eGFR) and albuminuria, however these biomarkers only offer modest risk prediction particularly in people with preserved levels of renal function [7] and are subject to intra-individual variability over time when hydration and medication use are involved. Additionally, albuminuria and eGFR can have a variable relationship, an example being the development of CKD (eGFR < 60 mL/min/1.73 m^2) without albuminuria [8, 9]. Several other pathways may be involved in CKD development including inflammation and endothelial function [3, 10]. Studies in cardiovascular disease (CVD) and metabolic syndrome, have benefited from the use of circulating biomarkers in risk prediction [11–13]. Unlike biomarkers in CVD, the list of prognostic biomarkers in CKD is in continuous growth and the concept of a multi-marker approach has been proposed as single biomarkers are unable to fully describe changes in renal function [14]. While multi-marker approach to predict CKD has been reported in whites [10], the predictive value of models incorporating multiple biomarkers in CKD prediction among African Americans is not well studied.

In a community-based sample of African Americans enrolled in the Jackson Heart Study (JHS), we sought to identify biomarkers of interest and evaluate their incremental predictive value from a multi-marker panel representing physiological pathways implicated in kidney diseases: adiposity (adiponectin and leptin); adrenal (aldosterone and cortisol); endothelial function (endothelin and homocysteine); inflammation (C - reactive protein, [CRP]); natriuretic (B-type Natriuretic Peptide [BNP]) and renin angiotensin (plasma renin activity, and renin mass). We conducted tests on model improvement using both the C-statistic and the newer measures of net reclassification index (NRI) and integrated discrimination index (IDI) [15, 16].

Methods
Study sample

The JHS is a single-site community-based prospective study designed to identify risk factors for cardiovascular disease in African Americans. The recruitment details have been summarized previously [17, 18]. Briefly, the study enrolled 5306 participants ≥21 years of age (clinic Exam 1, September 2000 to March 2004) from urban and rural areas of three counties (Hinds, Madison, and Rankin) that comprises a Jackson, Mississippi Metropolitan Statistical Area (MSA). Participants were asked to return for a second clinic Exam (October 2005 to December 2008) and third clinic Exam (February 2009 to January 2013). The 9 biomarkers studied in this analysis were measured at Exam 1, while serum creatinine was measured at Exam 1 and 3 (8.2 median follow-up years). Analysis was restricted to 2813 participants after we excluded participants who (i) were missing serum creatinine values measured at Exam 1 and clinic Exam 3, $n = 1548$; (ii) had prevalent CKD at baseline or reported being on dialysis, $n = 202$; and (iii) were missing biomarker data, $n = 743$. Data were imputed for 206 participants with missing covariates. The institutional review board at the University of Mississippi Medical Center, Jackson State University, and Tougaloo College approved the study. All participants provided informed written consent.

Definition of renal outcomes, biomarker selection and measurement

Incident CKD and RKFD, were both defined based on serum creatinine measured at Exams 1 and 3, as serum creatinine was not measured at the Exam 2. Serum creatinine was measured Exam 1 (2000–2004) and Exam 3 (2009–2013), serum creatinine was measured using a multipoint enzymatic spectrophotometric assay with the Vitros Ortho-Clinical Diagnostics Analyzer (Raritan, NJ). As part of the calibration study, measurement of serum creatinine were repeated for a random sample of 206 in 2006 using the enzymatic method on the Roche Modular P Chemistry Analyzer (Roche Diagnostics Corporation, Indianapolis, IN [19, 20]. Serum creatinine measured at Exam 1 was then calibrated to harmonize with serum creatinine measured at Exam 3 using isotope-dilution mass spectrometry traceable method [21]. We defined both endpoints based on the change between clinic Exams 1 and 3, and eGFR was estimated using Chronic Kidney Disease Epidemiology Collaboration (CKD-EPI) creatinine equation [21–23]. Incident CKD was defined as eGFR ≥60 mL/min/1.73 m^2 at Exam 1 (i.e., no CKD at baseline) and eGFR < 60 mL/min/1.73 m^2 at Exam 3 [24]. For RKFD, the difference expressed as a percentage of baseline eGFR represented progression if greater than 30% [2, 25]. Any eGFR > 120 mL/min/1.73 m^2 was truncated to 120 mL/min/1.73 m^2 to avoid large changes in those with high normal eGFRs [26, 27]. Positive values indicate a decline of eGFR from Exam 1 to Exam 3.

Nine biomarkers were selected because of the reported associations with kidney function, biologic plausibility and availability at first examination cycle. We measured high-sensitivity C-reactive protein (a marker of inflammation); adiponectin and leptin (adiposity); aldosterone, plasma renin activity, active renin mass concentration and B-type natriuretic peptide (markers of neuro-hormonal activity); homocysteine and endothelin (markers of endothelial function and oxidant stress). A detailed description of the standard assays were used for all biomarkers with coefficient of variations reported by Musani et al. [12]. Briefly, venous blood samples were withdrawn from study participants following 8-h fasting and stored at the JHS central repository in Minneapolis, MN, USA at -70 °C until assayed [19, 28].

Covariate assessments

The baseline examination included a complete medical history, physical examination and blood/urine collections. Prevalent diabetes was defined according to the American Diabetes Association (ADA) criteria as fasting (≥ 8 h) glucose ≥ 126 mg/dL, or hemoglobin A1c (HbA1C) $\geq 6.5\%$ or use of diabetic medication (actual or self-reported) within 2 weeks prior to the clinic visit). Body mass index (BMI) was defined as the weight in kilograms divided by the height in meters squared. Clinic blood pressure (BP) was measured using random zero sphygmomanometer (Hawksley and Sons Ltd., Lancing, UK) following appropriate procedure; whereby the participants' rested for 5 min in an upright position with their back and arms supported and a trained staff took two BP measurements in the right arm. The two clinic-measured BP were averaged to obtain the BP value used in the analysis. Fasting total and high-density lipoprotein (HDL) cholesterol were measured and quantified by an oxidase method and expressed as total to HDL ratio. Nephalometric immunoassay and enzymatic methods were used to quantify urinary albumin from a timed 24-h urine collection and a random spot morning urine collection [19]. Albuminuria was defined as a urinary-albumin-to-urinary-creatinine ratio (ACR) ≥ 30 mg/g using both methods. Current smoking status was defined as yes in participants who had smoked over 400 cigarettes in their lifetime and were actively smoking at the time of the baseline examination.

Statistical analysis

All biomarkers were naturally log-transformed and standardized (mean = 0 and variance = 1) within sex to normalize their skewed distributions and also to account for sex-related differences. We performed separate analyses for incident CKD and RKFD by fitting 2 different models: i) the traditional model that consisted of known independent risk factors for CKD such as systolic blood pressure, hypertension, use of antihypertensive medication, current smoking status, body mass index, total cholesterol to HDL ratio, and diabetes; and ii) the biomarker model that consisted of CKD traditional risk factors and biomarkers. For the biomarker model, we first tested the relation of the entire biomarker panel with each outcome, and if the biomarker panel was statistically significant, we used backward elimination to identify a parsimonious subset of biomarkers that remained significantly associated with incident CKD and RKFD. The retained biomarkers were thereafter used to construct weighted multi-marker score following the approach applied by Wang et al. [29]. The sum of sex-standardized log-biomarker concentration weighed by the estimated regression coefficients of each selected biomarker constituted the risk score on a continuous scale. We then used the risk score as a continuous predictor or categorized using quartiles to evaluate its association with each outcome. For secondary analyses, we stratified by obesity status in our effort to understand obesity's moderating effects on the association of biomarkers with the outcomes, considering that the Jackson Heart Study participants are on average obese (BMI > 30 kg/m^2). Additionally, we compared the biomarkers distributions between included versus excluded participants using Wilcoxon rank-sum test.

To understand the utility of the biomarkers in the prediction of incident CKD and RKFD we compared the performance of the biomarker model with the traditional model. We computed performance metrics that included change in the C-statistic to assess model discrimination, and Integrated discrimination index (IDI) and net reclassification index (NRI) [16, 30] to assess reclassification improvement. IDI and NRI quantifies the model's ability to predict outcome when biomarkers are included in addition to traditional risk factors. Calibration was evaluated with Hosmer-Lemeshow goodness-of-fit test with P-value < 0.05 indicating a poorly calibrated model. Data were imputed for participants with missing covariates ($n = 206$), with 20 data sets using fully conditional specification (FCS) [31]. In FCS, imputations are generated sequentially by specifying an imputation model for each variable given the other variables. In this way, FCS is suited for imputing data of variables with different scales and complex relations with each other. The percentage of missing for each variable included in the analysis was 0.07% for BMI, 0.11% for SBP, 5.65% for total cholesterol to HDL ratio, 0.78% for antihypertensive medication, 0.04% for diabetes and 0.78% for current cigarette smoking status. We used the SAS EG statistical software version 7.1 for all statistical tests and SAS macro developed by Kennedy and Pencina for model performance evaluation [32]. All statistical significance was defined as two-tailed $P \leq 0.05$. For analysis of the structure of association between biomarkers and outcome, we used Generalized Additive Models implemented in R to check for non-linearity.

Results

Baseline study characteristics

Demographic, clinical and biomarker distributions at exam 1 are presented in Table 1. We included 2813 JHS participants in our analytic cohort based on various inclusion criteria. A consort diagram of the exclusions performed in our analyses is shown in Fig. 1. Mean age of the study cohort at baseline was 54 years, 62.8% were women, the mean body mass index (BMI) was 31.9 ± 7.3, while 16.6% had diabetes and 47.5% reported taking blood pressure medications. The average estimated GFR at baseline was 98.08 ± 17.76 ml/min/1.73m^2. eGFR declined 9.93% (median 8.10; ranged from 0.00 to 18.00%) between Exam 1 and Exam 3 (8.2 median follow-up years).

Table 1 Baseline characteristics of study participants ($N = 2607$)

Characteristics	Mean ± SD
Age, years	53 ± 12
Female, % (n)	63 (1636)
BMI, kg/m^2	31.9 ± 7.3
SBP, mmHg	125.9 ± 15.7
Baseline eGFR, mL/min per 1.73 m^2	98.1 ± 17.7
Total cholesterol to HDL ratio	4.1 ± 1.3
Blood pressure medications, % (n)	47.5 (1238)
Diabetes, % (n)	16.6 (432)
Current smoking, % (n)	11.7 (306)
Biomarker level	Median (25th, 75th percentiles)
Adiponectin, ng/mL	4037.0 (2640.1, 6339.2)
Aldosterone, ng/mL	4.3 (2.5, 6.9)
BNP, pg/mL	6.7 (2.3, 14.8)
hsCRP, mg/dL	0.3 (0.1, 0.6)
Endothelin, pg/mL	1.2 (0.9, 1.6)
Homocysteine, μmol/dL	8.4 (7.2, 9.9)
Leptin, ng/mL	22.9 (10.1, 39.3)
Plasma renin activity, ng/mL/hr	0.4 (0.2, 1.0)
Active renin mass concentration, pg/mL	6.7 (5.1, 9.4)

Data presented as mean ± standard deviation (SD) for continuous variables and percentage (count) for dichotomous variables unless otherwise indicated
Abbreviations: *BMI* body mass index, *SBP* systolic blood pressure, *eGFR* estimated glomerular filtration rate, *HDL* high-density lipoprotein cholesterol, *hsCRP* high-sensitive c-reactive protein, *BNP* B-type natriuretic peptide

Association of multi-marker panel with incident CKD

During a median follow-up period of 8.2 years, 10.5% ($n = 178$ women) of participants developed incident CKD. We observed that the multi-marker panel was significantly associated with the development of CKD ($P = 0.004$) on follow-up. Upon backward elimination, continuous log plasma adiponectin ($P = 0.005$) and leptin concentrations ($P = 0.011$) were retained as significantly associated with incident CKD. We also tested the association of high levels (based on data derived quartiles) of plasma adiponectin and leptin with incident CKD. The multivariable adjusted odds ratios (ORs) and 95% confidence intervals (95% CI) are summarized in Table 2. High levels of log plasma adiponectin (OR, 1.66; 95% CI, 1.08–2.55) and leptin (OR, 2.00; 95% CI 2.00; *P*-value = 0.022); 95% CI, 1.18–3.38; *P*-value = 0.009) were significantly associated with incident CKD. In addition, moderate levels (second quartile) of plasma adiponectin were also significantly associated with incident CKD. When we combined adiponectin and leptin to form a multi-marker score, and found that the ORs almost doubled for the continuous multi-marker score. Both high and moderate levels of the multi-marker score were significantly associated with incident CKD. In Fig. 2a, the smoother splines show the structure of the multivariable relationship between plasma aldosterone with CKD. Moderate level of plasma aldosterone appeared to be protective against incident CKD development.

Association of multi-marker panel with rapid kidney function decline

During a median follow-up period of 8.2 years, 11.0% ($n = 202$ women) of participants developed RKFD, and the multi-marker panel was significantly associated with RKFD (*p*-value = 0.001). Adiponectin and aldosterone were retained as significant correlates of RKFD (Table 2). When divided into quartiles, with exception of aldosterone, which was protective (OR, 0.62; 95% CI, 0.43–0.89; *P*-value = 0.009), the highest quartile for adiponectin (OR, 1.49; 95% CI, 1.10–2.44; *P*-value =0.045) and medium quartile leptin level (OR, 1.64; 95% CI, 1.10–2.44; *P*-value = 0.015) were not significantly associated with RKFD. A multi-marker score that comprise the three biomarkers was significantly associated with the risk for RKFD both as a continuous and categorical states. A smoother splines, Fig. 2b depict the multivariable relationship between leptin with RKFD.

Secondary analyses

For secondary analyses, we compared the biomarkers distributions of participants included versus those

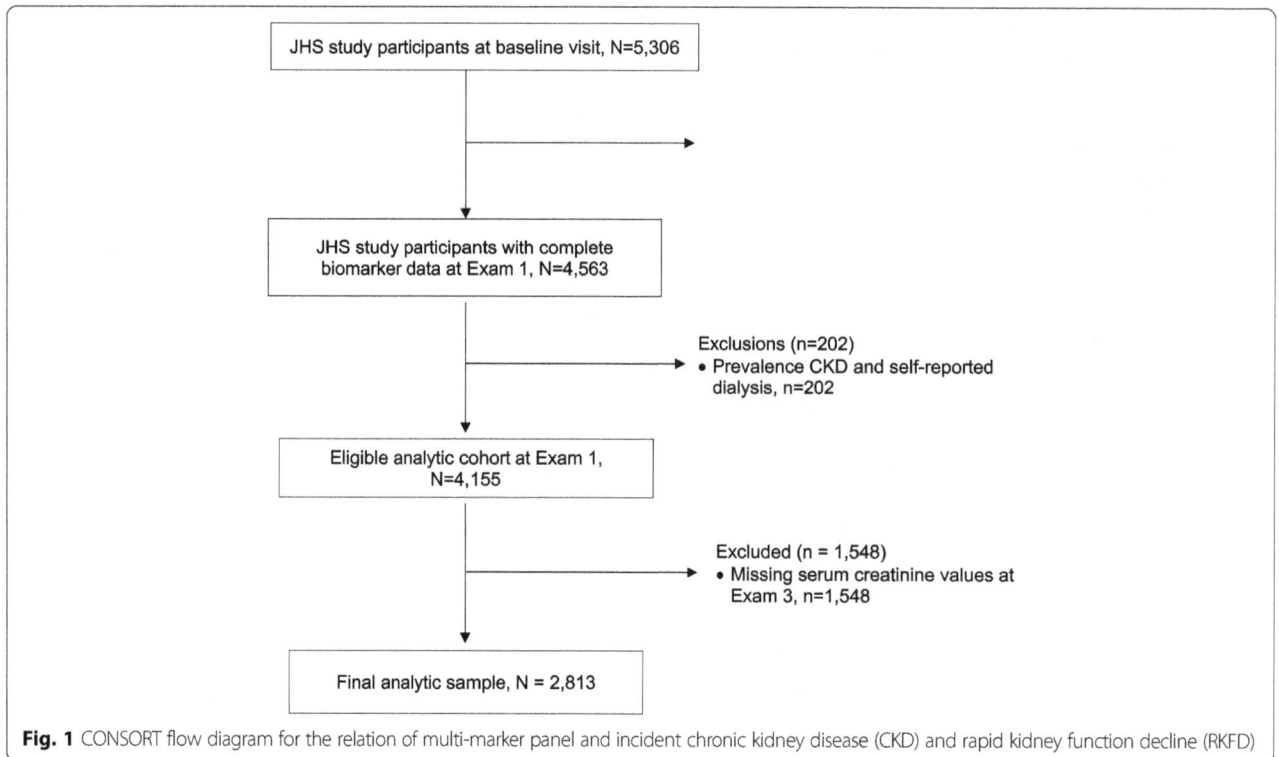

Fig. 1 CONSORT flow diagram for the relation of multi-marker panel and incident chronic kidney disease (CKD) and rapid kidney function decline (RKFD)

excluded from the analyses due and results are summarized on Additional file 1: Table S1. We also repeated the association analyses stratified by obesity status to assess whether obesity moderates the biomarker-incident CKD / RKFD relation. Only adiponectin concentrations interacted significantly with obesity status (P-value = 0.016). Results of the analysis stratified by obesity status, showed that high levels of both adiponectin and medium level of leptin were significantly associated with development of CKD among non-obese participants but not among obese participants. Similar results were evident for the multi-marker score combining adiponectin and leptin although among obese participants, the highest quartile (4th) of the risk score was also significantly associated with CKD. Stratified analyses of the association of adiponectin, aldosterone and leptin with RKFD showed a similar pattern as for incident CKD. In the leptin-RKFD relation however, the second quartile was significantly associated with RKFD but not the other quartiles suggesting possible non-linear relation (Additional file 1: Table S3).

Evaluation of model performance
The added predictive ability of the biomarker model in terms of improved discrimination and reclassification above the conventional CKD risk factors is shown in Table 3. The biomarker model exceeds the traditional CKD risk factor model by 1% in predicting incident

CKD and RKFD. With respect to reclassification improvement, the biomarker model reclassified 11% and 15% CKD and RKFD events, respectively compared to the traditional model. Moreover, the predicted mean probability of events was significantly different between biomarker and traditional CKD risk factor models, with the former performing better than the later.

Discussion
We investigated the relation of a multi-marker panel with the development of incident CKD and RKFD in a large community-based sample of African Americans. We observed that a panel consisting of nine circulating biomarkers (adiponectin, aldosterone, BNP, hsCRP, endothelin, homocysteine, leptin, PRA, ARM) representing several distinct biologic pathways was associated with development of CKD and RKFD. We identified a smaller subset of biomarkers representing adiposity (adiponectin, leptin); and RAS (aldosterone) pathways that were also associated with these outcomes. Plasma adiponectin and leptin were both associated with development of CKD while plasma aldosterone had a protective effects against both CKD development and RKFD. The addition of biomarkers only marginally improved model discrimination and reclassification compared to the model with traditional risk factors as demonstrated by the small change in C-statistic and reclassification indices. In secondary analyses stratified by obesity status, selected biomarkers were significantly associated with

Table 2 Associations of multi-marker panel, individuals' biomarkers and multi-marker scores with incident CKD and rapid kidney function decline

Biomarkers	Incident CKD			Rapid Kidney Function Decline (RKFD)		
	Cases/ # at risk	Multivariable Adjusted Odds Ratio (95% CI)	P-value	Cases/ # at risk	Multivariable Adjusted Odds Ratio (95% CI)	P-value
Entire panel		2.72 (1.63, 4.56)	0.001		2.61 (1.67, 4.08)	0.001
Adiponectin						
Continuous		1.24 (1.07, 1.44)	0.005		1.22 (1.06, 1.40)	0.006
Q1	54/703	Reference		63/703	Reference	
Q2	71/703	1.37 (0.89, 2.09)	0.151	78/703	1.20 (0.83, 1.75)	0.330
Q3	72/704	1.31 (0.85, 2.02)	0.217	72/704	1.14 (0.77, 1.67)	0.515
Q4	98/703	1.66 (1.08, 2.55)	0.022	97/703	1.49 (1.02, 2.18)	0.045
Leptin						
Continuous		1.31 (1.06, 1.61)	0.011		1.12 (0.93, 1.34)	0.234
Q1	54/698	Reference	...	67/698	Reference	...
Q2	79/711	1.37 (0.89, 2.11)	0.151	77/711	1.13 (0.77, 1.66)	0.525
Q3	73/699	1.52 (0.95, 2.42)	0.079	90/699	1.64 (1.10, 2.44)	0.015
Q4	89/705	2.00 (1.18, 3.38)	0.009	76/705	1.29 (0.80, 2.06)	0.295
hsCRP						
Continuous		1.13 (0.96, 1.33)	0.149		1.17 (1.01, 1.36)	0.031
Q1	53/700	Reference	...	56/700	Reference	...
Q2	88/707	1.22 (0.80, 1.87)	0.358	81/707	1.12 (0.76, 1.65)	0.572
Q3	85/705	1.32 (0.86, 2.02)	0.212	88/705	1.25 (0.85, 1.84)	0.258
Q4	69/701	1.13 (0.71, 1.80)	0.593	85/701	1.28 (0.85, 1.92)	0.230
Aldosterone						
Continuous		0.92 (0.8,1.06)	0.229		0.85 (0.74, 0.96)	0.012
Q1	77/698	Reference	...	93/698	Reference	...
Q2	68/720	0.82 (0.55, 1.23)	0.347	80/720	0.88 (0.62,1.24)	0.461
Q3	58/707	0.54 (0.35, 0.82)	0.004	66/707	0.66 (0.46, 0.95)	0.026
Q4	92/688	0.68 (0.46, 1.04)	0.077	71/688	0.62 (0.43, 0.89)	0.009
Multi-marker Score						
0	40/651	Reference		42/651	Reference	
1	53/652	1.48 (0.94–2.33)	0.093	54/652	1.12 (0.75–1.67)	0.586
2	73/652	2.02 (1.30–3.14)	0.002	74/652	1.62 (1.11–2.37)	0.001
3	90/652	2.45 (1.53–3.91)	<.001	95/652	2.04 (1.40–2.99)	<.001

Abbreviations: *Q1* quartile 1, *Q2* quartile 2, *Q3* quartile 3, *Q4* quartile 4, *hsCRP* high-sensitive C-reactive protein

Incident chronic kidney disease (CKD) was defined a decline from eGFR ≥60 mL/min/1.73 m² at exam1 to eGFR < 60 mL/min/1.73 m² at exam 3 follow-up (median follow-up duration: 8.0 years)

Rapid kidney function decline (RKFD) was defined as a decline in estimated glomerular filtration rate (eGFR) ≥ 30% from exam 1 to exam 3 (median follow-up duration: 8.0 years)

Multivariate model for the estimation of ORs were for adjusted for age, sex, baseline estimated glomerular filtration rate (eGFR), systolic blood pressure, hypertension, use of hypertension medication, smoking, body mass index (BMI), total cholesterol to high-density lipoprotein cholesterol (HDL) ratio and diabetes

incident CKD and RKFD in non-obese participants only, suggesting modification by obesity status.

In our study, adiponectin and leptin, two of the key cytokines secreted by adipocytes, predicted the development of incident CKD in a multivariable adjusted model. These findings are consistent with previous studies that investigated their association with CKD. In a case-control study among Chinese and Indian adults, patients with CKD had higher levels of leptin and adiponectin compared to controls [33]. Similar findings were also found in a patient population comprised of 60% African Americans in the greater New Orleans, Louisiana region, after adjusting for race and other risk factors associated with kidney disease [34]. To the contrary, other studies have also reported no difference in adiponectin levels [35–37]. The link between adipokines and changes in glomerular filtration rate has

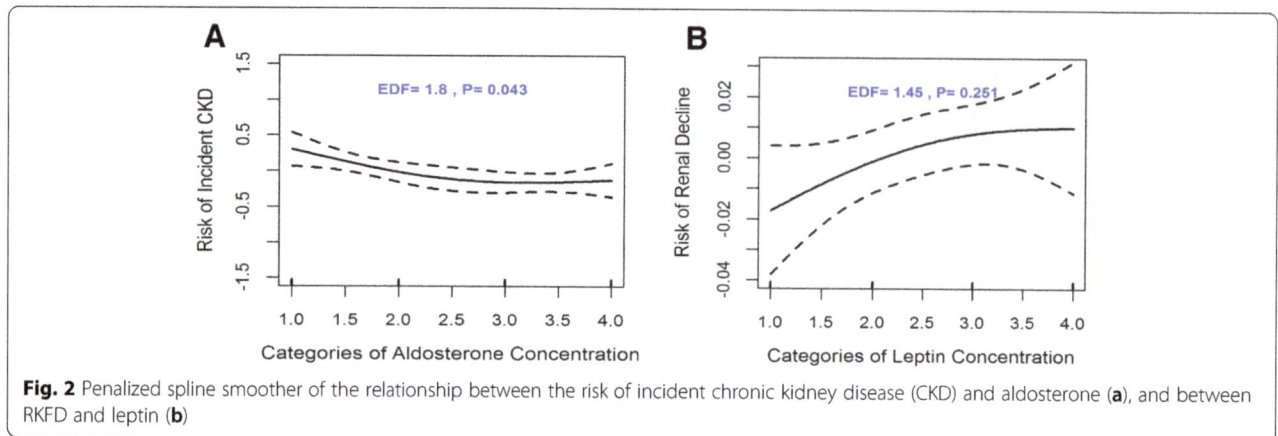

Fig. 2 Penalized spline smoother of the relationship between the risk of incident chronic kidney disease (CKD) and aldosterone (**a**), and between RKFD and leptin (**b**)

been reported previously [38]. Through endothelial dysfunction, oxidative stress and changes in immune response and inflammation, the adipokines are involved in kidney damage [39]. While serum aldosterone was reported to have weak but significant association with lower eGFR in Framingham Offspring Study, an inverse association where aldosterone appear to be protective was observed in this present study. Aldosterone's conflicting results are also reported in the Ohasama Study where the authors attributed the lack of association of aldosterone with eGFR to a high salt-intake resulting from high sodium dietary conditions [40, 41].

Studies on single biomarkers have reported on the relation of CRP and aldosterone with kidney function. Works by Fox and colleagues as well as Shankar and others showed that CRP is associated with prevalent CKD but not with the development of CKD [42, 43]. While previous studies both clinical and observational have demonstrated CRP's pathogenic role in renal

damage [44, 45], in the current analysis, CRP was not associated with the development of either CKD or RKFD. Hannemann and colleagues found an inverse association of plasma aldosterone concentration with eGFR in the general population [46]. In the present study, participants with medium level quartile and higher aldosterone level had 46% ($P = 0.004$) and 38% (P-value = 0.009) less likely to develop CKD or experience RKFD, respectively. When stratified by obesity status, biomarkers were associated with development of CKD and RKFD in non-obese, particularly for leptin and adiponectin. Biomarkers linkages to the development of CKD in the absence of obesity has been reported before even though the mechanism is poorly understood [38, 47].

Few community-based studies have evaluated kidney disease biomarkers to assess their usefulness in stratifying disease risk [3]. We undertook this study to address this gap in CKD literature. Data from the Framingham Heart Study (FHS) followed a multi-marker approach to

Table 3 Incremental predictive utility of biomarkers for incident chronic kidney disease (CKD), rapid kidney function decline (RKFD) showing C-statistics and reclassification metrics

	C-Statistics	NRI		IDI		Calibration Statistics[a] (χ^2, P)
		Events *correctly* reclassified	Non-Events *correctly* reclassified	Mean *probability* for events	Mean *probability* for non-events	
Chronic kidney disease (CKD)						
Model 1: age-sex-MV[b]	0.87	11%	5%	32%	7.4%	12.93 ($P = 0.11$)
Model 2: age-sex-MV-Biomarker[c]	0.88			33%	7.3%	14.26 ($P = 0.08$)
P-value comparing models 1 vs. 2	0.003	0.08	0.01	0.01		
Rapid kidney function decline						
Model 1: age-sex-MV	0.76	15%	11%	19.3%	9%	12.19 ($P = 0.14$)
Model 2: age-sex-MV-Biomarker[d]	0.77			20.3%	9%	18.42 ($P = 0.02$)
P-value comparing models 1 vs. 2	0.10	0.01	<.0001	0.0001		

Abbreviations: NRI net reclassification index, *IDI* integrated discrimination index
[a]A Hosmer-Lemeshow goodness-of-fit test indicate poor calibration if *P*-value < 0.05
[b]MV adjusted for age, sex, baseline estimated glomerular filtration rate (eGFR), systolic blood pressure, hypertension, use of hypertension medication, smoking, body mass index (BMI), total cholesterol to high-density lipoprotein cholesterol (HDL) ratio and diabetes
[c]In backward elimination of the biomarker panel, adiponectin and leptin are significant
[d]In backward elimination of the biomarker panel, adiponectin, high-sensitive C - reactive protein (CRP) and aldosterone are significant

predict incident CKD and microalbuminuria. A panel of seven biomarkers (C-reactive protein, aldosterone, renin, BNP, plasminogen-activator inhibitor type 1, fibrinogen, and homocysteine) was associated with the development of CKD with homocysteine and aldosterone retained as significant markers in the backward elimination model [10]. Our data extends these findings to a large community-based sample of African Americans in Mississippi. Unlike FHS where homocysteine and aldosterone were retained as significant markers for incident CKD prediction, in JHS adiponectin and leptin were the significant markers.

When comparing indices of model improvement the biomarker model was associated with the same change in C-statistic ($\Delta C = 0.01$) for prediction of incident CKD and RKFD. Researchers generally consider a change in C-statistic of at least 0.05 as indicative of a predictor with clinical significance [48]. While C statistics has been criticized for being insensitive to small changes in predictive accuracy [49], it was preferred here to permit easy comparison with findings in the literature, which often used the metric [50]. We also computed the NRI and IDI indices to complement C-statistic. Consistent with results based on C-statistics for the biomarker model, relative IDI had small but significant incremental predictive ability that was also higher than that reported in FHS. NRI though statistically non-significant was higher than that reported in FHS (JHS NRI = 16.1%, $P = 0.08$; FHS NRI = 6.9%, $P = 0.0004$). Though the metrics of model improvement are study/cohort specific, suffice it to say that they hold promise for CKD prediction in African Americans as is in white populations. The utility of biomarkers in improving disease prediction is highly successful in the area of cardiovascular medicine [50–52]; however, the yield has been relatively small in women and the elderly [53, 54]. With exception of Velagaleti et al. report on prediction of heart failure ($\Delta C = 0.02$) [55], most CVD research has reported lower incremental benefit compared to current analyses. This may be because CVD risk factors are well characterized and the existence of multiple risk-algorithms aid prediction, something which is lacking in CKD research.

Strengths and limitations

This study has some strengths and limitations. The analyses had a large sample size and a well-documented spectrum of biomarkers. We also adjusted for many CKD factors so the independent association between multi-marker panel and CKD development could be assessed. Some limitations require mentioning. Our sample was primarily African Americans, limiting generalizability to other ethnicities. JHS was designed to investigate CVD risk factors, thus the biomarkers collected were not specifically for CKD, although CVD is a

potent risk factor for CKD and CKD progression. Finally, with the study being observational in nature, it is possible that the CKD being detected might have developed at an earlier date.

Conclusions

In summary, while the predictive utility of biomarkers in these data were minimal, they do not exclude the role of using circulating biomarkers to provide insight into early development of CKD in this vulnerable population. Circulating adipokines (adiponectin, leptin), CRP and aldosterone biomarkers incrementally predicted incident CKD and RKFD in our large community-based sample.

Abbreviations
ACR: Albumin-creatinine ratio; ADA: American Diabetes Association; BMI: Body mass index; BNP: B-natriuretic peptide; BP: Blood pressure; CKD: Chronic kidney disease; CKD-EPI: Chronic Kidney Disease Epidemiology Collaboration creatinine equation; CVD: Cardiovascular disease; eGFR: Estimated glomerular filtration rate; FCS: Fully conditional specification; HDL: High-density lipoprotein; hsCRP: High sensitive C-reactive protein; IDI: Integrated discrimination index; JHS: Jackson Heart Study; NRI: Net reclassification index; RKFD: Rapid kidney function decline

Acknowledgements
The authors thank the participants and data collection staff of the Jackson Heart Study.

Funding
The Jackson Heart Study is supported by contracts HHSN268201300046C, HHSN268201300047C, HHSN268201300048C, HHSN268201300049C, HHSN268201300050C from the NHLBI and the NIMHD. This work was also supported by NIDDK grants R01 DK102134 (B.A.Y.) and R01HL117323 (P.M.). M.S. receives support through grants P60MD002249 and U54MD008176 from the NIMHD; 15SFDRN26140001 and P50HL120163 from the American Heart Association; and 1R01HL116446 from the NHLBI. B.A.Y. is also supported in part by funding from Veterans Affairs Puget Sound Health Care System. The funding sources have no role in the design and conduct of the study; collection, management, analysis, and interpretation of the data; preparation, review, or approval of the manuscript; or decision to submit the manuscript for publication.

Disclaimer
The views expressed in this manuscript are those of the authors and do not necessarily represent the views of the National Heart, Lung, and Blood Institute; the National Institutes of Health; or the U.S. Department of Health and Human Services.

Authors' contributions
SEM interpreted and drafted the manuscript. BY, AB, MS, and AC made substantial contributions to the interpretation of the data and critical revision of the manuscript. SKM was responsible for the study conception and design, data analysis, interpretation of the data and drafting and critical revision of the manuscript. All authors read and approved the final manuscript.

Competing interests
The authors declare that other than the disclosures and funding sources described herein, they have no competing interests.
The views expressed in this manuscript are those of the authors and do not

necessarily represent the views of the National Heart, Lung, and Blood Institute; the National Institutes of Health; the U.S. Department of Health and Human Services. The US Department of Veteran Affairs does not endorse any of the statement or opinions advocated by this article.

Author details

[1]Jackson Heart Study, Jackson State University, 350 W. Woodrow Wilson Ave., Suite 701, Jackson, MS 39213, USA. [2]Division of Nephrology, Kidney Research Institute University of Washington, Seattle, WA, USA. [3]Veterans Affairs Puget Sound Health Care System, Seattle, WA, USA. [4]Department of Medicine, University of Mississippi Medical Center, Jackson, MS, USA. [5]Department of Epidemiology and Biostatistics, School of Public Health, Indiana University, Bloomington, IN, USA.

References

1. Coresh J, Selvin E, Stevens LA, Manzi J, Kusek JW, Eggers P, Van Lente F, Levey AS. Prevalence of chronic kidney disease in the United States. JAMA. 2007;298(17):2038–47.
2. Young BA, Katz R, Boulware LE, Kestenbaum B, de Boer IH, Wang W, Fulop T, Bansal N, Robinson-Cohen C, Griswold M, et al. Risk factors for rapid kidney function decline among African Americans: the Jackson Heart Study (JHS). Am J Kidney Dis. 2016;68(2):229–39.
3. Zoccali C. Biomarkers in chronic kidney disease: utility and issues towards better understanding. Curr Opin Nephrol Hypertens. 2005;14(6):532–7.
4. Peralta CA, Katz R, Sarnak MJ, Ix J, Fried LF, De Boer I, Palmas W, Siscovick D, Levey AS, Shlipak MG. Cystatin C identifies chronic kidney disease patients at higher risk for complications. J Am Soc Nephrol. 2011;22(1):147–55.
5. Weekley CC, Peralta CA. Advances in the use of multimarker panels for renal risk stratification. Curr Opin Nephrol Hypertens. 2012;21(3):301–8.
6. Tarver-Carr ME, Powe NR, Eberhardt MS, LaVeist TA, Kington RS, Coresh J, Brancati FL. Excess risk of chronic kidney disease among African-American versus white subjects in the United States: a population-based study of potential explanatory factors. J Am Soc Nephrol. 2002;13(9):2363–70.
7. Dunkler D, Gao P, Lee SF, Heinze G, Clase CM, Tobe S, Teo KK, Gerstein H, Mann JF, Oberbauer R. Risk prediction for early CKD in type 2 diabetes. Clin J Am Soc Nephrol. 2015;10(8):1371–9.
8. Peters KE, Davis WA, Ito J, Winfield K, Stoll T, Bringans SD, Lipscombe RJ, Davis TME. Identification of novel circulating biomarkers predicting rapid decline in renal function in type 2 diabetes: the Fremantle diabetes study phase II. Diabetes Care. 2017;40(11):1548–55.
9. Looker HC, Colombo M, Hess S, Brosnan MJ, Farran B, Dalton RN, Wong MC, Turner C, Palmer CN, Nogoceke E, et al. Biomarkers of rapid chronic kidney disease progression in type 2 diabetes. Kidney Int. 2015;88(4):888–96.
10. Fox CS, Gona P, Larson MG, Selhub J, Tofler G, Hwang SJ, Meigs JB, Levy D, Wang TJ, Jacques PF, et al. A multi-marker approach to predict incident CKD and microalbuminuria. J Am Soc Nephrol. 2010;21(12):2143–9.
11. Gaggin HK, Januzzi JL Jr. Biomarkers and diagnostics in heart failure. Biochim Biophys Acta. 2013;1832(12):2442–50.
12. Musani SK, Vasan RS, Bidulescu A, Liu J, Xanthakis V, Sims M, Gawalapu RK, Samdarshi TE, Steffes M, Taylor HA, et al. Aldosterone, C-reactive protein, and plasma B-type natriuretic peptide are associated with the development of metabolic syndrome and longitudinal changes in metabolic syndrome components: findings from the Jackson Heart Study. Diabetes Care. 2013; 36(10):3084–92.
13. Ingelsson E, Pencina MJ, Tofler GH, Benjamin EJ, Lanier KJ, Jacques PF, Fox CS, Meigs JB, Levy D, Larson MG, et al. Multimarker approach to evaluate the incidence of the metabolic syndrome and longitudinal changes in metabolic risk factors: the Framingham offspring study. Circulation. 2007;116(9):984–92.
14. Mischak H, Delles C, Vlahou A, Vanholder R. Proteomic biomarkers in kidney disease: issues in development and implementation. Nat Rev Nephrol. 2015; 11(4):221–32.
15. Leening MJ, Vedder MM, Witteman JC, Pencina MJ, Steyerberg EW. Net reclassification improvement: computation, interpretation, and controversies: a literature review and clinician's guide. Ann Intern Med. 2014;160(2):122-131.
16. Pencina MJ, D'Agostino RB Sr, Steyerberg EW. Extensions of net reclassification improvement calculations to measure usefulness of new biomarkers. Stat Med. 2011;30(1):11–21.
17. Fuqua SR, Wyatt SB, Andrew ME, Sarpong DF, Henderson FR, Cunningham MF, Taylor HA Jr. Recruiting African-American research participation in the Jackson Heart Study: methods, response rates, and sample description. Ethn Dis. 2005;15(4 Suppl 6):S6-18-29.
18. Sempos CT, Bild DE, Manolio TA. Overview of the Jackson Heart Study: a study of cardiovascular diseases in african american men and women. Am J Med Sci. 1999;317(3):142-46.
19. Carpenter MA, Crow R, Steffes M, Rock W, Heilbraun J, Evans G, Skelton T, Jensen R, Sarpong D. Laboratory, reading center, and coordinating center data management methods in the Jackson Heart Study. Am J Med Sci. 2004;328(3):131–44.
20. Rebholz CM, Harman JL, Grams ME, Correa A, Shimbo D, Coresh J, Young BA. Association between endothelin-1 levels and kidney disease among blacks. J Am Soc Nephrol. 2017;28(11):3337-44.
21. Wang W, Young BA, Fulop T, de Boer IH, Boulware LE, Katz R, Correa A, Griswold ME. Effects of serum creatinine calibration on estimated renal function in african americans: the Jackson Heart Study. Am J Med Sci. 2015;349(5):379–84.
22. Inker LA, Schmid CH, Tighiouart H, Eckfeldt JH, Feldman HI, Greene T, Kusek JW, Manzi J, Van Lente F, Zhang YL, et al. Estimating glomerular filtration rate from serum creatinine and cystatin C. N Engl J Med. 2012;367(1):20–9.
23. Shlipak MG, Katz R, Kestenbaum B, Siscovick D, Fried L, Newman A, Rifkin D, Sarnak MJ. Rapid decline of kidney function increases cardiovascular risk in the elderly. J Am Soc Nephrol. 2009;20(12):2625–30.
24. Bash LD, Coresh J, Kottgen A, Parekh RS, Fulop T, Wang Y, Astor BC. Defining incident chronic kidney disease in the research setting: the ARIC study. Am J Epidemiol. 2009;170(4):414–24.
25. Coresh J, Turin TC, Matsushita K, Sang Y, Ballew SH, Appel LJ, Arima H, Chadban SJ, Cirillo M, Djurdjev O, et al. Decline in estimated glomerular filtration rate and subsequent risk of end-stage renal disease and mortality. Jama. 2014;311(24):2518–31.
26. Stevens LA, Schmid CH, Greene T, Zhang YL, Beck GJ, Froissart M, Hamm LL, Lewis JB, Mauer M, Navis GJ, et al. Comparative performance of the CKD epidemiology collaboration (CKD-EPI) and the modification of diet in renal disease (MDRD) study equations for estimating GFR levels above 60 mL/min/1.73 m2. Am J Kidney Dis. 2010;56(3):486–95.
27. Hiramoto JS, Katz R, Peralta CA, Ix JH, Fried L, Cushman M, Siscovick D, Palmas W, Sarnak M, Shlipak MG. Inflammation and coagulation markers and kidney function decline: the multi-ethnic study of atherosclerosis (MESA). Am J Kidney Dis. 2012;60(2):225–32.
28. Taylor HA Jr, Wilson JG, Jones DW, Sarpong DF, Srinivasan A, Garrison RJ, Nelson C, Wyatt SB. Toward resolution of cardiovascular health disparities in African Americans: design and methods of the Jackson Heart Study. Ethn Dis. 2005;15(4 Suppl 6):S6-4. 17
29. Wang TJ, Larson MG, Levy D, Benjamin EJ, Leip EP, Omland T, Wolf PA, Vasan RS. Plasma natriuretic peptide levels and the risk of cardiovascular events and death. N Engl J Med. 2004;350(7):655–63.
30. Pencina MJ, D'Agostino RB Sr, D'Agostino RB Jr, Vasan RS. Evaluating the added predictive ability of a new marker: from area under the ROC curve to reclassification and beyond. Stat Med. 2008;27(2):157–72. discussion 207-112
31. Liu Y, De A. Multiple imputation by fully conditional specification for dealing with missing data in a large epidemiologic study. Int J Stat Med Res. 2015;4(3):287–95.
32. Kennedy K, Pencina M: A SAS® macro to compute added predictive ability of new markers predicting a dichotomous outcome. SouthEeast SAS users group annual meeting proceedings 2010.
33. Lim CC, Teo BW, Tai ES, Lim SC, Chan CM, Sethi S, Wong TY, Sabanayagam C. Elevated serum leptin, adiponectin and leptin to adiponectin ratio is associated with chronic kidney disease in Asian adults. PLoS One. 2015; 10(3):e0122009.
34. Mills KT, Hamm LL, Alper AB, Miller C, Hudaihed A, Balamuthusamy S, Chen CS, Liu Y, Tarsia J, Rifai N, et al. Circulating adipocytokines and chronic kidney disease. PLoS One. 2013;8(10):e76902.
35. Guebre-Egziabher F, Bernhard J, Funahashi T, Hadj-Aissa A, Fouque D. Adiponectin in chronic kidney disease is related more to metabolic disturbances than to decline in renal function. Nephrol Dial Transplant. 2005;20(1):129–34.
36. Yaturu S, Reddy RD, Rains J, Jain SK. Plasma and urine levels of resistin and adiponectin in chronic kidney disease. Cytokine. 2007;37(1):1–5.

37. Becker B, Kronenberg F, Kielstein JT, Haller H, Morath C, Ritz E, Fliser D. Renal insulin resistance syndrome, adiponectin and cardiovascular events in patients with kidney disease: the mild and moderate kidney disease study. J Am Soc Nephrol. 2005;16(4):1091–8.

38. Briffa JF, McAinch AJ, Poronnik P, Hryciw DH. Adipokines as a link between obesity and chronic kidney disease. Am J Physiol Renal Physiol. 2013; 305(12):F1629–36.

39. Ruster C, Wolf G. Adipokines promote chronic kidney disease. Nephrol Dial Transplant. 2013;28(Suppl 4):iv8–14.

40. Terata S, Kikuya M, Satoh M, Ohkubo T, Hashimoto T, Hara A, Hirose T, Obara T, Metoki H, Inoue R, et al. Plasma renin activity and the aldosterone-to-renin ratio are associated with the development of chronic kidney disease: the Ohasama study. J Hypertens. 2012;30(8):1632–8.

41. Jurgens G, Graudal NA. Effects of low sodium diet versus high sodium diet on blood pressure, renin, aldosterone, catecholamines, cholesterols, and triglyceride. Cochrane Database Syst Rev. 2004;(1):Cd004022.

42. Fox ER, Benjamin EJ, Sarpong DF, Nagarajarao H, Taylor JK, Steffes MW, Salahudeen AK, Flessner MF, Akylbekova EL, Fox CS, et al. The relation of C--reactive protein to chronic kidney disease in African Americans: the Jackson Heart Study. BMC Nephrol. 2010;11(1).

43. Shankar A, Sun L, Klein BE, Lee KE, Muntner P, Nieto FJ, Tsai MY, Cruickshanks KJ, Schubert CR, Brazy PC, et al. Markers of inflammation predict the long-term risk of developing chronic kidney disease: a population-based cohort study. Kidney Int. 2011;80(11):1231–8.

44. Remuzzi G, Cattaneo D, Perico N. The aggravating mechanisms of aldosterone on kidney fibrosis. J Am Soc Nephrol. 2008;19(8):1459–62.

45. Del Vecchio L, Procaccio M, Vigano S, Cusi D. Mechanisms of disease: the role of aldosterone in kidney damage and clinical benefits of its blockade. Nat Clin Pract Nephrol. 2007;3(1):42–9.

46. Hannemann A, Rettig R, Dittmann K, Volzke H, Endlich K, Nauck M, Wallaschofski H. Aldosterone and glomerular filtration--observations in the general population. BMC Nephrol. 2014;15:44.

47. Stepien M, Stepien A, Wlazel RN, Paradowski M, Banach M, Rysz M, Rysz J. Obesity indices and adipokines in non-diabetic obese patients with early stages of chronic kidney disease. Med Sci Monit. 2013;19:1063–72.

48. May A, Wang TJ. Biomarkers for cardiovascular disease: challenges and future directions. Trends Mol Med. 2008;14(6):261–7.

49. Cook NR. Use and misuse of the receiver operating characteristic curve in risk prediction. Circulation. 2007;115(7):928–35.

50. Wang TJ, Gona P, Larson MG, Tofler GH, Levy D, Newton-Cheh C, Jacques PF, Rifai N, Selhub J, Robins SJ, et al. Multiple biomarkers for the prediction of first major cardiovascular events and death. N Engl J Med. 2006;355(25):2631–9.

51. Melander O, Newton-Cheh C, Almgren P, Hedblad B, Berglund G, Engstrom G, Persson M, Smith JG, Magnusson M, Christensson A, et al. Novel and conventional biomarkers for prediction of incident cardiovascular events in the community. JAMA. 2009;302(1):49–57.

52. Kavousi M, Desai CS, Ayers C, Blumenthal RS, Budoff MJ, Mahabadi AA, Ikram MA, van der Lugt A, Hofman A, Erbel R, et al. Prevalence and prognostic implications of coronary artery calcification in low-risk women: a meta-analysis. JAMA. 2016;316(20):2126–34.

53. Zethelius B, Berglund L, Sundstrom J, Ingelsson E, Basu S, Larsson A, Venge P, Arnlov J. Use of multiple biomarkers to improve the prediction of death from cardiovascular causes. N Engl J Med. 2008;358(20):2107–16.

54. Ridker PM, Buring JE, Rifai N, Cook NR. Development and validation of improved algorithms for the assessment of global cardiovascular risk in women: the Reynolds risk score. Jama. 2007;297(6):611–9.

55. Velagaleti RS, Gona P, Larson MG, Wang TJ, Levy D, Benjamin EJ, Selhub J, Jacques PF, Meigs JB, Tofler GH, et al. Multimarker approach for the prediction of heart failure incidence in the community. Circulation. 2010; 122(17):1700–6.

The National Kidney Foundation of Illinois KidneyMobile: a mobile resource for community based screenings of chronic kidney disease and its risk factors

Swati Lederer[1,2,3,4*], Laurie Ruggiero[6,7], Nicole M. Sisen[5], Nancy Lepain[5], Kate Grubbs O'Connor[5], Yamin Wang[6], Jinsong Chen[3], James P. Lash[3] and Michael J. Fischer[1,2,3]

Abstract

Background: Early detection and treatment of chronic kidney disease (CKD) and its risk factors improves outcomes; however, many high-risk individuals lack access to healthcare. The National Kidney Foundation of Illinois (NKFI) developed the KidneyMobile (KM) to conduct community-based screenings, provide disease education, and facilitate follow-up appointments for diabetes, hypertension, and CKD.

Methods: Cross-sectional design. Adults $\geq$ 18 years of age participated in NKFI KM screenings across Illinois between 2005 and 2011. Sociodemographic and medical history were self-reported using structured interviews; laboratory data and blood pressure were assessed using standard procedures.

Results: Among 20,770 participants, mean age was 53.5 years, 68% were female, 49% were African-American or Hispanic, 21% primarily spoke Spanish, and at least 27% lacked health insurance. Seventy-eight percent of participants with elevated blood pressure ($\geq$ 140/90 mmHg) were aware of having hypertension, 93% of participants with abnormal blood glucose (fasting glucose > 126 mg/dl or a random glucose of > 200 mg/dL) were aware of having diabetes, and 19% of participants with albuminuria (> 30 mg/gm) were aware of having CKD. In participants reporting hypertension, 47% had blood pressure $\geq$ 140/90 mmHg, and in those reporting diabetes, 56% had blood glucose $\geq$ 130 mg/dl (fasting) or $\geq$ 180 mg/dl (random). Among 4937 participants with abnormal screening findings that participated in follow-up interviews, 69% reported having further medical evaluation.

Conclusions: A high-risk disadvantaged population is being reached by the NKFI KidneyMobile and connected with healthcare services. A significant proportion of participants were newly informed of having abnormal results suggestive of diabetes, hypertension, and/or CKD or that their diabetes and hypertension were inadequately controlled.

Keywords: Kidney disease, Diabetes, Hypertension, Screening, Awareness

Background

Chronic kidney disease (CKD) is a common and costly disease affecting approximately 14% of the adult population in the United States and accounting for approximately 20% of Medicare Part A and B costs [1]. Despite the significant utilization of healthcare services among this patient population, CKD continues to be strongly associated with poorer patient outcomes including an increased risk of death, cardiovascular events, end-stage kidney disease (ESKD), and hospitalizations [1, 2].

Large screening initiatives such as the National Health and Nutrition Examination Survey (NHANES) and the Kidney Early Evaluation Program (KEEP) have found that most adults afflicted with CKD are unaware of their diagnosis [3–5]. Furthermore, awareness of comorbid conditions that increase risk of CKD, such as diabetes and hypertension, is also suboptimal. The under-recognition

* Correspondence: swati.lederer@va.gov
[1]Center of Innovation for Complex Chronic Healthcare, Jesse Brown VA Medical Center, Chicago, IL, USA
[2]Edward Hines Jr. VA Hospital, Hines, IL, USA
Full list of author information is available at the end of the article

and delayed treatment of CKD and its associated health problems hastens disease progression and contributes to the growth of the ESKD population [3, 5–10]. Studies also show that low socio-economic subgroups, African Americans, and Hispanics have lower disease awareness and carry a higher burden of ESKD compared to the general population [11–13]. These vulnerable populations may have barriers to accessing healthcare resulting in later diagnoses of medical conditions [11–14]. Improving awareness of CKD and its comorbid conditions allows patients to seek the appropriate medical management, obtain fundamental disease knowledge, and participate in disease management.

Mobile screening initiatives have been successful in identifying individuals who may not otherwise seek medical care and facilitating the early diagnosis of silent diseases (e.g., CKD, hypertension, diabetes, and breast cancer) [15–19]. While findings from broad screening initiatives for hypertension, diabetes, and kidney disease are well-known, community-based mobile screening programs targeting under-insured individuals without access to primary care providers have not been well characterized. In addition to facilitating early diagnoses, these initiatives often provide individuals with health education and primary care follow up. Community-based screening initiatives also help educate public health officials and health providers about the burden of disease within specific communities and may inform the development and implementation of targeted interventions.

The National Kidney Foundation of Illinois (NKFI) developed a KidneyMobile (KM) as a mobile screening vehicle in 2005 to enhance the detection of hypertension, diabetes, and kidney disease in high-risk and vulnerable communities across Illinois. Working with community partners, the NKFI KM has conducted almost 41,000 screenings for diabetes, hypertension, and kidney disease in underserved areas between the years of 2005–2014. The KM also provides interactive educational activities and facilitates healthcare provider follow up for participants with abnormal screening results who lack access to healthcare services. To characterize the population reached by screenings and to evaluate the impact of this program, we examined data collected from 20,770 participating individuals between the years of 2005–2011.

Methods
Study sample and design
We conducted a cross-sectional analysis of data from NKFI KM participants throughout Illinois between 2005 and 2011. A total of 23,166 adult participants over the age of 18 were voluntarily screened. The NKFI KM was developed to conduct free screenings, provide disease education (diabetes, hypertension, CKD), and facilitate healthcare appointments for participants. The NKFI

partnered with federally qualified health centers, health departments, and community hospitals in underserved areas to ensure that we targeted a high-risk population, characterized by substantial proportions of underinsured as well as uninsured adults without ready access to health care. Examples of such high-risk groups in our screenings included urban communities with significant percentages of African American and Hispanic adults subject to health disparities and rural communities with geographic barriers to health care services. Additionally, screening sites were selected based on their ability to provide resources for the screening day (e.g., volunteers, space, equipment) and post-screening follow up care.

A screening visit consisted of three stages and was led by a nurse who was assisted by trained healthcare volunteers. First, sociodemographic information, medical history, vital signs, anthropometric measures, and laboratory tests were obtained from participants. Second, educational information related to healthy living, hypertension, diabetes, and CKD was provided to participants. Third, participants with abnormal screening results met individually with a healthcare provider for further consultation. Those participants who had health insurance were directed back to their primary care provider, while those participants without health insurance were provided with a healthcare referral for a follow up appointment at a federally qualified health center or community hospital. Finally, attempts were made to reach participants with abnormal screening tests, by telephone for follow up to ensure that they had visited a healthcare provider following screening.

IRB approval from the University of Illinois at Chicago was obtained for analysis of these screening data, which had originally been obtained for non-research purposes.

Variables and data sources
Sociodemographic characteristics were self-reported by participants on a 19-item questionnaire at the initial screening visit. These characteristics included age, sex, race/ethnicity (white, African-American, Hispanic, Asian/Pacific Islander, other), primary language (English, Spanish, other), presence of health insurance and primary provider, and personal or family history of hypertension, diabetes, kidney disease. Height, weight, and manual blood pressure were measured by a trained nurse per standard protocols [20]. If the systolic blood pressure was greater than 160 mmHg, the reading was repeated. Blood glucose measurements were drawn and analyzed via the One Touch Ultra-2 device [21]. After collecting a clean catch midstream urine sample from all participants, a urine dipstick and a urine microalbumin were analyzed onsite by Clinitek device [22]. Any participant with albuminuria (defined below), personal history of diabetes, or an abnormal serum glucose testing was

offered a blood test to measure serum creatinine, either on site by the Abbott I-stat Chem 8+ or by a nearby hospital laboratory [23].

Definition of variables

We defined prevalent hypertension as participants who self-reported a history of hypertension, or those who had a systolic blood pressure ≥ 140 mmHg or a diastolic pressure ≥ 90 mmHg, while recognizing that a definitive diagnosis of hypertension cannot be made by a single blood pressure measurement. Among those participants with prevalent hypertension, awareness of hypertension was defined as an affirmative to the following questionnaire item: "Have you ever been told you have high blood pressure or hypertension?". Among participants who reported a history of hypertension, control of the disease was defined as having both a systolic blood pressure of < 140 mmHg and a diastolic blood pressure of < 90 mmHg.

We defined prevalent diabetes as participants who self-reported a history of diabetes, a fasting serum glucose ≥ 126 mg/dl or a non-fasting glucose ≥ 200 mg/dl, recognizing that a definitive diagnosis of diabetes cannot be made by a single blood glucose measurement and requires confirmatory testing [24]. Among participants with prevalent diabetes, awareness of diabetes was defined as an affirmative to the following questionnaire item: "Have you ever been told that you have diabetes or high blood sugar?". Among those participants reporting a history of diabetes, control of the disease was defined as a fasting blood glucose of < 130 mg/dl or a non-fasting blood glucose of < 180 mg/dl [24].

We defined prevalent chronic kidney disease as participants self-reporting a history of kidney disease or those with a urine albumin to creatinine ratio of ≥ 30 mg/gm, recognizing that diagnosis of kidney disease cannot be made by a single urine measurement [25]. Among those with prevalent CKD, awareness of the condition was defined as an affirmative to the following questionnaire item: "Have you ever been told you have kidney disease?"

A small subset of the total cohort underwent blood testing to measure serum creatinine. Among those participants, eGFR was calculated using the modification of diet in renal disease (MDRD) equation [26].

Statistical analysis

All sociodemographic, clinical and laboratory data from participants screened was organized into analytic datasets. Participant characteristics were summarized using means with standard error for continuous variables and frequency distribution with percentages for categorical variables. Characteristics were compared across strata of albuminuria by Chi-Squared or ANOVA testing as appropriate. Missing values occurred under the following circumstances: i) when a participant failed to answer a question on a reporting form, ii) when a physical measure was not obtained, iii) when a laboratory test was not performed. All statistical summaries were conducted using SAS, version 9.1 (Cary, NC, USA).

Results

Participant sociodemographic and clinical characteristics

Out of a total of 23,166 adults participating in Kidney-Mobile screenings across Illinois from 2005 to 2011, 20,770 had complete data regarding age, sex, and race/ethnicity, and were included in the final analytic cohort. Figure 1 illustrates the geographic distribution of the KM screening across Illinois. Nearly half of the participants (54%) were from the greater Chicago area, 44% were from the remainder of Illinois, and 2% were not known.

The mean age of participants was 53.5 years, approximately 68% were female, 58% were of non-White racial/ethnic background, and 21% reported Spanish as their primary language (Table 1). A large percentage of participants either lacked health insurance (27%) or were unsure if they had active insurance (13%), and 50% did not have or did not know if they had a primary care provider. While 39% of participants reported a history of hypertension, 20% and only 5% of participants reported a history of diabetes mellitus and kidney disease, respectively. A family history of hypertension (54%) and diabetes (43%) were common among participants, but a family history of kidney disease was reported by only 12%. Among all participants, 31% were overweight (BMI 25–29.9), 29% were obese (BMI 30–39.9), and 6% were morbidly obese (BMI > 40). The mean systolic and diastolic blood pressure among participants was 127.5 mmHg (se 0.13) and 76.6 mmHg (se 0.08), respectively. Most participants (72%) had fasting or non-fasting blood glucose levels within normal range.

Most participants (74%) had no evidence of albuminuria, whereas 20% were found to have between 30 and 300 mg/gm of albuminuria and 1.5% were found to have > 300 mg/gm of albuminuria. Approximately 4% of screening participants did not have a urine microalbumin screen. Participant characteristics differed substantially across strata of albuminuria (Table 1). Mean age was significantly higher with increasing albuminuria ($p < 0.001$). Participants with albuminuria (> 30 mg/gm) were more likely to report a personal history of hypertension, diabetes, and kidney disease compared to participants without albuminuria ($p < 0.001$). Albuminuria was also more common among participants who reported a family history of hypertension, diabetes, and kidney disease. Less consistent changes were observed with other sociodemographic characteristics.

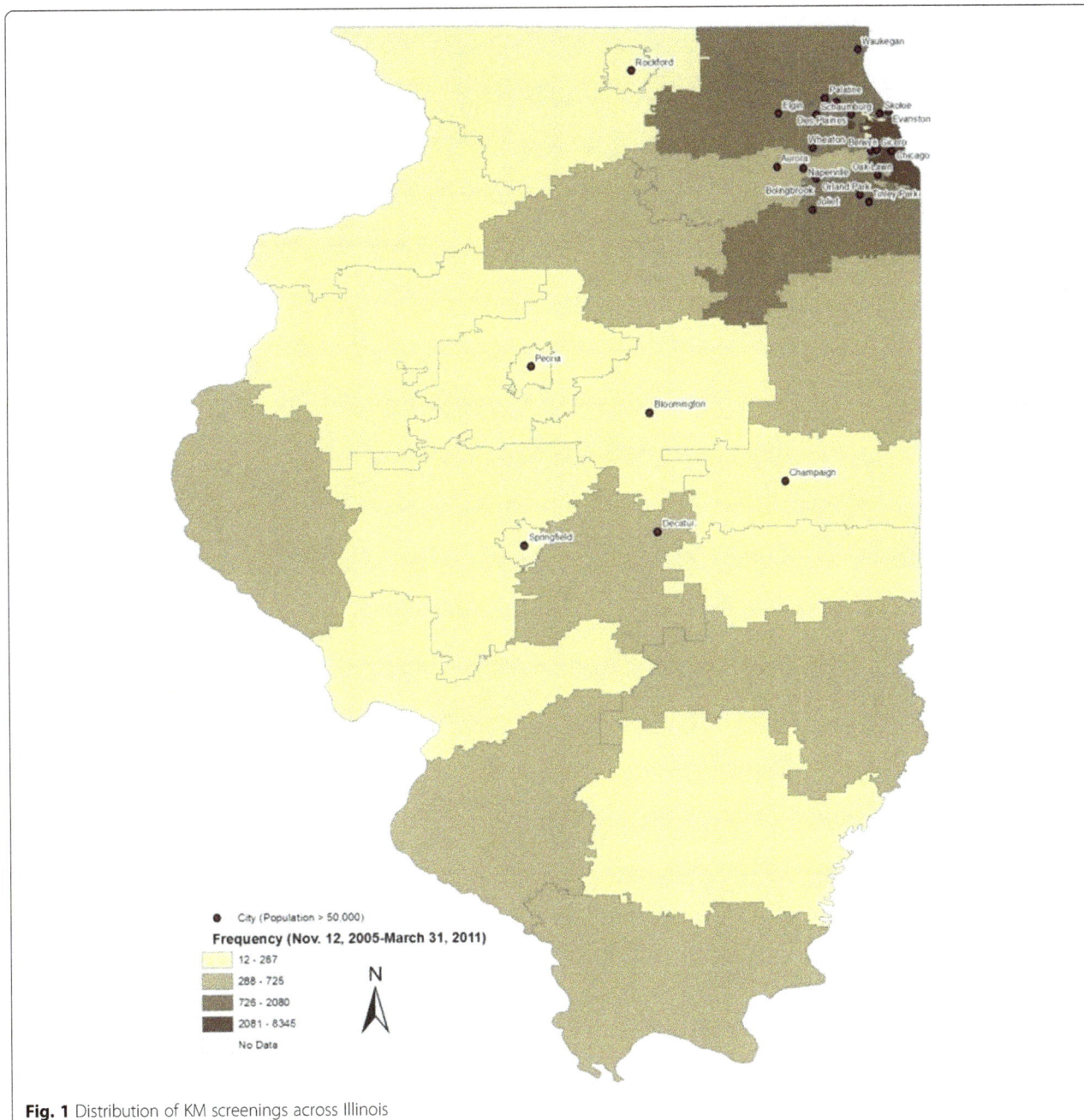

Fig. 1 Distribution of KM screenings across Illinois

Mean systolic and diastolic blood pressure increased significantly with higher albuminuria. The mean systolic blood pressure for participants without albuminuria was 126.3 mmHg, 130.8 mmHg for those with 30-300 mg/gm albuminuria, and 143.3 mmHg for those with > 300 mg/gm albuminuria (p-value < 0.001). Diastolic blood pressure also increased with higher albuminuria: 76.1 mmHg in participants without albuminuria, 77.8 mmHg among those with 30-300 mg/gm of albuminuria, and 80.4 mmHg among those with > 300 mg/gm of albuminuria (p-value < 0.001).

Increasing albuminuria was associated with poorer blood glucose control. Four percent of participants without albuminuria had a fasting blood glucose of > 126 mg/dl or a non-fasting glucose > 200, whereas 10% of participants with 30-300 mg/gm and 22% of those with > 300 mg/gm of albuminuria had abnormal blood glucose levels.

Estimated glomerular filtration rate among a subgroup of patients with abnormal screening results

A total of 4014 participants with albuminuria and either hypertension or diabetes underwent serum blood testing and calculation of eGFR (Table 2). There was a significant association between albuminuria and eGFR (p < 0.001).

Table 1 Participant Sociodemographic and Clinical Characteristics Stratified by Albuminuria

Characteristic	ALL N (%) or Mean (se)	Urine albumin/crt < 30 N (%)	Urine albumin/crt 30–300 N (%)	Urine albumin/crt > 300 N (%)	p-value	Unknown/Not tested N (%) or Mean (s.e.)
Total	20,770	15,396 (74.1)	4173 (20.1)	311 (1.5)		890 (4.3)
Age[a]	53.5 (0.12)	53.09 (0.13)	55.26 (0.27)	61.42 (0.94)	< 0.001	50.35 (0.58)
Sex					< 0.001	
Male	6717 (32.3)	5051 (32.8)	1246 (29.9)	120 (38.6)		300 (33.7)
Female	14,053 (67.7)	10,345 (67.2)	2927 (70.1)	191 (61.4)		590 (66.3)
Race/ethnicity					< 0.001	
White (non-Hispanic)	8801 (42.4)	6673 (43.3)	1693 (40.6)	144 (46.3)		291 (32.7)
African-American	4346 (20.9)	3062 (19.9)	1015 (24.3)	55 (17.7)		214 (24.04)
Hispanic	5838 (28.1)	4365 (28.4)	1130 (27.1)	78 (25.1)		265 (29.8)
Asian/Pacific Islander	934 (4.5)	713 (4.63)	156 (3.8)	20 (6.4)		45 (5.1)
Other/unknown	505 (2.43)	350 (2.3)	98 (2.4)	5 (1.6)		52 (5.8)
Primary language					< 0.001	
English	13,736 (66.1)	10,131 (65.8)	2944 (70.6)	222 (71.4)		439 (49.3)
Spanish	4417 (21.3)	3289 (21.36)	890 (21.3)	64 (20.6)		174 (19.6)
Other/unknown	2108 (10.15)	1580 (10.26)	250 (6.0)	11 (3.5)		267 (30.0)
Health insurance					0.1130	
Yes	12,524 (60.3)	9399 (61.1)	2583 (61.9)	184 (59.2)		358 (40.2)
No	5561 (26.8)	4171 (27.1)	1156 (27.7)	90 (28.9)		144 (16.2)
Unknown	2685 (12.9)	1826 (11.9)	434 (10.4)	37 (11.9)		388 (43.6)
Primary Provider					< 0.001	
Yes	10,311 (49.6)	7722 (50.2)	2118 (50.8)	164 (52.7)		307 (34.5)
No	3936 (19.0)	3027 (19.7)	733 (17.6)	38 (12.2)		138 (15.5)
Unknown	6523 (31.4)	4647 (30.2)	1322 (31.7)	109 (35.1)		445 (50.0)
Hypertension					< 0.001	
Yes	8053 (38.8)	5596 (36.4)	1968 (47.2)	204 (65.6)		285 (32.0)
No	11,742 (56.5)	9122 (59.3)	2048 (49.1)	95 (30.6)		477 (53.6)
Unknown	975 (4.7)	678 (4.4)	157 (3.8)	12 (3.9)		128 (14.4)
Diabetes					< 0.001	
Yes	4187 (20.2)	2752 (17.9)	1149 (27.5)	155 (49.8)		32 (3.6)
No	15,577 (75.0)	11,972 (77.8)	2853 (68.4)	145 (46.6)		524 (58.9)
Unknown	1006 (4.8)	672 (4.4)	171 (4.1)	11 (3.5)		334 (37.5)

Table 1 Participant Sociodemographic and Clinical Characteristics Stratified by Albuminuria (*Continued*)

Characteristic	ALL N (%) or Mean (se)	Urine albumin/crt < 30 N (%)	Urine albumin/crt 30–300 N (%)	Urine albumin/crt > 300 N (%)	p-value	Unknown/Not tested N (%) or Mean (s.e.)
Kidney disease						
Yes	990 (4.8)	625 (4.1)	272 (6.5)	61 (19.6)	< 0.001	32 (3.6)
No	18,065 (87.0)	13,696 (89.0)	3620 (86.8)	225 (72.4)		524 (58.9)
Unknown	1715 (8.2)	1075 (7.0)	281 (6.7)	25 (8.0)		334 (37.5)
Family history of hypertension						
Yes	11,183 (53.8)	8258 (53.6)	2358 (56.6)	181 (58.0)	< 0.001	386 (43.4)
No	6836 (32.9)	5153 (33.5)	1312 (31.4)	78 (25.1)		293 (32.9)
Unknown	2751 (13.2)	1985 (12.9)	503 (12.1)	52 (16.7)		211 (23.7)
Family history of diabetes						
Yes	8837 (42.5)	6466 (42.0)	1956 (46.9)	164 (52.7)	< 0.001	251 (28.2)
No	8116 (39.1)	6158 (40.0)	1620 (38.8)	97 (31.2)		241 (27.1)
Unknown	3817 (18.4)	2771 (18.0)	597 (14.3)	50 (16.7)		398 (44.7)
Family history of kidney disease, transplant, or dialysis						
Yes	2477 (11.9)	1846 (12.0)	507 (12.2)	59 (19.0)	< 0.001	65 (7.3)
No	13,070 (62.9)	9763 (63.4)	2757 (66.1)	179 (57.6)		371 (41.7)
Unknown	5223 (25.2)	3787 (24.6)	909 (21.8)	73 (23.5)		454 (51.0)
BMI[a]	29.4 (0.05)	29.2 (0.05)	30.1 (0.11)	29.6 (0.4)	< 0.001	29.1 (0.29)
BMI Category						
< 25	4865 (23.4)	3701 (24.0)	926 (22.2)	74 (23.8)	< 0.001	164 (18.4)
25–29.9	6470 (31.2)	5007 (32.5)	1189 (28.5)	88 (28.3)		186 (20.9)
30–39.9	6024 (29.0)	4447 (28.9)	1332 (31.9)	86 (27.7)		159 (17.9)
>=40	1273 (6.1)	871 (5.7)	342 (8.2)	24 (7.7)		36 (4.0)
Unknown	2138 (10.3)	1370 (8.9)	384 (9.2)	39 (12.5)		345 (38.8)
Systolic blood pressure, mm Hg[1]	127.5 (0.13)	126.3 (0.14)	130.8 (0.31)	143.3 (1.33)	< 0.001	126.2 (0.83)
Systolic blood pressure categories, mmHg						
< 120	6186 (29.8)	4868 (31.6)	1066 (25.6)	37 (11.9)	< 0.001	215 (24.2)
120–139	8513 (41.0)	6489 (42.2)	1706 (40.9)	99 (31.8)		219 (24.6)
140–159	3662 (17.6)	2609 (17.0)	866 (20.8)	86 (27.7)		101 (11.4)
160–179	952 (4.6)	591 (3.8)	290 (7.0)	49 (15.8)		22 (2.5)

Table 1 Participant Sociodemographic and Clinical Characteristics Stratified by Albuminuria (*Continued*)

Characteristic	ALL N (%) or Mean (se)	Urine albumin/crt < 30 N (%)	Urine albumin/crt 30–300 N (%)	Urine albumin/crt > 300 N (%)	p-value	Unknown/Not tested N (%) or Mean (s.e.)
>= 180	237 (1.1)	106 (0.7)	92 (2.2)	25 (8.0)		14 (1.6)
Unknown	1220 (5.9)	733 (4.8)	153 (3.7)	15 (4.8)		319 (35.8)
Diastolic blood pressure mm Hg[a]	76.6 (0.08)	76.1 (0.09)	77.8 (0.19)	80.4 (0.74)	< 0.001	77.6 (0.5)
Diastolic blood pressure categories						
<80	11,022 (53.1)	8468 (55.0)	2117 (50.7)	130 (41.8)	< 0.001	307 (34.5)
80–89	6023 (29.0)	4530 (29.4)	1220 (29.2)	91 (29.3)		182 (20.5)
90–99	2003 (9.6)	1417 (9.2)	480 (11.5)	47 (15.1)		59 (6.6)
>=100	575 (2.8)	317 (2.1)	203 (4.9)	26 (8.4)		29 (3.3)
Unknown	1147 (5.5)	664 (4.3)	153 (3.7)	17 (5.5)		313 (35.2)
Blood glucose level, gm/dL[b]						
F < 100 or NF < 140	15,013 (72.3)	11,596 (75.3)	2795 (67.0)	168 (54.0)	< 0.001	307 (34.5)
F = 100–126 or NF = 140–200	2488 (12.0)	1771 (11.5)	600 (14.4)	46 (14.8)		182 (20.5)
F > 126 or NF > 200	1138 (5.5)	607 (3.9)	432 (10.4)	68 (21.9)		59 (6.6)
Unknown	2123 (10.2)	1417 (9.2)	343 (8.2)	29 (9.3)		313 (35.2)

[a] mean (standard error)
[b] F = fasting, NF = non-fasting

Table 2 Estimated GFR among a subgroup of 4014 participants with abnormal lab results

	ALL N (%) or Mean (se)	Urine albumin/crt < 30 N (%)	Urine albumin/crt 30–300 N (%)	Urine albumin/crt > 300 N (%)	p-value	Unknown/Not tested N (%) or Mean (s.e.)
Total	4014	2873	982	311		70
eGFR, ml/min/1.73m^2						
>= 60	3203 (79.8)	2427 (84.5)	692 (70.5)	36 (40.4)	< 0.001	48
30–59	723 (18.0)	414 (14.4)	252 (25.7)	36 (40.4)		21
<= 29	88 (2.2)	32 (1.1)	38 (3.9)	17 (19.1)		1

Among participants without albuminuria, most (85%) had an eGFR >= 60 ml/min/1.73m^2, whereas 14% had an eGFR between 30 and 59 ml/min/1.73m^2 and 1% had an eGFR < 30 ml/min/1.73m^2. Twenty-six percent of participants with 30-300 mg/gm of albuminuria and 40 % of those with > 300 mg/gm of albuminuria had an eGFR between 30 and 59 ml/min/1.73m^2, and almost 20 % of participants with > 300 mg/gm of albuminuria had an eGFR of < 30 ml/min/1.73m^2.

Prevalence, awareness, and control of diabetes, hypertension, and kidney disease among participants

Fifty percent of participants had prevalent hypertension, as defined by self-reported history of hypertension, systolic blood pressure $\geq$ 140 mmHg, or a diastolic blood pressure $\geq$ 90 mmHg. Of those with hypertension, 78% were aware of a hypertension diagnosis prior to the screening. Among patients with a reported history of hypertension, about half (53%) were well-controlled with a systolic blood pressure of < 140 mmHg and a diastolic blood pressure of < 90 mmHg (Fig. 2).

Twenty-two percent of study participants had prevalent diabetes, as defined by a self-reported history of diabetes, a fasting blood glucose > 126 mg/dl, or a non-fasting blood glucose of > 200 mg/dl. Among those with diabetes, 93% reported awareness of diabetes diagnosis prior to the screening. Only 24% of participants who reported diabetes were well-controlled with a fasting BS < 130 or a non-fasting BS < 180 (Fig. 2).

Twenty-seven percent of participants had prevalent CKD, as defined by a reported history of CKD or a urine albumin/creatinine ratio of $\geq$ 30 mg/gm. Only 19% of participants with CKD were aware of this diagnosis prior to the screening. (Fig. 2).

Access to healthcare among participants with prevalent hypertension, diabetes, and CKD

Compared to all participants, access to healthcare was better among participants with hypertension and diabetes and similar among participants with CKD. Approximately 19% of participants with prevalent hypertension, 21% of those with diabetes, and 29% with CKD reported lacking health insurance, whereas approximately 27% of all participants reported not having health insurance. Eleven percent of participants with hypertension, 10% with diabetes, and 18% with CKD, reported not having a primary care provider, while 19% of all participants reported not having one (Fig. 3).

Post-screening telephone follow up

A total of 4937 participants with abnormal screening findings (e.g., elevated blood pressure, elevated blood glucose readings, and abnormal urine findings) were reached by telephone for a follow up interview after their screening. Of these participants, 3387 or 68.6% reported follow up with a healthcare provider, whereas 1138 participants (23.1%) reported no follow up. Of the participants who obtained healthcare post-screening,

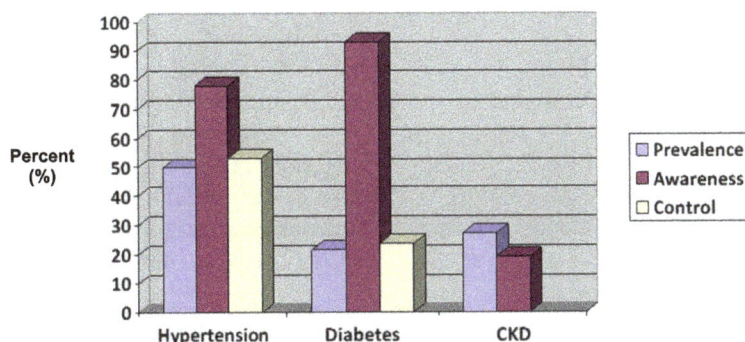

Fig. 2 Prevalence, awareness, and control of hypertension, diabetes, and chronic kidney disease

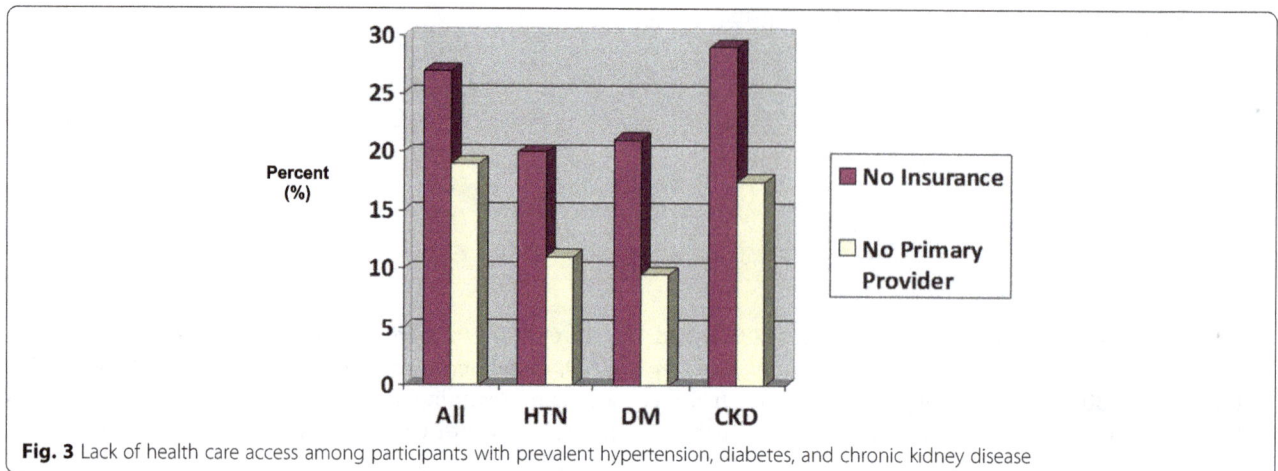

Fig. 3 Lack of health care access among participants with prevalent hypertension, diabetes, and chronic kidney disease

1580 (46.6%) had repeat testing and 1317 (38.9%) reported initiation of treatment for their condition.

Discussion

Among a diverse cohort of 20,770 adults across the state of Illinois who participated in health screenings by the NKFI KM, we found a significant prevalence of undetected and poorly controlled hypertension, diabetes, and kidney disease. At KM screenings, 78% of adults with prevalent hypertension were aware of their hypertension, 93% of participants with prevalent diabetes were aware of their diabetes, but only 19% of participants with prevalent CKD were aware of having the condition. Among those participants reporting hypertension, 53% had adequate blood pressure control as defined by $\leq 140/90$ mmHg, and in those reporting diabetes, 24% had adequate control, as defined by a fasting blood glucose ≤ 130 mg/dl or a non-fasting blood glucose < 180 mg/dl. The NKFI KM reached an underserved population as 27% of participants reported lacking health insurance and 19% did not have access to a healthcare provider. The NKFI KM assisted many underserved participants in addressing their healthcare needs. Among five thousand individuals with abnormal findings who participated in a post-screening interview, almost 70% had a healthcare provider appointment and further evaluation arranged through the NKFI.

Hypertension and diabetes comprise leading causes of CKD, and control of these conditions is needed to prevent CKD and related complications [1, 27, 28]. Studies have shown that adults who are provided with a diagnosis of hypertension and diabetes have better control of these conditions [16], which in turn reduces the incidence of CKD and slower progression of established CKD [27, 29–31]. Similarly, individuals who are made aware of a diagnosis of kidney disease are more likely to obtain CKD care, which may help reduce their incidence of ESKD and CKD related complications [6, 32]. The

positive impact of disease awareness on clinical outcomes underscores the importance of timely diagnosis of these conditions. However, it is important to note that there can be unintended results of screening, including unnecessary worry by participants, barriers to securing disability insurance for participants, and generation of additional testing and/or treatments that may not yield better outcomes. While large health screenings for diabetes, hypertension, and kidney disease such as the KEEP study are common, there are fewer examples of mobile health screenings such as the NKFI KM. Mobile health screenings offer specific advantages of being able to reach individuals without health insurance or a primary provider and who have less geographic mobility. In addition, mobile health screenings can target certain geographic areas overrepresented by disadvantaged and high-risk groups [16, 33, 34]. Our mobile screening initiative allowed us to reach a more vulnerable and disadvantaged population (e.g., lack primary provider, lack health insurance, racial/ethnic minority, non-English speaking) than that represented in broader screening initiatives such as NHANES and KEEP [35]. Furthermore, approximately 22% of KM participants were found to have albuminuria, which is markedly higher than that identified by KEEP (12%) or NHANES (10%) [35, 36].

We found a significant burden of undiagnosed hypertension, diabetes, and kidney disease among NKFI KM participants, consistent with findings from KEEP [37]. The KEEP initiative screened adult patients between the ages of 18–65 years, with either a personal or first-degree family history of diabetes, hypertension and/or chronic kidney disease across the United States. In contrast, the NKFI KidneyMobile screened all adult participants over the age of 18 irrespective of their personal or family health history throughout the state of Illinois. Among participants with abnormal screening results, KEEP investigators found that 35% of those with elevated blood pressure ($> = 140/90$), 2% with abnormal serum glucose ($> = 180$), 96% with albuminuria were unaware of a personal history of hypertension, diabetes, and/or kidney disease, respectively [37]. Using a more inclusive screening protocol, we found that 22% of participants with elevated blood pressure (> = 140/90), 7% of participants with elevated blood glucose (Fasting ≥ 126 mg/dl, Non-Fasting ≥ 200 mg/dl), and 81% of participants with albuminuria (> 30 mg/gm) were unaware of a personal history of hypertension, diabetes, and kidney disease, respectively.

It is well known that poor control of hypertension and diabetes leads to an increased risk of cardiovascular disease, ESKD, and death [27, 28]. However, control of hypertension and diabetes remains suboptimal per recent reports in representative American samples [38, 39]. Similar to our findings, other screening studies have also found suboptimal control of hypertension and diabetes among adults who have known disease. In KEEP, 64% of participants with known hypertension had elevated blood pressure (> = 140/90) and 35% of those with known diabetes had an elevated serum glucose level (glucose level ≥ 180 mg/dl) [37]. We found that 47% of participants with known hypertension had an elevated blood pressure (> = 140/90) and 76% of participants with known diabetes had inadequate control of blood glucose level (fasting > = 130 mg/dl, non-fasting > = 180 mg/dl).

While screening studies have assessed the prevalence of undetected and uncontrolled hypertension, diabetes, and kidney disease within high-risk communities [17, 40], few have coupled screening with disease education or examined the impact of screenings on participants likelihood to follow-up for further care [37, 40], All KM screenings involved interactive, nurse-led educational sessions pertaining to the prevention, detection, and management of silent chronic diseases (e.g., CKD, hypertension, diabetes, obesity, hyperlipidemia). Furthermore, as part of the NKFI KM mission, all participants were given the opportunity to obtain an on-site consultation with a healthcare professional. Individuals with abnormal anthropomorphic parameters or laboratory data also received assistance with obtaining follow up medical evaluation and treatment post-screening. Based on post-screening phone calls by the NKFI staff, these efforts appeared to be quite successful as many participants reached by phone (77%) reported having had an appointment with a healthcare provider after the NKFI KM screening, and of those, 47% reported having undergone repeat testing and 39% reported initiation of medical treatment. Although the impact of this follow-up care cannot be assessed by our study, it clearly provides an opportunity for intervening and reducing complications from these conditions. A future large study would be helpful to examine whether such screening and follow up

endeavors, such as the NKFI KM, affects clinical outcomes.

While our study involved a large diverse participant sample across the state of Illinois and employed detailed data collection strategies with rigorously trained study personnel, it does have limitations. First, like other screening studies such as KEEP and NHANES, only a single anthropomorphic and laboratory measurement for diabetes, hypertension, and kidney disease were done and this does not allow for a diagnosis. Repeated measurements of blood pressure and laboratory tests are generally recommended to support a new diagnosis of hypertension, diabetes, or chronic kidney disease, which underscores the importance of the NKFI KM's coordination of medical follow up for participants with abnormal values. Also, because HbA1C was rarely performed at screening, we relied on capillary blood glucose levels to assess presence and control of diabetes, and these values may vary greatly depending on timing of meals and anti-glycemic agent, and therefore allows for possible misclassification of diabetes prevalence and control [24]. Second, we encountered missing sociodemographic, medical history, and laboratory data that may bias our results. However, missing data occurred rarely and comprised a minority of all data. Third, serum creatinine values were only obtained in participants who had urine studies positive for albumin so we may have missed participants with non-proteinuric kidney disease and underreported the prevalence of kidney disease in this screening cohort. Also, given the mobile nature and time period of the screening initiative, measurement of serum creatinine was not calibrated or standardized in a central laboratory to IDMS, which could introduce error into reported eGFR values. Fourth, as with many screening initiatives, motivational bias may have resulted in individuals participating in more than one free screening and/or attracted individual with existing health concerns, which limits the generalizability of the results.

Conclusion

In summary, we found a high prevalence of hypertension, diabetes, and kidney disease among participants without known disease as well as poor control of these chronic conditions in participants with known disease. Additionally, the screening and follow up procedures of the NKFI KM appear to be connecting many adults with undiagnosed and uncontrolled conditions to much needed healthcare services. These results reinforce the continued need for mobile disease screening units like the NKFI KM to reach high-risk populations who often lack regular access to healthcare. Additional studies are needed to examine the impact of such mobile screening facilities on important and well-recognized clinical outcomes over time.

Abbreviations

CKD: Chronic Kidney Disease; eGFR: Estimated Glomerular Filtration Rate; ESKD: End-Stage Kidney Disease; KM: KidneyMobile; NKFI: National Kidney Foundation of Illinois; VA: United States Department of Veteran Affairs

Acknowledgements

We thank Anne Black and Mara Lidacis for their administrative support at the NKFI and Weihan Zhao, PhD for his help with statistical analyses. The contents presented in this paper are those of the authors and do not represent the views of the U.S. Department of Veterans Affairs or the United States Government.

Funding

Funding for data analysis for this study was provided by National Kidney Foundation of Illinois. Additional support was provided from the VA Office of Academic Affiliations, Advance Fellowship Program in Health Services Research (Swati Lederer). Dr. Lash is supported by K24-DK092290.

Authors' contributions

SL: data analyses, drafted manuscript, contributed to critical revision of the manuscript, approved the final version of the manuscript. LR: study design, data analyses, contributed to critical revision of the manuscript, approved the final version of the manuscript. NMS: data collection, contributed to critical revision of the manuscript, approved the final version of the manuscript. NL: data collection, contributed to critical revision of the manuscript, approved the final version of the manuscript. KGO: data collection, contributed to critical revision of the manuscript, approved the final version of the manuscript. YW: data analyses, contributed to critical revision of the manuscript, approved the final version of the manuscript. JC: data analyses, contributed to critical revision of the manuscript, approved the final version of the manuscript. JPL: data analyses, contributed to critical revision of the manuscript, approved the final version of the manuscript. MJF: study design, data analyses, contributed to critical revision of the manuscript, approved the final version of the manuscript.

Competing interests

The authors declare that they have no competing interests.

Author details

[1]Center of Innovation for Complex Chronic Healthcare, Jesse Brown VA Medical Center, Chicago, IL, USA. [2]Edward Hines Jr. VA Hospital, Hines, IL, USA. [3]Department of Medicine, University of Illinois at Chicago, College of Medicine, Chicago, IL, USA. [4]Department of Medicine, VA North Texas Healthcare System, 4500 South Lancaster Ave, MC 111G1, Dallas, TX 75216, USA. [5]National Kidney Foundation of Illinois, Chicago, IL, USA. [6]Community Health Sciences Division/Institute for Health Research and Policy, School of Public Health, University of Illinois at Chicago, Chicago, IL, USA. [7]Behavioral Health and Nutrition, College of Health Sciences, University of Delaware, Newark, DE, USA.

References

1. Saran R, Li Y, Robinson B, Ayanian J, Balkrishnan R, Bragg-Gresham J, Chen JT, Cope E, Gipson D, He K, et al. US renal data system 2014 annual data report: epidemiology of kidney disease in the United States. Am J Kidney Dis. 2015;65(6 Suppl 1):A7.
2. Go AS, Chertow GM, Fan D, McCulloch CE, Hsu CY. Chronic kidney disease and the risks of death, cardiovascular events, and hospitalization. N Engl J Med. 2004;351(13):1296-305.
3. Nickolas TL, Frisch GD, Opotowsky AR, Arons R, Radhakrishnan J. Awareness of kidney disease in the US population: findings from the National Health and nutrition examination survey (NHANES) 1999 to 2000. Am J Kidney Dis. 2004;44(2):185-97.
4. Whaley-Connell A, Shlipak MG, Inker LA, Kurella Tamura M, Bomback AS, Saab G, Szpunar SM, McFarlane SI, Li S, Chen SC, et al. Awareness of kidney disease and relationship to end-stage renal disease and mortality. Am J Med. 2012;125(7):661-9.
5. Vassalotti JA, Li S, McCullough PA, Bakris GL. Kidney early evaluation program: a community-based screening approach to address disparities in chronic kidney disease. Semin Nephrol. 2010;30(1):66-73.

6. Tuot DS, Plantinga LC, Hsu CY, Jordan R, Burrows NR, Hedgeman E, Yee J, Saran R, Powe NR, Centers for Disease Control Chronic Kidney Disease Surveillance T. Chronic kidney disease awareness among individuals with clinical markers of kidney dysfunction. Clin J Am Soc Nephrol. 2011;6(8):1838-44.
7. National Kidney F. K/DOQI clinical practice guidelines for chronic kidney disease: evaluation, classification, and stratification. Am J Kidney Dis. 2002;39(2 Suppl 1):S1-266.
8. Martínez-Ramírez HR, Cortés-Sanabria L, Rojas-Campos E, Hernández-Herrera A, Cueto-Manzano AM. Multidisciplinary strategies in the management of early chronic kidney disease. Arch Med Res. 2013;44(8):611-5.
9. Nwankwo T, Yoon SS, Burt V, Gu Q. Hypertension among adults in the United States: National Health and nutrition examination survey. NCHS Data Brief. 2011-2012;2013(133):1-8.
10. National Diabetes Statistics Report: Estimate of Diabetes and its Burden in the United States. Atlanta, GA. Center for Disease Control and Prevention, US Department of Health and Human Services. 2015.
11. Crews DC, Pfaff T, Powe NR. Socioeconomic factors and racial disparities in kidney disease outcomes. Semin Nephrol. 2013;33(5):468-75.
12. Palmer Alves T, Lewis J. Racial differences in chronic kidney disease (CKD) and end-stage renal disease (ESRD) in the United States: a social and economic dilemma. Clin Nephrol. 2010;74(Suppl 1):S72-7.
13. Perneger TV, Whelton PK, Klag MJ. Race and end-stage renal disease. Socioeconomic status and access to health care as mediating factors. Arch Intern Med. 1995;155(11):1201-8.
14. Nzerue CM, Demissochew H, Tucker JK. Race and kidney disease: role of social and environmental factors. J Natl Med Assoc. 2002;94(8 Suppl):28S-38S.
15. McCullough PA, Brown WW, Gannon MR, Vassalotti JA, Collins AJ, Chen SC, Bakris GL, Whaley-Connell AT. Sustainable community-based CKD screening methods employed by the National Kidney Foundation's kidney early evaluation program (KEEP). Am J Kidney Dis. 2011;57(3 Suppl 2):S4-8.
16. Victor RG, Ravenell JE, Freeman A, Leonard D, Bhat DG, Shafiq M, Knowles P, Storm JS, Adhikari E, Bibbins-Domingo K, et al. Effectiveness of a barber-based intervention for improving hypertension control in black men: the BARBER-1 study: a cluster randomized trial. Arch Intern Med. 2011;171(4):342-50.
17. Abdelsatir S, Al-Sofi A, Elamin S, Abu-Aisha H. The potential role of nursing students in the implementation of community-based hypertension screening programs in Sudan. Arab J Nephrol Transplant. 2013;6(1):51-4.
18. Santoyo-Olsson J, Cabrera J, Freyre R, Grossman M, Alvarez N, Mathur D, Guerrero M, Delgadillo AT, Kanaya AM, Stewart AL. An innovative multiphased strategy to recruit underserved adults into a randomized trial of a community-based diabetes risk reduction program. Gerontologist. 2011;51(Suppl 1):S82-93.
19. Aitaoto N, Braun KL, Estrella J, Epeluk A, Tsark J. Design and results of a culturally tailored cancer outreach project by and for Micronesian women. Prev Chronic Dis. 2012;9:E82.
20. Chobanian AV, Bakris GL, Black HR, Cushman WC, Green LA, Izzo JL, Jones DW, Materson BJ, Oparil S, Wright JT, et al. Seventh report of the joint National Committee on prevention, detection, evaluation, and treatment of high blood pressure. Hypertension. 2003;42(6):1206-52.
21. OneTouch Ultra 2 [http://www.onetouch.com/onetouch-ultra2]. Accessed 10 Oct 2018.
22. Point of Care Testing [http://usa.healthcare.siemens.com/point-of-care]. Accessed 10 Oct 2018.
23. Abbott Point of Care [https://www.abbottpointofcare.com/products-services/istat-handheld]. Accessed 10 Oct 2018.
24. American Diabetes A. Standards of medical care in diabetes--2014. Diabetes Care. 2014;37(Suppl 1):S14-80.
25. Group KDIGOKCW. KDIGO 2012 clinical practice guideline for the evaluation and Management of Chronic Kidney Disease. Kidney Int. 2013;3:1-150.
26. Levey AS, Coresh J, Greene T, Stevens LA, Zhang YL, Hendriksen S, Kusek JW, Van Lente F, Chronic Kidney Disease Epidemiology C. Using standardized serum creatinine values in the modification of diet in renal disease study equation for estimating glomerular filtration rate. Ann Intern Med. 2006;145(4):247-54.
27. Hemmingsen B, Lund SS, Gluud C, Vaag A, Almdal TP, Hemmingsen C, Wetterslev J. Targeting intensive glycaemic control versus targeting conventional glycaemic control for type 2 diabetes mellitus. Cochrane Database Syst Rev. 2013;11:CD008143.

The National Kidney Foundation of Illinois KidneyMobile: a mobile resource for community based screenings...

129

28. Bakris GL, Ritz E. The message for world kidney day 2009: hypertension and kidney disease: a marriage that should be prevented. Kidney Int. 2009;75(5):449–52.

29. Hsu CY, McCulloch CE, Darbinian J, Go AS, Iribarren C. Elevated blood pressure and risk of end-stage renal disease in subjects without baseline kidney disease. Arch Intern Med. 2005;165(8):923–8.

30. Ohkubo Y, Kishikawa H, Araki E, Miyata T, Isami S, Motoyoshi S, Kojima Y, Furuyoshi N, Shichiri M. Intensive insulin therapy prevents the progression of diabetic microvascular complications in Japanese patients with non-insulin-dependent diabetes mellitus: a randomized prospective 6-year study. Diabetes Res Clin Pract. 1995;28(2):103–17.

31. Coresh J, Wei GL, McQuillan G, Brancati FL, Levey AS, Jones C, Klag MJ. Prevalence of high blood pressure and elevated serum creatinine level in the United States: findings from the third National Health and nutrition examination survey (1988-1994). Arch Intern Med. 2001;161(9):1207–16.

32. Wouters OJ, O'Donoghue DJ, Ritchie J, Kanavos PG, Narva AS. Early chronic kidney disease: diagnosis, management and models of care. Nat Rev Nephrol. 2015;11(8):491–502.

33. Willis J, Lloyd L, Jenkins W. Undergraduate students trained to provide basic health care screening in an underserved community: a door-to-door campaign. Work. 2012;41(3):277–84.

34. Saffar D, Perkins DW, Williams V, Kapke A, Mahan M, Milberger S, Brady M, Wisdom K. Screening for diabetes in an African American community: identifying characteristics associated with abnormal blood glucose readings. J Natl Med Assoc. 2011;103(3):190–3.

35. Agrawal V, Jaar BG, Frisby XY, Chen SC, Qiu Y, Li S, Whaley-Connell AT, McCullough PA, Bomback AS, Investigators K. Access to health care among adults evaluated for CKD: findings from the kidney early evaluation program (KEEP). Am J Kidney Dis. 2012;59(3 Suppl 2):S5–15.

36. Chronic Kidney Disease Surveillance System—United States. [http://www.cdc.gov/ckd]. Accessed 10 Oct 2018.

37. Brown WW, Peters RM, Ohmit SE, Keane WF, Collins A, Chen SC, King K, Klag MJ, Molony DA, Flack JM. Early detection of kidney disease in community settings: the kidney early evaluation program (KEEP). Am J Kidney Dis. 2003;42(1):22–35.

38. Ong KL, Cheung BM, Man YB, Lau CP, Lam KS. Prevalence, awareness, treatment, and control of hypertension among United States adults 1999-2004. Hypertension. 2007;49(1):69–75.

39. Ong KL, Cheung BM, Wong LY, Wat NM, Tan KC, Lam KS. Prevalence, treatment, and control of diagnosed diabetes in the U.S. National Health and nutrition examination survey 1999-2004. Ann Epidemiol. 2008;18(3):222–9.

40. Wee LE, Koh GC, Yeo WX, Chin RT, Wong J, Seow B. Screening for cardiovascular disease risk factors in an urban low-income setting at baseline and post intervention: a prospective intervention study. Eur J Prev Cardiol. 2013;20(1):176–88.

13

Long-term survival in Japanese renal transplant recipients with Alport syndrome: a retrospective study

Ai Katsuma[1], Yasuyuki Nakada[1], Izumi Yamamoto[1]*(iD), Shigeru Horita[2], Miyuki Furusawa[3], Kohei Unagami[3], Haruki Katsumata[1], Masayoshi Okumi[3], Hideki Ishida[3], Takashi Yokoo[1], Kazunari Tanabe[3] and Japan Academic Consortium of Kidney Transplantation (JACK)

Abstract

Background: Patients with Alport syndrome (AS) develop progressive kidney dysfunction due to a hereditary type IV collagen deficiency. Survival of the kidney allograft in patients with AS is reportedly excellent because AS does not recur. However, several studies have implied that the type IV collagen in the GBM originates from podocytes recruited from the recipient's bone marrow-derived cells, suggesting the possibility of AS recurrence. Limited data are available regarding AS recurrence and graft survival in the Japanese population; the vast majority were obtained from living related kidney transplantation (LRKTx).

Methods: In this retrospective study, twenty-one patients with AS were compared with 41 matched patients without AS from 1984 to 2015 at two centers using propensity scores. Nineteen of the 21 patients with AS underwent LRKTx. The mean post-transplant follow-up period was 83 months in the AS group and 110 months in the control group. Histopathological AS recurrence was assessed by immunoreactivity of α5 (type IV collagen) antibody and electron microscopy.

Results: The graft survival rate was equivalent between patients with and without AS (86.7% vs. 77.1% and 69.3% vs. 64.2% at 5 and 10 years; $p = 0.16$, log-rank test). Immunoreactivity to α5 antibody showed strong linear positivity with no focal defect in six patients. Electron microscopy showed no GBM abnormalities in two patients who were exhibiting long-term kidney allograft survival.

Conclusions: We confirmed that α5 and the GBM structure were histopathologically maintained in the long term after kidney transplantation. The patient and graft survival rates were equivalent between Japanese patients with and without AS.

Keywords: Alport syndrome, Kidney transplantation, Type IV collagen

Background

Alport syndrome (AS) is an inherited nephropathy characterized by sensorineural hearing loss and typical ocular abnormalities. It is caused by a hereditary type IV collagen deficiency [1–3]. In 85% of patients with AS, the collagen deficiency exhibits X-linked inheritance (COL4A5 gene), and the remaining 15% show autosomal recessive and rarely autosomal dominant inheritance (COL4A3 or COL4A4 genes). Histopathologically, these genetic alterations reflect glomerular basement membrane (GBM) thickening and lamellation, leading to focal segmental glomerulosclerosis and resultant global sclerosis and/or hyalinosis [1]. With respect to therapy, several studies have demonstrated the efficacy of angiotensin-converting enzyme inhibitors as the first-choice medications [4, 5], with angiotensin II receptor blockers and spironolactone as alternatives [6]. However, these medications are not always satisfactory, and there are no disease-specific medications. For these reasons, AS commonly progresses gradually

* Correspondence: izumi26@jikei.ac.jp
[1]Division of Nephrology and Hypertension, Department of Internal Medicine, The Jikei University School of Medicine, 3-25-8, Nishi-Shimbashi, Minato-ku, Tokyo 105-8461, Japan
Full list of author information is available at the end of the article

from childhood, resulting in end-stage renal disease at a young age [3]. Indeed, according to the United States Renal Data System, the median age at which renal replacement therapy was initiated in AS from 2005 to 2009 was 33.7 years [7].

Patients with AS account for >1% of all patients undergoing kidney transplantation [8]. Kidney allograft survival in patients with AS is excellent despite the fact that AS recipients can develop anti-GBM disease, which can induce allograft loss at a high rate early after kidney transplantation. These excellent results have been reported in several countries. These reasons were mainly explained by the lack of risk factors for chronic kidney disease (hypertension and diabetes mellitus), the absence of AS recurrence, and the very low rate of anti-GBM disease (only 1.9%) [9]. However, the clinical outcomes of renal allografts in the Japanese population, the vast majority of whom have undergone living related kidney transplantation (LRKTx), have not yet been investigated.

Another aim of this study was to evaluate the recurrence of AS in recipients of kidney transplantation. This topic was investigated for the following three reasons. First, the type IV collagen α3α4α5 heterotrimer in the GBM originates only from podocytes [10]. Second, there is evidence that allograft podocytes are produced from turnover of the recipient's bone marrow-derived cells [11]. Third, experimental evidence has shown that the transplantation of wild-type bone marrow into irradiated Alport mice results in the recruitment of podocytes, which produce type IV collagen α5 within the damaged glomerulus [12, 13]. We hypothesized that recurrence of AS occurs locally and influences the clinical abnormalities of patients with AS.

To address these clinical and histopathological issues, we investigated the graft survival and histopathological changes in patients with AS as well as the expression of GBM type IV collagen α5 and electron microscopy findings in renal allograft recipients with AS in the Japanese population.

Methods

We used the clinical, laboratory, and pathological data from recipients who underwent kidney transplantation at the Department of Urology, Tokyo Women's Medical University, and the Division of Nephrology and Hypertension, Department of Internal Medicine, The Jikei University School of Medicine, from February 1984 to February 2015. Twenty-one recipients had AS as the primary renal disease leading to end-stage renal disease. Controls included patients who underwent transplantation with end-stage renal disease due to a condition other than AS. The two groups of patients were matched for recipient and donor age, number of renal transplants, presence of donor-specific antibodies, donor resources,

and era of transplantation using propensity-score analysis. Endpoints were graft loss or patients death.

Immunosuppressive regimens and desensitization protocols

All of the recipients were administered a triple immunosuppressive protocol comprising calcineurin inhibitors (CNI), antimetabolite drugs, and methylprednisolone (MP). Patients transplanted between 1989 and 1997 received cyclosporine and azathioprine (AZA), those transplanted between 1998 and 2000 received tacrolimus (TAC) and AZA, and those transplanted after 2001 received TAC and mycophenolate mofetil (MMF). After 2002, all patients received basiliximab perioperativelly. Splenectomy was performed at the time of transplantation between 1989 and 2004, and thereafter as an alternative to splenectomy, one dose of rituximab was administered 5–7 days before transplantation [14].

Histopathology

Two independent observers performed histological evaluation of formalin-fixed paraffin sections stained with hematoxylin and eosin, periodic acid-Schiff, Masson's trichrome, and periodic acid methenamine. All biopsies were evaluated based on the Banff 2013 classification.

Immunofluorescence

Immunohistochemistry was performed on cold acetone-fixed frozen sections using fluorescein isothiocyanate-conjugated anti-α5 (IV) (H53 and B51) and Texas red-conjugated anti-α2 (IV) (H51) (Shigei Medical Research Institute, Okayama, Japan). The immunoreactivities of type IV collagen α2 and α5 were observed and photographed by fluorescence microscopy (DP-70; Olympus, Tokyo, Japan). To evaluate histological recurrence of AS, we selected all recipients who underwent allograft biopsy more than one year after kidney transplantation. We could not obtain frozen biopsy specimens from some of those patients because the biopsy performed long before. As a result, we could assess frozen specimens obtained from six recipients. We evaluated two to three glomeruli per patient to identify focal or diffuse defects of type IV collagen α5 immunoreactivities in the GBM.

Electron microscopy

We observed the electron microscopic structure of the GBM in six patients of whom we could survey the allograft specimens in the long term more than one year after transplantation (Case1, 11, 12, 15, 16, 19). Among them we evaluated the electron microscopic figure of the GBM in two patients of whom we could survey the allograft specimens in particularly long term (101 and 110 months after kidney transplantation). For each, a total of 10 GBM measurements were evaluated on 10 randomly selected glomerular capillaries to determine the average (arithmetic mean) GBM thickness. Each electron micrograph was reviewed to determine whether foci of splitting or lamellation of the GBM was present.

Biopsy and definition of AS recurrence

Graft biopsy was performed based on episodic hematuria and proteinuria or worsening renal function. The other protocol biopsies were performed at 3 months, 1 year, and 3 years after kidney transplantation. We defined the recurrence of AS as either focal or diffuse defects of immunoreactivities of type IV collagen $\alpha 5$ chains in the GBM. On electron microscopy, we defined the recurrence of AS as the significant progression of irregular thinning and thickening of the GBM with splitting and lamellation of the lamina densa.

Statistical analyses

The baseline characteristics are presented as median with range or mean with standard deviation. We used Fisher's exact test to compare categorical variables between groups and the Mann–Whitney test to compare continuous variables. Allograft and patient survival were evaluated using the Kaplan–Meier method and compared between groups using the log-rank test. A two-tailed p-value of < 0.05 was considered statistically significant.

Results

Patient characteristics

The characteristics of patients with AS and without AS are listed in Table 1. None of the variables except donor sex was significantly different between the two groups. The median age of the recipients was not significantly different between the AS and control groups [22 (range, 15–56) and 23 (range, 9–71) years, respectively; $p =$ 0.94]. The median follow-up period was 99.5 months (range, 0–348 months) and was not significantly different between the two groups ($p = 0.78$). A total of 71.4% (15/21) of the patients in the AS group and 65.9% (27/41) in the control group were male. Most patients underwent their first kidney transplantation (AS vs. control, 95.2% vs. 97.5%, respectively), and the rates of LRKTx were not significantly different between the two groups (90.5% in AS group vs. 92.7% in control group, $p = 1.0$). In our institutes, LRKTx occupy large majority of kidney transplantation. Among them, a few deceased donor kidney transplantation (DDKTx) were performed, which were 2/21(9.5%) and 3/41(7.3%) in each Alport group and control group. Average age of recipient and donor were 29/20 and 53/28 respectively in each group (Alport group/control group). In DDKTx cases, number of renal transplants, presence of donor-specific antibodies, and era of transplantation were comparable in

Table 1 Baseline characteristics in AS and control groups

Variables	Alport group	Matched Control group	p value
N	21	41	
Recipient age	22 (15–56)	23 (9–71)	0.94
Recipient gender (Male)	15 (71.4%)	27 (65.9%)	0.78
Recipient BMI	18.3 (14.4–22.9)	20.2 (14.6–27.2)	0.083
Time on Dialysis (month)	12 (0–193)	25 (0–137)	0.070
RRT modality (HD)	17 (81.0%)	33 (80.5%)	1.0
Donor age	52 (40–65)	50 (16–78)	0.42
Donor gender (Male)	15 (71.4%)	15 (37.5%)	0.015*
No. of Transplantation			
first	20 (95.2%)	40 (97.5%)	1.00
second	1 (4.8%)	1 (2.4%)	NA
third	0 (0.0%)	0 (0.0%)	
HLA-mismatch			
Class I	1.33 ± 0.73	1.46 ± 0.71	0.46
Class II	0.62 ± 0.59	0.78 ± 0.42	0.17
ABO incompatible	5 (23.8%)	9 (22.0%)	1.0
Graft weight	170 (125–280)	175 (120–270)	0.50
WIT (min)	5 (0–15)	5 (0–24)	0.67
TIT (min)	73 (39–660)	67.5 (44–2233)	0.55
Preformed DSA[a]			
HLA-Class I	0/9 (0.0%)	5/21 (23.8%)	0.30
HLA-Class II	0/6 (0.0%)	3/19 (15.8%)	1.0
Graft failure	6 (28.6%)	19 (45.2%)	0.27
Chronic rejection	4	14	0.89
Non-compliance	1	1	0.073
Unknown	1	4	NA
Follow up period (month)	83 (5–315)	110 (0–348)	0.78
Living donor RTx	19 (90.5%)	38 (92.7%)	1.0
Era of transplantation			
-1989	3 (14.3%)	5 (12.2%)	1.0
1990–1999	4 (19.0%)	11 (26.8%)	0.55
2000–2009	6 (28.5%)	18 (43.9%)	0.28
2010-	8 (38.1%)	7 (17.1%)	0.12
Hematuria[b]	2/18 (11.1%)	5/25 (20.0%)	0.69

DSA: donor-specific antibody, RTx: renal transplantation, TCMR: T cell-mediated rejection, ABMR: Antibody-mediated rejection

[a]Preformed DSA was evaluated by HLA-antibody single antigen test (Luminex method). This test for HLA-Class I was performed to nine cases in AS and twenty-one cases in control, and for HLA-Class II to six cases in AS and nineteen cases in control

[b]Hematuria displays the number of recipients who had hematuria more than (1+) at the latest examination/total recipients who could be obtained the information of latest urine examination

*p-value was < 0.05

both groups, without any significant difference. Human leukocyte antigen mismatch, ABO compatibility, pre-formed donor-specific antibody, and the era of kidney transplantation were not significantly different between the two groups. The primary disease in 10 patients (24.4%) in the control group ($N = 41$) was predominantly reflux nephropathy, followed by IgA nephropathy in 5 patients (12.2%), focal segmental glomerulosclerosis in 3 (7.3%), diabetic nephropathy in 1 (2.4%), other conditions in 12 (29.3%), and unknown in 6 (14.6%) (Table 2). Fifteen of 21 recipients were male, and the donors comprised 10 fathers, 3 mothers, and 2 cadavers in AS group. Six female recipients underwent donations from three fathers, two mothers, and one husband (Table 3). We could obtain the information of hematuria in 43 recipients (69.3%, Alport group: 18cases, matched control group: 25cases) at the latest urine sample. Only few patients showed positive hematuria at the latest urine examination. There was no statistical difference in patients who showed positive hematuria between Alport group (2/18: 11.1%) and matched control group (5/25: 20.0%). We investigated the episodes of rejection in Alport group and control group. The rate of cases who underwent rejection were 8/17 (47.1%), 20/33 (60.6%) in Alport group and Control group, respectively. The results were not significantly different in both groups.

Patients and graft survival in AS and matched control groups

The cumulative patient survival rate was not significantly different between the two groups ($p = 0.11$, log-rank test) (Fig. 1). The 10-year patient survival rate after transplantation was 100% in the AS group and 94.6% in the matched control group. The cumulative graft survival rate was higher in the AS group (100%, 86.7%, and 69.3% at 1, 5, and 10 years, respectively) than that in the control group (95.1%, 77.1%, and 64.2% at 1, 5, and 10 years, respectively), but the difference was not significant ($p = 0.16$, log-rank test) (Fig 2). Five patients (28.6%) in the AS group and 19 (45.2%) in the matched control group developed allograft failure mainly caused

Table 2 Primary disease in control group

Primary disease	Number (%)
Reflux nephropathy	10 (24.4%)
IgA nephropathy	5 (12.2%)
FSGS	3 (7.3%)
Hypoplastic kidney	2 (4.9%)
RPGN	2 (4.9%)
Diabetic nephropathy	1 (2.4%)
Others	12 (29.3%)
Unknown	6 (14.6%)

by chronic rejection (66.7% in AS group vs. 73.7% in control group) or by non-compliance (16.0% in AS group vs. 5.3% in control group). There were no cases of recurrent nephropathy in the AS group.

Long-term immunoreactivity of type IV collagen in GBM of AS allograft specimens after kidney transplantation

We evaluated the graft specimens in 6 of 21 patients in the AS group who underwent allograft biopsy more than 1 year after kidney transplantation (Table 3). The median age of these patients at the time of kidney transplantation was 24 years (range, 21–27 years), and five of the six patients were male. The median duration of time from kidney transplantation to allograft biopsy was 23.5 months (range, 12–110 months). Type IV collagen $\alpha 5$ chains in the GBM of all patients were maintained linearly, and even focal depletion was not observed (Fig. 3). In one patient with chronic active antibody-mediated rejection, the $\alpha 2$ chains showed thickening in the GBM that extended to subendothelial lesions (Fig. 3, Case 12).

Long-term electron microscopic findings of GBM in allograft specimens of AS recipients after kidney transplantation

We assessed the electron microscopic findings of six patients who underwent allograft biopsy. Cases 11 and 16 (data not shown) showed a focally thin basement membrane in the GBM, suggesting the transmission of thin basement membrane disease. Among these patients, we evaluated detailed long-term data after kidney transplantation (101 and 110 months after transplantation in Cases 11 and 12, respectively). We found no significant changes, such as splitting or lamination of the GBM, in both cases. Case 11 showed a thickness of 275 nm at 101 months after kidney transplantation 339 nm at 0 h. Case 12 showed a thickness of 220 nm at 110 months after transplantation and 146 nm at 0 h, suggesting the transmission of thin basement membrane disease. This case was characterized by chronic antibody-mediated rejection by light microscopy and showed a double-countered GBM with extended edema of the subendothelial lesion and fusion of foot process, suggesting endothelial and podocyte injury.

Discussion

This study is the first to demonstrate patient and graft survival in the Japanese population of patients with AS. We retrospectively reviewed the long-term outcomes of 21 patients with AS who underwent kidney transplantation with a mean follow-up duration of 83 months and found that the cumulative patient and graft survival rates in the AS group were not significantly different from those of a well-matched control group (Figs. 1 and 2). Our data as well as those reported by Yilmaz from

Table 3 Twenty-one kidney transplantation recipients with Alport syndrome

Case No.	Living/Cadaver	ABO-compatibility	Recipient Age	Donor Type/Relation	Donor Age	f/u period (month)	UP[a]	Hematuria[b]	Latest creatinine in serum	Recurrence of AS[c]	Graft loss	Causes of graft loss
1	Living	Incompatible	26–30	Father	56–60	36	(+)	(−)	Loss	(−)	(+)	CR
2	Living	Compatible	26–30	Father	46–50	131	(−)	(−)	1.59		(−)	
3	Living	Incompatible	16–20	Father	41–45	5	(−)	unknown	1.16		(−)	
4	Living	Compatible	56–60	Husband	56–60	12	(−)	(−)	0.78		(−)	
5	Living	Incompatible	16–20	Mother	46–50	110	(−)	unknown	Loss		(+)	CR
6	Living	Compatible	26–30	Mother	56–60	5	(−)	(+)	1.06		(−)	
7	Living	Compatible	21–25	Father	46–50	290	(+)	(−)	Loss		(+)	CR
8	Living	Compatible	26–30	Father	56–60	276	(−)	(−)	1.95		(−)	
9	Living	Compatible	21–25	Father	56–60	239	(+)	(−)	1.62		(−)	
10	Living	Compatible	16–20	Father	46–50	216	(−)	unknown	1.4		(−)	
11	Living	Compatible	21–25	Father	56–60	180	(−)	(−)	2.17	(−)	(−)	
12	Living	Compatible	22–25	Father	56–60	120	(+)	(−)	Loss	(−) TBMD	(+)	CR
13	Living	Compatible	31–35	Father	56–60	83	(−)	(−)	1.31		(−)	
14	Living	Incompatible	21–25	Father	51–55	47	(−)	(−)	1.32		(−)	
15	Living	Incompatible	21–25	Father	46–50	24	(−)	(−)	1.16	(−)	(−)	
16	Living	Compatible	21–25	Father	46–50	11	(−)	(−)	1.44	(−) TBMD	(−)	
17	Living	Compatible	16–20	Mother	51–55	204	(−)	(−)	1.35		(−)	
18	Living	Compatible	21–25	Mother	46–50	39	(+)	(−)	Loss		(+)	NC
19	Living	Compatible	21–25	Mother	46–50	56	(−)	(+)	1.58	(−)	(−)	
20	Cadaver	Compatible	16–20	Other	36–40	315	(+)	(−)	Loss		(+)	unknown
21	Cadaver	Compatible	41–45	Other	61–65	35	(−)	(−)	1.92		(−)	

KTx kidney transplantation, *Bx* allograft biopsy, *AS* Alport syndrome, *N.D.* no data, *f/u* follow up, *UP* urine proteinuria, *NC* non-compliance, *CR* chronic rejection, *TBMD* thin basement membrane disease. [a]Positive of urine proteinuria was defined as more than one plus by urinary qualitative examination. [b]Positive hematuria was defined as more than one plus at the latest examination. [c]Recurrence of AS was defined as no appearance of a deficiency of collagen α5 in glomerular basement membrane

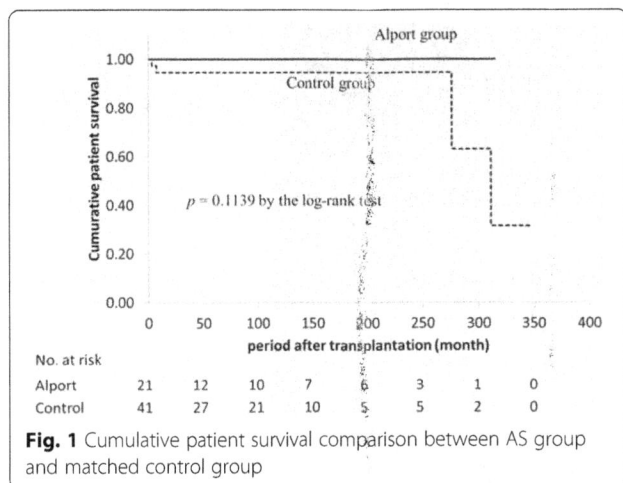

Fig. 1 Cumulative patient survival comparison between AS group and matched control group

Turkey showed no difference between patients with and without AS [15]. In contrast, Temme showed better graft survival (HR, 0.75; 95% CI, 0.60–0.93; $p = 0.008$) and patient survival (HR, 0.46; 95% CI, 0.30–0.59; $p = 0.001$) in patients with AS using the ERA-EDTA Registry data [7]. The only difference in the patients' characteristics was the rate of deceased donors (63.0% in the ERA-EDTA data, 32.0% in Yilma's data, and 9.5% in our data). Notably, the author demonstrated that the patient and graft survival rates were better in deceased donors than in controls, but not in living donors. This finding suggests that living donors with AS could negatively affect patient and graft survival. In line with this, Gross from Germany observed six cases of living donor kidney transplantation in AS from relatives with mild urinary abnormalities and found that three of the six donors developed new-onset hypertension and two of the six donors developed new-onset proteinuria. The author pointed out that, genetically, AS may also affect other family members, and physicians should be aware of an increased risk of renal failure in both the donor and the recipient [16]. In this context, in countries with a donor shortage, such as Japan (in which almost 90% of transplantations are living donor kidney transplantations), careful evaluation and monitoring of both donors and recipients with AS are necessary. In the present study, 13 of 21 patients received kidneys from a father, suggesting that most donations were from an unaffected father with X-linked (COL4A5 gene) AS. However, we found at least two patients (Cases 12 and 16) with a relatively thin GBM on electron microscopy, suggesting possible transmission of thin basement membrane disease from autosomal-recessive (COL4A3 or COL4A4 gene) affected relatives [17, 18]. For example, in Case 16, we confirmed that type IV collagen α5 staining of the recipient's native kidney biopsy revealed positive in the basement membrane of Bowman's capsule but negative in GBM, suggesting autosomal-recessive AS associated with COL4A3/4 gene abnormality. Of note, previous report showed that about 40% of TBMD patients have heterozygous mutations at the COL4A3/4 locus [19]. Therefore, the donor in Case 16 could be heterozygous carrier with autosomal-recessive AS, resulting in TBMD shown in baseline allograft biopsy. These two patients had stable kidney function and did not show proteinuria or hematuria. These results suggest that living donor kidney transplantation from relatives with AS is acceptable if the donors and recipients are carefully evaluated. Another important factor associated with patient and graft outcomes is the occurrence of anti-GBM disease. Anti-GBM disease induces graft failure in the early stage of kidney transplantation in recipients with AS, but the incidence is generally very low at 1.9% [9]. Fortunately, no recipients in the AS group developed anti-GBM disease within the observation. Among patients with AS, the risk factors associated with graft loss in patients other than living donors and those with anti-GBM disease have not been fully evaluated. In the present study, 6 of 21 (28.6%) recipients with AS developed graft loss. Of these, four (66.6%) were due to chronic rejection, one (16.7%) was due to noncompliance with medication, and another was of unknown cause. These results are comparable with the causes of graft loss in the matched control group.

Another main finding of this study is that no patients developed recurrence of AS. To the best of our knowledge, this is the first study to evaluate the recurrence of AS in detail using histopathological methods. Generally, recurrent glomerulonephritis or glomerulopathy may cause graft loss in kidney transplantation, but most nephrologists believe that patients with AS do not develop recurrence. However, several recent clinical and experimental studies have implied that GBM type IV collagen originates from podocytes recruited from the recipient's bone marrow-derived cells, suggesting the possibility of recurrence of AS. For example, Abrahamson clearly demonstrated that

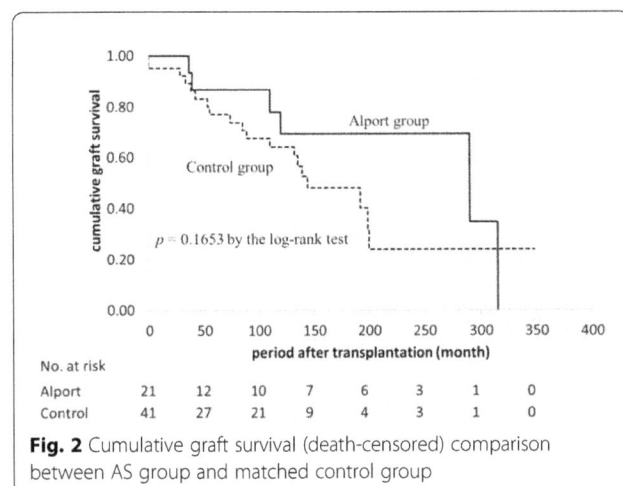

Fig. 2 Cumulative graft survival (death-censored) comparison between AS group and matched control group

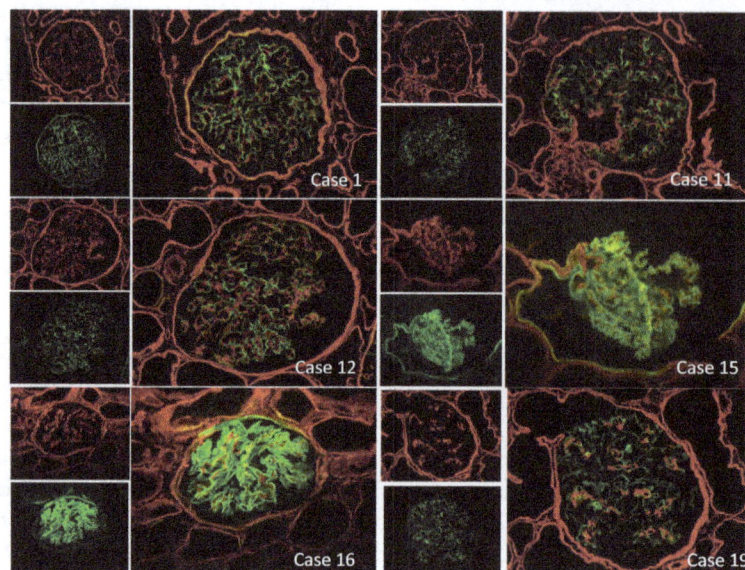

Fig. 3 Immunofluorescence staining of type IV collagen α5 chain. Immunofluorescence staining of type IV collagen α2 chain (red), α5 chain (green), and merged images (combined red and green) of GBM on allograft biopsy specimens of AS recipients performed more than 1 year after transplantation (patient characteristics are shown in Table 3). In all cases, the type IV collagen α5 chain was stained linearly in the GBM without defects. Case1: A 27-year-old woman. Allograft biopsy specimen at 33 months after transplantation. The pathological diagnosis was chronic active antibody-mediated rejection. Case 11: A 21-year-old man. Allograft biopsy specimen at 101 months after transplantation. The pathological diagnosis was arteriolar hyalinosis. Case 12: A 21-year-old man. Allograft biopsy specimen at 110 months after transplantation. The pathological diagnoses were chronic active antibody-mediated rejection and IF/TA, moderate. The immunoreactivity of type IV collagen α2 chain was slightly increased in the mesangial and subendothelial regions compared with that in the other cases. Case 15: A 26-year-old man. Allograft biopsy specimen at 12 months after transplantation. The pathological diagnosis was minimally aggressive tubulointerstitial rejection, mild. Case 16: A 26-year-old man. Allograft biopsy specimen at 12 months after transplantation. The pathological diagnosis was no evidence of rejection. Case 19: A 23-year-old man. Allograft biopsy specimen at 14 months after transplantation. The pathological diagnosis was IF/TA, mild

α3α4α5 chains are produced only by podocytes, as evidenced by immunoelectron microscopic examination [10]. In human kidney transplantation research, Becker showed that recipient-derived podocytes were found in 4 of 8 biopsies, representing 3 of 6 patients, and that 5 of the 740 podocytes examined in the female-donated allograft were male-derived, using fluorescence in situ hybridization for the X and Y chromosomes [11]. In addition, Sugimoto et al. reported that bone marrow transplantation from wild-type mice to Alport model mice (COL4A3 −/−) improved the symptoms of AS and the level of protein produced from bone marrow-derived cells [12]. Therefore, we initially hypothesized that the podocytes of allografts can be replaced by recipient-derived podocytes that cannot synthesize α3α4α5 chains, resulting in deficiency of the GBM of allograft. However, we found that the structure of the GBM remained normal and that no deficiencies of the α5 chains in the GBM occurred, even long after kidney transplantation, suggesting that AS does not recur histologically. We speculated following two mechanisms for this phenomenon:1) a very small number of donor derived podocytes were replaced by recipient derived ones [11], or 2) podocytes injury is rare in recipients with AS, and both podocytes and

GBM turnover was not evident [20–22]. Additionally, only few recipients in Alport group showed hematuria in the latest examination (11.1%, Table 1), which further strengthen no histological recurrence of AS because electron microscopy might underestimate the presence of GBM changes of AS due to sampling bias.

The strengths of this study include the selection of controls (propensity-score analysis with matching of six factors: recipient and donor age, number of transplants, donor-specific antibody positivity, donor resources, and era of transplantation) and longer observational periods than in previous reports (99.5 vs. 75.4 months) [15]. Limitations include the retrospective design, small sample size due to the rarity of AS, lack of genetic information, and performance of few allograft biopsies because the allograft function was relatively good, even long after kidney transplantation, in recipients with AS.

Conclusion

Our data demonstrate that graft survival in patients with AS is similar to that in patients with other primary diseases in the Japanese population. Careful selection of living donors is necessary for the successful management of kidney transplantation in patients with AS. Neither deficiency of the α5 chains (type IV collagen) nor GBM abnormalities were detected in the kidney allograft biopsies, indicating that AS recurrence was not present or was very limited in recipients with AS. Further pathological analysis with a longer follow-up to evaluate the possible recurrence of AS and transmission of thin basement membrane disease from affected relatives will contribute to a better understanding of kidney transplantation in patients with AS.

Abbreviations

ABMR: antibody-mediated rejection; AS: Alport syndrome; DDKTx: deceased donor kidney transplantation; GBM: glomerular basement membrane; IF/TA: interstitial fibrosis and tubular atrophy; KTx: kidney transplantation; LRKTx: living related kidney transplantation

Acknowledgments

We appreciate the support provided by Katsunori Shimada, PhD (STATZ Institute, Inc., Tokyo, Japan), who provided expert assistance with the statistical analysis.

Funding

Astellas Pharma Inc. (Tokyo, Japan) supported this study with a grant. The sponsor was not involved in the study design, patient enrollment, data collection, data analysis, data interpretation, or preparation of the manuscript.

Author's contributions

AK and YN designed this study and drafted the article. SH embedded, cut, and stained the renal biopsies. HK, MF, KU corrected the clinical data. IY proposed the research design and corrected the article. MO and HI provided those clinical data and closely examined the article. TY and KT closely examined and corrected the article. All the authors contributed to preparation of the manuscript. In addition, all authors have read and approved the final manuscript.

Competing interest

The authors declare that they have no competing interests.

Author details

[1]Division of Nephrology and Hypertension, Department of Internal Medicine, The Jikei University School of Medicine, 3-25-8, Nishi-Shimbashi, Minato-ku, Tokyo 105-8461, Japan. [2]Department of Medicine, Kidney center, Tokyo Women's Medical University, Tokyo, Japan. [3]Department of Urology, Tokyo Women's Medical University, Tokyo, Japan.

References

1. Hudson BG, Tryggvason K, Sundaramoorthy M, Neilson EG. Alport's syndrome, Goodpasture's syndrome, and type IV collagen. N Engl J Med. 2003;348(25):2543–56.
2. Heidet L, Cai Y, Guicharnaud L, Antignac C, Gubler MC. Glomerular expression of type IV collagen chains in normal and X-linked Alport syndrome kidneys. Am J Pathol. 2000;156(6):1901–10.
3. Kruegel J, Rubel D, Gross O. Alport syndrome--insights from basic and clinical research. Nat Rev Nephrol. 2013;9(3):170–8.
4. Gross O, Licht C, Anders HJ, Hoppe B, Beck B, Tonshoff B, Hocker B, Wygoda S, Ehrich JH, Pape L, Konrad M, Rascher W, Dotsch J, Muller-Wiefel DE, Hoyer P, Study group members of the Gesellschaft fur Padiatrische Nephrologie, Knebelmann B, Pirson Y, Grunfeld JP, Niaudet P, Cochat P, Heidet L, Lebbah S, Torra R, Friede T, Lange K, Muller GA, Weber M. Early angiotensin-converting enzyme inhibition in Alport syndrome delays renal failure and improves life expectancy. Kidney Int. 2012;81(5):494–501.
5. Kashtan CE, Ding J, Gregory M, Gross O, Heidet L, Knebelmann B, Rheault M, Licht C, Collaborative ASR. Clinical practice recommendations for the treatment of Alport syndrome: a statement of the Alport syndrome research collaborative. Pediatr Nephrol. 2013;28(1):5–11.
6. Savige J, Gregory M, Gross O, Kashtan C, Ding J, Flinter F. Expert guidelines for the management of Alport syndrome and thin basement membrane nephropathy. J Am Soc Nephrol. 2013;24(3):364–75.
7. Temme J, Kramer A, Jager KJ, Lange K, Peters F, Muller GA, Kramar R, Heaf JG, Finne P, Palsson R, Reisaeter AV, Hoitsma AJ, Metcalfe W, Postorino M, Zurriaga O, Santos JP, Ravani P, Jarraya F, Verrina E, Dekker FW, Gross O. Outcomes of male patients with Alport syndrome undergoing renal replacement therapy. Clin J Am Soc Nephrol. 2012;7(12):1969–76.
8. Gross O, Kashtan CE, Rheault MN, Flinter F, Savige J, Miner JH, Torra R, Ars E, Deltas C, Savva I, Perin L, Renieri A, Ariani F, Mari F, Baigent C, Judge P, Knebelman B, Heidet L, Lagas S, Blatt D, Ding J, Zhang Y, Gale DP, Prunotto M, Xue Y, Schachter AD, Morton LC, Blem J, Huang M, Liu S, Vallee S, Renault D, Schifter J, Skelding J, Gear S, Friede T, Turner AN, Lennon R. Advances and unmet needs in genetic, basic and clinical science in Alport syndrome: report from the 2015 international workshop on Alport syndrome. Nephrol Dial Transplant. 2017;32(6):916–24.
9. Byrne MC, Budisavljevic MN, Fan Z, Self SE, Ploth DW. Renal transplant in patients with Alport's syndrome. Am J Kidney Dis. 2002;39(4):769–75.
10. Abrahamson DR, Hudson BG, Stroganova L, Borza DB, St John PL. Cellular origins of type IV collagen networks in developing glomeruli. J Am Soc Nephrol. 2009;20(7):1471–9.
11. Becker JU, Hoerning A, Schmid KW, Hoyer PF. Immigrating progenitor cells contribute to human podocyte turnover. Kidney Int. 2007;72(12):1468–73.
12. Sugimoto H, Mundel TM, Sund M, Xie L, Cosgrove D, Kalluri R. Bone-marrow-derived stem cells repair basement membrane collagen defects and reverse genetic kidney disease. Proc Natl Acad Sci U S A. 2006;103(19):7321–6.
13. Prodromidi EI, Poulsom R, Jeffery R, Roufosse CA, Pollard PJ, Pusey CD, Cook HT. Bone marrow-derived cells contribute to podocyte regeneration and amelioration of renal disease in a mouse model of Alport syndrome. Stem Cells. 2006;24(11):2448–55.
14. Okumi M, Toki D, Nozaki T, Shimizu T, Shirakawa H, Omoto K, Inui M, Ishida H, Tanabe K. ABO-incompatible living kidney transplants: evolution of outcomes and immunosuppressive management. Am J Transplant. 2016;16:886–96.
15. Yilmaz VT, Dinckan A, Yilmaz F, Suleymanlar G, Kocak H. Outcomes of renal transplantation in patients with Alport syndrome. Transplant Proc. 2015; 47(5):1377–81.
16. Gross O, Weber M, Fries JW, Müller GA. Living donor kidney transplantation from relatives with mild urinary abnormalities in Alport syndrome: long-term risk, benefit and outcome. Nephrol Dial Transplant. 2009 May;24(5): 1626–30.
17. Ivanyi B, Pap R, Ondrik Z. Thin basement membrane nephropathy: diffuse and segmental types. Arch Pathol Lab Med. 2006 Oct;130(10):1533–7.
18. Pierides A, Voskarides K, Athanasiou Y, Ioannou K, Damianou L, Arsali M, Zavros M, Pierides M, Vargemezis V, Patsias C, Zouvani I, Elia A, Kyriacou K, Deltas C. Clinico-pathological correlations in 127 patients in 11 large pedigrees, segregating one of three heterozygous mutations in the COL4A3/ COL4A4 genes associated with familial haematuria and significant late progression to proteinuria and chronic kidney disease from focal segmental glomerulosclerosis. Nephrol Dial Transplant. 2009;24(9):2721–9.
19. Haas M. Alport syndrome and thin glomerular basement membrane nephropathy: a practical approach to diagnosis. Arch Pathol Lab Med. 2009 Feb;133(2):224–32.
20. Wanner N, Hartleben B, Herbach N, Goedel M, Stickel N, Zeiser R, Walz G, Moeller MJ, Grahammer F, Huber TB. Unraveling the role of podocyte turnover in glomerular aging and injury. J Am Soc Nephrol. 2014;25:707–16.
21. Price RG, Spiro RG. Studies on the metabolism of the renal glomerular basement membrane. Turnover measurements in the rat with the use of radiolabeled amino acids. J Biol Chem. 1977;252:8597–602.
22. Walker F. The origin, turnover and removal of glomerular basement-membrane. J Pathol. 1973;110:233–44.

14

Onset and progression of diabetes in kidney transplant patients receiving everolimus or cyclosporine therapy: an analysis of two randomized, multicenter trials

Claudia Sommerer[1*], Oliver Witzke[2], Frank Lehner[3], Wolfgang Arns[4], Petra Reinke[5], Ute Eisenberger[6], Bruno Vogt[6], Katharina Heller[7], Johannes Jacobi[7], Markus Guba[8], Rolf Stahl[9], Ingeborg A. Hauser[10], Volker Kliem[11], Rudolf P. Wüthrich[12], Anja Mühlfeld[13], Barbara Suwelack[14], Michael Duerr[15], Eva-Maria Paulus[16], Martin Zeier[1], Martina Porstner[16†] and Klemens Budde[15†] on behalf of the ZEUS and HERAKLES study investigators

Abstract

Background: Conversion from calcineurin inhibitor (CNI) therapy to a mammalian target of rapamycin (mTOR) inhibitor following kidney transplantation may help to preserve graft function. Data are sparse, however, concerning the impact of conversion on posttransplant diabetes mellitus (PTDM) or the progression of pre-existing diabetes.

Methods: PTDM and other diabetes-related parameters were assessed post hoc in two large open-label multicenter trials. Kidney transplant recipients were randomized (i) at month 4.5 to switch to everolimus or remain on a standard cyclosporine (CsA)-based regimen (ZEUS, $n = 300$), or (ii) at month 3 to switch to everolimus, remain on standard CNI therapy or convert to everolimus with reduced-exposure CsA (HERAKLES, $n = 497$).

Results: There were no significant differences in the incidence of PTDM between treatment groups (log rank $p = 0.97$ [ZEUS], $p = 0.90$ [HERAKLES]). The mean change in random blood glucose from randomization to month 12 was also similar between treatment groups in both trials for patients with or without PTDM, and with or without pre-existing diabetes. The change in eGFR from randomization to month 12 showed a benefit for everolimus versus comparator groups in all subpopulations, but only reached significance in larger subgroups (no PTDM or no pre-existing diabetes).

Conclusions: Within the restrictions of this post hoc analysis, including non-standardized diagnostic criteria and limited glycemia laboratory parameters, these data do not indicate any difference in the incidence or severity of PTDM with early conversion from a CsA-based regimen to everolimus, or in the progression of pre-existing diabetes.

Keywords: Diabetes, Everolimus, Kidney transplantation, TOR inhibitor, PTDM, Post-transplant

* Correspondence: claudia.sommerer@med.uni-heidelberg.de
†Martina Porstner and Klemens Budde contributed equally to this work.
[1]Department of Nephrology, University of Heidelberg, Im Neuenheimer Feld 162, 69120 Heidelberg, Germany
Full list of author information is available at the end of the article

Background

Diabetic nephropathy is now the most frequent indication for kidney transplantation, accounting for approximately a third of kidney transplants in the US [1], and is set to grow in frequency as the prevalence of diabetes continues to grow [2, 3]. Additionally, under conventional immunosuppressive regimens, up to 20% of kidney transplant recipients develop posttransplant diabetes mellitus (PTDM) [4–6]. Both pre-existing diabetes [7, 8] and PTDM [9] are associated with an increased risk of cardiovascular events [9, 10] and inferior long-term survival, as well as morbidity from diabetes-related complications [7, 11]. The diabetogenic effect of calcineurin inhibitors (CNIs), particularly tacrolimus [4, 12] and steroids [5], can be compounded by maintenance steroid therapy, especially pulsed steroid therapy for the treatment of rejection [13]. In this unfavorable context, novel immunosuppressive regimens must be carefully evaluated in terms of their diabetogenic potential.

The mammalian target of rapamycin (mTOR) inhibitor agents sirolimus and everolimus have been widely assessed within a variety of regimens for de novo or delayed initiation following kidney transplantation [14]. mTOR inhibitors offer the potential for CNI sparing, which might be expected to lower the risk for PTDM [15]. However, results from the early era of sirolimus therapy in kidney transplantation raised concerns that the class may have an inherent diabetogenic effect [16, 17]. In a large randomized trial of sirolimus published in 2006, Vitko et al. reported an increased rate of PTDM in patients randomized to a loading dose (6 mg) and a fixed dose of 2 mg/day versus mycophenolate mofetil when both were administered in combination with standard-dose tacrolimus and steroids [18]. Although smaller trials using fixed sirolimus dosing [19, 20] or high sirolimus exposure targets [21] did not demonstrate any effect, an analysis of United States Renal Data System data from over 20,000 patients undergoing kidney transplantation during 1995–2003 concluded that patients treated with sirolimus were at increased risk of PTDM whether administered in combination with a CNI or an antimetabolite [22]. In contrast, a large meta-analysis published in 2006 found that use of mTOR inhibitors was not associated with any increased risk of developing insulin-treated PTDM compared to antimetabolite therapy [23].

As experience with mTOR inhibitors has grown, fixed dosing has been replaced by progressively lower trough concentration targets, and concomitant CNI exposure has been reduced [14]. Loading doses for sirolimus have typically become smaller, and no loading dose is required for everolimus due to its shorter half-life. In large, randomized trials undertaken recently, no increase in the rate of PTDM was observed in the sirolimus [24, 25] or everolimus [26, 27] treatment arms.

Conversion to an mTOR inhibitor from CNI therapy after the first 3–12 months post-transplant is an appealing immunosuppressive strategy, harnessing the potent immunosuppressive effect of CNIs during the period of highest risk for rejection but taking advantage of the reduced nephrotoxicity associated with mTOR inhibitors [28]. To date, no analyses are available concerning the impact of conversion to an mTOR inhibitor on PTDM or the progression of pre-existing diabetes. We report here a post hoc analysis of diabetic parameters in two large, multicenter trials (ZEUS [29] and HERAKLES [30]) in which de novo kidney transplant recipients were randomized to either convert to everolimus in a CNI-free regimen or to remain on a standard cyclosporine (CsA)-based regimen, or in one study to alternatively switch to everolimus with reduced-exposure CsA.

Methods

Study design and conduct

This was a post hoc analysis of data from two 12-month, prospective, open-label, multicenter, randomized trials of de novo kidney transplant recipients (ZEUS [29] and HERAKLES [30]).The objective of the analysis was to compare the incidence and severity of PTDM, and progression of pre-existing diabetes, to month 12 post-transplant in patients receiving everolimus-based CNI-free maintenance immunosuppression versus those who continued to receive a standard CsA-based regimen or everolimus with reduced-exposure CsA. In both studies, patients received standard-exposure CsA with enteric-coated mycophenolate sodium (EC-MPS) and steroids from time of transplant, and were randomized to continue the CsA-based regimen or convert to everolimus at 4.5 months (ZEUS) [29] or 3 months (HERAKLES) [30] post-transplant. In one of the studies (HERAKLES), there was a third treatment arm in which patients received reduced-exposure CsA with everolimus targeting a lower exposure range.

Patients

The inclusion and exclusion criteria in the two studies were identical other than a lower maximum age for recipients and donors in the ZEUS study (65 years) versus the HERAKLES study (70 years). The minimum recipient and donor ages were 18 and 5 years, respectively, in both studies. Key exclusion criteria at time of study entry were more than one previous kidney transplant, loss of a previous graft due to immunological reasons, multiorgan transplantation, donation after cardiac death, and previous or current panel reactive antibodies > 25%. At the time of randomization, additional exclusion criteria were graft loss, severe (Banff grade ≥ III), recurrent or steroid-resistant rejection prior to randomization, proteinuria > 1 g/day and dialysis dependency. In both studies, patients with uncontrolled diabetes mellitus that in the opinion of the investigator would interfere with the appropriate conduct of the study were excluded. A full list of inclusion and exclusion criteria is shown in Additional file 1: Table S1.

Immunosuppression

All patients received induction with basiliximab (Simulect®, Novartis Pharma, Nürnberg, Germany). CsA (Sandimmun Optoral®, Novartis Pharma, Germany) was administered to all patients, with a target trough concentration in both studies of 150–220 ng/mL from the time of transplant to randomization. All patients received EC-MPS 1440 mg/day (myfortic®, Novartis Pharma, Germany), and steroids administered according to local practice from the time of transplant to month 12.

For patients in the standard-CsA arms, CsA target trough concentrations after randomization were 120–180 ng/mL to month 6, and 100–150 ng/mL thereafter; EC-MPS was continued to month 12. In the CNI-free everolimus arms of both studies, everolimus was initiated at a dose of 1.5 mg then adjusted to target a trough concentration of 5–10 ng/mL, and EC-MPS was continued to month 12. In the ZEUS study, conversion from CsA to everolimus took place stepwise over a period of up to four weeks starting at month 4.5. In the HERAKLES study, conversion took place at month 3 and was completed within 24 h. In the patients randomized to everolimus with reduced-exposure CsA in the HERAKLES study, EC-MPS was discontinued and everolimus was started on the day of randomization with CsA dose unchanged, then on the following day CsA dose was adjusted to target 50–75 ng/mL thereafter. In this group, the everolimus target range was 3–8 ng/mL.

Evaluation

This post hoc analysis compared the following outcomes between treatment groups up to month 12 post-transplant within the ZEUS and HERAKLES trials: the incidence of PTDM; requirement for hypoglycemic therapy (insulin or non-insulin); change in random blood glucose; estimated GFR (eGFR) at month 12 and the change in eGFR from randomization to month 12. Other than eGFR at month 12, none of these endpoints were pre-specified in the study protocols. Data were analyzed according to whether patients did or did not have pre-existing diabetes and subsequently did or did not develop PTDM. PTDM was defined as diabetes reported by the investigator as an adverse event at any point after transplantation in a patient not categorized as diabetic at baseline (i.e. at time of transplant). Patients were categorized as diabetic if diabetes was listed in the medical history by the investigator at the time of study entry. There were no pre-specified laboratory criteria for PTDM or

pre-existing diabetes. Data on the use of insulin or other antidiabetic therapies were obtained via standard reporting procedures for concomitant medication at each study visit. If treatment with such drugs was started, investigators were required to document any adverse events, as per Good Clinical Practice guidelines. Both trials were fully monitored by an external medical monitor.

Blood glucose was measured at routine visits and are random values.

Biopsy-proven acute rejection (BPAR) was graded according to Banff criteria [31].

The primary efficacy endpoint of the ZEUS study was the adjusted eGFR estimated by the Nankivell formula (eGFR, [32]) at month 12. The primary efficacy endpoint in the HERAKLES study was change in eGFR (Nankivell formula) from randomization (month 3) to month 12.

Statistical analysis

All analyses are reported for the safety populations, comprising all patients who received at least one dose of study drug after study entry. Data on the incidence of PTDM across both studies in patients randomized to everolimus-based CNI-free therapy or standard CsA-based therapy were pooled.

Last observation carried forward (LOCF) method was applied for missing 12-month values for immunosuppression drug doses, drug concentrations, and eGFR. Continuous variables (e.g. drug dose, drug exposure) were compared between groups using the two-sample Wilcoxon rank-sum test of the F-test. The incidence of categorical events in each study and in the pooled analysis was compared between groups using Fisher's test. Kaplan-Meier estimates of time to events were compared between groups using the log rank test. The change in eGFR from randomization to month 12 was analyzed by an ANCOVA model with treatment, center, donor type as factors and eGFR value at randomization as covariate.

All tests were two-sided. P values < 0.05 were considered significant.

Results

Patient population and risk factors for diabetes

In total, 300 patients in the ZEUS study and 497 patients in the HERAKLES study were included in the current analysis. Patients were categorized according to whether they developed PTDM or whether they had pre-existing diabetes (Fig. 1).

In both studies, demographic factors, body mass index (BMI), hepatitis C (HCV) status and baseline random blood glucose concentration, generally showed no marked differences between the treatment arms among patients with PTDM, no PTDM or pre-existing diabetes (Table 1). There were significant differences between the

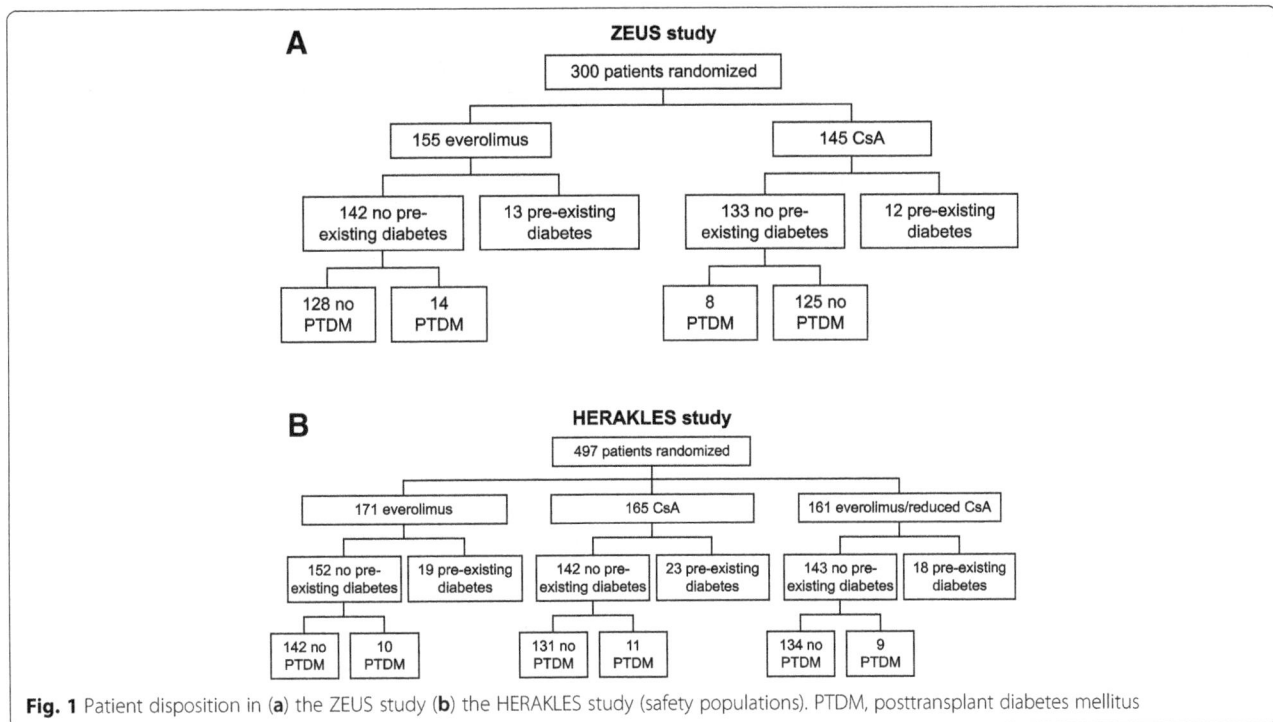

Fig. 1 Patient disposition in (a) the ZEUS study (b) the HERAKLES study (safety populations). PTDM, posttransplant diabetes mellitus

everolimus and CsA cohorts of ZEUS for recipient age among patients with pre-existing diabetes, and for BMI at time of transplant in patients without PTDM and without pre-existing diabetes (Table 1). Almost all patients in both studies were white (97.5% [268/275] in ZEUS, 93.6% [409/437] in HERAKLES).

Immunosuppression

CsA exposure was comparable between treatment groups at randomization in both trials (Table 2). Oral steroid doses were generally slightly higher after randomization in the everolimus-based CNI-free groups than in CsA-containing regimens within the subpopulations of both trials, with the difference reaching significance in the 'no PTDM' and 'no pre-existing diabetes' groups of ZEUS (Table 2). Use of intravenous steroids to treat rejection before or after randomization was similar between treatment group arms prior to randomization in both trials, and any observed percentage differences within the PTDM and pre-existing diabetes cohorts arose from very small absolute numbers.

Post-transplant diabetes mellitus

In the ZEUS study, PTDM was present at randomization (i.e. month 4.5 post-transplant) in 9.2% (13/142) everolimus-treated patients and 5.3% (7/133) of CsA-treated patients; corresponding values at month 12 were 9.9% (14/142) and 6.0% (8/133). In the HERAKLES trial, the incidence of PTDM was 4.6% (7/152), 6.3% (9/142) and 4.2% (6/143) at randomization (i.e. month 3 post-transplant) in

the everolimus, CsA and everolimus/reduced CsA groups, respectively, compared to 6.6% (10/152), 7.8% (11/142) and 6.3% (9/143) at month 12. Thus, after randomization, there were only a total of two new cases of PTDM in the ZEUS study and eight new cases in the HERAKLES trial, distributed equally across treatment groups. Kaplan-Meier estimates showed that there were no significant differences in the incidence of PTDM between treatment groups in either trial (Fig. 2).

When data from both studies were pooled, the incidence of PTDM at month 12 among patients without pre-existing diabetes was 8.2% (24/294) in patients randomized to everolimus without CNI therapy, compared to 6.9% (19/275) in those randomized to standard CsA therapy ($p = 0.64$).

The use of antihyperglycemic therapy was similar between groups for patients with PTDM (everolimus 13/14 [11 insulin, 9 non-insulin therapies] patients, CsA 6/8 [6 insulin, 2 non-insulin therapies] patients) in the ZEUS study, and in the HERAKLES study (everolimus 9/10 [5 insulin, 6 non-insulin therapies], CsA 10/11 [7 insulin, 6 non-insulin therapies], everolimus/reduced CsA 9/9 [8 insulin, 6 non-insulin therapies]).

Pre-existing diabetes

At time of transplant, pre-existing diabetes was present in 8.4% and 8.3% of the everolimus-treated and CsA-treated patients in the ZEUS trial, and in 11.1%, 13.9% and 11.2% of the patients randomized to everolimus, CsA or everolimus/reduced CsA in the HERAKLES

Table 1 Risk factors for diabetes in (a) the ZEUS study (b) the HERAKLES study

(a) ZEUS

	PTDM		No PTDM[a]		Pre-existing diabetes		No pre-existing diabetes	
	EVR (n = 14)	CsA (n = 8)	EVR (n = 128)	CsA (n = 125)	EVR (n = 13)	CsA (n = 12)	EVR (n = 142)	CsA (n = 133)
Recipient age at time of Tx (years)	52.9 (10.7)	57.4 (7.1)	45.8 (12.0)	45.1 (11.7)	50.7 (6.3)	56.2 (7.7)[b]	46.5 (12.0)	45.8 (11.8)
Male gender, n (%)	10 (71.4)	6 (75.0)	82 (64.1)	73 (58.4)	10 (76.9)	7 (58.3)	92 (64.8)	79 (59.4)
White recipient, n (%)	14 (100.0)	7 (87.5)	126 (98.4)	121 (96.8)	12 (92.3)	11 (91.7)	140 (98.6)	128 (96.2)
BMI (kg/m²)								
Time of Tx	27.4 (3.0)	26.1 (3.4)	25.1 (3.9)	24.1 (3.9)[c]	28.8 (3.7)	26.9 (4.1)	25.3 (3.9)	24.2 (3.9)[d]
Time of RDN (month 4.5)	26.9 (3.1)	28.4 (5.6)	25.7 (4.2)	25.0 (4.1)	29.1 (4.5)	27.0 (4.2)	25.8 (4.1)	25.1 (4.1)
HCV+, n/N (%)	1/13 (7.7)	0/8 (0.0)	3/127 (2.4)	0/122 (0.0)	0/13 (0.0)	0/12 (0.0)	4/140 (2.9)	0/130 (0.0)
Random blood glucose, mmol/L								
Time of Tx	6.3 (1.7)	6.6 (1.1)	5.4 (1.3)	5.1 (1.1)	8.9 (3.3)	9.3 (2.7)	5.5 (1.3)	5.2 (1.1)
Time of RDN (month 4.5)	7.5 (3.9)	5.6 (1.8)	5.1 (1.0)	5.2 (1.0)	7.4 (3.2)	7.7 (3.6)	5.3 (1.3)	5.2 (1.1)
IV. treatment for rejection before RDN, n (%)	4 (28.6)	1 (12.5)	12 (9.4)	21 (16.8)	2 (15.4)	2 (16.7)	17 (12.0)	22 (16.5)

(b) HERAKLES

	PTDM			No PTDM[a]			Pre-existing diabetes			No pre-existing diabetes		
	EVR (n = 10)	CsA (n = 11)	EVR/reduced CsA (n = 9)	EVR (n = 142)	CsA (n = 131)	EVR/reduced CsA (n = 134)	EVR (n = 19)	CsA (n = 23)	EVR/reduced CsA (n = 18)	EVR (n = 152)	CsA (n = 142)	EVR/reduced CsA (n = 143)
Recipient age at Tx (years)	49.4 (12.3)	58.2 (6.9)	51.7 (10.9)	48.3 (12.6)	48.7 (11.9)	47.8 (12.6)	58.2 (8.1)	56.5 (9.7)	57.5 (7.1)	48.3 (12.5)	49.4 (11.8)	48.0 (12.5)
Male gender, n (%)	5 (50.0)	4 (36.4)	2 (22.2)	84 (59.2)	80 (61.1)	84 (62.7)	13 (68.4)	16 (69.6)	14 (77.8)	89 (58.6)	84 (59.2)	86 (60.1)
White recipient, n (%)	10 (100.0)	11 (100.0)	9 (100.0)	132 (93.0)	126 (96.2)	121 (90.3)	16 (84.2)	23 (100.0)	17 (94.4)	142 (93.4)	137 (96.5)	130 (90.9)
BMI (kg/m²)												
Time of Tx	25.0 (3.4)	28.2 (4.8)	28.2 (6.1)	24.9 (3.9)	25.3 (4.0)	25.4 (4.1)	28.8 (5.6)	30.2 (4.8)	29.4 (4.3)	24.9 (3.8)	25.5 (4.2)	25.5 (4.3)
Time of RDN (month 3)	25.3 (3.4)	28.0 (4.5)	29.3 (7.0)	25.3 (3.6)	25.4 (3.9)	25.5 (4.3)	28.7 (5.8)	29.5 (5.1)	29.2 (3.9)	25.3 (3.6)	25.6 (4.0)	25.7 (4.6)
HCV+, n/N (%)	–	–	–	1 (0.7)	3 (2.3)	2 (1.5)	–	–	–	1 (0.7)	3 (2.1)	2 (1.4)
Random blood glucose (mmol/L)												
Time of Tx	5.3 (0.9)	6.0 (1.4)	5.8 (1.1)	5.4 (1.1)	5.2 (0.8)	5.4 (1.2)	6.4 (2.7)	8.7 (3.6)	6.0 (0.9)	5.4 (1.1)	5.2 (0.9)	5.4 (1.2)
Time of RDN (month 3)	6.3 (1.7)	5.8 (0.9)	6.3 (2.4)	5.3 (1.1)	5.2 (1.1)	5.2 (1.0)	7.0 (2.4)	7.6 (3.2)	7.9 (4.1)	5.4 (1.2)	5.3 (1.1)	5.3 (1.2)
IV. treatment for rejection before RDN, n (%)	–	1 (9.1)	2 (22.2)	14 (9.9)	7 (5.3)	12 (9.0)	4 (21.1)	4 (17.4)	1 (5.6)	14 (9.2)	8 (5.6)	14 (9.8)

[a] And no pre-existing diabetes
[b] p = 0.038 for everolimus versus CsA (Fisher's test)
[c] p = 0.027 for everolimus versus CsA (Fisher's test)
[d] p = 0.010 for everolimus versus CsA (Fisher's test)
All differences between the everolimus and CsA groups are not significant unless stated otherwise
Continuous variables are shown as mean (SD)
BMI body mass index, CsA cyclosporine, EVR everolimus, HCV+ hepatitis C virus positive, PTDM posttransplant diabetes mellitus, RDN randomization, SD standard deviation, Tx transplantation

Table 2 Immunosuppression in (a) the ZEUS study and (b) the HERAKLES study

(a) ZEUS

	PTDM		No PTDM[a]		Pre-existing diabetes		No pre-existing diabetes	
	EVR (n = 14)	CsA (n = 8)	EVR (n = 128)	CsA (n = 125)	EVR (n = 13)	CsA (n = 12)	EVR (n = 142)	CsA (n = 133)
Everolimus C_0 (ng/mL)								
RDN[b]	—	—	—	—	—	—	—	—
M12	6.2 (1.4)	—	6.5 (2.1)	—	7.7 (2.8)	—	6.5 (2.0)	—
CsA C_0 (ng/mL), mean (SD)								
At RDN (month 3)	158 (25)	142 (38)	153 (51)	147 (50)	138 (63)	159 (40)	154 (49)	147 (50)
M12	—	141 (85)	—	118 (33)	—	130 (40)	—	120 (37)
EC-MPS dose (mg/day), mean (SD)								
RDN (month 3)	1234 (366)	1035 (449)	1317 (284)	1294 (289)	1246 (431)	1110 (419)	1309 (293)	1278 (305)
M12	1108 (452)	1080 (465)	1193 (363)	1234 (340)	1135 (385)	1211 (333)	1186 (371)	1226 (347)
Oral steroids(mg/day)								
BL to RDN (month 3)	21.3 (5.1)	16.3 (4.2)[c]	17.7 (5.7)	17.9 (5.7)	18.1 (6.2)	15.4 (4.8)	18.1 (5.7)	17.8 (5.6)
RDN to M12	10.7 (7.9)	10.2 (3.2)	7.6 (2.8)	7.2 (4.3)[c]	10.3 (10.9)	6.3 (3.1)	7.9 (3.7)	7.4 (4.3)[c]
I.V. steroids to treat rejection, n (%)								
BL to RDN (month 3)	4 (28.6)	1 (12.5)	13 (10.2)	21 (16.8)	2 (15.4)	2 (16.7)	17 (12.0)	22 (16.5)
RDN to M12	3 (21.4)	1 (12.5)	12 (9.4)	11 (8.8)	1 (7.7)	2 (16.7)	15 (10.6)	12 (9.0)

(b) HERAKLES

	PTDM			No PTDM[a]			Pre-existing diabetes			No pre-existing diabetes		
	EVR (n = 10)	CsA (n = 11)	EVR/reduced CsA (n = 9)	EVR (n = 142)	CsA (n = 131)	EVR/reduced CsA (n = 134)	EVR (n = 19)	CsA (n = 23)	EVR/reduced CsA (n = 18)	EVR (n = 152)	CsA (n = 142)	EVR/reduced CsA (n = 143)
Everolimus C_0 (ng/mL)												
RDN (month 4.5)	5.6 (3.0)	—	4.5 (2.1)	6.1 (3.2)	—	7.0 (12.6)	5.7 (2.1)	—	6.1 (2.2)	6.1 (3.1)	—	6.8 (12.2)
M12	7.2 (2.9)	—	5.7 (2.4)	6.6 (2.2)	—	6.3 (2.7)	7.2 (1.8)	—	5.2 (2.2)	6.6 (2.3)	—	6.3 (2.7)
CsA C_0 (ng/mL)												
RDN (month 4.5)	155 (29)	167 (48)	157 (38)	154 (46)	164 (55)	161 (72)	169 (61)	167 (50)	157 (42)	154 (45)	164 (54)	161 (70)
M12	—	138 (56)	126 (34)	—	119 (29)	80 (34)	—	116 (36)	59 (22)	—	120 (32)	83 (35)
EC-MPS dose (mg/day)												
RDN (month 4.5)	1305 (268)	1360 (240)	1440 (0)	1345 (246)	1375 (214)	1287 (314)	1357 (216)	1271 (288)	1305 (413)	1342 (246)	1374 (215)	1296 (307)
M12	1183 (342)	1280 (317)	—	1171 (345)	1266 (335)	—	1260 (306)	1239 (336)	—	1172 (343)	1267 (332)	—
Oral steroids(mg/day)												
BL to RDN (month 4.5)	21.4 (4.4)	19.7 (5.5)[c]	20.9 (2.6)	19.2 (5.6)	19.2 (5.6)	19.3 (5.3)	16.6 (4.4)	18.4 (5.4)	18.8 (5.3)	19.4 (5.0)	19.3 (5.6)	19.4 (5.2)
RDN to M12	8.2 (3.4)	7.4 (3.2)	6.0 (2.7)	7.4 (3.6)	6.8 (3.7)	6.9 (3.1)	7.3 (4.0)	7.1 (4.2)	6.5 (1.7)	7.4 (3.6)	6.9 (3.6)	6.9 (3.1)

Table 2 Immunosuppression in (a) the ZEUS study and (b) the HERAKLES study (*Continued*)

	PTDM		No PTDM[a]			Pre-existing diabetes			No pre-existing diabetes		
I.V. steroids to treat rejection, n (%)											
BL to RDN (month 4.5)	0	2 (22.2)	12 (8.5)	7 (5.3)	11 (8.2)	4 (21.1)	1 (4.3)	1 (5.6)	12 (7.9)	7 (4.9)	13 (9.1)
RDN to M12	1 (10.0)	2 (18.2)	13 (9.2)	10 (7.6)	12 (9.0)	4 (21.1)	2 (8.7)	1 (5.6)	14 (9.2)	12 (8.5)	13 (9.1)

[a]And no pre-existing diabetes

[b]Not recorded at RDN

[c]$p < 0.05$ for everolimus vs CsA (two-sample Wilcoxon rank-sum test of the F-test)

Continuous variables are shown as mean (SD)

Last observation carried forward (LOCF) method applied to month 12 values. All differences versus the standard CsA groups were not significant unless stated otherwise

BL baseline, C_0 trough concentration, *CsA* cyclosporine, *EC-MPS* enteric-coated mycophenolate sodium, *EVR* everolimus, *I.V.* intravenous, *M12* month 12, *M6* month 6, *PTDM* posttransplant diabetes mellitus, *RDN* randomization, *SD* standard deviation

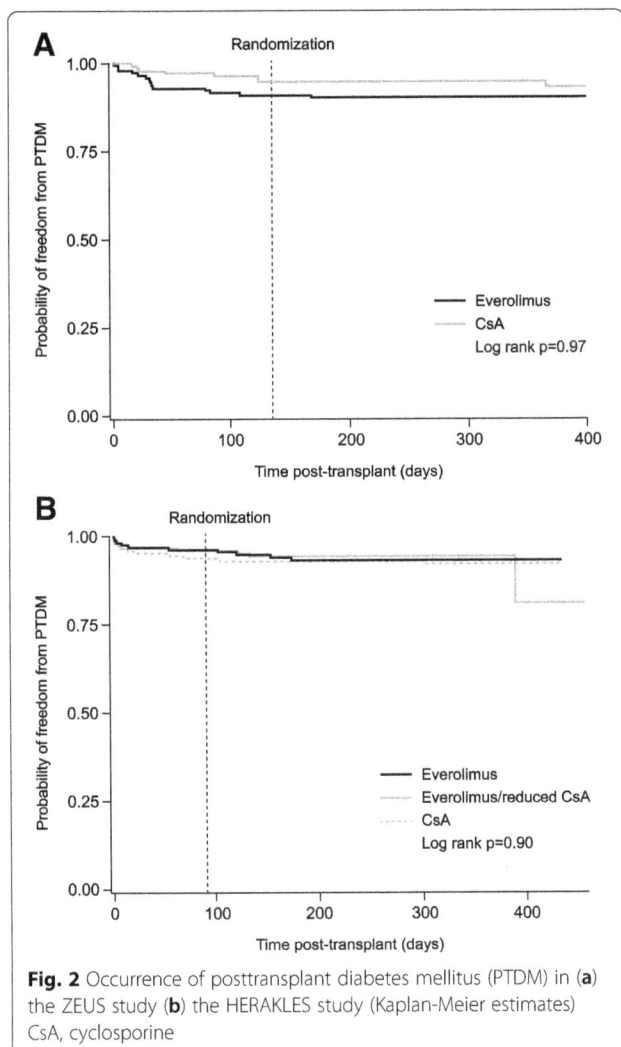

Fig. 2 Occurrence of posttransplant diabetes mellitus (PTDM) in (**a**) the ZEUS study (**b**) the HERAKLES study (Kaplan-Meier estimates) CsA, cyclosporine

study, respectively. There was no apparent difference in progression of random glucose concentrations between the two treatment groups to month 12 for patients with pre-existing diabetes (Fig. 3). From randomization to month 12, the mean (SD) change in random glucose concentration was 1.1 (3.4) mmol/L versus 1.5 (4.5)mmol/L in the everolimus versus CsA groups in the ZEUS study (p = 0.52). In the HERAKLES study, the mean (SD) change was 2.2 (3.0) mmol/L, 0.5 (4.9) mmol/L and – 0.2 (3.7) mmol/L in the everolimus, CsA and everolimus/reduced CsA arms, respectively (p = 0.24).

Among patients with pre-existing diabetes, use of antihyperglycemic therapy was similar between groups in the ZEUS trial (everolimus 12/13 patients [12 insulin, 3 non-insulin therapies], CsA 12/12 [12 insulin, 4 non-insulin therapies]) and the HERAKLES trial (everolimus 16/19 [16 insulin, 3 non-insulin], CsA 22/23 [20 insulin, 9 non-insulin], everolimus/reduced CsA17/18 [17 insulin, 6 non-insulin]).

Blood glucose concentrations

The mean (SD) change in random blood glucose from randomization to month 12 among patients with PTDM was similar in the everolimus group versus the CsA group for the ZEUS study (p = 0.10) and the HERAKLES study (p = 0.38). Mean random blood glucose levels also remained similar between treatment groups in both trials for patients who did not develop PTDM (Fig. 3). As expected, patients with PTDM clearly had higher glucose values compared to patients without PTDM (Fig. 3).

Biopsy-proven acute rejection

The higher rate of mild BPAR (Grade I) in the overall ZEUS study population was reflected in the cohorts without PTDM or pre-existing diabetes (Additional file 1: Table S2). In the HERAKLES study, there were no significant differences in the incidence of BPAR between treatment groups in any subpopulation (Additional file 1: Table S2).

Renal function

The change in eGFR from randomization to month 12 was significantly in favor of everolimus in the two largest subpopulations (no PTDM and no pre-existing diabetes) for both trials (Table 3). In the subpopulations with PTDM or pre-existing diabetes, the differences between groups were of a similar order of magnitude to those seen in the larger subpopulations, but in these small cohorts statistical significance was not reached.

Discussion

Results from this post hoc analysis of two large randomized studies do not suggest any difference in the incidence or severity of PTDM in patients who were converted early post-transplant from a CsA-based regimen to everolimus, or in the progression of pre-existing diabetes. Kaplan-Meier estimates showed comparable rates of PTDM in the different treatment cohorts after randomization in both studies to month 12, with similar patterns of random blood glucose concentration over time in the subpopulations with or without PTDM or pre-existing diabetes. The number of patients who developed PTDM after randomization was identical in the everolimus group or the standard CsA group, but absolute numbers were very low, even within this large pooled cohort, so firm conclusions cannot be drawn.

The progressive renal deterioration which is frequently associated with diabetes in the general population has also been documented in patients with PTDM [33, 34], so any potential benefit for preservation of renal function may be particularly relevant in this subpopulation. Here, the change in eGFR from randomization to month 12 in patients receiving everolimus within a CNI-free

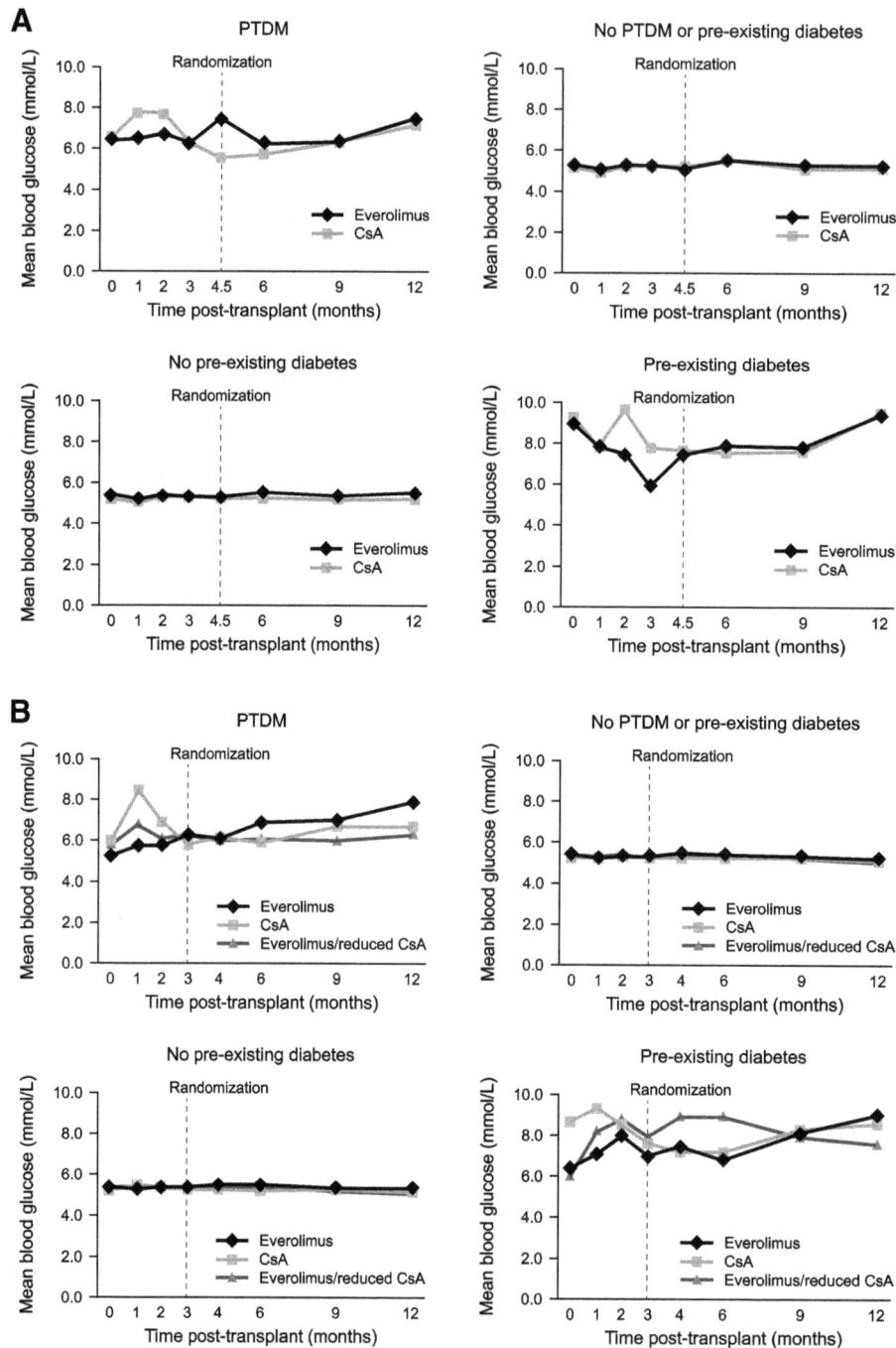

Fig. 3 Mean random blood glucose concentrations from time of transplant to month 12 in (**a**) the ZEUS study and (**b**) the HERAKLES study. CsA, cyclosporine; PTDM, posttransplant diabetes mellitus

regimen which was achieved in the overall study populations at month 12 [29, 30] was also observed in the subpopulation of patients with PTDM, although the small numbers of patients precluded any statistical differences. Mean eGFR in patients randomized to CNI-free therapy with everolimus in patients with PTDM improved by 14 mL/min/1.73m^2 in the ZEUS

study and by 4.9 mL/min/1.73m^2 in HERAKLES by month 12. Among patients with pre-existing diabetes, there was a numerically greater improvement in renal function from randomization to month 12 in the CNI-free cohorts of both trials versus the comparator groups.

Certain aspects of the analysis should be taken into account. First, PTDM was included from the time of

Table 3 Estimated GFR (Nankivell formula [32]) (mL/min/1.73m²) in (a) the ZEUS study (b) the HERAKLES study. Values are shown as mean (SD)

(a) ZEUS study	PTDM		No PTDM[a]		Pre-existing diabetes		No pre-existing diabetes	
	EVR (n = 14)	CsA (n = 8)	EVR (n = 128)	CsA (n = 125)	EVR (n = 13)	CsA (n = 12)	EVR (n = 142)	CsA (n = 133)
RDN (month 3)	64.8 (13.8)	54.3 (23.0)	63.3 (17.6)	63.0 (14.7)	67.6 (22.4)	64.4 (19.7)	63.4 (17.2)	62.5 (15.2)
P value vs CsA[b]	0.31	–	0.92	–	0.50	–	0.85	–
M12	78.5 (17.9)	49.2 (16.3)	70.4 (18.7)	61.6 (16.1)	73.1 (22.1)	65.7 (22.2)	71.1 (18.7)	61.0 (16.2)
P value vs CsA[b]	0.008	–	< 0.001	–	0.22	–	< 0.001	–
Change from RDN to M12	14.0 (11.4)	−9.2 (15.9)	7.5 (10.5)	−1.5 (9.6)	5.5 (5.9)	0.7 (10.0)	8.2 (10.8)	−1.8 (10.0)
P value vs CsA[c]	Not available[d]	–	< 0.001	–	0.87	–	< 0.001	–

(b) HERAKLES study	PTDM			No PTDM[a]			Pre-existing diabetes			No pre-existing diabetes		
	EVR (n = 10)	CsA (n = 11)	EVR/reduced CsA (n = 9)	EVR (n = 142)	CsA (n = 131)	EVR/reduced CsA (n = 134)	EVR (n = 19)	CsA (n = 23)	EVR/reduced CsA (n = 18)	EVR (n = 152)	CsA (n = 142)	EVR/reduced CsA (n = 143)
RND (month 4.5)	70.6 (22.1)	62.4 (16.7)	59.4 (23.4)	64.9 (14.6)	61.2 (15.1)	62.8 (14.1)	71.3 (17.9)	65.1 (13.6)	67.6 (15.2)	65.3 (15.2)	61.3 (15.2)	62.6 (14.8)
P value vs CsA[b]	0.34	–	0.81	0.05	–	0.39	0.41	–	0.59	0.03	–	0.43
M12	75.5 (29.9)	60.5 (26.3)	56.4 (28.1)	70.8 (18.3)	62.2 (16.1)	63.1 (18.9)	76.5 (20.8)	65.5 (16.8)	70.5 (19.8)	71.1 (19.2)	62.1 (17.0)	62.7 (19.5)
P value vs CsA[b]	0.19	–	1.0	< 0.001	–	0.61	0.11	–	0.50	< 0.001	–	0.63
Change from RDN to M12	4.9 (16.7)	−1.9 (15.8)	−3.0 (10.1)	5.9 (13.9)	1.0 (11.1)	0.4 (12.8)	5.3 (12.9)	2.8 (11.8)	0.1 (11.7)	5.8 (14.0)	0.7 (11.5)	0.1 (12.7)
P value vs CsA[c]	0.11	–	0.86	< 0.001	–	< 0.001	0.17	–	0.78	< 0.001	–	< 0.001

[a]And no pre-existing diabetes
[b]P values based on the two-sample Wilcoxon rank-sum test of the F-test
[c]P values based on ANCOVA model with treatment, center, donor type as factors and estimated GFR value at randomization as covariate
[d]Numbers too low to permit a meaningful ANCOVA analysis
Last observation carried forward (LOCF) method applied to month 12 values
CsA cyclosporine, EVR everolimus, GFR glomerular filtration rate, M12 month 12, PTDM posttransplant diabetes mellitus, RDN randomization

transplant, with few events in either group after randomization, and the onset of PTDM was collected by standard adverse event reporting, with no pre-specified criteria. In the DIRECT study [4], in which data on HbA1$_c$, insulin level and oral glucose tolerance testing were collected prospectively to month 6 in patients receiving a standard CsA-based regimen, the incidence of treated PTDM was 7.4% but a further 7.4% had untreated PTDM based on American Diabetes Association criteria (14.8% overall) [35]. Based on the 6.8–8.0% incidence of PTDM reported by 12 months in the current studies, it is likely that the standard reporting adverse event techniques did not capture all cases of PTDM. However, since it seems reasonable to assume that centers applied the same procedures for monitoring and defining PTDM regardless of patients' immunosuppressive treatment, it is unlikely that this will have biased diagnosis rates between treatment arms. Second, oral glucose tolerance tests were not recorded and HbA1$_c$ levels were not measured, with the only available laboratory test being random blood glucose levels. This is a weakness of the analysis. The presence of hyperglycemia could be recorded as an adverse event by investigators, but no strict reporting checks for this value were in place, hence reporting of hyperglycemia is not fully reliable. Information on antidiabetic therapy was captured by standard documentation of concomitant medication, and may have been incomplete despite the strict external monitoring. Third, the analysis does not address the relative diabetogenic effect of everolimus and CsA during the very early post-transplant period (up to month 3), when the rate of onset of glucose metabolism disturbances, hyperglycemia and onset of PTDM can be highest [4, 36]. Fourth, the results presented here apply only to conversion from CsA (not tacrolimus) to everolimus after the initial weeks post-transplant. Tacrolimus, now the dominant CNI, is widely regarded to be more diabetogenic than CsA [37, 38]. Fifth, the studies were not powered to detect differences within subpopulations for the primary endpoint (eGFR at month 12) or to detect differences in any of the endpoints which were specified post hoc. Indeed, even with this large pooled dataset, the number of patients who developed PTDM after randomization was very small, restricting interpretation. Lastly, the follow-up period (a maximum of nine months after randomization) was too short to assess any long-term effect of CNI administration on late-onset PTDM or progression of pre-existing diabetes.

Conclusions

Within the limitations of this post hoc analysis, including an absence of pre-specified diagnostic criteria for PTDM or extensive laboratory data, conversion from a CsA-based regimen to everolimus in combination with mycophenolic acid and steroids within the first six months after kidney

transplantation does not appear to affect the subsequent risk of developing PTDM, or adversely affect the progression of pre-existing diabetes. This finding from the subgroup analysis adds to the observed benefit on renal function after switching to everolimus-based therapy with CNI-withdrawal seen from the main study analyses.

Abbreviations

BMI: Body mass index; BPAR: Biopsy-proven acute rejection; CNI: Calcineurin inhibitor; CsA: Cyclosporine; EC-MPS: Enteric-coated mycophenolate sodium; eGFR: Estimated glomerular filtration rate; HCV: Hepatitis C virus; LOCF: Last observation carried forward; mTOR: Mammalian target of rapamycin; PTDM: Posttransplant diabetes mellitus; SD: Standard deviation

Acknowledgements

The authors would like to thank Caroline Dunstall for editorial support and Elisabeth Grünewald for statistical support.

Funding

The ZEUS and HERAKLES studies were funded by Novartis Pharma GmbH, Nürnberg, Germany. The company contributed to the design of the study and to the analysis of data, and reviewed the manuscript before submission. All data collection was undertaken by the investigators.

Authors' contributions

CS guided the analysis, developed the PTDM post hoc analysis study design presented here, analyzed the data and wrote the manuscript. CS, OW, FL, WA, PR, UE, BV, KH, JJ, MG, RS, IAH, VK, RPW, AM, BS, MD, MZ, and KB recruited patients and acquired data. CS, E-MP, MP and KB provided medical input, and analyzed the data. CS and MP wrote the manuscript. All authors were involved in drafting the manuscript or revising it critically for important intellectual content. All authors read and approved the final manuscript.

Competing interests

Claudia Sommerer has received honoraria from Novartis, Chiesi and Sanofi, and her institution has received research funding from Chiesi, Astellas and Novartis.
Oliver Witzke has received research funds and/or honoraria from Alexion, Astellas, Bristol-Myers Squibb, Chiesi, Janssen-Cilag, MSD, Novartis, Pfizer, Roche and Shire.
Frank Lehner has received research funds and/or honoraria from Astellas, Bristol-Myers Squibb, Chiesi, Fresenius, Hexal, Novartis, Pfizer and Roche Pharma.
Wolfgang Arns has received research funds and/or honoraria from Alexion, Astellas, Chiesi and Novartis.
Petra Reinke has received research funds, honoraria, advisory board from Teva, ThermoFisher, Pfizer, Astellas, Amgen, Baxalta; MSD and Pluriste.
Ute Eisenberger has received honoraria and/or travel expenses from Novartis Pharma, Astellas and Amgen.
Bruno Vogt has no conflicts of interest to declare.
Katharina Heller has no conflicts of interest to declare.
Johannes Jacobi has received honoraria from Roche.
Markus Guba has no conflicts of interest to declare.
Rolf Stahl has no conflicts of interest to declare.
Ingeborg A Hauser has received honoraria from Alexion, Astellas, Chiesi, Fresenius, Hexal, Novartis, Roche, Sanofi and Teva.
Volker Kliem has received honoraria and fees from Astellas, Novartis, Raptor and Fresenius.
Rudolf P Wüthrich has received fees for scientific advice from Astellas, Novartis, Roche and Wyeth (now Pfizer).
Anja Mühlfeld has no conflicts of interest to declare.
Barbara Suwelack has no conflicts of interest to declare .
Michael Duerr has received research funds from Bristol–Myers Squibb and travel grants from Novartis and Roche.
Martin Zeier has received research funding from Dietmar Hopp-Stiftung.
Martina Porstner is an employee of Novartis Pharma GmbH.

Eva-Maria Paulus is employee of Novartis Pharma GmbH and holds stock options.
Klemens Budde has received research funds and/or honoraria from Abbvie, Alexion, Astellas, Bristol-Myers Squibb, Chiesi, Fresenius, Genentech, Hexal, Novartis, Otsuka, Pfizer, Roche, Shire, Siemens, and Veloxis Pharma.

Author details
[1]Department of Nephrology, University of Heidelberg, Im Neuenheimer Feld 162, 69120 Heidelberg, Germany. [2]Department of Infectious Diseases, University Duisburg-Essen, Essen, Germany. [3]Department of General, Visceral and Transplantation Surgery, Hannover Medical School, Hannover, Germany. [4]Department of Nephrology and Transplantation, Cologne Merheim Medical Center, Cologne, Germany. [5]Department of Nephrology and Intensive Care, Charité Campus Virchow, Charité-Universitätsmedizin Berlin, Berlin, Germany. [6]Department of Nephrology and Hypertension, University of Bern, Inselspital, Bern, Switzerland. [7]Department of Nephrology and Hypertension, University of Erlangen-Nuremberg, Erlangen, Germany. [8]Department of General-, Visceral- and Transplantation Surgery, Munich University Hospital, Campus Grosshadern, Munich, Germany. [9]Division of Nephrology, University Medical Center Hamburg-Eppendorf, Hamburg, Germany. [10]Med. Klinik III, Department of Nephrology, UKF, Goethe University, Frankfurt, Germany. [11]Department of Internal Medicine and Nephrology, Kidney Transplant Center, Nephrological Center of Lower Saxony, Klinikum Hann, Münden, Germany. [12]Division of Nephrology, University Hospital, Zürich, Switzerland. [13]Division of Nephrology and Immunology, University Hospital RWTH Aachen, Aachen, Germany. [14]Department of Internal Medicine - Transplant Nephrology, University Hospital of Münster, Münster, Germany. [15]Department of Nephrology, Charité Universitätsmedizin Berlin, Berlin, Germany. [16]Novartis Pharma GmbH, Nürnberg, Germany.

References
1. https://optn.transplant.hrsa.gov/data/about-data/optn-database/ (Organ Procurement and Transplantation Network [OPTN] National Data Reports, Waiting list, Organ by diagnosis) Accessed 13 Mar 2016.
2. Adeghate E, Schattner P, Dunn E. An update on the etiology and epidemiology of diabetes mellitus. Ann N Y Acad Sci. 2006;1084:1–29.
3. Herman WH, Zimmet P. Type 2 diabetes: an epidemic requiring global attention and urgent action. Diabetes Care. 2012;35(5):943–4.
4. Vincenti F, Friman S, Scheuermann E, et al. DIRECT (Diabetes Incidence after Renal Transplantation: Neoral C Monitoring Versus Tacrolimus) Investigators. Results of an international, randomized trial comparing glucose metabolism disorders and outcome with cyclosporine versus tacrolimus. Am J Transplant. 2007;7(6):1506–14.
5. Chadban SJ. New-onset diabetes after transplantation--should it be a factor in choosing an immunosuppressant regimen for kidney transplant recipients. Nephrol Dial Transplant. 2008;23(6):1816–8.
6. Sarno G, Muscogiuri G, De Rosa P. New-onset diabetes after kidney transplantation: prevalence, risk factors, and management. Transplantation. 2012;93(12):1189–95.
7. Boucek P, Saudek F, Pokorna E, et al. Kidney transplantation in type 2 diabetic patients: a comparison with matched non-diabetic subjects. Nephrol Dial Transplant. 2002;17(9):1678–83.
8. Rømming Sørensen V, Schwartz Sørensen S, Feldt-Rasmussen B. Long-term graft and patient survival following renal transplantation in diabetic patients. Scand J Urol Nephrol. 2006;40(3):247–51.
9. Hjelmesaeth J, Hartmann A, Leivestad T, et al. The impact of early-diagnosed new-onset post-transplantation diabetes mellitus on survival and major cardiac events. Kidney Int. 2006;69(3):588–91.
10. Cosio FG, Kudva Y, van der Velde M, et al. New onset hyperglycemia and diabetes are associated with increased cardiovascular risk after kidney transplantation. Kidney Int. 2005;67(6):2415–21.
11. Burroughs TE, Swindle J, Takemoto S, et al. Diabetic complications associated with new-onset diabetes mellitus in renal transplant recipients. Transplantation. 2007;83(8):1027–34.
12. Heisel O, Heisel R, Balshaw R, Keown P. New onset diabetes mellitus in patients receiving calcineurin inhibitors: a systematic review and meta-analysis. Am J Transplant. 2004;4(4):583–95.
13. Vesco L, Busson M, Bedrossian J, Bitker MO, Hiesse C, Lang P. Diabetes mellitus after renal transplantation: characteristics, outcome, and risk factors. Transplantation. 1996;61(10):1475–8.
14. Weir MR, Diekmann F, Flechner SM, et al. mTOR inhibition: the learning curve in kidney transplantation. Transpl Int. 2010;23(5):447–60.
15. Sharif A, Shabir S, Chand S, Cockwell P, Ball S, Borrows R. Meta-analysis of calcineurin-inhibitor-sparing regimens in kidney transplantation. J Am Soc Nephrol. 2011;22(11):2107–18.
16. Sharif A, Hecking M, de Vries AP, et al. Proceedings from an international consensus meeting on posttransplantation diabetes mellitus: recommendations and future directions. Am J Transplant. 2014;14(9):1992–2000.
17. Liefeldt L, Budde K. Risk factors for cardiovascular disease in renal transplant recipients and strategies to minimize risk. Transpl Int. 2010;23(12):1191–204.
18. Vitko S, Wlodarczyk Z, Kyllönen L, et al. Tacrolimus combined with two different dosages of sirolimus in kidney transplantation: results of a multicenter study. Am J Transplant. 2006;6(3):531–8.
19. Sampaio EL, Pinheiro-Machado PG, Garcia R, et al. Mycophenolate mofetil vs. sirolimus in kidney transplant recipients receiving tacrolimus-based immunosuppressive regimen. Clin Transpl. 2008;22(2):141–149.
20. Machado PG, Felipe CR, Hanzawa NM, et al. An open-label randomized trial of the safety and efficacy of sirolimus vs. azathioprine in living related renal allograft recipients receiving cyclosporine and prednisone combination. Clin Transpl. 2004;18(1):28–38.
21. Groth CG, Bäckman L, Morales JM, et al. Sirolimus (rapamycin)-based therapy in human renal transplantation: similar efficacy and different toxicity compared with cyclosporine. Sirolimus European Renal Transplant Study group. Transplantation. 1999;67(7):1036–42.
22. Johnston W, Rose CL, Webster AC, Gill JS. Sirolimus is associated with new-onset diabetes in kidney transplant recipients. J Am Soc Nephrol. 2008;19(7):1411–8.
23. Webster AC, Lee VWS, Chapman JR, Craig JC. Target of rapamycin inhibitors (sirolimus and everolimus) for primary immunosuppression of kidney transplant recipients: a systematic review and meta-analysis of randomized trials. Transplantation. 2006;81(9):1234–48.
24. Flechner SM, Glyda M, Cockfield S, et al. The ORION study: comparison of two sirolimus-based regimens versus tacrolimus and mycophenolate mofetil in renal allograft recipients. Am J Transplant. 2011;11(8):1633–44.
25. Ekberg H, Tedesco-Silva H, Demirbas A, et al. ELITE-Symphony Study. Reduced exposure to calcineurin inhibitors in renal transplantation. N Engl J Med. 2007;357(25):2562–75.
26. Tedesco Silva H Jr, Cibrik D, Johnston T, et al. Everolimus plus reduced-exposure CsA versus mycophenolic acid plus standard-exposure CsA in renal-transplant recipients. Am J Transplant. 2010;10(6):1401–13.
27. Qazi Y, Shaffer D, Kaplan B, et al. Efficacy and safety of everolimus plus low-dose tacrolimus versus mycophenolate mofetil plus standard-dose tacrolimus in de novo renal transplant recipients: 12-month data. Am J Transplant. 2017;17(5):1358–69.
28. Rostaing L, Kamar N. mTOR inhibitor/proliferation signal inhibitors: entering or leaving the field? J Nephrol. 2010;23(2):133–42.
29. Budde K, Becker T, Arns W, Sommerer C, Reinke P, Eisenberger U. Everolimus-based, calcineurin-inhibitor-free regimen in recipients of de-novo kidney transplants: an open-label, randomised, controlled trial. Lancet. 2011;377(9768):837–47.
30. Budde K, Zeier M, Witzke O, et al. Everolimus with cyclosporine withdrawal or low-exposure cyclosporine in kidney transplantation from month 3: a multicentre, randomized trial. Nephrol Dial Transplant. 2017;32(6):1060–70.
31. Racusen LC, Solez K, Colvin RB, et al. The Banff 97 working classification of renal allograft pathology. Kidney Int. 1999;55(2):713–23.
32. Nankivell BJ, Gruenewald SM, Allen R, Chapman JR. Predicting glomerular filtration rate after kidney transplantation. Transplantation. 1995;59(12):1683–9.
33. Madhav D, Ram R, Dakshinamurty KV. Posttransplant diabetes mellitus: analysis of risk factors, effects on biochemical parameters and graft function 5 years after renal transplantation. Transplant Proc. 2010;42(10):4069–71.
34. Pietrzak-Nowacka M, Safranow K, Dziewanowski K, et al. Impact of posttransplant diabetes mellitus on graft function in autosomal dominant polycystic kidney disease patients after kidney transplantation. Ann Acad Med Stetin. 2008;54(1):41–8.
35. American Diabetes Association. Expert Committee on the Diagnosis and Classification of Diabetes Mellitus.Report of the expert committee on the diagnosis and classification of diabetes mellitus. Diabetes Care. 2003;26(Suppl 1):S5–20.

36. Luan FL, Stuckey LJ, Ojo AO. Abnormal glucose metabolism and metabolic syndrome in non-diabetic kidney transplant recipients early after transplantation. Transplantation. 2010;89(8):1034–9.

37. Wissing KM, Abramowicz D, Weekers L, et al. Prospective randomized study of conversion from tacrolimus to cyclosporine A to improve glucose metabolism in patients with posttransplant diabetes mellitus after renal transplantation. Am J Transplant. 2018;18(7):1726–34

38. Knoll GA, Bell RC. Tacrolimus versus cyclosporin for immunosuppression in renal transplantation: meta-analysis of randomised trials. BMJ. 1999; 318(7191):1104–7.

15

Risk factors, mortality and acute kidney injury outcomes in cirrhotic patients in the emergency department

Paulo Ricardo Gessolo Lins[1]* (iD), Wallace Stwart Carvalho Padilha[1], Carolina Frade Magalhaes Giradin Pimentel[2], Marcelo Costa Batista[1] and Aécio Flávio Teixeira de Gois[2]

Abstract

Background: Acute kidney injury (AKI) is common in cirrhotic patients and is associated with negative outcomes. The aim of this study was to evaluate the presence of AKI and its progression according to KDIGO (Kidney Disease: Improving Global Outcomes) criteria in cirrhotic patients admitted to the emergency department and to determine the association of AKI with hospital mortality.

Methods: This retrospective study included 258 cirrhotic patients admitted to the emergency department of a university hospital from March 2015 to February 2017. AKI was diagnosed and classified according to the KDIGO criteria.

Results: The overall incidence of AKI in cirrhotic patients was 53.9%, and the overall hospital mortality was 28.4%. Mortality was associated with the presence, stage, and progression of AKI. Patients with AKI stage 1 and sCr < 1.5 mg/dl (KDIGO 1a) had a lower mortality rate than patients with AKI stage 1 and sCr > 1.5 mg/dl (KDIGO 1b). In the logistic regression analysis, three variables were independently associated with hospital mortality: cancer, AKI and progression of AKI.

Conclusions: According to the data presented, a single measure of creatinine is not enough, and there is a need for meticulous follow-up of the renal function of patients with hepatic cirrhosis hospitalized in an emergency unit. In addition, this study reinforces the need for subclassification of KDIGO 1 in cirrhotic patients, since patients with acute renal injury and creatinine greater than 1.5 mg/dL present a worse clinical outcome.

Keywords: Liver cirrhosis, Acute kidney injury, Hospital mortality, KDIGO, Progression of AKI

Background

Acute kidney injury (AKI) is a common complication in patients with liver cirrhosis who are admitted to the emergency department, and it is related to significantly higher mortality rates among this population [1–8]. AKI pathogenesis in cirrhotic patients is intimately related to hemodynamic changes secondary to liver failure and to a self-perpetuating process that ultimately leads to renal and splenic vasoconstriction, promoting decoupling between renal supply and demand and ultimately promoting AKI [9].

Over time, different definitions of AKI have been proposed for cirrhotic patients [10]. In 2012, a universal definition of acute renal injury was proposed by the KDIGO group [11]. However, although this definition is widely applied in different populations, there are few validation studies of KDIGO in cirrhotic patients [2, 12], and such studies rarely consider the context of the emergency department [4].

In addition, an attempt to better describe and identify cirrhotic patients with AKI, is to implement a substratification of KDIGO stage 1 into 1a and 1b, with a creatinine value of 1.50 mg/dL as the discriminatory threshold [7].

* Correspondence: pr.lins@uol.com.br
[1]Discipline of Nephrology, Federal University of São Paulo, Rua Botucatu, 591 - 15 ° andar - Cj153 - Vila Clementino, São Paulo, SP 04023-062, Brazil
Full list of author information is available at the end of the article

Such stratification proposes that those patients belonging to subgroup 1a would present a short-term mortality similar to the patients in the non-AKI group, which is different from those in subgroup 1b, who would present a higher odds ratio for mortality when compared to those in the non-AKI control group [2]. Another important tool is to evaluate the progression of AKI since patients who do not show improvement or stabilization of renal function will have a worse prognosis [13].

This study aimed to characterize a population of cirrhotic patients treated at the emergency department based on risk factors associated with worse prognosis for mortality and development of AKI. We also applied the KDIGO criteria for AKI within the first 7 days of hospitalization, testing the possible correlation between mortality and substratification of the KDIGO 1 group in stages 1a and 1b, and finally, looking for an association between progression of AKI with mortality in this population.

Methods

All hospitalizations from the Emergency Department of the São Paulo Hospital, a university hospital linked to the Federal University of São Paulo, Brazil, between March 2015 and February 2017, were retrospectively evaluated. The inclusion criteria were a clinical diagnosis of hepatic cirrhosis, age above 18 years and a minimum hospital stay of 48 h. Exclusion criteria included renal and/or hepatic transplant patients, pregnant women and patients with chronic kidney disease who previously underwent dialysis. For those who were admitted to the emergency department more than one time within the specified period above, we only included data from the first admission. For the characterization and evaluation (incidence and mortality outcome) of AKI, the KDIGO 2012 criteria were applied, comparing peak creatinine and baseline creatinine (Fig. 1). Baseline creatinine was defined as the one prior to admission up to 3 months

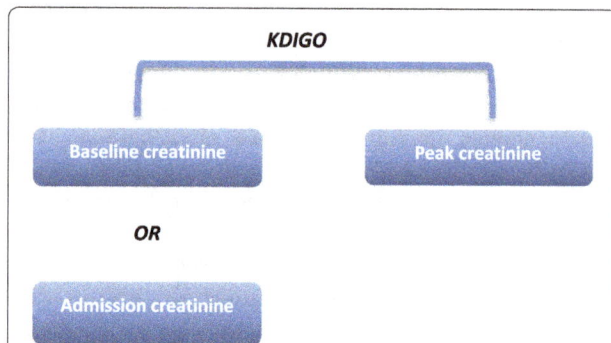

Fig. 2 Flowchart of KDIGO Classification for AKI Progression. Baseline creatinine: previous value within the last 3 months of hospital admission. MDRD 75: Calculated creatinine value considering an eGFR of 75 ml/min/1.73m^2 using the MDRD formula. Peak creatinine: highest value within the first 7 days of hospital stay. Progressors defined if KDIGO B > KDIGO A

before hospitalization, which was obtained from the electronic medical record, or, in its absence, was considered to be the admission value, according to the guidance of the International Club of Ascites [14]. According to the common and widespread use in the literature, the final stage of AKI was defined by peak creatinine (the highest value obtained during the first 7 days of hospital admission) [2, 14, 15]. Diuresis data were not considered because of the difficulty of measuring diuresis in the emergency department, resulting in the absence of these data for most patients, and because it is not a very accurate measurement to evaluate kidney function in cirrhotic patients [14, 16, 17].

For the analysis of the progression of AKI from admission to the first 7 days and its correlation with mortality,

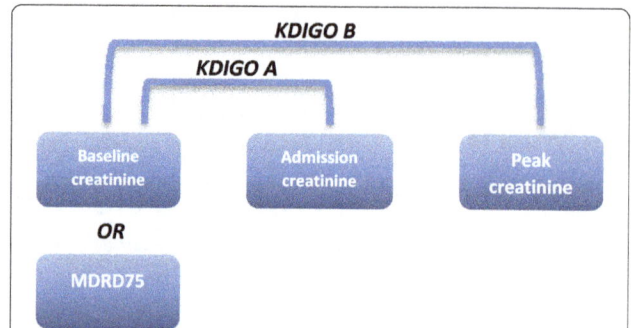

Fig. 1 Flowchart of KDIGO Classification for AKI definition and Mortality Assessment. Baseline creatinine: previous value within the last 3 months of hospital admission. Peak creatinine: highest value within the first 7 days of hospital stay

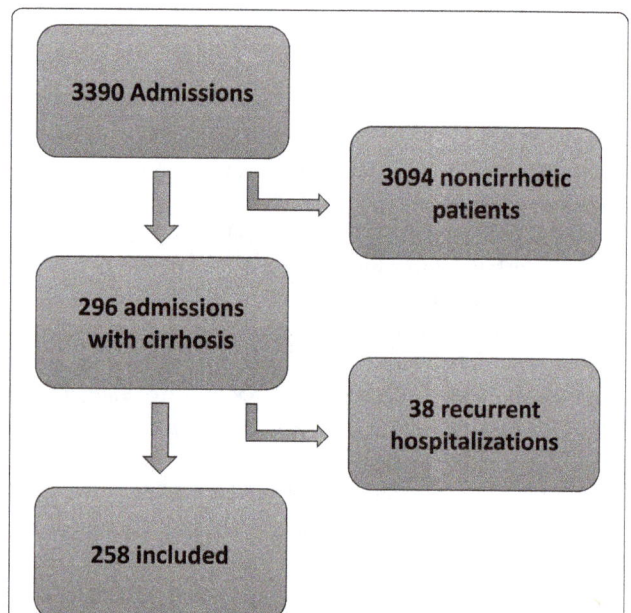

Fig. 3 Derivation of the study cohort

Table 1 Demographic, clinical and laboratory data among survivors and non-survivors

	Total	Survivors	Non-survivors	p
Patients, %	258	185 (71.7)	73 (28.4)	
Age, years (median, IQR)	59 (52;65)	57.9 (12.2)	58.7 (12.2)	0.681
Gender, male / female (%)	185 (71.7) / 73 (28.3)	130 (70.3) / 55 (75.3)	55 (29.7) / 18 (24.7)	0.447
Etiology, n (%)				
Alcohol	125 (48.4)	93 (50.3)	32 (43.8)	0.407
Viral	100 (38.8)	68 (36.8)	32 (43.8)	0.322
Non-viral and Non-alcohol	54 (20.9)	40 (21.6)	14 (19.2)	0.736
Days of hospitalization (median, IQR)	7 (3;13)	6 (3;11)	12 (6;23)	< 0.001
ICU admission (%)	78 (30.2)	35 (18.9)	43 (58.9)	< 0.001
admission MELD score (median, IQR)	18 (14;23)	17 (13;22)	19 (16;26)	0.002
admission APACHE II (median, IQR)	16 (12;22)	15 (12;20)	18 (14;23)	0.015
admission MAP (mmHg), (median, IQR)	89 (75;100)	91 (74;102)	84 (76;95)	0.036
Comorbidities, n (%)				
Hypertension	114 (44.2)	88 (47.6)	26 (35.6)	0.095
Diabetes	82 (31.8)	67 (36.2)	15 (20.5)	0.017
Smoking (present or past)	69 (26.7)	46 (24.9)	23 (31.5)	0.279
Cancer	57 (22.1)	32 (17.3)	25 (34.2)	0.004
Hepatocarcinoma	41 (70.7)	24 (72.7)	17 (68)	0.775
Non-hepatocarcinoma	17 (29.3)	9 (27.3)	8 (32)	
Heart failure	26 (10.1)	20 (10.8)	6 (8.2)	0.649
Cause of hospitalization, n (%)				
Infection	138 (53.5)	92 (66.7)	46 (33.3)	0.071
Non-infection	120 (46.5)	93 (77.5)	27 (22.5)	
AKI, n (%)				
Yes	139 (53.9)	80 (57.6)	59 (42.4)	< 0.001
No	119 (46.1)	105 (82.2)	14 (11.8)	
Progression of AKI, n (%)				
Yes	39 (27.9)	16 (41)	23 (59)	< 0.001
No	101 (72.1)	77 (76.2)	24 (23.8)	
Baseline eGFR (ml/min/1.73m^2) (median, IQR)	57 (35;80)	59 (37;82)	52 (31;72)	0.055
Laboratory				
Hemoglobin, g/dL (mean, SD)	11.2 (2.75)	11.2 (2.7)	11.1 (2.8)	0.894
Albumin, g/dL (mean, SD)	2.9 (0.6)	3 (0.6)	2.7 (0.6)	0.008
Leucocytes, 1000/uL (median, IQR)	8.8 (5.7;12.4)	8.1 (5.4;11.0)	10.7 (7.3;14.1)	< 0001
Platelets, 1000/uL (median, IQR)	126 (80;186)	122 (74;180)	143 (94;195)	0.158
INR (median, IQR)	1.4 (1.2;1.6)	1.4 (1.2;1.6)	1.5 (1.3;1.7)	0.022
Total Bilirrubin, mg/dL (median, IQR)	2.2 (1.0;4.7)	1.7 (0.8;3.5)	2.9 (1.2;7.6)	0.002
Baseline Creatinine, mg/dL (median, IQR)	1.04 (0.80; 1.58)	1.02 (0.76;1.50)	1.10 (0.87;1.74)	0.054
Admission Creatinine, mg/dL (median,IQR)	1.40 (0.85; 2.34)	1.24 (0.80; 2.31)	1.61 (0.96; 2.50)	0.086
Peak Creatinine, mg/dL (median, IQR)	1.9 (1.01; 2.98)	1.47 (0.92; 2.48)	2.86 (1.93; 4.10)	< 0.001
Sodium mEq/L (median, IQR)	136 (132; 139)	137 (133;139)	136 (132;139)	0.197
Urea, mg/dL (median, IQR)	61 (34;99)	52 (33;89)	76 (38;104)	0.022

AKI Acute Kidney Injury. *MAP* Mean Arterial Pressure. *eGFR* Estimated Glomerular Filtration Rate. MELD and APACHE II were obtained from admission data

we performed a second classification of AKI according to the KDIGO criteria, comparing admission creatinine to the previous creatinine of hospitalization (baseline creatinine). Because we had no previous creatinine value for 109 patients (42% of total), we used the back calculation of creatinine considering a MDRD of 75 ml/min/1.73 m^2 (MDRD-75) for these patients [16]. Both classifications were compared, admission and peak, in order to analyze the progression of AKI [18]. Progression of AKI was defined as the increase from lower stages of AKI to higher stages, such as AKI stage 1 to stage 2 or 3 or from stage 2 to stage 3 during the first week or until discharge [13] (Fig. 2).

Statistical analysis was performed with SPSS statistics software version 23.0 for Windows. Quantitative variables were represented by mean and standard deviation

Table 2 Demographic, clinical and laboratory data among AKI and non-AKI groups

	Total	Non-AKI	AKI	p
Patients, %	258	119 (46.1)	139 (53.9)	
Age, years (median, IQR)	59 (52;65)	59 (52;66)	60 (53;65)	0.630
Gender, male / female (%)	185 (71.7) / 73 (28.3)	83 (69.7) / 36 (30.3)	102 (73.4) / 37 (26.6)	0.580
Etiology, n (%)				
Alcohol	125 (48.4)	55 (46.2)	70 (50.4)	0.534
Viral	100 (38.8)	41 (34.5)	59 (42.4)	0.202
Non-viral and Non-alcohol	54 (20.9)	30 (25.2)	24 (17.3)	0.127
Days of hospitalization (median, IQR)	7 (3;13)			
ICU admission (%)	78 (30.2)	19 (16)	59 (42.4)	< 0.001
admission MELD score (median, IQR)	18 (14;23)	16 (11;19)	19 (16;25)	< 0.001
admission APACHE II (median, IQR)	16 (12;22)	14 (11;18)	19 (14;23)	< 0.001
admission MAP (mmHg), (median, IQR)	89 (75;100)	89 (76;100)	87 (74;100)	0.679
Comorbidities, n (%)				
Hypertension	114 (44.2)	51 (42.9)	63 (45.3)	0.708
Diabetes	82 (31.8)	36 (30.3)	46 (33.1)	0.688
Smoking (present or past)	69 (26.7)	30 (25.2)	39 (28.1)	0.673
Cancer	57 (22.1)	26 (21.8)	31 (22.3)	1
Hepatocarcinoma	41 (70.7)	19 (70.4)	22 (71)	1
Non-hepatocarcinoma	17 (29.3)	8 (29.6)	9 (29)	
Heart failure	26 (10.1)	11 (9.2)	15 (10.8)	0.836
Cause of hospitalization, n (%)				
Infection	138 (53.5)	52 (37.7)	86 (62.3)	0.004
Non-infection	120 (46.5)	67 (55.8)	53 (44.2)	
Baseline eGFR (ml/min/1.73m^2) (median, IQR)	57 (35;80)	66 (35;89)	56 (35;73)	0.073
Laboratory				
Hemoglobin, g/dL (mean, SD)	11.2 (2.75)	11.3 (2.72)	11.1 (2.78)	0.493
Albumin, g/dL (mean, SD)	2.9 (0.6)	2.9 (0.6)	2.8 (0.6)	0.070
Leucocytes, 1000/uL (median, IQR)	8.8 (5.7;12.4)	7.7 (5.2;11)	10 (6.7;13.5)	0.001
Platelets, 1000/uL (median, IQR)	126 (80;186)	108.5 (70.5;174.5)	137 (88;192)	0.036
INR (median, IQR)	1.4 (1.2;1.6)	1.4 (1.2;1.6)	1.5 (1.3;1.7)	0.009
Total Bilirrubin, mg/dL (median, IQR)	2.2 (1.0;4.7)	2 (0.8;4)	2 (1;4.6)	0.370
Baseline Creatinine, mg/dL (median, IQR)	1.04 (0.80; 1.58)	0.96 (0.70;1.56)	1.05 (0.85;1.59)	0.081
Admission Creatinine, mg/dL (median,IQR)	1.40 (0.85; 2.34)	0.98 (0.72;1.60)	1.80 (1.13;2.77)	< 0.001
Peak Creatinine, mg/dL (median, IQR)	1.9 (1.01; 2.98)	0.99 (0.75;1.56)	2.55 (1.93;3.85)	< 0.001
Sodium (median, IQR)	136 (132; 139)	137 (133;140)	136 (132;139)	0.078
Urea, mg/dL (median, IQR)	61 (34;99)	39 (27;70)	78 (46;108)	< 0.001

AKI Acute Kidney Injury. *MAP* Mean Arterial Pressure. *eGFR* Estimated Glomerular Filtration Rate. MELD and APACHE II were obtained from admission data if the distribution was normal (Kolmogorov-Smirnov test) and were compared by Student's T test. When a nonnormal distribution was characterized, median and interquartile range values were expressed, and the comparison was tested by the Wilcoxon test. Categorical variables were compared by the χ^2 test (or Fischer exact test, when applicable). Possible risk factors for mortality that were identified in the univariate analysis with p value < 0.1 were included in models of logistic regression analysis. The data were presented as odds ratios and 95% confidence intervals. Values of $p < 0.05$ (2-tailed) were considered statistically significant.

Regarding the variables with missing data, we did not have previous creatinine values of 109 patients, as previously mentioned, and we did not have albumin values of 31 patients (12%). For the missing albumin data, we used the multiple imputation method to perform the necessary analysis.

This study was approved by the Ethics in Research Committee of the Federal University of São Paulo, and formal informed consent was waived because of the observational nature of the study.

Results

The population studied included 258 patients (Fig. 3). From 3390 hospitalizations at the University Hospital Emergency Department, 3094 were noncirrhotic patients. Among the remaining 296 cirrhotic patients, 38 had recurrent hospitalizations, and only the first admission was considered for statistical analysis.

Clinical, laboratory, and demographic characteristics of patients included in the study are presented in Tables 1 and 2. These tables include the main comorbidities of patients in descending order of prevalence, mean length of hospital stay, ICU admission rate, APACHE II score from admission, MELD score from admission and admission mean arterial pressure (MAP). Regarding the etiology of cirrhosis, it was classified in three groups (viral, alcoholic and nonviral non-alcoholic), according to the two main causes of cirrhosis worldwide. The reason for admission to the emergency room was similarly divided into two groups, considering both infectious and noninfectious causes.

The overall mortality rate was 28.4%, with no significant difference in relation to the mean age ($p = 0.681$), sex ($p = 0.447$), the etiology of cirrhosis (alcoholic $p = 0.407$, viral $p = 0.322$, nonviral and non-alcoholic $p = 0.736$) or hospitalization due to infectious causes ($p = 0.071$). However, the nonsurvivor group had the highest median APACHE II admission (18 vs 15 $p = 0.015$), the highest median MELD score (19 vs 17 $p = 0.002$) and the highest ICU admission rate (58.9% vs 18.9% $p = < 0.01$). Among the comorbidities presented, patients with cancer

presented higher mortality when compared to noncancer patients (34.2% vs 17.3% $p = 0.004$), but this difference was not statistically significant when the primary site was evaluated as hepatocarcinoma ($p = 0.775$) versus non-hepatocarcinoma tumors.

In multivariate analysis, variables with $p < 0.1$ according to univariate analysis were included in the model. Independent risk factors for in-hospital mortality are shown in Table 3.

When the criteria for AKI were applied for evaluation related to the first 7 days, 139 (53.9%) patients presented AKI: 55 (39.5%) patients with KDIGO 1, 35

Table 3 Logistic Regression – Risk Factors for In-Hospital Mortality

Variable	OR	95% CI	p
MODEL 1			
AKI	4.66	1.94–11.17	< 0.001
Cancer	3.94	1.74–8.89	< 0.001
Length of stay in hospital	1.07	1.03–1.10	< 0.001
Leukocytes	1.08	1.01–1.15	0.016
Diabetes	0.31	0.11–0.80	0.016
MAP	0.98	0.96–1.00	0.126
Age	1.02	0.98–1.05	0.195
MELD	1.04	0.97–1.11	0.247
APACHE II	0.97	0.88–1.05	0.427
Suspected infection	0.76	0.35–1.63	0.483
Baseline eGFR	1.07	0.77–1.47	0.694
Male Sex	1.16	0.51–2.59	0.726
Hypertension	0.89	0.37–2.09	0.788
Urea	0.99	0.98–1.01	0.868
MODEL 2			
Progression of AKI	12.05	3.29–44.07	< 0.001
Cancer	10.27	2.73–38.47	< 0.001
Age	1.08	1.02–1.14	0.006
MELD	1.15	1.03–1.26	0.006
Length of stay in hospital	1.08	1,02 - 1,13	0.007
Urea	1.01	0.99–1.02	0.073
MAP	0.98	0.95–1.00	0.090
APACHE II	0.93	0.82–1.05	0.240
Baseline eGFR	0.81	0.55–1.17	0.273
Hypertension	0.53	0.14–1.87	0.322
Leukocytes	1.04	0.95–1.13	0.367
Male Sex	1.26	0.38–4.10	0.702
Diabetes	0.89	0.26–2.99	0.852
Suspected infection	1.09	0.34–3.46	0.882

We considered the following units: per day for Length of stay in hospital, per year for Age, per 1 mg/dL for Urea, per 1 mmHg for MAP, per 1 ml/min/ 1.73m^2 for eGFR, per 1 × 10^3/μL. *AKI* Acute Kidney Injury. *MAP* Mean Arterial Pressure. *eGFR* Estimated Glomerular Filtration Rate. MELD and APACHE II were obtained from admission data

(25.1%) with KDIGO 2 and 49 (35.2%) with KDIGO 3. Of the 49 patients with KDIGO 3, 18 (36.7%) required dialysis treatment. Among the patients with AKI, a higher admission rate in the ICU (42.4% vs 16%), higher APACHE II value (19 vs 14), higher MELD score (19 vs 16) and a higher incidence of infectious causes (62.3% vs. 37.7%) when compared to the non-AKI group were observed. There was no difference in relation to the etiology of cirrhosis or the presence of comorbidities between the groups. The overall mortality of the AKI group was 42.4%, and it was 11.8% in the non-AKI group.

The AKI subgroups of the KDIGO classification and the relationship with mortality are presented in Fig. 4 and Table 4. Within the KDIGO 1 group, 28 fulfill only elevation in creatinine ≥0.3 mg/dL in 48 h; the other 27 patients matched the criteria of elevation of 1.5× baseline creatinine at 7 days. Among these patients, 16 (29.1%) were KDIGO 1a and 39 (70.9%) KDIGO 1B. Differences in mortality with statistical significance were observed for the groups 2 and 3 when compared to group without AKI. In the analysis of KDIGO 1 subgroups, mortality was 12.5% and 33.3% for 1a and 1b, respectively, with significance only for subgroup 1b. There was no significant difference in mortality between the KDIGO 2 and 3 groups. The final model was adjusted for age, sex, hypertension, diabetes, APACHE II and MELD scores.

Logistic regression methods are shown in 2 models to mitigate collinearity between AKI admission diagnosis and AKI progression status (Table 3) - MODEL 1 consider admission criteria of AKI plus all covariates that presents with $p < 0.1$ in univariate analysis. MODEL 2 shows criteria of Progression of AKI plus all covariates that present with $p < 0.1$ in univariate analysis. In model 1, admission criteria of AKI, cancer diagnosis, length of stay in hospital, and leukocyte count (per 103 increase) are shown as risk factors for mortality. About model 2, the risk factors for mortality present as Progression of AKI, cancer diagnosis, Age (per year), MELD score at admission and length of stay in hospital.

Finally, the progression of AKI occurred in 39 patients (27.9% of those with AKI). In those who progressed, mortality was 59% and was 23.8% in the nonprogression group ($p < 0.001$) (Table 4).

Discussion

This study presented the evaluation of 258 cirrhotic patients admitted to an emergency unit. In general, the mortality rate (28.4%) was similar to that reported for similar cohorts [1, 6–8, 12, 15]. The most common etiology was similar to that of national and international cohorts [17], with alcoholic cirrhosis being the most common followed by viral etiology (mainly secondary to hepatitis C). Due to the unavailability of the level of ascites in electronic records of some patients and the heterogeneous classification of hepatic encephalopathy, a Child-Pugh-Turcotte classification was not possible, but we inferred from clinical and laboratory data that the majority of patients would be classified as having at least Child B liver cirrhosis with a mortality similar to that reported in the literature [8].

This investigation has shown that patients with AKI in progression have an increasing mortality according to the classification of renal impairment (Fig. 4), which reinforces the need for a temporal and progressive evaluation of renal function. In addition, in this population, the presence of progression of AKI and peak creatinine in the first 7 days of admission presented better performance when compared to the isolated creatinine value of entry, regarding mortality. Surprisingly, the baseline eGFR prior to hospital admission did not present as a risk factor for mortality or acute kidney injury during hospitalization, as widely established in the

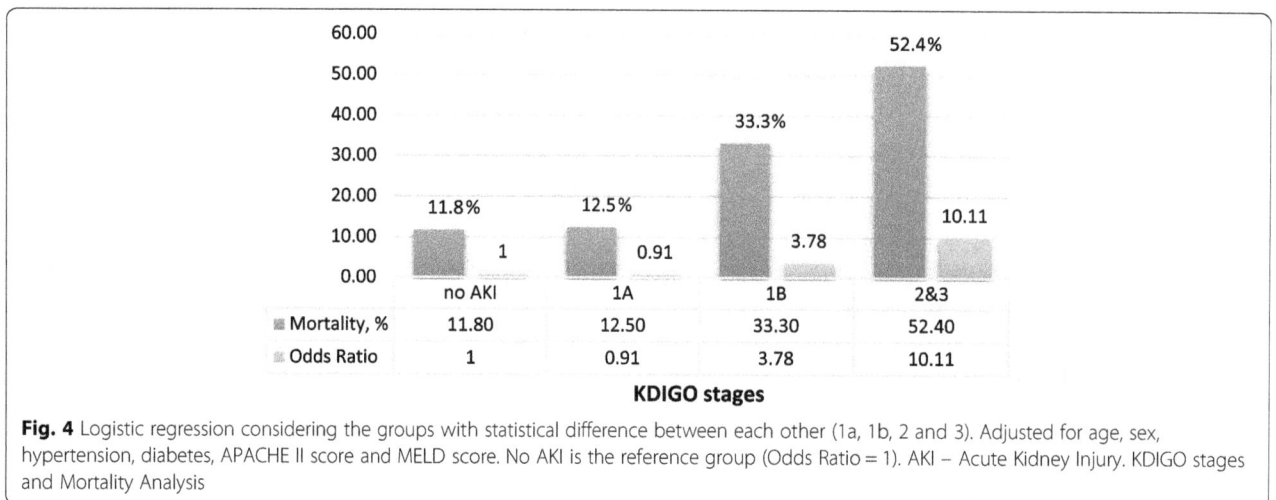

	no AKI	1A	1B	2&3
Mortality, %	11.80	12.50	33.30	52.40
Odds Ratio	1	0.91	3.78	10.11

KDIGO stages

Fig. 4 Logistic regression considering the groups with statistical difference between each other (1a, 1b, 2 and 3). Adjusted for age, sex, hypertension, diabetes, APACHE II score and MELD score. No AKI is the reference group (Odds Ratio = 1). AKI – Acute Kidney Injury. KDIGO stages and Mortality Analysis

Table 4 AKI Stages and Mortality Outcome

Stages of AKI	Total	Mortality, %	Unadjusted			Adjusted[b]		
			OR	IC 95%	p	OR	IC 95%	p
no AKI[a]	119	11.8	1			1		
AKI	139	42.2						
KDIGO 1	55	27.3	2.81	1.24–6.35	0.013			
1a	16	12.5	1.07	0.22–5.21	0.932	0.91	0.18–4.60	0.916
1b	39	33.3	3.75	1.57–8.93	0.003	3.78	1.47–9.70	0.006
KDIGO 2 and 3	84	52.4				10.11	4.36–23.43	< 0.001
KDIGO 2	35	40.0	5.00	2.08–12.01	< 0.001			
KDIGO 3	49	61.2	11.84	5.31–26.37	< 0.001			

[a]Reference group. [b]Adjusted for age, sex, hypertension, diabetes, APACHE II score and MELD score. AKI, acute kidney injury

literature of noncirrhotic patients [18]; however, there are already clinical trials in cirrhotic patients with results similar to our study [6].

Multivariate analysis showed that both AKI diagnosis at admission and AKI Progression criteria are major risk factors for mortality; this information suggests that cirrhotic patients with less severe AKI (KDIGO 1) need a special approach and structured care. Surprisingly, the APACHE II score lost its power of discrimination on both models in multivariate analysis. Another study found similar results [19] and presented a possible explanation that the Apache II score lacks a liver-specific prognostic factor in its calculator, so it is probable that the Apache II score will lose its strength when compared with another specific variables. In model 1, the MELD score lost its ability to predict mortality risk probably because of collinearity between the admission creatinine and calculated admission MELD.

As shown in Table 4, the presence of AKI KDIGO 1b was shown to be a risk factor for mortality, different from the presence of AKI KDIGO 1a. This fact corroborates the subclassification proposed by the International Club of Ascites [13], which reinforces that small elevations in the value of creatinine, especially when they exceed 1.50 mg / dL, have a great impact on the morbidity and mortality of patients with cirrhosis.

No significant difference in mortality was found between the stages without AKI and KDIGO 1a, and the KDIGO stages 2 and 3. It is possible to identify three major progressive mortality groups: KDIGO 1a, KDIGO 1b and KDIGO 2/3, with the prognosis of the first group comparable to the absence of AKI, reinforcing previous data [15].

There are several limitations of our study. Although the present investigation was based on a retrospective cohort, it presents an analysis of a considerably large number of patients, regarding this specific population of cirrhotic patients in an emergency department, which ought to be considered innovative in the literature. Due to missing clinical data, we were not able to achieve a Child-Pugh classification or include the etiology of AKI. Since we designed this study to assess only the first week in the hospital, we did not evaluate the occurrence of late AKI (after 7 days). Another limitation is the lack of data on AKI duration, since patients who improve within 48 h may represent a phenotype of AKI with a better prognosis. Final limitation is the possible misclassification of chronic kidney disease as AKI when analyzing progression of AKI, since those patients without previous creatinine value were considered as having a eGFR of 75 ml/min/1.73m^2.

Conclusions

According to the data presented above, a single measure of creatinine is not enough in this population, as this paper reinforces the need for meticulous follow-up of the renal function of patients with hepatic cirrhosis hospitalized in an emergency unit, in view of the correlation of renal function with clinical outcomes. In addition, in agreement with the current literature, the data reinforce the need for subclassification of KDIGO 1 in cirrhotic patients, demonstrating that patients with acute renal injury and creatinine greater than 1.5 mg/dL present a worse clinical outcome.

Abbreviations
AKI: Acute Kidney Injury; eGFR: Estimated Glomerular Filtration Rate; ICU: Intensive Care Unit; KDIGO: Kidney Disease: Improving Global Outcomes; MAP: Mean Arterial Pressure; MDRD: Modification of Diet in Renal Disease Formula for eGFR

Acknowledgements
We thank Dr. Daniel Ribeiro da Rocha, Dr. Sarah Pontes de Barros Leal, Dr. Klaus Nunes Ficher and Dr. Raphael Costa Bandeira de Melo for their contributions.

Authors' contributions

PRGL and AFTG designed the study. PRGL and WSCP contributed to the implementation of the research, data collection, statistical work, to the analysis of the results and to the writing of the manuscript. WSCP designed the tables and figures. AFTG, CFGM and MCB verified the analytical methods and aided in interpreting the results. All authors discussed the results and contributed to the final manuscript. All authors read and approved the final manuscript

Competing interests

The authors declare that they have no competing interests.

Author details

[1]Discipline of Nephrology, Federal University of São Paulo, Rua Botucatu, 591 - 15 ° andar - Cj153 - Vila Clementino, São Paulo, SP 04023-062, Brazil. [2]Discipline of Medicine of Urgency and Evidence-Based Medicine from the Department of Medicine, Federal University of São Paulo, Rua Napoleão de Barros, 865 - Vila Clementino, São Paulo, SP 04023-090, Brazil.

References

1. Alsultan MA, Alrshed RS, Aljumah AA, Baharoon SA, Arabi YM, Aldawood AS. In-hospital mortality among a cohort of cirrhotic patients admitted to a tertiary hospital. Saudi J Gastroenterol. 2011;17(6):387–90.
2. Piano S, Rosi S, Maresio G, Fasolato S, Cavallin M, Romano A, et al. Evaluation of the acute kidney injury network criteria in hospitalized patients with cirrhosis and ascites. J Hepatol. 2013;59(3):482–9.
3. Wong F, Bernardi M, Balk R, Christman B, Moreau R, Garcia-Tsao G, et al. Sepsis in cirrhosis: report on the 7th meeting of the international ascites Club. Gut. 2005;54(5):718–25.
4. Ximenes RO, Farias AQ, Scalabrini Neto A, Diniz MA, Kubota GT, MMA-A I, et al. Patients with cirrhosis in the ED: early predictors of infection and mortality. Am J Emerg Med. 34(1):25–9.
5. Pant C, Olyaee M, Gilroy R, Pandya PK, Olson JC, Oropeza-Vail M, et al. Emergency department visits related to cirrhosis: a retrospective study of the Nationwide emergency department sample 2006 to 2011. Medicine. 2015;94(1):e308.
6. Belcher JM, Garcia-Tsao G, Sanyal AJ, Bhogal H, Lim JK, Ansari N, et al. Association of AKI with mortality and complications in hospitalized patients with cirrhosis. Hepatology (Baltimore), Md. 2013;57(2):753–62.
7. Fagundes C, Barreto R, Guevara M, Garcia E, Sola E, Rodriguez E, et al. A modified acute kidney injury classification for diagnosis and risk stratification of impairment of kidney function in cirrhosis. J Hepatol. 2013;59(3):474–81.
8. Scott RA, Austin AS, Kolhe NV, McIntyre CW, Selby NM. Acute kidney injury is independently associated with death in patients with cirrhosis. Frontline gastroenterology. 2013;4(3):191–7.
9. Ginès P, Schrier RW. Renal failure in cirrhosis. N Engl J Med. 2009;361(13): 1279–90.
10. Sherman DS, Fish DN, Teitelbaum I. Assessing renal function in cirrhotic patients: problems and pitfalls. Am J Kidney Dis. 2003;41(2):269–78.
11. Nadim MK, Kellum JA, Davenport A, Wong F, Davis C, Pannu N, et al. Hepatorenal syndrome: the 8(th)international consensus conference of the acute Dialysis quality initiative (ADQI) group. Crit Care. 2012;16(1):R23–R.
12. Pan H-C, Chien Y-S, Jenq C-C, Tsai M-H, Fan P-C, Chang C-H, et al. Acute kidney injury classification for critically ill cirrhotic patients: a comparison of the KDIGO, AKIN, and RIFLE classifications. Sci Rep. 2016;6:23022.
13. Belcher JM, Garcia-Tsao G, Sanyal AJ, Thiessen-Philbrook H, Peixoto AJ, Perazella MA, et al. Urinary biomarkers and progression of AKI in patients with cirrhosis. Clin J Am Soc Nephrol. 2014;9(11):1857–67.
14. Angeli P, Ginès P, Wong F, Bernardi M, Boyer TD, Gerbes A, et al. Diagnosis and management of acute kidney injury in patients with cirrhosis: revised consensus recommendations of the International Club of Ascites. J Hepatol. 62(4):968–74.
15. Huelin P, Piano S, Sola E, Stanco M, Sole C, Moreira R, et al. Validation of a staging system for acute kidney injury in patients with cirrhosis and association with acute-on-chronic liver failure. Clin Gastroenterol Hepatol. 2017;15(3):438–45.e5.
16. Angeli P, Gines P, Wong F, Bernardi M, Boyer TD, Gerbes A, et al. Diagnosis and management of acute kidney injury in patients with cirrhosis: revised consensus recommendations of the International Club of Ascites. J Hepatol. 2015;62(4):968–74.
17. Wong F, Nadim MK, Kellum JA, Salerno F, Bellomo R, Gerbes A, et al. Working party proposal for a revised classification system of renal dysfunction in patients with cirrhosis. Gut. 2011;60(5):702–9.
18. Wang HE, Jain G, Glassock RJ, Warnock DG. Comparison of absolute serum creatinine changes versus kidney disease: improving global outcomes consensus definitions for characterizing stages of acute kidney injury. Nephrol Dial Transplant. 2013;28(6):1447–54.
19. Fang JT, Tsai MH, Tian YC, Jenq CC, Lin CY, Chen YC, et al. Outcome predictors and new score of critically ill cirrhotic patients with acute renal failure. Nephrol Dial Transplant. 2008;23(6):1961–9.

16

Inadequate dietary energy intake associates with higher prevalence of metabolic syndrome in different groups of hemodialysis patients: a clinical observational study in multiple dialysis centers

Tuyen Van Duong[1], Te-Chih Wong[2], Hsi-Hsien Chen[3,4], Tzen-Wen Chen[4], Tso-Hsiao Chen[4,5], Yung-Ho Hsu[4,6], Sheng-Jeng Peng[7], Ko-Lin Kuo[8], Hsiang-Chung Liu[9], En-Tzu Lin[10], Chi-Sin Wang[1], I-Hsin Tseng[1], Yi-Wei Feng[1], Tai-Yue Chang[1], Chien-Tien Su[11,12] and Shwu-Huey Yang[1,13,14]* [iD]

Abstract

Background: Metabolic syndrome (MetS) has been established as a risk for cardiovascular diseases and mortality in hemodialysis patients. Energy intake (EI) is an important nutritional therapy for preventing MetS. We examined the association of self-reported dietary EI with metabolic abnormalities and MetS among hemodialysis patients.

Methods: A cross-sectional study design was carried out from September 2013 to April 2017 in seven hemodialysis centers. Data were collected from 228 hemodialysis patients with acceptable EI report, 20 years old and above, underwent three hemodialysis sessions a week for at least past 3 months. Dietary EI was evaluated by a three-day dietary record, and confirmed by 24-h dietary recall. Body compositions were measured by bioelectrical impedance analysis. Biochemical data were analyzed using standard laboratory tests. The cut-off values of daily EI were 30 kcal/kg, and 35 kcal/kg for age ≥ 60 years and < 60 years, respectively. MetS was defined by the American Association of Clinical Endocrinologists (AACE-MetS), and Harmonizing Metabolic Syndrome (HMetS). Logistic regression models were utilized for examining the association between EI and MetS. Age, gender, physical activity, hemodialysis vintage, Charlson comorbidity index, high sensitive C-reactive protein, and interdialytic weight gains were adjusted in the multivariate analysis.

(Continued on next page)

* Correspondence: sherry@tmu.edu.tw
[1]School of Nutrition and Health Sciences, Taipei Medical University, No. 250 Wuxing Street, Taipei 110, Taiwan
[13]Research Center of Geriatric Nutrition, Taipei Medical University, Taipei, Taiwan
Full list of author information is available at the end of the article

(Continued from previous page)

Results: The prevalence of inadequate EI, AACE-MetS, and HMetS were 60.5%, 63.2%, and 53.9%, respectively. Inadequate EI was related to higher proportion of metabolic abnormalities and MetS ($p < 0.05$). Results of the multivariate analysis shows that inadequate EI was significantly linked with higher prevalence of impaired fasting glucose (OR = 2.42, $p < 0.01$), overweight/obese (OR = 6.70, $p < 0.001$), elevated waist circumference (OR = 8.17, $p < 0.001$), AACE-MetS (OR = 2.26, $p < 0.01$), and HMetS (OR = 3.52, $p < 0.01$). In subgroup anslysis, inadequate EI strongly associated with AACE-MetS in groups of non-hypertension (OR = 4.09, $p = 0.004$), and non-cardiovascular diseases (OR = 2.59, $p = 0.012$), and with HMetS in all sub-groups of hypertension (OR = 2.59~ 5.33, $p < 0.05$), diabetic group (OR = 8.33, $p = 0.003$), and non-cardiovascular diseases (OR = 3.79, $p < 0.001$).

Conclusions: Inadequate EI and MetS prevalence was high. Energy intake strongly determined MetS in different groups of hemodialysis patients.

Keywords: Hemodialysis patients, Inadequate dietary energy intake, Metabolic syndrome, AACE, HMetS

Introduction

The prevalence of treated end-stage renal disease (ESRD) has steadily increased from 2001 to 2014 in all countries, and become a burden to every nation and healthcare system [1]. In 2014, the prevalence of ESRD patients undergoing dialysis in Taiwan was 3093 patients per million population, about 90% of them receiving in-center hemodialysis treatment [1]. It was summarized that nutritional factor was implicated as a risk factor for the development of metabolic in chronic kidney disease, especially in ESRD patients [2].

Nutritional therapy is recognized as an effective approach to prevent metabolic abnormalities and unfavorable outcomes in people with chronic conditions [3–8]. Increased dietary energy intake is mentioned in the National Kidney Foundation-Kidney Disease Outcomes Quality Initiative (K/DOQI) guidelines [9]. It is recommended that consuming enough energy daily guarantees the nitrogen balance and prevents protein catabolism and tissue destruction, which could optimize the nutritional status and hemodialysis outcomes [9]. However, the daily intake of macro-nutrients and micro-nutrients are largely inadequate in hemodialysis patients [10]. More than a half of hemodialysis patients had problems to follow the healthy diet guidelines (related to energy and nutrients intakes) which related behaviors, technical difficulties, physical conditions, time, and food preparation [11]. Inadequate dietary intake is also a possible result of a significant lifestyle change while receiving dialysis treatment. On the other hand, adherence to a complicated and restrictive dietary intake further exacerbates nutrient deficits in this group of patients [9, 12–14].

The prevalence of metabolic syndrome was high in the ESRD patients undergoing hemodialysis [15]. The MetS has been implicated as a risk factor for the development of diabetes, cardiovascular disease, cancer, and all-cause mortality [16–19]. The prevalence of metabolic syndrome varied by different assessment criteria, e.g. 51%, 66.3%, and 75.3% according to National Cholesterol

Education Program Adult Treatment Panel III (NCEP ATP III), International Diabetes Federation (IDF), and Harmonizing the Metabolic Syndrome (HMetS) criteria, respectively [20]. This indicated that there was not yet a single definition that could reflect the real spectrum of the epidemiology of MetS. Therefore, in the current study, two definitions were used with different focuses to assess the MetS: The American Association of Clinical Endocrinologists (AACE) definition, focused on hyperglycosemia, was glucocentric [21]; and Harmonizing Metabolic Syndrome definition was agreed by Joint statement from the IDF, American Heart Association (AHA) and the National Heart, Lung, and Blood Institute (NHLBI), the World Heart Federation, the International Atherosclerosis Society, and the International Association for the Study of Obesity, which relayed on collection of abdominal obesity and related CVD risk factors [22].

There were few studies investigated dietary intake among hemodialysis patients. One study compared the dietary intake status between 54 HD patients, and 47 non-HD patients, and between dialysis day and non-dialysis day among elderly people in Brazil [23]. The other study in the United States only examined the association between dietary energy intake and body composition changes in 13 HD patients [24]. In addition, the dietary approach was found as an effective therapy to decrease most of the risks for MetS in a randomized controlled trial [25]. However, hemodialysis patients were with high metabolic syndrome prevalence, and generally have difficulties achieving recommended energy intakes. In our knowledge, the role of dietary energy intake on metabolic disorders among hemodialysis patients remains to be investigated.

This study was to examine the association of inadequate dietary energy intake with metabolic abnormalities and metabolic syndrome among patients who receiving hemodialysis treatment from seven hemodialysis centers. It was hypothesized that hemodialysis patients with reported inadequate dietary energy intake (IDEI) more likely had metabolic abnormalities or metabolic syndrome.

Methods

Study design and setting

A cross-sectional study design was carried out from September 2013 to April 2017. We collected data from 492 patients from hemodialysis centers in seven hospitals. The study sample consisted 165 from Taipei Medical University Hospital, 91 from Taipei Medical University – Wan Fang Hospital, 39 from Taipei Medical University – Shuang Ho Hospital, 41 from Cathay General Hospital, 57 from Taipei Tzu-Chi Hospital, 49 from Wei-Gong Memorial Hospital, and 50 from Lotung Poh-Ai Hospital.

Sample size

The sample size in a cross-sectional design is calculated using the formula: $n = \frac{Z^2 P(1-P)}{d^2}$ Where n (sample size), Z (level of confidence), P (expected prevalence), and d (precision, corresponding to effect size) [26]. The sample of 92 was calculated with $Z = 1.96$ for type I error of 5%, $P = 0.745$ as the prevalence of MetS was 74.5% in hemodialysis patients [27], and $d = 0.1$ as suggested for a medical study [28]. In the current study, the final sample of 228 patients is adequate for analysis and depicted in Fig. 1.

Patient recruitment criteria

The study patients in the current study fulfilled the recruitment criteria as mentioned elsewhere [29–31].

Data collection procedure

The physicians and nurses in each hospital screened for qualified patients who satisfied the recruitment criteria. The interviewers (Registered Dietitians) then contacted the eligible patients and asked for their voluntary participation.

The eligible patients signed the informed consent form before participating in the face-to-face or telephone interviews which conducted by registered dietitians (three-day dietary intake, physical activity). The medical charts were reviewed after the interviews. Anthropometric, and energy expenditure values were also measured. Licensed nurses collected blood samples at the first dialysis session during the study week, biochemical data was then analyzed using available laboratory test kits, the procedure was described in details elsewhere [32].

Measures

Patients' characteristics

The information regarding age, gender, hemodialysis vintage, comorbidities calculated using the Charlson comorbidity index [33], history of hypertension, cardiovascular diseases, and type 2 diabetes mellitus (T2DM), body mass index, BMI (kg/m^2), pre-dialysis systolic (SBP) and diastolic (DBP) blood pressure were also assessed using medical records. The waist circumference (WC), body fat mass (FM) were assessed using the bio-electrical impedance analysis device (InBody S10, Biospace, Seoul, Korea), the detailed procedure was described elsewhere [34]. Elevated body fat mass was defined as FM ≥ 25% for men, FM ≥ 30% for women, respectively [35]. Interdialytic

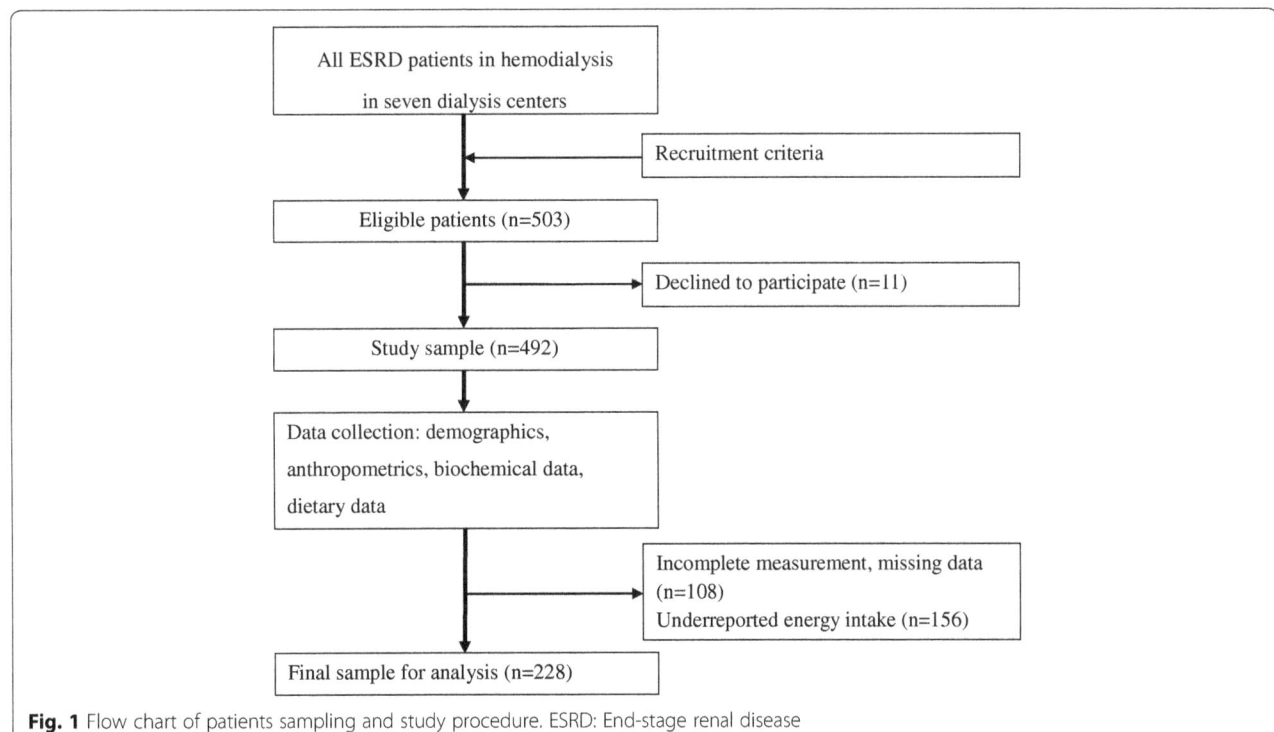

Fig. 1 Flow chart of patients sampling and study procedure. ESRD: End-stage renal disease

weight gains (IDWG) was also calculated. Higher IDWG linked with higher BP in hemodialysis patients [36].

Physical activity

The short version of the International Physical Activity Questionnaire was used to evaluate physical activity level. Patients were asked about their time spent (days per week, and minutes per day) on different levels of physical intensity (vigorous, moderate, walking, and sitting), questionnaire took 4 to 15 min to complete [37]. The overall physical activity score was calculated as the sum of minutes spent on activities at different levels of vigorous, moderate, walking, and sitting over last seven days multiplied by 8.0, 4.0, and 3.3, 1.0, respectively [38]. The common method using metabolic equivalent task scored in minute per week (named as MET- min/wk) was used to represent the physical activity [39].

Dietary energy intake

We used three-day dietary intake record to assess patient's intake, and confirmed data by a 24-h dietary recall, the details were mentioned elsewhere [32, 40]. In brief, the information related to names of food, brand, ingredients, cooking methods, portion or weight, meal location and time were collected. The e-Kitchen software, a nutrient analysis software (Nutritionist Edition, Enhancement plus 3, version 2009, Taichung, Taiwan) was used for analyzing nutrients.

The recommended daily dietary energy intake was ≥ 35 kcal/kg for patients younger than 60 years old, and ≥ 30 kcal/kg for those who 60 years old or older, respectively [9]. Inadequate dietary energy intake was defined as patients consumed less than the recommended levels. In order to enhance the reliability of measures and analysis, the under-reported dietary energy intake (EI) data were excluded from the final analysis if the ratio of EI:REE < 1.27 [41]. The results of the analysis were not affected by excluding the under-reporters in the study [42]. The resting energy expenditure (REE) was assessed using a hand-held indirect calorimeter, named MedGem (Microlife USA, Dunedin, FL). A modified Weir equation together with a fixed respiratory exchange ratio of 0.85 were used to estimate carbon dioxide production. Patients wore a nose clip and a mouthpiece, then breathe normally for about 7–10 min, or until the volume of oxygen is stable. The MedGem has been validated against several metabolic calorimeters such as Douglas Bag method [43], and metabolic cart systems [44, 45]. This device has the similar accuracy of commonly used prediction equations such as the WHO/FAU/UNU, Mifflin, or Harris–Benedict equations [46], and used in hemodialysis patients [47].

The biochemical values

Fasting blood glucose (FPG), fasting plasma insulin (FPI), total cholesterol (TC), triglyceride (TG), high-density lipoprotein cholesterol (HDL-C), low-density lipoprotein cholesterol (LDL-C), high sensitive C-reactive protein (hs-CRP), Creatinine, Albumin, intact parathyroid hormone (iPTH), the normalized protein nitrogen appearance (nPNA) was estimated using the formula: nPNA = Pre-BUN/[25.8 + 1.15*(eKt/V) + 56.4/(eKt/V)] + 0.168, where pre-BUN is pre-dialysis blood urea nitrogen (mg/dL), post-BUN is post-dialysis blood urea nitrogen (mg/dl), and equilibrated Kt/V is dialysis quality [48].

Diagnosis of metabolic syndrome (MetS)

The MetS was classified by American Association of Clinical Endocrinologists (AACE), hereafter referred as AACE-MetS [21]. Patients were identified as MetS if they had (1) and any of the criteria (2), or (3), or (4). (1) Impaired fasting glucose (IFG) which patients had FPG $\geq$ 100 mg/dL, or previously diagnosed T2DM [49]. (2) Overweight or obese (BMI ≥ 24.0 kg/m^2 for Taiwanese) [50]. (3) TG ≥ 150 mg/dL, HDL-C < 40 mg/dL for men or HDL-C < 50 mg/dL for women. (4) SBP ≥ 130 mmHg or DBP ≥ 85 mmHg.

To affirm the non-spurious association, the Harmonizing Metabolic Syndrome definition (HMetS) was also used to evaluate MetS. Patients were classified as MetS if they have three or more abnormalities (WC ≥ 90 cm for men, WC ≥ 80 cm for women, TG ≥ 150 mg/dL, low HDL-C, high BP, or IFG) [22].

Other biochemical value classifications

The lipid profile (LDL-C ≥ 100 mg/dL, and TC ≥ 200 mg/dL) [51], inflammation maker (high sensitive-CRP > 0.5 mg/dL) [52], elevated insulin (FPI ≥ 12 mU/L) [53, 54], iPTH ≥ 300 pg/mL [55]. In addition, the poor nutritional status including nPNA < 1.0 g/kg, serum albumin (Alb) $\leq$ 3.5 mg/dL, and serum creatinine (Cr) ≤ 7.5 mg/dL [56].

Statistical analysis

The study sample was described using mean ± standard deviation (SD), or median (interquartile range), or frequency (percentage). The continuous variables were tested for normality by using a Shapiro-Wilk's test [57, 58], and histograms, box plots, and normal Q-Q plots were examined. The ANOVA, Mann-Whitney U test, or Chi-Square test were recruited in order to compare characteristics and metabolic parameters of the adequate and inadequate EI groups. The bivariate logistic regression models were recruited for examining associations of patients' characteristics, dietary intake with metabolic abnormalities and MetS. The multivariate logistic regression analyses were then utilized for examining the association of inadequate dietary intake of nutrients with metabolic abnormalities and MetS. The sub-group analyses were performed in different groups of diabetes mellitus, hypertension, and cardiovascular diseases. Patients' gender, age, physical activity, hemodialysis vintage, Charlson comorbidity index (CCI), hs-CRP, and IDWG were controlled in the multivariate analyses as they showed the associations with metabolic syndrome [59–63]. The analyses were performed for both diagnosed criteria of MetS (AACE-MetS and H-MetS) to affirm the non-spurious association. The IBM SPSS software version 20.0 for Windows (IBM Corp., New York, USA) was used for all analyses. The statistically significant level was set at P value < 0.05.

Results

The mean ± SD of age, hemodialysis vintage, physical activity, CCI, and interdialytic weight gains were 59.4 ± 11.3, 5.5 ± 5.0, 4831.3 ± 1893.1, 4.6 ± 1.5, and 3.0 ± 1.7, respectively. Of study sample, there were 64.9% men, 38.2% diabetes, 48.2% hypertension, and 29.8% cardiovascular diseases, 28.5% with an elevated level of hs-CRP, 54.5% elevated body fat mass. The REE was lower in patients with inadequate EI (1014.5 ± 280.4) than those with adequate EI (1100.9 ± 274.7), with p = 0.023. Regarding metabolic abnormalities, the prevalence of IFG, overweight or obese, elevated WC, high BP, high TG, and low HDL-C were 64.9%, 36.4%, 26.3%, 81.6%, 39.0%, and 61.0%, respectively. The prevalence of metabolic syndrome was 63.2% as diagnosed by AACE criteria, and 53.9% as diagnosed by HMetS criteria. The prevalence of the metabolic abnormalities (not hypertension) and syndromes were statistically significantly higher in hemodialysis patients with inadequate EI than those who with adequate EI (Table 1). Out of patients, 60.5% reported less than the recommendation level of dietary energy intake. Patients with inadequate EI more likely consumed inadequate protein and fat, but consumed less mineral, water, and vitamin than those with adequate EI (Table 2).

The results of bivariate logistic regression analyses presented that higher age associated with higher prevalence of IFG and AACE-MetS with odd ratio, OR = 1.03, 95% confidence interval, 95%CI, 1.00–1.05, p < 0.05, and OR = 1.03, 95%CI, 1.01–1.06, p < 0.05, respectively. Men experienced higher prevalence of overweight or obesity (OR = 1.85, 95%CI, 1.03–3.33, p < 0.05), but lower prevalence of elevated waist circumference (OR = 0.32, 95%CI, 0.17–0.59, p < 0.001) than women. Hemodialysis vintage was negatively associated with IFG (OR = 0.91, 95%CI, 0.86–0.97, p < 0.001), Overweight/obese (OR = 0.92, 95%CI, 0.86–0.98, p < 0.05), high TG (OR = 0.94, 95%CI, 0.89–0.99, p < 0.05), low HDL-C (OR = 0.95, 95%CI, 0.90–0.99, p < 0.05), AACE-MetS (OR = 0.90, 95%CI, 0.85–0.96, p < 0.001), and HMetS (OR = 0.94, 95%CI, 0.89–0.99, p < 0.05), respectively. Charlson

comorbidity index was positively associated with IFG (OR = 1.38, 95%CI, 1.14–1.67, p < 0.001), Overweight/obese (OR = 1.21, 95%CI, 1.01–1.45, p < 0.05), AACE-MetS (OR = 1.44, 95%CI, 1.19–1.74, p < 0.001), and HMetS (OR = 1.28, 95%CI, 1.07–1.53, p < 0.01), respectively. Interdialytic weight gains was positively linked with IFG (OR = 1.21, 95%CI, 1.03–1.43, p < 0.05), AACE-MetS (OR = 1.22, 95%CI, 1.04–1.43, p < 0.05), and HMetS (OR = 1.24, 95%CI, 1.06–1.46, p < 0.01), respectively (Table 3).

Reported inadequate dietary energy intake associated with 1.83–6.20 folds of metabolic abnormalities or metabolic syndrome. It was significantly linked to higher prevalence of IFG (OR = 2.50, 95%CI, 1.43–4.37, p < 0.001), overweight/obese (OR = 6.10, 95%CI, 3.10–11.99, p < 0.001), elevated waist circumference (OR = 6.20, 2.78–13.84, p < 0.001), high triglyceride (OR = 1.90, 95%CI, 1.09–3.34, p < 0.05), low HDL-C (OR = 1.83, 95%CI, 1.06–3.15, p < 0.05), AACE -MetS (OR = 2.34, 95%CI, 1.35–4.06, p < 0.01), and HMetS (OR = 3.24, 95%CI, 1.86–5.63, p < 0.001), respectively. The sodium and fluid intake were not associated with metabolic abnormalities or MetS (Table 3).

The associations of inadequate energy intake with metabolic abnormalities, AACE-MetS, and HMetS were stronger by 2.26 to 8.17 folds after adjusted for gender, age, physical activity, hemodialysis vintage, Charlson comorbidity index (CCI), hs-CRP, and IDWG in multivariate analyses. Inadequate energy intake did not show the significant association with high TG, low HDL-C or high blood pressure (Table 4). On the other hand, the consumption of MUFA greater or equal to 20% of EI is associated with higher likelihood of having IFG (OR = 2.85, 95%CI, 1.39–5.87, p < 0.01), and AACE-MetS (OR = 3.01, 95%CI, 1.45–6.26, p < 0.01, Table 4).

In sub-group analyses, inadequate EI showed an significant association with higher prevalence of AACE-MetS in non-hypertension group (OR = 4.09, 95%CI, 1.55–10.77, p = 0.004), and non-cardiovascular disease group (OR = 2.59, 95%CI, 1.23–5.42, p = 0.012); and associated with HMetS in group of diabetes (OR = 8.33, 95%CI, 2.08–33.37, p = 0.003), non-hypertension (OR = 5.33, 95%CI, 1.97–14.40, p = 0.001), hypertension (OR = 2.59, 95%CI, 1.05–6.37, p = 0.038), and non-CVD (OR = 3.79, 95%CI, 1.80–7.97, p < 0.001, Table 5).

Discussion

In the present study, results elucidated that reported inadequate dietary energy intake (IDEI) associated with more MetS abnormalities, and a higher proportion of MetS. The reported IDEI strongly determined 2.26 to 8.17 folds of metabolic abnormalities and MetS diagnosed either by AACE or HMetS criteria. In hemodialysis patients, IDEI disrupts the energy balance, and the nitrogen balance, increases the tissue destruction, and protein catabolism

Table 1 Characteristics, and metabolic parameters, and other biochemical values in hemodialysis patients[a]

Variables	Total sample (n = 228)	Adequate EI (n = 90)	Inadequate EI (n = 138) [b]	P value [c]
Characteristics				
Age, years	59.4 ± 11.3	59.9 ± 10.8	59.1 ± 11.6	0.630
Gender, male	148 (64.9)	57 (63.3)	91 (65.9)	0.687
Hemodialysis vintage, years	5.5 ± 5.0	6.9 ± 5.9	4.5 ± 4.0	< 0.001
CCI	4.6 ± 1.5	4.7 ± 1.5	4.5 ± 1.6	0.327
Diabetes mellitus	87 (38.2)	24 (26.7)	63 (45.7)	0.004
Hypertension	110 (48.2)	45 (50.0)	65 (47.1)	0.669
Cardiovascular diseases	68 (29.8)	26 (28.9)	42 (30.4)	0.803
Physical activity, MET score	4831.3 ± 1893.1	4984.9 ± 2033.2	4732.6 ± 1798.1	0.330
Height, cm	162.4 ± 8.3	161.4 ± 7.0	163.0 ± 9.0	0.149
Weight, kg	61.4 ± 12.3	55.1 ± 8.9	65.4 ± 12.6	0.000
IDWG, %	3.0 ± 1.7	2.9 ± 2.0	3.1 ± 1.5	0.227
FM, %	27.2 ± 10.0	23.4 ± 9.1	29.7 ± 9.9	< 0.001
Elevated FM	122 (54.5)	34 (38.2)	88 (65.2)	< 0.001
REE, kcal/day	1048.6 ± 280.8	1100.9 ± 274.7	1014.5 ± 280.4	0.023
Metabolic abnormalities				
FPG	105.3 (90.5, 145.2)	97.3 (90.3, 134.0)	114.0 (93.6, 153.8)	0.025
IFG	148 (64.9)	47 (52.2)	101 (73.2)	0.001
BMI, kg/m^2	23.2 ± 3.8	21.1 ± 2.6	24.5 ± 3.9	< 0.001
BMI ≥ 24 (kg/m^2)	83 (36.4)	13 (14.4)	70 (50.7)	< 0.001
WC, cm	81.1 ± 10.4	75.7 ± 7.5	87.6 ± 36.4	0.002
Elevated WC	60 (26.3)	8 (8.9)	52 (37.7)	< 0.001
TG, mg/dL	115.0 (82.9, 202.6)	99.1 (78.0, 155.4)	136.8 (85.0, 250.5)	0.004
High TG ≥ 150 (mg/dL)	89 (39.0)	27 (30.0)	62 (44.9)	0.024
HDL-C, mg/dL	41.6 ± 22.1	45.8 ± 21.0	38.9 ± 22.4	0.021
Low HDL-C	139 (61.0)	47 (52.2)	92 (66.7)	0.029
SBP, mmHg	146.5 ± 22.7	149.5 ± 24.0	144.3 ± 21.3	0.089
DBP, mmHg	80.0 ± 18.2	79.8 ± 19.0	79.9 ± 17.6	0.959
High BP	186 (81.6)	73 (81.1)	113 (81.9)	0.883
AACE-MetS [d]	144 (63.2)	46 (51.1)	98 (71.0)	0.002
HMetS[e]	123 (53.9)	33 (36.7)	90 (65.2)	< 0.001
Other biochemical values				
TC, mg/dL	168.3 ± 37.9	163.8 ± 33.7	170.7 ± 40.0	0.178
TC ≥ 200 mg/dL	39 (17.1)	10 (11.1)	29 (21.0)	0.052
LDL-C, mg/dL	102.1 ± 32.5	98.0 ± 31.0	104.6 ± 32.9	0.130
LDL-C ≥ 100 mg/dL	41 (18.0)	13 (14.4)	28 (20.3)	0.261
FPI, µU/mL	15.2 (7.9, 31.9)	12.7 (6.8, 26.5)	18.6 (9.3, 35.7)	0.004
FPI ≥ 12 µU/mL	142 (62.3)	47 (52.2)	95 (68.8)	0.011
hs-CRP, mg/dL	0.3 (0.1, 0.6)	0.2 (0.1, 0.5)	0.3 (0.1, 0.6)	0.277
hs-CRP ≥ 0.5 mg/dL	65 (28.5)	23 (25.6)	42 (30.4)	0.425
iPTH, pg/mL	225.2 (80.6, 409.1)	231.0 (68.5, 441.2)	223.9 (94.4, 382.7)	0.916
iPTH ≥300 pg/mL	93 (40.8)	38 (42.2)	55 (39.9)	0.722
Creatinine, mg/dL	11.1 ± 1.9	10.8 ± 1.7	11.3 ± 2.1	0.077
Creatinine ≤7.5 mg/dL	8 (3.5)	6 (6.7)	2 (1.4)	0.036

Table 1 Characteristics, and metabolic parameters, and other biochemical values in hemodialysis patients[a] *(Continued)*

Variables	Total sample ($n = 228$)	Adequate EI ($n = 90$)	Inadequate EI ($n = 138$) [b]	P value [c]
Albumin, mg/dL	4.0 ± 0.4	4.0 ± 0.4	4.0 ± 0.4	0.992
Albumin ≤3.5 mg/dL	24 (10.5)	8 (8.9)	16 (11.6)	0.515
Pre-BUN, mg/dL	72.9 ± 20.9	76.7 ± 21.2	70.2 ± 20.7	0.023
Post-BUN, mg/dL	19.9 ± 7.8	19.0 ± 7.6	20.7 ± 7.9	0.106
eKt/V	1.6 ± 0.3	1.8 ± 0.4	1.5 ± 0.3	< 0.001
nPNA, g/kg	1.4 ± 0.4	1.4 ± 0.4	1.3 ± 0.4	< 0.001
nPNA < 1.0 g/kg	29 (12.7)	7 (7.8)	22 (15.9)	0.071

CCI: Charlson comorbidity index, MET: metabolic equivalent minute/week, IDWG, interdialytic weight gains, FM: fat mass, IFG: Impaired fasting glucose, BMI: body mass index, WC: waist circumference, TG: triglyceride, HDL-C: high-density lipoprotein cholesterol, BP: blood pressure, SBP: systolic blood pressure, DBP: diastolic blood pressure, TC: total cholesterol, LDL-C: low-density lipoprotein cholesterol, FPI: fasting plasma insulin, hs-CRP: high sensitive C-reactive protein, iPTH, intact parathyroid hormone, nPNA = normalized protein nitrogen appearance
[a]Categorical data is shown as n (%). Continuous data is presented as mean ± SD, or median (interquartile range)
[b]Inadequate energy intake was classified as EI < 30 kcal/kg/day for age 60 and above; < 35 for age less than 60
[c]Independent-samples T-test, Mann-Whitney U test, or Chi-square tests are performed
[d]Metabolic syndrome diagnosed by American Association of Clinical Endocrinologists (IFG plus any other abnormality: overweight/obese, high TG, low HDL, high blood pressure)
[e]Metabolic syndrome diagnosed by Harmonizing Metabolic Syndrome (three or more abnormalities: Elevated WC, IFG, low HDL, high TG, high blood pressure)

which cause the MetS and exacerbate the dialysis outcomes [64]. On the other hand, the MetS was found to be a high-risk for many chronic health problems such as obesity, T2DM, cardiovascular diseases, cancer, and all-cause of death [16–19]. Therefore, the early MetS identification and nutritional therapy were highly recommended to reduce above adverse health problems [25, 65]. In addition, patients who consumed adequate energy-rich-protein can improve the balance of body protein, body composition which further improve hemodialysis outcomes [66].

The current study showed that about 60% of hemodialysis patients consumed low dietary energy intake. This was in the line with a reliable previous publication in which patients had at most 75% of the energy and protein intake as recommended by K/DOQI guidelines [9]. MetS prevalence was high in the present study (63.2% AACE-MetS, 53.9% HMetS), and in previous studies in Southern Taiwan was 61.0% measured by NCEP-ATP III criteria [15]. In comparison with previous studies, the prevalence of MetS was lower in the current study than that in a study in Brazil (74.5%) using the HMetS criteria [27], and in United States (69.3%) using the NCEP-ATP III criteria [67].

The consumption of PUFA and SFA did not show the significant association with MetS and its abnormalities, while the consumption of MUFA equal or greater than 20% demonstrated the association with higher IFG and AACE-MetS in the current study. In a previous study, no association between PUFA, or SFA, and MetS was found [68]. Inconsistently, a number of previous studies suggested that the consumption of dietary MUFA improves insulin sensitivity. In addition, MUFA intake as a substitution for SFA demonstrated the benefit for reducing the metabolic syndrome [69, 70]. The discrepancy

between the findings of this study and other studies could be explained by the cross-sectional design of the current study, the causal relationship is not generated. In addition, the 24-h dietary recall is subject to reporting bias from patients. In practical application, the MUFA was with high density in the Mediterranean dietary pattern (MDP). Strong evidence from several studies and trials proved that the MDP was inversely associated with the incidence of MetS, cardiovascular diseases [71–74]. Therefore, this MDP can be still encouraged and adopted in various population and cultures, with cost-effective serve for preventing the MetS and its components [75]. However, the application is with precaution and more studies are suggested to intensively investigate the MDP effect on the MetS in hemodialysis patients.

The current results illustrated that the inadequate dietary EI was associated with high prevalence of HMetS in different sub-groups. In a study conducted in Italy, the authors found that patients with MetS reported lower energy intake than those without MetS [76]. This suggested that MetS diagnosed by Harmonizing Metabolic Syndrome criteria is more sensitive than AACE-MetS in relation to energy intake. In practice, in order to improve the hemodialysis outcomes, the adequate dietary EI is recommended by the K/DOQI guidelines which can reduce the risks of MetS [9].

The present study demonstrated that the higher prevalence of IFG and AACE-MetS was observed in older patients. The association was also found in previous studies on the general population in Norway, which MetS was diagnosed by either NCEP- ATP III, or IDF criteria [60], and in individuals in the United States [61]. This emphasized that the old people are more likely to have metabolic abnormalities, risks for CVD, and type 2

Table 2 Dietary intake among hemodialysis patients[a]

Daily dietary intake [b]	Total sample (n = 228)	Adequate EI (n = 90)	Inadequate EI (n = 138) [c]	P value [d]
Macronutrients				
Energy intake, kcal	1885.0 ± 477.2	2182.6 ± 448.9	1690.9 ± 387.7	< 0.001
Energy intake, kcal/kg	31.5 ± 8.8	39.8 ± 7.0	26.1 ± 4.6	< 0.001
Protein, g/kg IBW	1.2 ± 0.3	1.4 ± 0.3	1.1 ± 0.3	< 0.001
Protein < 1.2 g/kg IBW	132 (57.9)	28 (31.1)	104 (75.4)	< 0.001
Protein, (%EI)	15.0 ± 3.0	14.6 ± 2.7	15.2 ± 3.2	0.090
Protein < 15% EI	118 (51.8)	52 (57.8)	66 (47.8)	0.142
Carbohydrate, g	222.1 ± 68.8	252.9 ± 71.5	202.0 ± 59.1	< 0.001
Carbohydrate, (%EI)	47.6 ± 8.6	46.5 ± 8.2	48.3 ± 8.9	0.138
Carbohydrate < 45%EI	80 (35.1)	33 (36.7)	47 (34.1)	0.687
Total fat, g	78.3 ± 27.0	92.5 ± 26.5	69.0 ± 23.0	< 0.001
Total fat, (%EI)	37.1 ± 7.8	38.2 ± 7.4	36.4 ± 8.1	0.100
SFA (%EI)	13.4 (8.0, 69.4)	10.6 (8.0, 62.9)	37.9 (8.5, 73.7)	0.083
SFA ≥10% EI	143 (62.7)	53 (58.9)	90 (65.2)	0.334
MUFA (%EI)	18.0 (10.6, 76.0)	13.4 (9.8, 73.4)	41.8 (11.3, 80.2)	0.024
MUFA ≥20% EI	109 (47.8)	34 (37.8)	75 (54.3)	0.014
PUFA (%EI)	17.6 (8.7, 60.6)	12.2 (7.6, 52.0)	32.8 (9.6, 62.9)	0.015
PUFA ≥10% EI	155 (68.0)	55 (61.1)	100 (72.5)	0.072
SFA/UFA ratio	0.5 ± 0.2	0.5 ± 0.2	0.5 ± 0.2	0.869
UFA/SFA ratio	2.3 ± 0.7	2.3 ± 0.6	2.3 ± 0.8	0.426
Micronutrients				
Mineral and Water				
Sodium, mg/d	1254.8 ± 897.6	1576.9 ± 1108.9	1044.6 ± 650.7	< 0.001
Sodium > 1800 mg/d	43 (18.9)	29 (32.2)	14 (10.1)	< 0.001
Fluid, mL/d	1382.6 ± 480.5	1493.7 ± 506.7	1310.2 ± 449.8	0.005
Fluid > 1500 mL/d	78 (34.2)	38 (42.2)	40 (29.0)	0.039
Potassium, mg/d	1445.2 ± 582.6	1616.3 ± 575.7	1333.6 ± 561.5	< 0.001
Phosphate, mg/d	694.9 ± 257.9	799.7 ± 270.2	626.6 ± 225.6	< 0.001
Calcium, mg/d	291.3 ± 177.2	336.9 ± 190.7	261.6 ± 161.6	0.002
Iron, mg/d	8.6 ± 4.6	9.7 ± 5.3	7.8 ± 4.0	0.003
Zinc, mg/d	8.1 ± 3.8	9.3 ± 4.0	7.3 ± 3.5	< 0.001
Vitamins				
Vitamin B1 (thiamin), mg/d	0.8 ± 0.6	1.0 ± 0.6	0.8 ± 0.6	0.008
Vitamin B2 (riboflavin), mg/d	0.9 ± 0.5	1.0 ± 0.6	0.8 ± 0.5	0.001
Niacin (B3), mg/d	11.8 ± 6.3	13.9 ± 7.0	10.5 ± 5.5	< 0.001
Vitamin B6 (pyridoxine), mg/d	1.2 ± 0.9	1.4 ± 1.0	1.0 ± 0.7	0.015
Vitamin B12, µg/d	3.8 ± 3.7	4.5 ± 4.1	3.4 ± 3.4	0.022
Vitamin C, mg/d	90.6 ± 63.5	95.6 ± 59.7	87.3 ± 65.8	0.335
Vitamin E, mg/d [†]	12.6 ± 10.3	12.9 ± 11.1	12.6 ± 10.3	0.717

EI: energy intake, IBW: ideal body weight, SFA: saturated fatty acid, MUFA: mono-unsaturated fatty acid, PUFA: poly-unsaturated fatty acid, UFA: unsaturated fatty acid

[a]Categorical data is shown as n (%). Continuous data is presented as mean ± SD, or median (interquartile range)

[b]Target values recommended by Standing Committee on the Scientific Evaluation of Dietary Reference Intakes, Food and Nutrition Board, Institute of Medicine; the European Best Practice Guideline on Nutrition and Chronic Kidney Disease; and Clinical Practice Guidelines for Nutrition in Chronic Renal Failure

[c]Inadequate energy intake was classified as EI < 30 kcal/kg/day for age 60 and above; < 35 for age less than 60

[d]Independent-samples T-test, Mann-Whitney U test, or Chi-square tests are performed

Table 3 Bivariate analysis the effects of personal factors and dietary intake on metabolic abnormalities and metabolic syndrome

	Metabolic abnormalities						AACE-MetS [a]	HMetS [b]
	IFG	Overweight/Obese	Elevated WC	High TG	Low HDL-C	High BP		
	OR (95% CI)	OR (95% CI)	OR (95% CI)	OR (95% CI)	OR (95% CI)	OR (95% CI)	OR (95% CI)	OR (95% CI)
Age, years	1.03 (1.00, 1.05)*	1.01 (0.99, 1.04)	1.00 (0.98, 1.03)	1.00 (0.98, 1.03)	1.01 (0.98, 1.03)	1.00 (0.97, 1.03)	1.03 (1.01, 1.06)*	1.01 (0.98, 1.03)
Male gender	1.18 (0.67, 2.07)	1.85 (1.03, 3.33)*	0.32 (0.17, 0.59)***	1.20 (0.68, 2.10)	1.25 (0.72, 2.18)	1.69 (0.86, 3.34)	1.13 (0.65, 1.99)	1.18 (0.69, 2.04)
Hemodialysis vintage, years	0.91 (0.86, 0.97)***	0.92 (0.86, 0.98)*	0.97 (0.91, 1.03)	0.94 (0.89, 0.99)*	0.95 (0.90, 0.99)*	1.01 (0.95, 1.09)	0.90 (0.85, 0.96)***	0.94 (0.89, 0.99)*
CCI	1.38 (1.14, 1.67)***	1.21 (1.01, 1.45)*	1.07 (0.88, 1.29)	1.11 (0.94, 1.33)	1.14 (0.95, 1.36)	1.12 (0.89, 1.39)	1.44 (1.19, 1.74)***	1.28 (1.07, 1.53)**
Physical activity, (10% MET increment)	1.07 (0.97, 1.18)	0.99 (0.90, 1.08)	0.92 (0.83, 1.02)	0.96 (0.87, 1.05)	0.93 (0.85, 1.03)	1.07 (0.95, 1.20)	1.06 (0.97, 1.17)	0.99 (0.91, 1.09)
hs-CRP > 0.5 mg/dL	1.45 (0.78, 2.70)	1.63 (0.90, 2.93)	1.37 (0.72, 2.58)	1.16 (0.64, 2.08)	1.36 (0.75, 2.49)	0.66 (0.33, 1.35)	1.20 (0.66, 2.19)	1.41 (0.79, 2.53)
IDWG, %	1.21 (1.03, 1.43)*	1.00 (0.85, 1.16)	1.10 (0.93, 1.31)	1.12 (0.96, 1.32)	1.13 (0.97, 1.32)	1.05 (0.87, 1.28)	1.22 (1.04, 1.43)*	1.24 (1.06, 1.46)**
Dietary intake								
Inadequate EI	2.50 (1.43, 4.37)***	6.10 (3.10, 11.99)***	6.20 (2.78, 13.84)***	1.90 (1.09, 3.34)*	1.83 (1.06, 3.15)*	1.05 (0.53, 2.08)	2.34 (1.35, 4.08)**	3.24 (1.86, 5.63)***
Protein < 1.2 g/kg IBW	1.20 (0.69, 2.08)	0.85 (0.50, 1.47)	0.93 (0.52, 1.70)	1.12 (0.65, 1.92)	1.31 (0.76, 2.23)	0.92 (0.47, 1.82)	1.05 (0.61, 1.81)	1.32 (0.78, 2.23)
Carbohydrate < 45%EI	1.42 (0.79, 2.54)	1.08 (0.61, 1.89)	1.95 (1.07, 3.57)*	0.83 (0.48, 1.46)	0.87 (0.50, 1.51)	1.44 (0.69, 3.00)	1.46 (0.82, 2.59)	1.25 (0.72, 2.16)
SFA ≥10% EI	1.41 (0.81, 2.46)	0.85 (0.49, 1.48)	0.64 (0.35, 1.17)	0.94 (0.54, 1.62)	0.91 (0.53, 1.58)	1.91 (0.97, 3.75)	1.45 (0.84, 2.53)	0.92 (0.54, 1.57)
MUFA ≥20% EI	2.25 (1.28, 3.94)**	1.11 (0.64, 1.90)	0.71 (0.39, 1.30)	0.89 (0.52, 1.52)	1.12 (0.66, 1.91)	1.44 (0.73, 2.84)	2.19 (1.26, 3.81)**	1.17 (0.69, 1.97)
PUFA ≥10% EI	1.04 (0.58, 1.85)	0.96 (0.54, 1.72)	1.02 (0.54, 1.93)	1.14 (0.64, 2.02)	1.14 (0.64, 2.00)	1.58 (0.79, 3.15)	1.10 (0.62, 1.95)	1.12 (0.64, 1.95)
SFA/UFA ratio	0.67 (0.13, 3.43)	0.30 (0.05, 1.80)	0.33 (0.05, 2.41)	0.49 (0.09, 2.64)	2.23 (0.41, 12.15)	2.50 (0.27, 23.46)	0.86 (0.17, 4.42)	0.53 (0.11, 2.62)
UFA/SFA ratio	1.11 (0.75, 1.63)	1.37 (0.93, 2.01)	1.51 (1.00, 2.28)	1.28 (0.88, 1.86)	1.08 (0.74, 1.58)	0.81 (0.51, 1.29)	1.05 (0.72, 1.55)	1.46 (0.99, 2.14)
Sodium > 1800 mg	0.62 (0.32, 1.22)	1.04 (0.53, 2.08)	0.82 (0.38, 1.78)	1.16 (0.59, 2.27)	1.61 (0.79, 3.29)	0.99 (0.42, 2.31)	0.68 (0.35, 1.34)	0.98 (0.50, 1.90)
Fluid > 1500 mL	0.68 (0.38, 1.19)	1.73 (0.99, 3.04)	1.55 (0.84, 2.85)	1.34 (0.76, 2.33)	1.45 (0.82, 2.57)	0.92 (0.46, 1.86)	0.70 (0.40, 1.23)	1.16 (0.67, 2.02)

IFG: Impaired fasting glucose, WC: waist circumference, TG: triglyceride, HDL-C: high-density lipoprotein cholesterol, BP: blood pressure, CCI: Charlson comorbidity index, MET: metabolic equivalent minute/week, hs-CRP: high sensitive C-reactive protein, IDWG: interdialytic weight gains; BF: body fat; IBW: ideal body weight, SFA: saturated fatty acid, MUFA: mono-unsaturated fatty acid, PUFA: polyunsaturated fatty acid, UFA: unsaturated fatty acid

[a] Metabolic syndrome diagnosed by American Association of Clinical Endocrinologists (IFG plus any other abnormality: overweight/obese, high TG, low HDL-C, high BP)

[b] Metabolic syndrome diagnosed by Harmonizing Metabolic Syndrome (three or more abnormalities: elevated WC, IFG, low HDL-C, high TG, high BP)

Significant level at * $p < 0.05$, ** $p < 0.01$, *** $p < 0.001$

Table 4 Associations of dietary intake and metabolic abnormalities and metabolic syndrome via multivariate logistic regression analyses [a]

Dietary intake	Metabolic abnormalities						AACE-MetS [b]	HMetS [c]
	IFG	Overweight/Obese	Elevated WC	High TG	Low HDL-C	High BP		
	OR (95% CI)	OR (95% CI)	OR (95% CI)	OR (95% CI)	OR (95% CI)	OR (95% CI)	OR (95% CI)	OR (95% CI)
Inadequate EI	2.42 (1.30, 4.51)**	6.70 (3.25, 13.81)***	8.17 (3.33, 20.01)***	1.72 (0.95, 3.10)	1.67 (0.94, 2.98)	1.18 (0.57, 2.43)	2.26 (1.21, 4.23)*	3.52 (1.91, 6.50)**
Protein < 1.2 g/kg IBW	0.94 (0.51, 1.74)	0.74 (0.41, 1.33)	0.81 (0.42, 1.56)	0.95 (0.54, 1.69)	1.14 (0.64, 2.02)	0.99 (0.48, 2.04)	0.78 (0.42, 1.46)	1.15 (0.64, 2.04)
Carbohydrate <45%EI	1.30 (0.69, 2.46)	1.12 (0.61, 2.05)	1.88 (0.97, 3.66)	0.86 (0.48, 1.56)	0.90 (0.50, 1.62)	1.57 (0.72, 3.43)	1.30 (0.69, 2.45)	1.33 (0.73, 2.41)
SFA ≥10% EI	1.70 (0.87, 3.31)	0.94 (0.50, 1.77)	0.90 (0.45, 1.80)	1.22 (0.66, 2.28)	1.22 (0.66, 2.29)	2.01 (0.93, 4.32)	1.88 (0.96, 3.70)	1.25 (0.66, 2.34)
MUFA ≥20% EI	2.85 (1.39, 5.87)**	1.20 (0.63, 2.30)	1.09 (0.52, 2.26)	1.07 (0.56, 2.03)	1.59 (0.83, 3.04)	1.40 (0.62, 3.16)	3.01 (1.45, 6.26)**	1.55 (0.81, 2.99)
PUFA ≥10% EI	0.99 (0.52, 1.90)	1.07 (0.58, 1.98)	1.27 (0.64, 2.51)	1.30 (0.71, 2.38)	1.33 (0.73, 2.44)	1.60 (0.77, 3.32)	1.09 (0.57, 2.09)	1.32 (0.72, 2.45)
SFA/UFA ratio	1.03 (0.17, 6.15)	0.47 (0.07, 3.05)	0.46 (0.06, 3.46)	0.82 (0.14, 4.71)	5.13 (0.79, 33.43)	3.07 (0.31, 30.62)	1.54 (0.26, 9.37)	1.12 (0.20, 6.24)
UFA/SFA ratio	0.98 (0.63, 1.52)	1.24 (0.82, 1.88)	1.34 (0.86, 2.10)	1.11 (0.74, 1.66)	0.89 (0.59, 1.35)	0.80 (0.49, 1.31)	0.90 (0.58, 1.39)	1.24 (0.81, 1.89)
Sodium > 1800 mg	0.63 (0.30, 1.31)	0.96 (0.47, 1.97)	0.96 (0.42, 2.20)	1.16 (0.57, 2.34)	1.66 (0.79, 3.51)	0.95 (0.39, 2.31)	0.73 (0.35, 1.52)	0.99 (0.49, 2.01)
Fluid > 1500 mL	0.60 (0.32, 1.15)	1.68 (0.91, 3.10)	1.76 (0.89, 3.46)	1.22 (0.67, 2.23)	1.30 (0.70, 2.40)	0.79 (0.37, 1.66)	0.61 (0.32, 1.17)	0.97 (0.52, 1.78)

IFG: Impaired fasting glucose, WC: waist circumference, TG: triglyceride, HDL-C: high-density lipoprotein cholesterol, BP: blood pressure, EI: energy intake, IBW: ideal body weight, SFA: saturated fatty acid, MUFA: monounsaturated fatty acid, PUFA: polyunsaturated fatty acid, UFA: unsaturated fatty acid

[a] The analysis was adjusted for age, gender, hemodialysis vintage, Charlson comorbidity index, physical activity, high sensitive C-reactive protein, and interdialytic weight gains

[b] Metabolic syndrome diagnosed by American Association of Clinical Endocrinologists (IFG plus any other abnormality: overweight/obese, high TG, low HDL-C, high BP)

[c] Metabolic syndrome diagnosed by Harmonizing Metabolic Syndrome (three or more abnormalities: elevated WC, IFG, low HDL-C, high TG, high BP)

Significant level at * $p < 0.05$, ** $p < 0.01$, *** $p < 0.001$

Table 5 Association between inadequate energy intake and metabolic syndrome in subgroups of medical history[a]

| | Inadequate EI | | AACE-MetS [b] | | | HMetS [c] | |
	(n = 138)	n	OR (95% CI)	p	n	OR (95% CI)	p
Non-DM (n = 141)	75	35	1.15 (0.54, 2.47)	0.718	35	1.91 (0.88, 4.15)	0.101
DM (n = 87)	63	63	N/A		55	8.33 (2.08, 33.37)	0.003
Non-HTN (n = 118)	73	51	4.09 (1.55, 10.77)	0.004	44	5.33 (1.97, 14.40)	0.001
HTN (n = 110)	65	47	1.33 (0.51, 3.51)	0.560	46	2.59 (1.05, 6.37)	0.038
Non-CVD (n = 160)	96	68	2.59 (1.23, 5.42)	0.012	62	3.79 (1.80, 7.97)	< 0.001
CVD (n = 68)	42	30	1.48 (0.33, 6.75)	0.612	28	3.64 (0.99, 13.36)	0.052

EI: energy intake, DM: diabetes mellitus, HTN: hypertension, CVD: cardiovascular diseases
[a]The analysis was adjusted for age, gender, hemodialysis vintage, Charlson comorbidity index, physical activity, high sensitive C-reactive protein, and interdialytic weight gains
[b]Metabolic syndrome diagnosed by American Association of Clinical Endocrinologists (IFG plus any other abnormality: overweight/obese, high TG, low HDL-C, high BP)
[c]Metabolic syndrome diagnosed by Harmonizing Metabolic Syndrome (three or more abnormalities: elevated WC, IFG, low HDL-C, high TG, high BP)

diabetes. Therefore, the MetS definitions should be specifically classified for elderly people, as in need of comprehensive assessment for risk factors. On the other hand, men more likely experienced overweight/obesity, but less likely had elevated waist circumference in comparison with women. This could be explained that men have greater abdominal visceral adipose tissue (likely corresponding to BMI), but less abdominal subcutaneous adipose tissue (likely corresponding to waist circumference) than women [77].

The study conducted on 153 hemodialysis patients in three dialysis centers in Tehran demonstrated that the prevalence of MetS among women was higher than that among men [62]. However, in the current study, gender was significantly associated with metabolic abnormalities, but not with AACE MetS or HMetS. This suggests that gender should take into consideration when assessing or treating patients with MetS, the presence of metabolic disorders in men or women may depend on their specific lifestyles and behaviors.

The longer hemodialysis vintage has shown the protective impact on MetS among studied hemodialysis patients. This somehow expressed the quality of hemodialysis in dialysis centers in Taiwan which reflected the effectiveness of multi-disciplinary care program in hospitals since 2003 to combat chronic kidney disease and related comorbidities [78]. In addition, the full reimbursement of dialysis costs by National Health Insurance in Taiwan medical system could further optimize the quality of care [79], which in turn reduced the prevalence of metabolic disorders in this study.

Physical activity was not associated with metabolic abnormalities or MetS in the present study. However, a review of several randomized trials concluded that the physical activity decreased the likelihood of development of MetS; if there were no contraindications, more intensive physical exercise or resistance training should be considered to prevent and treat MetS [63]. In addition,

patients who performed regular exercise had better dialysis outcomes and health benefits as reported in an international study on hemodialysis patients [80].

Finally, the elevated level of hs-CRP did not show the association with MetS and its components. Inconsistently, the association was existed in the previous study, that inflammatory biomarkers had a correlation with MetS in hemodialysis patients [62]. An elevated level of hs-CRP may be a key independent predictor of adverse outcomes in hemodialysis patients with MetS. Therefore, reducing serum hs-CRP level should be considered for preventing MetS, CVD, and finally mortality among hemodialysis patients.

There was some limitations in the current study. Firstly, the causality cannot be proved between dietary EI and metabolic abnormalities and MetS in a cross-sectional design. In addition, the application of adequate EI but less MUFA intake was not clearly addressed because of the nature of the cross-sectional study design, and unavoidable reporting bias. More in-depth longitudinal studies and trials are required. The self-reported dietary assessment using food records and recalls had impacts on energy underreporting, appropriate interpretations of the results are recommended [81]. In the current study, we excluded those patients underreported their energy intake in order to avoid the bias and improve the reliability of findings [42]. However, the sample size is relatively small for subgroup analysis. Further investigation should be conducted on larger sample, to enhance the reliability of finding. The present study demonstrated a number of strengths that patients' body composition was measured precisely and directly using the BIA, while biochemical data were assessed by using standard laboratory tests. Two MetS definitions reflecting the glucocentric, obesity, and CVD risk factors were used to assure the non-spuriousness of the relationships. Future longitudinal studies or trials were recommended to confirm the relationship between dietary intake and MetS and impacts of nutritional interventions on dialysis outcomes.

Conclusions

This was the first study exploring the association of the reported dietary EI with metabolic abnormalities and MetS diagnosed by AACE and Harmonizing Metabolic Syndrome criteria in hemodialysis patients. We found that inadequate EI was high prevalence and associated with up to 2.26–8.17 folds of MetS and its components. Promoting adequate dietary energy intake following the K/DOQI guidelines could help to improve dialysis quality, prevent MetS, minimize the negative effects of metabolic disorders and their consequences, in turn, optimize the quality of care, and improve the quality of life of HD patients. Future studies are suggested for carefully exploring the mechanism, and evaluating the effect of dietary energy interventions.

Abbreviations
AACE-MetS: Metabolic syndrome diagnosed by American Association of Clinical Endocrinologists; BIA: Bioelectrical impedance analysis; BMI: Body mass index; BP: Blood pressure; CCI: Charlson comorbidity index; CVD: Cardiovascular diseases; DBP: Diastolic blood pressure; EI: Energy intake; ESRD: End-stage renal disease; FPG: Fasting plasma glucose; HDL: High-density lipoprotein; HDL-C: High-density lipoprotein cholesterol; HMetS: Metabolic syndrome diagnosed by Harmonizing Metabolic Syndrome defined by Joint statement from the International Diabetes Federation (IDF), American Heart Association (AHA) and the National Heart, Lung, and Blood Institute (NHLBI), the World Heart Federation, the International Atherosclerosis Society, and the International Association for the Study of Obesity; hs-CRP: High sensitive C-reactive protein; IBW: Ideal body weight; IFG: Impaired fasting glucose; iPTH: Intact parathyroid hormone; LDL-C: Low-density lipoprotein cholesterol; MET: Metabolic equivalent minute/ week; MUFA: Mono-unsaturated fatty acid; NCEP- ATP III: National Cholesterol Education Program-Adult Treatment Panel-III definition; NKF-KDOQI: National Kidney Foundation-Kidney Disease Outcomes Quality Initiative; nPNA: Normalized protein nitrogen appearance; PUFA: Poly-unsaturated fatty acid; SBP: Systolic blood pressure;; SFA: Saturated fatty acid; TC: Total cholesterol; TG: Triglyceride; UFA: Unsaturated fatty acid; WC: Waist circumference

Acknowledgments
The authors express the appreciation to medical staff and patients from Taipei Medical University Hospital, Wan-Fang Hospital, Shuang Ho Hospital, Cathay General Hospital, and Taipei Tzu-Chi Hospital, Wei-Gong Memorial Hospital, and Lotung Poh-Ai Hospital.

Funding
The research was funded by Ministry of Science and Technology in Taiwan (NSC-102-2320-B-038-026; MOST 105-2320-B-038-033-MY3). The funder had no role in the decision to collect data, data analysis, or reporting of the results.

Authors' contributions
TVD contributed to conception and design, analysis and interpretation of data, and drafted the manuscript. TCW, HHC, TWC, THC, YHH, SJP, KLK, HCL, ETL, CTS contributed to study design, acquisition of data, and involved in drafting the manuscript. CSW, IHT, YWF, TYZ contributed to acquisition of data, interpretation of data and the discussion. SHY contributed to overall study design and conception, critically revised the manuscript. All authors have read and approved the final version and the submission of the manuscript.

Competing interest
The authors have no competing interests to be declared.

Author details
[1]School of Nutrition and Health Sciences, Taipei Medical University, No. 250 Wuxing Street, Taipei 110, Taiwan. [2]Department of Nutrition and Health Sciences, Chinese Culture University, Taipei, Taiwan. [3]Department of Nephrology, Taipei Medical University Hospital, Taipei, Taiwan. [4]School of Medicine, Taipei Medical University, Taipei, Taiwan. [5]Department of Nephrology, Taipei Medical University- Wan Fang Hospital, Taipei, Taiwan. [6]Division of Nephrology, Department of Internal Medicine, Taipei Medical University- Shuang Ho Hospital, Taipei, Taiwan. [7]Division of Nephrology, Cathay General Hospital, Taipei, Taiwan. [8]Division of Nephrology, Taipei Tzu-Chi Hospital, Taipei, Taiwan. [9]Department of Nephrology, Wei Gong Memorial Hospital, Miaoli, Taiwan. [10]Department of Nephrology, Lotung Poh-Ai Hospital, Yilan, Taiwan. [11]School of Public Health, Taipei Medical University, Taipei, Taiwan. [12]Department of Family Medicine, Taipei Medical University Hospital, Taipei, Taiwan. [13]Research Center of Geriatric Nutrition, Taipei Medical University, Taipei, Taiwan. [14]Nutrition Research Center, Taipei Medical University Hospital, Taipei, Taiwan.

References
1.   United States Renal Data System: International comparisons. The 2016 Annual data report: epidemiology of kidney disease in the United States: volume 2 – end-stage renal disease (ESRD) in the United States. In. USRDS Coordinating Center: National Institutes of Health, National Institute of Diabetes and Digestive and Kidney Diseases; 2016.
2.   Slee AD. Exploring metabolic dysfunction in chronic kidney disease. Nutr Metab (Lond). 2012;9(1):36.
3.   Qian F, Korat AA, Malik V, Hu FB. Metabolic effects of monounsaturated fatty acid–enriched diets compared with carbohydrate or polyunsaturated fatty acid–enriched diets in patients with type 2 diabetes: a systematic review and meta-analysis of randomized controlled trials. Diabetes Care. 2016;39(8):1448–57.
4.   Kent PS, MP MC, Burrowes JD, Mc Cann L, Pavlinac J, Goeddeke-Merickel CM, Wiesen K, Kruger S, Byham-Gray L, Pace RC, et al. Academy of nutrition and dietetics and National Kidney Foundation: revised 2014 standards of practice and standards of professional performance for registered dietitian nutritionists (competent, proficient, and expert) in nephrology nutrition. J Acad Nutr Diet. 2014;114(9):1448–57.e45.
5.   Schoenaker DAJM, Mishra GD, Callaway LK, Soedamah-Muthu SS. The role of energy, nutrients, foods, and dietary patterns in the development of gestational diabetes mellitus: a systematic review of observational studies. Diabetes Care. 2015;39(1):16–23.
6.   Beto JA, Ramirez WE, Bansal VK. Medical nutrition therapy in adults with chronic kidney disease: integrating evidence and consensus into practice for the generalist registered dietitian nutritionist. J Acad Nutr Diet. 2014; 114(7):1077–87.
7.   Fouque D, Guebre-Egziabher F. An update on nutrition in chronic kidney disease. Int Urol Nephrol. 2007;39(1):239–46.
8.   Kistler BM, Benner D, Burrowes JD, Campbell KL, Fouque D, Garibotto G, Kopple JD, Kovesdy CP, Rhee CM, Steiber A, et al. Eating during hemodialysis treatment: a consensus statement from the International Society of Renal Nutrition and Metabolism. J Ren Nutr. 2018;28(1):4–12.
9.   Kopple JD. National Kidney Foundation K/DOQI clinical practice guidelines for nutrition in chronic renal failure. Am J Kidney Dis. 2001;37(1 Suppl 2):S66–70.
10. Stark S, Snetselaar L, Hall B, Stone RA, Kim S, Piraino B, Sevick MA. Nutritional intake in adult hemodialysis patients. Top Clin Nutr. 2011;26(1):45–56.
11. St-Jules DE, Woolf K, Pompeii ML, Sevick MA. Exploring problems in following the hemodialysis diet and their relation to energy and nutrient intakes: the BalanceWise study. J Ren Nutr. 2016;26(2):118–24.

12. The National Kidney Foundation Kidney Disease Outcomes Quality Initiative (K/DOQI) Workgroup. KDOQI clinical practice guidelines and clinical practice recommendations for diabetes and chronic kidney disease. Am J Kidney Dis. 2007;49(2):S12–S154.

13. Kidney Disease Outcomes Quality Initiative (K/DOQI) Group. K/DOQI clinical practice guidelines for management of dyslipidemias in patients with kidney disease. Am J Kidney Dis. 2003;41(4 Suppl 3):S1–S91.

14. The National Kidney Foundation Kidney Disease Outcomes Quality Initiative (K/DOQI) Workgroup. K/DOQI clinical practice guidelines on hypertension and antihypertensive agents in chronic kidney disease. Am J kidney dis. 2004;43. Supplement. 1:11–3.

15. Tu S-F, Chou Y-C, Sun C-A, Hsueh S-C, Yang T. The prevalence of metabolic syndrome and factors associated with quality of Dialysis among hemodialysis patients in southern Taiwan. Glob J Health Sci. 2012;4(5):53–62.

16. Mottillo S, Filion KB, Genest J, Joseph L, Pilote L, Poirier P, Rinfret S, Schiffrin EL, Eisenberg MJ. The metabolic syndrome and cardiovascular risk. A Systematic Review and Meta-Analysis J Am Coll Cardiol. 2010; 56(14):1113–32.

17. Sattar N, McConnachie A, Shaper AG, Blauw GJ, Buckley BM, de Craen AJ, Ford I, Forouhi NG, Freeman DJ, Jukema JW, et al. Can metabolic syndrome usefully predict cardiovascular disease and diabetes? Outcome data from two prospective studies. Lancet. 2008;371(9628):1927–35.

18. Kastorini CM, Panagiotakos DB, Georgousopoulou EN, Laskaris A, Skourlis N, Zana A, Chatzinikolaou C, Chrysohoou C, Puddu PE, Tousoulis D, et al. Metabolic syndrome and 10-year cardiovascular disease incidence: the ATTICA study. Nutr Metab Cardiovasc Dis. 2016;26(3):223–31.

19. Harding J, Sooriyakumaran M, Anstey KJ, Adams R, Balkau B, Briffa T, Davis TME, Davis WA, Dobson A, Giles GG, et al. The metabolic syndrome and cancer: is the metabolic syndrome useful for predicting cancer risk above and beyond its individual components? Diabetes Metab. 2015;41(6):463–9.

20. Vogt BP, Souza PL, Minicucci MF, Martin LC, Barretti P, Caramori JT. Metabolic syndrome criteria as predictors of insulin resistance, inflammation, and mortality in chronic hemodialysis patients. Metab Syndr Relat Disord. 2014;12(8):443–9.

21. Einhorn D, Reaven GM, Cobin RH, Ford E, Ganda OP, Handelsman Y, Hellman R, Jellinger PS, Kendall D, Krauss RM, et al. American College of Endocrinology position statement on the insulin resistance syndrome. Endocr Pract. 2003;9(3):237–52.

22. Alberti KGMM, Eckel RH, Grundy SM, Zimmet PZ, Cleeman JI, Donato KA, Fruchart J-C, James WPT, Loria CM, Smith SC, et al. Harmonizing the metabolic syndrome: a joint interim statement of the international diabetes federation task force on epidemiology and prevention; National Heart, Lung, and Blood Institute; American Heart Association; world heart federation; international atherosclerosis society; and International Association for the Study of obesity. Circulation. 2009;120(16):1640–5.

23. Martins AM, Dias Rodrigues JC, de Oliveira Santin FG, Barbosa Brito FdS, Bello Moreira AS, Lourenço RA, Avesani CM. Food intake assessment of elderly patients on hemodialysis. J Ren Nutr 2015;25(3):321–326.

24. Shah A, Bross R, Shapiro BB, Morrison G, Kopple JD. Dietary energy requirements in relatively healthy maintenance hemodialysis patients estimated from long-term metabolic studies. Am J Clin Nutr. 2016; 103(3):757–65.

25. Azadbakht L, Mirmiran P, Esmaillzadeh A, Azizi T, Azizi F. Beneficial effects of a dietary approaches to stop hypertension eating plan on features of the metabolic syndrome. Diabetes Care. 2005;28(12):2823–31.

26. Daniel WW, Cross CL. Biostatistics: A Foundation for analysis in the health sciences. 10th ed. New York, United States of America: John Wiley & Sons; 2013.

27. Vogt BP, Ponce D, Caramori JCT. Anthropometric indicators predict metabolic syndrome diagnosis in maintenance hemodialysis patients. Nutr Clin Pract. 2016;31(3):368–74.

28. Pourhoseingholi MA, Vahedi M, Rahimzadeh M. Sample size calculation in medical studies. Gastroenterol Hepatol Bed Bench. 2013;6(1):14–7.

29. Wong T-C, Chen Y-T, Wu P-Y, Chen T-W, Chen H-H, Chen T-H, Hsu Y-H, Yang S-H. Ratio of dietary ω-3 and ω-6 fatty acids—independent determinants of muscle mass—in hemodialysis patients with diabetes. Nutrition. 2016;32(9):989–94.

30. Duong TV, Wong T-C, Chen H-H, Chen T-W, Chen T-H, Hsu Y-H, Peng S-J, Kuo K-L, Wang C-S, Tseng IH, et al. The cut-off values of dietary energy intake for determining metabolic syndrome in hemodialysis patients: a clinical cross-sectional study. PLoS One. 2018;13(3):e0193742.

31. Duong TV, Wong T-C, Su C-T, Chen H-H, Chen T-W, Chen T-H, Hsu Y-H, Peng S-J, Kuo K-L, Liu H-C, et al. Associations of dietary macronutrients and micronutrients with the traditional and nontraditional risk factors for cardiovascular disease among hemodialysis patients: a clinical cross-sectional study. Medicine (Baltimore). 2018;97(26):e11306.

32. Wong T-C, Su H-Y, Chen Y-T, Wu P-Y, Chen H-H, Chen T-H, Hsu Y-H, Yang S-H. Ratio of C-reactive protein to albumin predicts muscle mass in adult patients undergoing hemodialysis. PLoS One. 2016;11(10):e0165403.

33. Hemmelgarn BR, Manns BJ, Quan H, Ghali WA. Adapting the Charlson comorbidity index for use in patients with ESRD. Am J Kidney Dis. 2003; 42(1):125–32.

34. Wong T-C, Chen Y-T, Wu P-Y, Chen T-W, Chen H-H, Chen T-H, Yang S-H. Ratio of dietary n-6/n-3 polyunsaturated fatty acids independently related to muscle mass decline in hemodialysis patients. PLoS One. 2015;10(10): e0140402.

35. Okorodudu DO, Jumean MF, Montori VM, Romero-Corral A, Somers VK, Erwin PJ, Lopez-Jimenez F. Diagnostic performance of body mass index to identify obesity as defined by body adiposity: a systematic review and meta-analysis. Int J Obes. 2010;34:791–9.

36. Ipema KJR, Kuipers J, Westerhuis R, Gaillard CAJM, van der Schans CP, Krijnen WP, Franssen CFM. Causes and consequences of Interdialytic weight gain. Kidney Blood Press Res. 2016;41(5):710–20.

37. Liou YM, Jwo CJC, Yao KG, Chiang L-C, Huang L-H. Selection of appropriate Chinese terms to represent intensity and types of physical activity terms for use in the Taiwan version of IPAQ. J Nurs Res. 2008;16(4):252–63.

38. Craig CL, Marshall AL, Sjöström M, Bauman AE, Booth ML, Ainsworth BE, Pratt M, Ekelund U, Yngve A, Sallis JF, et al. International physical activity questionnaire: 12-country reliability and validity. Med Sci Sports Exerc. 2003; 35(8):1381–95.

39. Lee PH, Macfarlane DJ, Lam TH, Stewart SM. Validity of the international physical activity questionnaire short form (IPAQ-SF): a systematic review. Int J Behav Nutr Phys Act. 2011;8:115.

40. Chiu Y-F, Chen Y-C, Wu P-Y, Shih C-K, Chen H-H, Chen H-H, Chen T-H, Yang S-H. Association between the hemodialysis eating index and risk factors of cardiovascular disease in hemodialysis patients. J Ren Nutr. 2014;24(3):163–71.

41. Shapiro BB, Bross R, Morrison G, Zadeh K, Kopple JD. Self-reported, interview-assisted diet records underreport energy intake in maintenance hemodialysis patients. J Ren Nutr. 2015;25(4):357–63.

42. Hirvonen T, Männistö S, Roos E, Pietinen P. Increasing prevalence of underreporting does not necessarily distort dietary surveys. Eur J Clin Nutr. 1997;51(5):297–301.

43. McDoniel SO. Systematic review on use of a handheld indirect calorimeter to assess energy needs in adults and children. Int J Sport Nutr Exerc Metab. 2007;17(5):491–500.

44. Nieman DC, Trone GA, Austin MD. A new handheld device for measuring resting metabolic rate and oxygen consumption. J Am Diet Assoc. 2003; 103(5):588–92.

45. St-Onge M-P, Rubiano F, Jones A, Heymsfield SB. A new hand-held indirect calorimeter to measure postprandial energy expenditure. Obes Res. 2004; 12(4):704–9.

46. Hasson RE, Howe CA, Jones BL, Freedson PS. Accuracy of four resting metabolic rate prediction equations: effects of sex, body mass index, age, and race/ethnicity. J Sci Med Sport. 2011;14(4):344–51.

47. Wu P-Y, Yang S-H, Wong T-C, Chen T-W, Chen H-H, Chen T-H, Chen Y-T. Association of Processed Meat Intake with hypertension risk in hemodialysis patients: a cross-sectional study. PLoS One. 2015;10(10):e0141917.

48. Daugirdas JT. Simplified equations for monitoring Kt/V, PCRn, eKt/V, and ePCRn. Adv Ren Replace Ther. 1995;2(4):295–304.

49. Shaw JE, Zimmet PZ, Alberti KGMM. Point: impaired fasting glucose: the case for the new American Diabetes Association criterion. Diabetes Care. 2006;29(5):1170–2.

50. Hwang L-C, Bai C-H, Chen C-J. Prevalence of obesity and metabolic syndrome in Taiwan. J Formos Med Assoc. 2006;105(8):626–35.

51. Expert Panel on Detection Evaluation and Treatment of High Blood Cholesterol in Adults. Executive summary of the third report of the national cholesterol education program (NCEP) expert panel on detection, evaluation, and treatment of high blood cholesterol in adults (adult treatment panel III). JAMA. 2001;285(19):2486–97.

52. Omae K, Kondo T, Tanabe K. High preoperative C-reactive protein values predict poor survival in patients on chronic hemodialysis undergoing nephrectomy for renal cancer. Urol Oncol 2015;33(2):67.e9-.e13.

53. McAuley KA, Williams SM, Mann JI, Walker RJ, Lewis-Barned NJ, Temple LA, Duncan AW. Diagnosing insulin resistance in the general population. Diabetes Care. 2001;24(3):460–4.

54. Ascaso JF, Pardo S, Real JT, Lorente RI, Priego A, Carmena R. Diagnosing insulin resistance by simple quantitative methods in subjects with normal glucose metabolism. Diabetes Care. 2003;26(12):3320–5.

55. Kidney Disease. Improving global outcomes (KDIGO) CKD–MBD work group. KDIGO clinical practice guideline for the diagnosis, evaluation, prevention, and treatment of chronic kidney disease–mineral and bone disorder (CKD–MBD). Kidney Int. 2009;76(Suppl 113):S1–S130.

56. Lopes AA, Bragg-Gresham JL, Elder SJ, Ginsberg N, Goodkin DA, Pifer T, Lameire N, Marshall MR, Asano Y, Akizawa T, et al. Independent and joint associations of nutritional status indicators with mortality risk among chronic hemodialysis patients in the Dialysis outcomes and practice patterns study (DOPPS). J Ren Nutr. 2010;20(4):224–34.

57. Shapiro SS, Wilk MB. An analysis of variance test for normality (complete samples). Biometrika. 1965;52(3/4):591–611.

58. Razali NM, Wah YB. Power comparisons of shapiro-wilk, kolmogorov-smirnov, lilliefors and Anderson-darling tests. Journal of Statistical Modeling and Analytics. 2011;1(1):21–3.

59. Sicras-Mainar A, Ruíz-Beato E, Navarro-Artieda R, Maurino J. Comorbidity and metabolic syndrome in patients with multiple sclerosis from Asturias and Catalonia, Spain. BMC Neurol. 2017;17:134.

60. Hildrum B, Mykletun A, Hole T, Midthjell K, Dahl AA. Age-specific prevalence of the metabolic syndrome defined by the international diabetes federation and the National Cholesterol Education Program: the Norwegian HUNT 2 study. BMC Public Health. 2007;7:220–9.

61. Razzouk L, Muntner P. Ethnic, gender, and age-related differences in patients with the metabolic syndrome. Curr Hypertens Rep. 2009;11(2):127–32.

62. Shahrokh S, Heydarian P, Ahmadi F, Saddadi F, Razeghi E. Association of Inflammatory Biomarkers with metabolic syndrome in hemodialysis patients. Ren Fail. 2012;34(9):1109–13.

63. Lakka TA, Laaksonen DE. Physical activity in prevention and treatment of the metabolic syndrome. Appl Physiol Nutr Metab. 2007;32(1):76–88.

64. Cuppari L, Ikizler TA. Energy balance in advanced chronic kidney disease and end-stage renal disease. Semin Dial. 2010;23(4):373–7.

65. Beto JA, Bansal VK. Medical nutrition therapy in chronic kidney failure: integrating clinical practice guidelines. J Am Diet Assoc. 2004;104(3):404–9.

66. Veeneman JM, Kingma HA, Boer TS, Stellaard F, De Jong PE, Reijngoud D-J, Huisman RM. Protein intake during hemodialysis maintains a positive whole body protein balance in chronic hemodialysis patients. Am J Physiol Endocrinol Metab. 2003;284(5):E954–E65.

67. Young DO, Lund RJ, Haynatzki G, Dunlay RW. Prevalence of the metabolic syndrome in an incident dialysis population. Hemodial Int. 2007;11(1):86–95.

68. Um Y-J, Oh S-W, Lee C-M, Kwon H-T, Joh H-K, Kim Y-J, Kim H-J, Ahn S-H. Dietary fat intake and the risk of metabolic syndrome in Korean adults. Korean J Fam Med. 2015;36(5):245–52.

69. Gillingham LG, Harris-Janz S, Jones PJH. Dietary monounsaturated fatty acids are protective against metabolic syndrome and cardiovascular disease risk factors. Lipids. 2011;46(3):209–28.

70. Riccardi G, Giacco R, Rivellese AA. Dietary fat, insulin sensitivity and the metabolic syndrome. Clin Nutr. 2004;23(4):447–56.

71. Esposito K, Maiorino MI, Ceriello A, Giugliano D. Prevention and control of type 2 diabetes by Mediterranean diet: a systematic review. Diabetes Res Clin Pract. 2010;89(2):97–102.

72. Koloverou E, Esposito K, Giugliano D, Panagiotakos D. The effect of Mediterranean diet on the development of type 2 diabetes mellitus: a meta-analysis of 10 prospective studies and 136,846 participants. Metabolism. 2014;63(7):903–11.

73. Martínez-González MÁ, Martín-Calvo N. The major European dietary patterns and metabolic syndrome. Rev Endocr Metab Disord. 2013;14(3):265–71.

74. Calton EK, James AP, Pannu PK, Soares MJ. Certain dietary patterns are beneficial for the metabolic syndrome: reviewing the evidence. Nutr Res. 2014;34(7):559–68.

75. Kastorini C-M, Milionis HJ, Esposito K, Giugliano D, Goudevenos JA, Panagiotakos DB. The Effect of Mediterranean Diet on Metabolic Syndrome and its Components: A Meta-Analysis of 50 Studies and 534,906 Individuals. J Am Coll Cardiol. 2011;57(11):1299–313.

76. Buscemi S, Verga S, Donatelli M, D'Orio L, Mattina A, Tranchina MR, Pizzo G, Mulè G, Cerasola G. A low reported energy intake is associated with metabolic syndrome. J Endocrinol Investig. 2009;32(6):538–41.

77. Maki KC, Rains TM, Bell M, Reeves MS, Farmer MV, Yasunaga K. Fat mass, abdominal fat distribution, and C-reactive protein concentrations in overweight and obese men and women. Metab Syndr Relat Disord. 2011;9(4):291–6.

78. Chen Y-R, Yang Y, Wang S-C, Chiu P-F, Chou W-Y, Lin C-Y, Chang J-M, Chen T-W, Ferng S-H, Lin C-L. Effectiveness of multidisciplinary care for chronic kidney disease in Taiwan: a 3-year prospective cohort study. Nephrol Dial Transplant. 2013;28(3):671–82.

79. Cheng T-M. Reflections on the 20th anniversary of Taiwan's single-payer National Health Insurance System. Health Aff. 2015;34(3):502–10.

80. Tentori F, Elder SJ, Thumma J, Pisoni RL, Bommer J, Fissell RB, Fukuhara S, Jadoul M, Keen ML, Saran R, et al. Physical exercise among participants in the Dialysis outcomes and practice patterns study (DOPPS): correlates and associated outcomes. Nephrol Dial Transplant. 2010;25(9):3050–62.

81. Subar AF, Freedman LS, Tooze JA, Kirkpatrick SI, Boushey C, Neuhouser ML, Thompson FE, Potischman N, Guenther PM, Tarasuk V, et al. Addressing current criticism regarding the value of self-report dietary data. J Nutr. 2015;145(12):2639–45.

17

Prognostic value of inflammation-based prognostic scores on outcome in patients undergoing continuous ambulatory peritoneal dialysis

Lu Cai[1,2†], Jianwen Yu[1,2†], Jing Yu[1,2], Yuan Peng[1,2], Habib Ullah[1,2], Chunyan Yi[1,2], Jianxiong Lin[1,2], Xiao Yang[1,2] and Xueqing Yu[1,2,3*] (iD)

Abstract

Background: Inflammation-based prognostic scores have been used as outcome predictors in patients with cancer or on hemodialysis. However, their role in patients on continuous ambulatory peritoneal dialysis (CAPD) remains unclear. This study aimed to examine the prognostic value of inflammation-based composite scores for mortality in CAPD patients.

Methods: This study was conducted in CAPD patients enrolled from January 1, 2006 to December 31, 2014 and followed until December 31, 2016. Three inflammation-based prognostic scores, including Glasgow prognostic score (GPS), prognostic nutritional index (PNI), and prognostic index (PI), were conducted in this study. The associations between these scores and all-cause or cardiovascular mortality were evaluated by Kaplan–Meier method and Cox proportional hazards models. The areas under the curve (AUC) of receiver-operating characteristic (ROC) analysis were used to determine the predictive values of mortality.

Results: A total of 1501 patients were included. During a median follow-up of 38.7 (range, 21.6–62.3) months, 346 (23. 1%) patients died, of which 168 (48.6%) were due to cardiovascular diseases (CVD). After adjustment for confounders, the results showed that elevated GPS, PNI, and PI scores were all independently associated with all-cause [GPS: Score 1: hazard ratio(HR) 3.94, 95% confidence interval(CI) 2.90–5.35; Score 2: HR 7.56, 95% CI 5.35–10.67; PNI: HR 1.82, 95% CI 1. 36–2.43; PI: Score 1: HR 2.08, 95% CI 1.63–2.65; Score 2: HR 3.03, 95% CI 2.00–4.60)] and CVD mortality(GPS: Score 1: HR 4.41, 95% CI 2.76–7.03; Score 2: HR 9.64, 95% CI 5.72–16.26; PNI: HR 1.63, 95% CI 1.06–2.51; PI: Score 1: HR 2.57, 95% CI 1. 81–3.66, Score 2: HR 3.85, 95% CI 1.99–7.46).The AUC values of GPS score were 0.798 (95% CI0.770–0.826) for all-cause mortality and 0.781 (95% CI 0.744–0.817) for CVD mortality, both of which significantly higher than those of PNI and PI scores ($P < 0.001$, respectively).

Conclusions: All elevated GPS, PNI, and PI scores were independently associated with all-cause and CVD mortality. The GPS score showed better predictive value than PNI and PI scores in CAPD patients.

Keywords: Inflammation-based prognostic scores, Continuous ambulatory peritoneal dialysis, All-cause mortality, Cardiovascular mortality

* Correspondence: yuxq@mail.sysu.edu.cn
†Lu Cai and Jianwen Yu contributed equally to this work.
[1]Department of Nephrology, The First Affiliated Hospital of Sun Yat-sen University, Guangzhou 510080, China
[2]Key Laboratory of Nephrology, Ministry of Health and Guangdong Province, Guangzhou, China
Full list of author information is available at the end of the article

Background

Peritoneal dialysis (PD) has been established as a successful treatment modality of renal replacement therapy over decades [1]. However, the mortality of PD patients remains much higher compared to general population, nearly half of which are caused by cardiovascular disease (CVD) [2, 3]. Numerous risk factors have been identified to be associated with CVD [4–7]. Among them, systemic inflammation is well recognized for its close relationship to cardiovascular morbidity and mortality [8]. We and others found that elevated C-reactive protein (CRP) levels, especially its elevated trend over time, could be independently predictive of mortality in PD population [9–11]. Importantly, inflammation drives the development of malnutrition, which may in turn amplify systemic inflammation responses, leading to a vicious cycle [12, 13]. Recently, International Society for Peritoneal Dialysis (ISPD) cardiovascular and metabolic guidelines suggest that PD patients with persistently elevated CRP should be investigated for any treatable cause of inflammation and nutritional status should be assessed within 6–8 weeks after commencement of PD for reducing the risk of CVD mortality [2]. Therefore, comprehensive assessment of inflammatory and nutritional status will help to identify patients at high risk and are crucial in the management of PD cohorts. However, standardized methods or systems available for this purpose remain to be explored.

Inflammation-based prognostic scores have been developed since last decade and successfully used to monitor patients' status and predict outcomes in cancer management [14–20]. The Glasgow prognostic score (GPS), composed of serum CRP and albumin, has been reported as a powerful predictor for mortality in many cancer patients [14–16]. The prognostic nutritional index (PNI), which was originally developed to monitor nutritional status of perioperative patients, can predict long-term outcomes in patients with a variety of malignancy [17–19]. The prognostic index (PI), based on CRP and white blood cell (WBC) count, has also been shown to be associated with survival in advanced lung cancer patients [20]. However, few studies have investigated the association of these composite scores with outcomes in continuous ambulatory peritoneal dialysis (CAPD) patients. Therefore, the purpose of this study was to evaluate the prognostic values of these scores in CAPD patients.

Methods
Study participants

Patients were enrolled from PD center of The First Affiliated Hospital of Sun Yat-sen University from January 1, 2006 to December 31, 2014. Patients who had received CAPD for more than 3 months were included. Patients

who were younger than 18 years old, undergone CAPD for less than 3 months, transferred from hemodialysis (HD), with a history of renal transplantation or malignancy before PD, or without data of serum CRP, albumin, or WBC count, were excluded from this study. The study was approved by the Ethics Committee of The First Affiliated Hospital of Sun Yat-sen University. All participants provided their written informed consent for this study.

Data collection and laboratory measurements

This work was a retrospective cohort study. Baseline demographic and clinical data, including age, gender, a history of smoke, diabetes, hypertension, cardiovascular disease, were collected at the start of CAPD treatment. Diabetes and hypertension were recorded as previously defined [21]. Baseline biochemical parameters were collected 1–3 months after the initiation of PD therapy, including blood pressure (BP), hemoglobin, WBC count, serum CRP, albumin, total triglycerides, total cholesterol, low-density lipoprotein cholesterol (LDL-C), high-density lipoprotein cholesterol (HDL-C), uric acid, and creatinine. Residual renal function, in ml/min/1.73m^2, was estimated from mean values of creatinine clearance and urea clearance and adjusted for body surface area calculated with the Gehan and George equation [6]. All measurements of biochemical parameters were performed in the biochemical laboratory of The First Affiliated Hospital of Sun Yat-sen University. The constituents of three inflammation-based prognostic scores (GPS, PNI and PI) were listed in Table 1.

Table 1 Inflammation-based prognostic scores

Scoring systems	Score
GPS	
CRP ≤ 10 mg/L and ALB ≥ 35 g/L	0
CRP > 10 mg/L or ALB < 35 g/L	1
CRP > 10 mg/L and ALB < 35 g/L	2
PNI	
10 × serum albumin value (g/dl) + 0.005 × peripheral lymphocyte count (/ul) ≥ 45	0
10 × serum albumin value (g/dl) + 0.005 × peripheral lymphocyte count (/ul) < 45	1
PI	
CRP ≤ 10 mg/L and WBC ≤ 11 × 10^9/L	0
CRP ≤10 mg/L and WBC > 11 × 10^9/L	1
CRP > 10 mg/L and WBC ≤ 11 × 10^9/L	1
CRP > 10 mg/L and WBC > 11 × 10^9/L	2

Abbreviations: GPS Glasgow Prognostic Score, CRP C-reactive protein, ALB albumin, PNI prognostic nutritional index, PI prognostic index, WBC white blood cell

Table 2 Baseline characteristics of 1501 CAPD patients

Characteristics	Values
Age (years)	46.4 ± 15.1
Gender (Male)	887 (59.1%)
Smoke	253 (16.9%)
Body mass index (kg/m^2)	21.5 ± 3.7
Systolic BP (mmHg)	136.2 ± 20.6
Diastolic BP (mmHg)	84.9 ± 14.4
Hypertension	605 (40.3%)
Diabetes mellitus	326 (21.7%)
Cardiovascular disease	249 (16.6%)
Serum albumin (g/L)	36.4 ± 5.0
Calcium (mmol/L)	2.2 ± 0.3
Phosphorus (mmol/L)	1.7 ± 0.6
iPTH (pg/mL)	289.0 (144.4–455.5)
CRP (mg/L)	1.6 (0.8–5.5)
WBC (× 10^9/L)	6.9 ± 2.4
Lymphocyte (× 10^9//L)	1.4 ± 0.6
Hemoglobin (g/L)	89.8 ± 22.8
Total cholesterol (mmol/L)	5.1 ± 1.4
Total triglycerides (mmol/L)	1.6 ± 1.1
HDL-C (mmol/L)	1.2 ± 0.4
LDL-C (mmol/L)	3.0 ± 1.1
Plasma uric acid (µmol/L)	430.3 ± 101.0
Plasma creatinine (µmol/L)	766.7 ± 277.5
RRF (ml/min/1.73m^2)	3.7 ± 3.0

Abbreviations: *CAPD* continuous ambulatory peritoneal dialysis, *BP* blood pressure, *iPTH* intact parathyroid hormone, *CRP* C-reactive protein, *WBC* white blood cell, *HDL-C* high-density lipoprotein cholesterol, *LDL-C* low-density lipoprotein cholesterol, *RRF* residual renal function

Outcomes

The primary endpoint of this study was all-cause mortality, and the second endpoint was CVD mortality. CVD mortality was defined as death caused by events including acute myocardial infarction, cardiac arrhythmia, congestive heart failure, atherosclerotic heart disease, cardiomyopathy, cardiac arrest, intracranial hemorrhage, cerebral infarction and peripheral vascular disease [22]. All participants were followed up until death, cessation of PD, or December 31, 2016.

Statistical analysis

The data were presented as mean ± standard deviation for normally distributed continuous variables, median (interquartile range) for skewed continuous variables, and number (proportion) for categorical variables. The Kaplan-Meier curve was used to calculate survival rate followed by log-rank test to compare differences among groups. Univariate and multivariate Cox proportional hazards models were used to analyze the associations between prognostic scores and all-cause and CVD mortality. The multivariate Cox regression model was constructed by adjusting covariates using a backward stepwise selection procedure with a stay criterion of 0.10 (the selection cut-off value was from default in SPSS software system as well as the importance of clinical concern). Receiver-operating characteristic (ROC) analysis was performed and the area under the curve (AUC) was calculated to determine the predictive power of prognostic scores for mortality. Comparison of AUC values among groups was determined using MedCalc software version 15.0 (Broekstraat, Mariakerke, Belgium) [23]. All other statistical analyses were performed using SPSS version 22.0 for Windows (SPSS, Chicago, IL, USA). $P < 0.05$ was considered statistically significant using two-tailed tests.

Table 3 Distribution of inflammation-based prognostic scores among groups

Prognostic score	All patients ($n = 1501$)	Survival patients ($n = 1155$)	All-cause mortality ($n = 346$)	CVD mortality ($n = 168$)
GPS				
0	909 (60.6%)	845 (73.2%)	64 (18.5%)	26 (15.5%)
1	456 (30.4%)	272 (23.5%)	184 (53.2%)	89 (53.0%)
2	136 (9.1%)	38 (3.3%)	98 (28.3%)	53 (31.5%)
PNI				
0	604 (40.2%)	537 (46.5%)	67 (19.4%)	29 (17.3%)
1	897 (59.8%)	618 (53.5%)	279 (80.6%)	139 (82.7%)
PI				
0	1213 (80.8%)	1016 (88.0%)	197 (56.9%)	89 (53.0%)
1	253 (16.9%)	130 (11.3%)	123 (35.6%)	68 (40.5%)
2	35 (2.3%)	9 (0.8%)	26 (7.5%)	11 (6.5%)

Abbreviations: *GPS* Glasgow Prognostic Score, *PNI* prognostic nutritional index, *PI* prognostic index, *CVD* cardiovascular disease

Table 4 Comparison of inflammation-based prognostic scores between diabetic and non-diabetic patients

Prognostic score	All patients (n = 1501)	Diabetic patients (n = 326)	Non-diabetic Patients (n = 1175)	P value
GPS				
0	909 (60.6%)	104 (31.9%)	805 (68.5%)	< 0.001
1	456 (30.4%)	175 (53.7%)	281 (23.9%)	
2	136 (9.1%)	47 (14.4%)	89 (7.6%)	
PNI				
0	604 (40.2%)	75 (23.0%)	529 (45.0%)	< 0.001
1	897 (59.8%)	251 (71.0%)	646 (55.0%)	
PI				
0	1213 (80.8%)	233 (71.5%)	980 (83.4%)	< 0.001
1	253 (16.9%)	79 (24.2%)	174 (14.8%)	
2	35 (2.3%)	14 (4.3%)	21 (1.8%)	

Abbreviations: *GPS* Glasgow Prognostic Score, *PNI* prognostic nutritional index, *PI* prognostic index, *CVD* cardiovascular disease

Results

Baseline demographic and clinical characteristics

Baseline demographic and clinical characteristics of the cohort study are given in Table 2. A total of 1501 eligible CAPD patients were included in this study. The mean age was 46.4 ± 15.1 years, 59.1% were male, 21.7% had a history of diabetes mellitus. The leading cause of ESRD was primary glomerulonephritis (928, 61.8%), followed by diabetic nephropathy (292, 19.5%), hypertension (135, 9.0%) and others (146, 9.7%). The median vintage of PD was 38.7 (range, 21.6–62.3) months.

During the follow-up period, 318 (21.2%) patients underwent renal transplantation, 185 (12.3%) were transferred to HD, 59 (3.9%) were transferred to other centers, 36 (2.4%) were lost to follow-up, and finally, 903 (60.2%) were followed up until the end of the study.

Inflammation-based prognostic scores

According to the GPS scoring system, 909 (60.6%) of the 1501 patients showed a score of 0, while 456 (30.4%) and 136 (9.1%) patients had a score of 1 and 2, respectively. PNI classification revealed that 897 (59.8%) patients had a

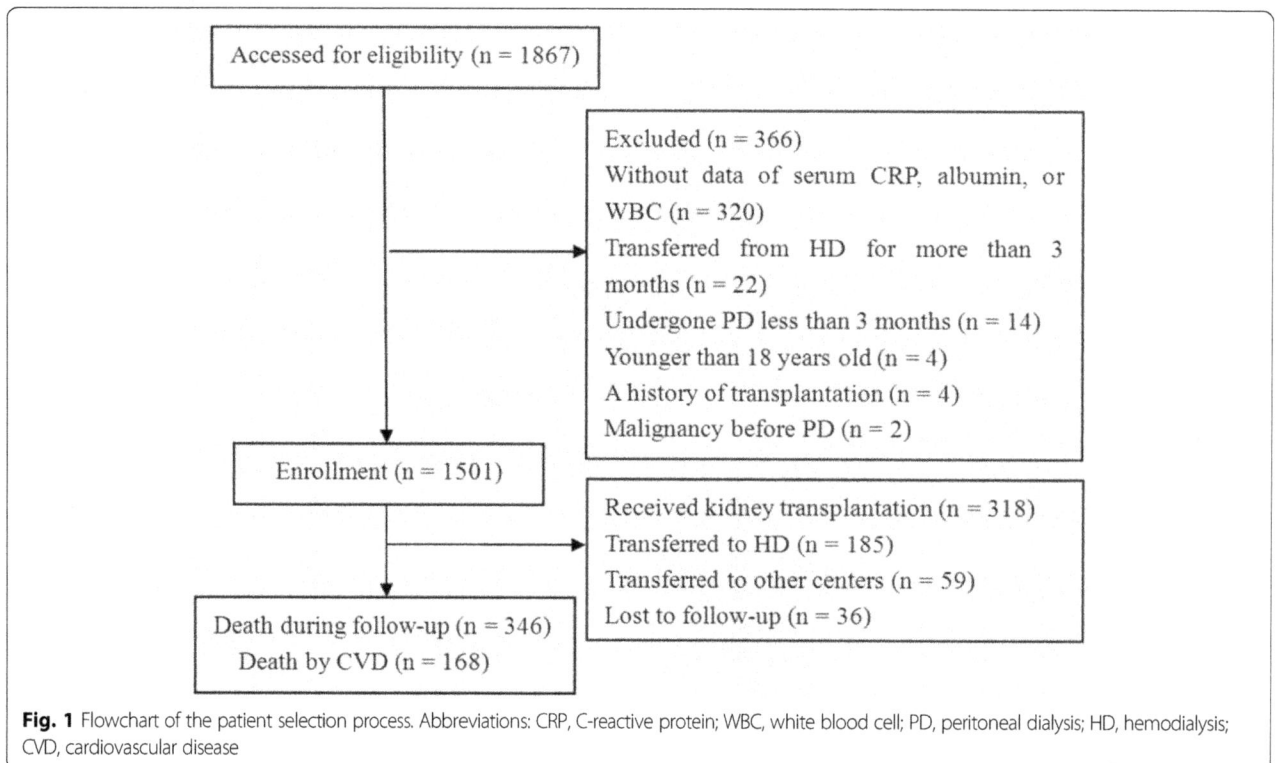

Fig. 1 Flowchart of the patient selection process. Abbreviations: CRP, C-reactive protein; WBC, white blood cell; PD, peritoneal dialysis; HD, hemodialysis; CVD, cardiovascular disease

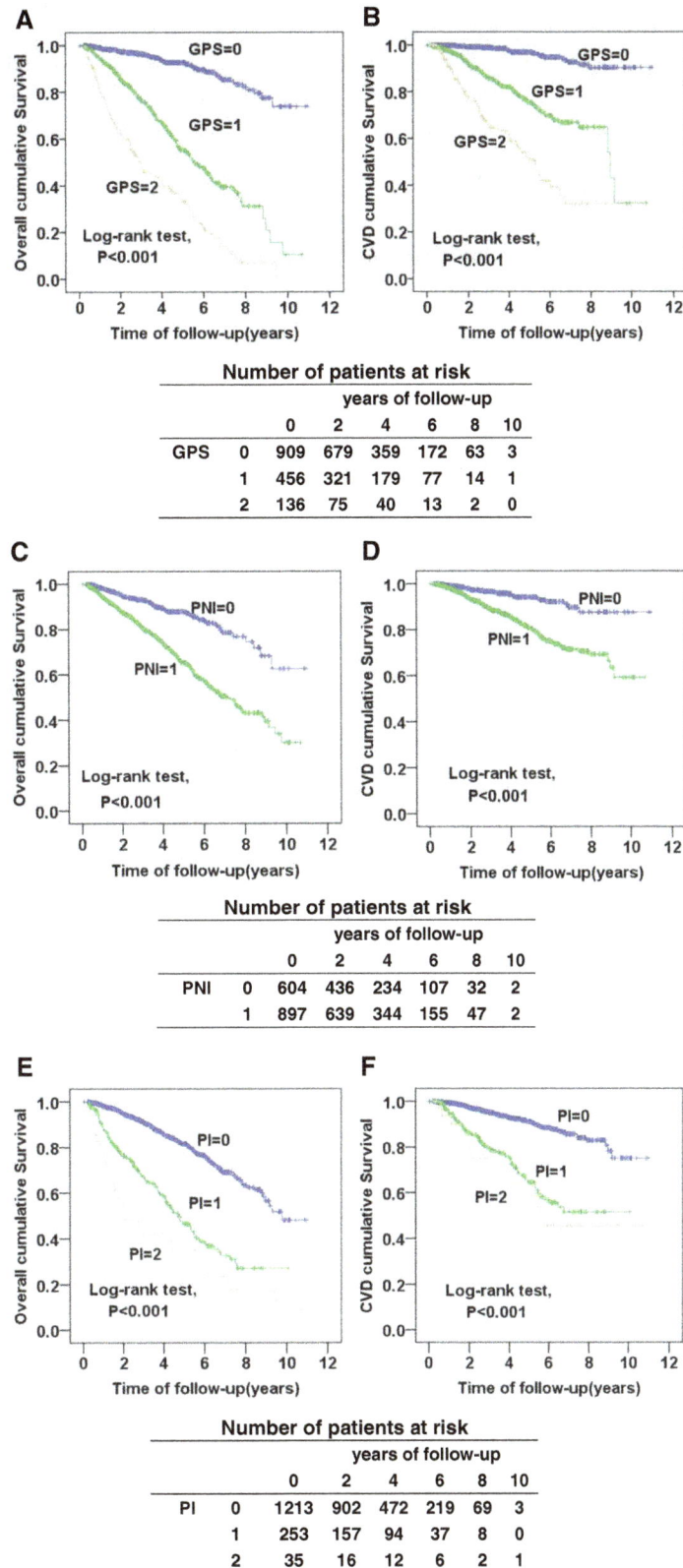

Fig. 2 Kaplan–Meier estimates of cumulative overall (**a**, **c**, **e**) and CVD-free (**b**, **d**, **f**) survival rate according to different prognostic scores. Abbreviations: CVD, cardiovascular disease; GPS, Glasgow Prognostic Score; PNI, prognostic nutritional index; PI, prognostic index

score of 1. With regard to PI, there were 253 (16.9%) and 35 (2.3%) patients who displayed a score of 1 and 2, respectively. In mortality population, larger proportions of patients were categorized into higher score groups (Table 3). Compared with non-diabetic patients, diabetic patients presented with higher scores (Table 4).

Patient survival

A total of 346 deaths (23.1%) occurred, of which 168 (48.6%) were attributed to CVD (Fig. 1). Kaplan-Meier analyses indicated that the cumulative overall survival rates of patients with a GPS score of 0, 1, 2, were 93.0%, 59.6%, 27.9%, respectively (log-rank test, $P < 0.001$); the CVD survival rates were also significantly lower in patients with higher scores (score 1: 80.5%; score 2: 61.0%) than those with a score of 0 (97.1%) (log-rank test, $P < 0.001$). Elevated PNI and PI scores were also shown to be associated with reduced all-cause and CVD survival rates (Fig. 2).

Univariate cox hazards analysis revealed that increased GPS, PNI and PI scores were all significantly related to

Table 5 Univariate cox proportional analysis for all-cause and CVD mortality

	Univariate (All-cause mortality)		Univariate (CVD mortality)	
	HR (95%CI)	P value	HR (95%CI)	P value
Age	1.06 (1.05–1.07)	< 0.001	1.07 (1.06–1.08)	< 0.001
Gender (Male)	0.92 (0.74–1.13)	0.429	0.96 (0.71–1.30)	0.790
Smoke	1.16 (0.88–1.52)	0.300	1.18 (0.80–1.73)	0.401
Body mass index(kg/m^2)	1.06 (1.03–1.09)	< 0.001	1.07 (1.03–1.12)	0.002
Systolic BP (mmHg)	1.01 (1.00–1.01)	0.013	1.01 (1.00–1.02)	0.003
Diastolic BP (mmHg)	0.98 (0.97–0.98)	< 0.001	0.98 (0.97–0.99)	< 0.001
Hypertension	2.86 (2.29–3.56)	< 0.001	3.92 (2.81–5.48)	< 0.001
Diabetes mellitus	3.35 (2.71–4.14)	< 0.001	4.45 (3.29–6.03)	< 0.001
Cardiovascular disease	3.54 (2.84–4.43)	< 0.001	4.96 (3.65–6.73)	< 0.001
Infection	3.46 (2.43–4.94)	< 0.001	2.64 (1.50–4.66)	0.001
Residual renal function	0.97 (0.92–1.01)	0.12	0.94 (0.88–1.01)	0.09
Calcium (mmol/L)	0.31 (0.21–0.45)	< 0.001	0.28 (0.16–0.49)	< 0.001
Phosphorus (mmol/L)	1.01 (0.85–1.20)	0.902	0.94 (0.73–1.20)	0.610
iPTH (pg/mL)	1.00 (1.00–1.00)	0.229	1.00 (1.00–1.00)	0.626
Hemoglobin (g/L)	0.99 (0.99–1.00)	0.001	0.99 (0.98–0.99)	< 0.001
Total cholesterol (mmol/L)	1.04 (0.97–1.13)	0.257	1.12 (1.02–1.23)	0.022
Total triglycerides (mmol/L)	1.12 (1.03–1.21)	0.008	1.16 (1.04–1.29)	0.007
HDL-C (mmol/L)	0.58 (0.44–0.77)	< 0.001	0.62 (0.42–0.93)	0.021
LDL-C (mmol/L)	1.05 (0.95–1.16)	0.341	1.12 (0.99–1.28)	0.070
Serum uric acid (μmol/L)	1.00 (1.00–1.00)	0.069	1.00 (1.00–1.00)	0.007
Serum creatinine (μmol/L)	1.00 (1.00–1.00)	< 0.001	1.00 (1.00–1.00)	< 0.001
GPS				
0	reference		Reference	
1	6.37 (4.79–8.48)	< 0.001	7.46 (4.81–11.56)	< 0.001
2	14.66 (10.68–20.13)	< 0.001	19.09 (11.91–30.57)	< 0.001
PNI				
0	reference		Reference	
1	2.84 (2.17–3.70)	< 0.001	3.27 (2.19–4.88)	< 0.001
PI				
0	reference		Reference	
1	3.48 (2.78–4.37)	< 0.001	4.26 (3.10–5.85)	< 0.001
2	5.29 (3.51–7.98)	< 0.001	5.08 (2.71–9.53)	< 0.001

Abbreviations: *HR* hazard ratio, *CI* confidence interval, *CAPD* continuous ambulatory peritoneal dialysis, *BP* blood pressure, *iPTH* intact parathyroid hormone, *CRP* C-reactive protein, *WBC* white blood cell, *HDL-C* high-density lipoprotein cholesterol, *LDL-C* low-density lipoprotein cholesterol, *RRF* residual renal function, *GPS* Glasgow Prognostic Score, *PNI* prognostic nutritional index, *PI* prognostic index, *CVD* cardiovascular disease

all-cause and CVD mortality (Table 5). After adjusting for covariates including age, BP, diabetes, hypertension, cardiovascular disease, infection, hemoglobin, total triglycerides, total cholesterol, LDL-C, HDL-C, uric acid, and creatinine, the patients with increased GPS scores still had a significant increased risk for overall [Score 1: hazard ratio(HR) 3.94, 95% confidence interval(CI) 2.90–5.35, $P < 0.001$; Score 2: HR 7.56, 95% CI 5.35–10.67, $P < 0.001$] and CVD mortality (Score 1: HR 4.41, 95% CI 2.76–7.03, $P < 0.001$; Score 2: HR 9.64, 95% CI 5.72–16.26, $P < 0.001$). Increased PNI and PI values were also independently predictive of all-cause and CVD mortality (Table 6).

Comparison of prognostic values of inflammation-based scores

When all-cause mortality was used as an endpoint, the area under the curve (AUC) was 0.798 (95% CI 0.770–0.826, $P < 0.001$) for GPS, 0.636 (95% CI 0.604–0.667, $P < 0.001$) for PNI, 0.658 (95% CI 0.622–0.694, $P < 0.001$) for PI. The AUC values for CVD mortality were 0.781 (95% CI 0.744–0.817, $P < 0.001$) for GPS, 0.629 (95% CI 0.589–0.670, $P < 0.001$) for PNI and 0.658 (95% CI 0.609–0.706, $P < 0.001$) for PI. By comparison of AUC values among groups, the GPS score showed a better distinguishing power for predicting all-cause and CVD mortality compared with PNI and PI ($P < 0.001$, respectively) (Fig. 3 & Table 7).

Discussion

In this retrospective cohort study of 1501 CAPD patients with a median follow-up of 38.7 months, we demonstrated

Table 6 Multivariate cox proportional analysis for all-cause and CVD mortality

	Multivariate (All-cause mortality)		Multivariate (CVD mortality)	
	HR (95%CI)	P value	HR (95%CI)	P value
GPS				
0	reference		Reference	
1	3.94 (2.90–5.35)	< 0.001	4.41 (2.76–7.03)	< 0.001
2	7.56 (5.35–10.67)	< 0.001	9.64 (5.72–16.26)	< 0.001
PNI				
0	Reference		reference	
1	1.82 (1.36–2.43)	< 0.001	1.63 (1.06–2.51)	0.027
PI				
0	reference		reference	
1	2.08 (1.63–2.65)	< 0.001	2.57 (1.81–3.66)	< 0.001
2	3.03 (2.00–4.60)	< 0.001	3.85 (1.99–7.46)	< 0.001

Adjustments were made for variables from the predictor variables of Table 5 using a backward stepwise cox proportional hazards model with a stay criterion of 0.10

Abbreviations: *GPS* Glasgow Prognostic Score, *PNI* prognostic nutritional index, *PI* prognostic index, *CVD* cardiovascular disease

that increased GPS, PNI, and PI scores were all significantly related to all-cause and CVD mortality after adjustment for confounders. ROC analysis indicated that GPS had the best predictive value among these three scores system for CAPD patients.

Inflammation is prevalent in PD patients [8]. Besides acute episodes of peritonitis, micro-inflammation also constitutes an important component of systemic inflammation responses [8, 9, 12]. Micro-inflammation in PD patients may be attributed to accumulation of uremic toxins, catheter implantation, bioincompatible dialysis solution, and so on [8]. Infections in the occult areas may also play a role, such as periodontal problems [24]. Systemic inflammation status is closely related to malnutrition and atherosclerosis. These three factors interrelate with each other and form a vicious cycle, eventually leading to increased cardiovascular morbidity and mortality [9, 12, 13]. In our study, although a minor population (62/1501) had active infection during data collection period, most patients did not present obvious signs of infection. The median level of CRP of the whole cohort was in the normal range, which may support the importance of micro-inflammation.

GPS, comprising CRP and serum albumin, is a concise prognostic score that may reflect presence of both the systemic inflammatory response and deteriorating nutritional status. Inamoto et al. found the GPS was an independent prognostic factor for cancer-specific survival and overall survival after surgery with curative intent for localized upper tract urothelial carcinoma [10]. A study based on regular HD patients showed that elevated GPS was independently predictive of all-cause mortality and hospitalization during 42-month follow-up [25]. Consistent to these reports, our results showed that raised GPS values consistently related to both overall and CVD mortality in CAPD patients. The strong power for outcome prediction of this score may be attributed to the combined effects of its components. Both markers, CRP and serum albumin, have been demonstrated to be strongly associated with all-cause and CVD mortality in patients on PD [9–11, 26, 27]. However, ROC analysis revealed that GPS had the higher value than hypoalbuminemia or increased CRP alone (data not shown), which may indicate a reciprocal interaction between these two factors.

The PNI score, which is based on serum albumin and total lymphocyte count, has been developed mainly to assess the nutritional status of patients [17–19]. In this study we found that elevated PNI score was independently associated with increased risk for overall and CVD mortality in CAPD patients. To our knowledge, another 2 studies have explored the predictive effect of PNI in PD cohorts [28, 29]. One study was limited to Korean subjects and showed that the PNI score was significantly related to all-cause mortality in PD patients, which is in agreement with our result [28]. The other

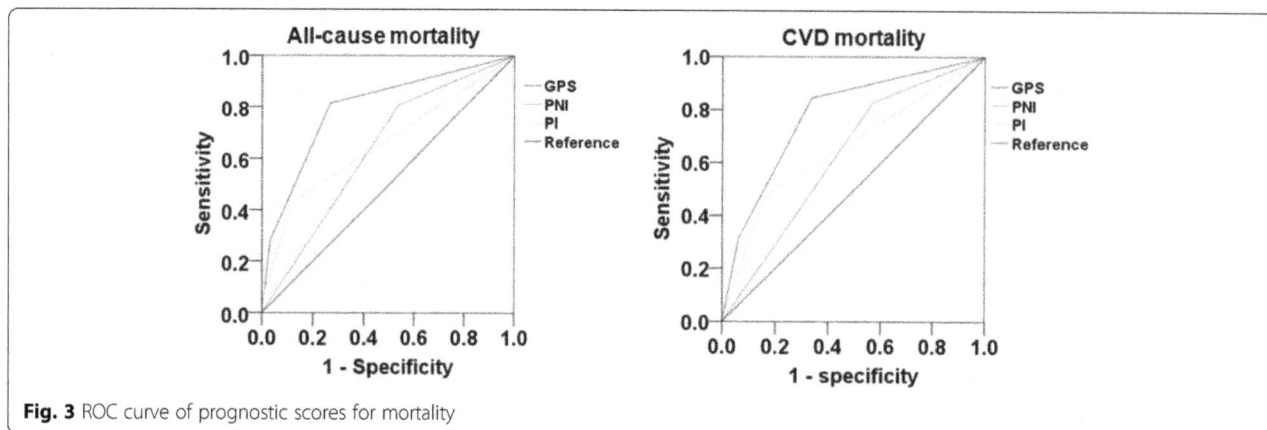

Fig. 3 ROC curve of prognostic scores for mortality

study reported that PNI was associated with increased risk for CVD mortality but not all-cause mortality in 345 Chinese PD patients, which is partly conflicting with our findings [29]. The discrepancy may be due to differences in sample size, definition of PNI thresholds, or confounders chosen for adjustment. The PI score is composed of CRP and WBC count and has been validated as a useful predictive factor in lung and colon cancer [20, 30]. It is also suggested that PI was related to all-cause mortality in patients on regular HD [24]. Our study added new evidence that elevated PI scores were also independently predictive of overall and CVD mortality in a large population of CAPD patients.

The prognostic values of these prognostic scores in CAPD patients were compared in our study. Results indicated that the GPS consistently exhibited a higher AUC value compared with PNI and PI scores and showed an excellent discriminatory performance for the CAPD patients. These findings were consistent with Akihiko's report [24], in which the GPS score had the best predictive power for prognosis

Table 7 Area under the ROC curve of prognostic scores for all-cause and CVD mortality

Prognostic score	Area under the ROC curve	95% CI	P value (vs. GPS)
All-cause mortality			
GPS	0.798	0.770–0.826	
PNI	0.636	0.604–0.667	< 0.001
PI	0.658	0.622–0.694	< 0.001
CVD mortality			
GPS	0.781	0.744–0.817	
PNI	0.629	0.589–0.670	< 0.001
PI	0.658	0.609–0.706	< 0.001

Abbreviations: *ROC* receiver-operating characteristic analysis, *HR* hazard ratio, *CI* confidence interval, *CAPD* continuous ambulatory peritoneal dialysis, *BP* blood pressure, *iPTH* intact parathyroid hormone, *CRP* C-reactive protein, *WBC* white blood cell, *HDL-C* high-density lipoprotein cholesterol, *LDL-C* low-density lipoprotein cholesterol, *RRF* residual renal function, *GPS* Glasgow Prognostic Score, *PNI* prognostic nutritional index, *PI* prognostic index, *CVD* cardiovascular disease

of HD patients. The GPS score was a combination of suitable markers for inflammation and malnutrition, while the other two were inclined to isolated aspects. These comparisons thus imply that a comprehensive monitor of both inflammatory and nutritional status may help better improve outcomes in dialysis patients. In addition, these inflammation-based prognostic scores consist of components which are routinely available with low cost.

There are some limitations in the present study. Firstly, this was a retrospective study conducted in one single center and may thus have potential selection bias. Secondly, a large number of patients without certain blood test results were excluded, making those enrolled may not be well representative for the PD population. Thirdly, we calculated the values of these scoring systems at baseline, while a time-averaged score may be better for outcome prediction. Last but not the least, a minor population of patients with active infection were included in our cohort. Although our results showed the existence of infection did not affect the prognostic significance of scoring systems, we could not exclude the possibility of other confounding effects that deranged CRP or albumin levels during infection may produce.

Conclusions

In conclusion, the present study demonstrated that three well-standardized prognostic scores, GPS, PNI, and PI, are all independently associated with all-cause and CVD mortality in CAPD patients. In particularly, the GPS score shows the better predictive power for mortality compared to the other two scores. The GPS score may thus represent a simple and feasible tool for outcome prediction in CAPD patients.

Abbreviations
AUC: The area under the curve; BP: Blood pressure; CAPD: Continuous ambulatory peritoneal dialysis; CI: Confidence interval; CRP: C-reactive protein; CVD: Cardiovascular disease; GPS: Glasgow Prognostic Score; HD: Hemodialysis; HDL-C: high-density lipoprotein cholesterol; HR: Hazard

ratio; LDL-C: Low-density lipoprotein cholesterol; PD: Peritoneal dialysis; PI: Prognostic index; PNI: Prognostic nutritional index; ROC: Receiver-operating characteristic analysis; WBC: White blood cell

Acknowledgments
We are grateful to all nephrologists and nurses in our PD center for their helpful assistance.

Funding
This work was supported by National Key Research and Development Program (Grant no. 2016YFC0906101), the National Natural Science Foundation of China (Grant no. 81600592, 81774069, 81570614), the Guangdong Science Foundation of China (Grant no. 2014A030313139, 2017A050503003, 2017B020227006), Foundation of Guangdong Key Laboratory of Nephrology (Grant no. 2014B030301023), the Guangdong Committee of Science and Technology (Grant no. 2014B020212020,2017A050503003,2017B020227006) and Guangzhou Municipal Program of Science and Technology (Grant no. 2014Y2–00543, 201704020167).

Authors' contributions
LC and JWY contributed equally to the study. They proposed the design of work, did the data collection and analysis, drafted and revised the manuscript. JY, YP, CYY and JXL contributed substantially to data collection and analysis. HU and XY provided efforts in data analysis and revision of the manuscript. XQY conceived and designed the study, wrote the manuscript and provided final supervision. All authors proofread the manuscript critically and approved the final version of the manuscript to be published.

Competing interests
The authors declare that they have no competing interests.

Author details
[1]Department of Nephrology, The First Affiliated Hospital of Sun Yat-sen University, Guangzhou 510080, China. [2]Key Laboratory of Nephrology, Ministry of Health and Guangdong Province, Guangzhou, China. [3]Institute of Nephrology, Guangdong Medical University, Zhanjiang, China.

References
1. Yu X, Yang X. Peritoneal dialysis in China: meeting the challenge of chronic kidney failure. Am J Kidney Dis. 2015;65(1):147–51.
2. Wang AY, Brimble KS, Brunier G, Holt SG, Jha V, Johnson DW, et al. ISPD cardiovascular and metabolic guidelines in adult peritoneal dialysis patients part II - management of various cardiovascular complications. Perit Dial Int. 2015;35(4):388–96.
3. Collins AJ, Foley RN, Chavers B, Gilbertson D, Herzog C, Ishani A, et al. US renal data system 2013 annual data report. Am J Kidney Dis. 2014;63:A7.
4. Kendrick J, Chonchol MB. Nontraditional risk factors for cardiovascular disease in patients with chronic kidney disease. Nat Clin Pract Nephol. 2008;4(12):672–81.
5. Xia X, He F, Wu X, Peng F, Huang F, Yu X. Relationship between serum uric acid and all-cause and cardiovascular mortality in patients treated with peritoneal Dialysis. Am J Kidney Dis. 2014;64(2):257–64.
6. Xia X, Zhao C, Peng FF, Luo QM, Zhou Q, Lin ZC, et al. Serum uric acid predicts cardiovascular mortality in male peritoneal dialysis patients with diabetes. Nutr Metab Cardiovasc Dis. 2016;26(1):20–6.
7. Peng F, Li Z, Yi C, Guo Q, Yang R, Long H, et al. Platelet index levels and cardiovascular mortality in incident peritoneal dialysis patients: a cohort study. Platelets. 2017;28(6):576–84.
8. Li PK, Ng JK, Mcintyre CW. Inflammation and peritoneal Dialysis. Semin Nephrol. 2017;37(1):54–65.
9. Ducloux D, Bresson-Vautrin C, Kribs M, Abdelfatah A, Chalopin JM. C-reactive protein and cardiovascular disease in peritoneal dialysis patients. Kidney Int. 2002;62(4):1417–22.
10. Wang AY, Woo J, Lam CW, Wang M, Sea MM, Lui SF, et al. Is a single time point C-reactive protein predictive of outcome in peritoneal dialysis patients? J Am Soc Nephrol. 2003;14(7):1871–9.
11. Li W, Xiong L, Fan L, Wang Y, Peng X, Rong R, et al. Association of baseline, longitudinal serum high-sensitive C-reactive protein and its change with mortality in peritoneal dialysis patients. BMC Nephrol. 2017;18(1):211.
12. He T, An X, Mao H, Wei X, Chen J, Guo N, et al. Malnutrition-inflammation score predicts long-term mortality in Chinese PD patients. Clin Nephrol. 2013;79(6):477–83.
13. Shahab I, Nolph KD. MIA syndrome in peritoneal dialysis: prevention and treatment. Contrib Nephrol. 2006;150:135–43.
14. Inamoto T, Matsuyama H, Sakano S, Ibuki N, Takahara K, Komura K, et al. The systemic inflammation-based Glasgow prognostic score as a powerful prognostic factor in patients with upper tract urothelial carcinoma. Ont Dent. 2017;8(68):113248–57.
15. Okimoto S, Kobayashi T, Tashiro H, Kuroda S, Ishiyama K, Ide K, et al. Significance of the Glasgow prognostic score for patients with colorectal liver metastasis. Int J Surg. 2017;42:209–14.
16. McMillan DC. The systematic inflammation-based Glasgow prognostic score: a decade of experience in patients with cancer. Cancer Treat Rev. 2013; 39(5):534–40.
17. Kanda M, Fujii T, Kodera Y, Nagai S, Takeda S, Nakao A. Nutritional predictors of postoperative outcome in pancreatic cancer. Br J Surg. 2011;98(7):268–74.
18. Sakurai K, Tamura T, Toyokawa T, Amano R, Kubo N, Tanaka H, et al. Low preoperative prognostic nutritional index predicts poor survival post-gastrectomy in elderly patients with gastric cancer. Ann Surg Oncol. 2016; 23(11):3669–76.
19. Mohri T, Mohri Y, Shigemori T, Takeuchi K, Itoh Y, Kato T. Impact of prognostic nutritional index on long-term out-comes in patients with breast cancer. World J Surg Oncol. 2016;14(1):170.
20. Kasymjanova G, MacDonald N, Agulnik JS, Cohen V, Pepe C, Kreisman H, et al. The predictive value of pre-treatment inflammatory markers in advanced non-small-cell lung cancer. Curr Oncol. 2010;17(14):52–8.
21. He F, Wu X, Xia X, Peng F, Huang F, Yu X. Pneumonia and mortality risk in continuous ambulatory peritoneal dialysis patients with diabetic nephropathy. PLoS One. 2013;8(4):e61497.
22. Peng F, Li Z, Zhong Z, Luo Q, Guo Q, Huang F, et al. An increasing of red blood cell distribution width was associated with cardiovascular mortality in patients on peritoneal dialysis. Int J Cardiol. 2014;176(3):1379–81.
23. Gao Y, Liu JJ, Zhu SY, Yi X. The diagnostic accuracy of ultrasonography versus endoscopy for primary nasopharyngeal carcinoma. PLoS One. 2014;9(6):e99679.
24. Kocyigit I, Yucel HE, Cakmak O, Dogruel F, Durukan DB, et al. An ignored cause of inflammation in patients undergoing continuous ambulatory peritoneal dialysis: periodontal problems. Int Urol Nephrol. 2014;46(10):2021–8.
25. Kato A, Tsuji T, Sakao Y, Ohashi N, Yasuda H, Fujimoto T, et al. Comparison of Systemic Inflammation-Based Prognostic Scores in Patients on Regular Hemodialysis. Nephron Extra. 2013;3(1):91–100.
26. Jones CH, Newstead CG, Wills EJ, Davison AM. Serum albumin and survival in CAPD patients: the implications of concentration trends over time. Nephrol Dial Transplant. 1997;12(3):554–8.
27. Kang SH, Cho KH, Park JW, Yoon KW, Do JY. Risk factors for mortality in stable peritoneal dialysis patients. Ren Fail. 2012;34(2):149–54.
28. Kang SH, Cho KH, Park JW, Yoon KW, Do JY. Onodera's prognostic nutritional index as a risk factor for mortality in peritoneal Dialysis patients. J Korean Med Sci. 2012;27(11):1354–8.
29. Peng F, Chen W, Zhou W, Li P, Niu H, Chen Y, et al. Low prognostic nutritional index associated with cardiovascular disease mortality in incident peritoneal dialysis patients. Int Urol Nephrol. 2017;49(6):1095–101.
30. Petersen VC, Baxter KJ, Love SB, Shepherd NA. Identification of objective pathological prognostic determinants and models of prognosis in Dukes' B colon cancer. Gut. 2002;51(1):65–9.

18

Trends in anemia care in non-dialysis-dependent chronic kidney disease (CKD) patients in the United States (2006–2015)

Haesuk Park[1]* (iD), Xinyue Liu[1], Linda Henry[1], Jeffrey Harman[2] and Edward A. Ross[3]

Abstract

Background: The objective of the study was to examine overall anemia management trends in non-dialysis patients with chronic kidney disease (CKD) from 2006 to 2015, and to evaluate the impact of Trial to Reduced Cardiovascular Events with Ananesp Therapy (TREAT)'s study results (October 2009) and the US Food and Drug Administration (FDA)'s (June 2011) safety warnings and guidelines on the use of ESA therapy in the current treatment of anemia.

Methods: A retrospective cohort analysis of anemia management in CKD patients using Truven MarketScan Commercial and Medicare Supplemental databases was conducted. Monthly rates and types of anemia treatment for post-TREAT and post-FDA safety warning periods were compared to pre-TREAT period. Anemia management included ESA, intravenous iron, and blood transfusion. A time-series analysis using Autoregressive Integrated Moving Average (ARIMA) model and a Generalized Estimating Equation (GEE) model were used.

Results: Between 2006 and 2015, CKD patients were increasingly less likely to be treated with ESAs, more likely to receive intravenous iron supplementation, and blood transfusions. The adjusted probabilities of prescribing ESAs were 31% (odds ratio (OR) = 0.69, 95% confidence interval (CI): 0.67–0.71) and 59% (OR = 0.41, 95% CI: 0.40, 0.42) lower in the post-TREAT and post-FDA warning periods compared to pre-TREAT period. The probability of prescribing intravenous iron was increased in the post-FDA warning period (OR = 1.11, 95% CI: 1.03–1.19) although the increase was not statistically significant in the post-TREAT period (OR = 1.03, 95% CI: 0.94–1.12). The probabilities of prescribing blood transfusion during the post-TREAT and post-FDA warning periods increased by 14% (OR = 1.14, 95% CI: 1.06–1.23) and 31% (OR = 1.31, 95% CI: 1.22–1.39), respectively. Similar trends of prescribing ESAs and iron supplementations were observed in commercially insured CKD patients but the use of blood transfusions did not increase.

Conclusions: After the 2011 FDA safety warnings, the use of ESA continued to decrease while the use of iron supplementation continued to increase. The use of blood transfusions increased significantly in Medicare patients while it remained stable in commercially insured patients. Results suggest the TREAT publication had effected treatment of anemia prior to the FDA warning but the FDA warning solidified TREAT's recommendations for anemia treatment for non- dialysis dependent CKD patients.

Keywords: Erythropoiesis-stimulating agent (ESA), Chronic kidney disease (CKD), Anemia, FDA safety warnings

* Correspondence: hpark@cop.ufl.edu
[1]Department of Pharmaceutical Outcomes and Policy, University of Florida College of Pharmacy, HPNP Building Room 3325, 1225 Center Drive, Gainesville, FL 32610, USA
Full list of author information is available at the end of the article

Introduction

The Centers for Disease Prevention and Control (CDC) estimate that one in every ten adults in the US are currently living with chronic kidney disease (CKD) with varying levels of severity [1]. Patients with moderate to severe cases of CKD typically develop anemia (National Kidney Foundation definition of anemia: adult males < 13.5 g/dL and adult females < 12.0 g/dL) treated with iron supplements, erythropoiesis stimulating agents (ESAs), and or blood transfusions dependent on patient symptoms [2, 3].

In 1997, the first set of comprehensive guidelines for the treatment of CKD-associated anemia was published by the National Kidney Disease Outcomes Quality Initiative (KDOQI) [4]. In these guidelines, KDOQI endorsed using ESAs to avoid exposure to blood transfusions especially in potential transplant candidates [4]. However, in recent years, several studies raised concerns about the use of ESA's in treating anemia among CKD non-dialysis patients.

Three studies in particular, CHOIR (Correction of Hemoglobin and Outcomes in Renal Insufficiency, 2006) [5], CREATE (Cardiovascular Risk Reduction by Early Anemia Treatment with Epoetin Beta, 2006) [6], and TREAT (Trial to Reduced Cardiovascular Events with Ananesp Therapy, 2009) [7], demonstrated that ESA's failed to reach their stated endpoints of reducing mortality and cardiovascular events in CKD patients [5–7]. In addition, the landmark study, TREAT, reported that treatment with darbepoetin did not reduce mortality or cardiovascular events, but its use resulted in a 2-fold higher stroke rate in CKD patients not undergoing dialysis [7].

Though there were significant design differences between the three studies, the results of all studies suggested that aiming for higher hemoglobin levels with higher doses of ESA agents may be the main contributors to the adverse outcomes of these studies. On the negative side, patients who received placebo agents were exposed significantly more to red blood cell transfusions and its associated risks [8].

Nonetheless, as a result of these studies, regulatory and reimbursement changes occurred which reduced the suggested ESA dose and lowered the target hemoglobin concentrations. Following these study results in June 2011, the US Food and Drug Administration's (FDA) officially changed ESA's labeling to recommended that the ESA should no longer be prescribed to obtain a target hemoglobin concentration range (10 to 12 g/dL), but should only be used for patients whose hemoglobin concentrations were below 10 g/dL, were symptomatic, and to avoid blood transfusions [9], which was followed by Kidney Disease Improving Global Outcomes (KDIGO) clinical practice guideline in 2012 [10].

However, little is known about the trends of anemia treatment in patients with non-dialysis-dependent CKD following the release of TREAT study results and the 2011 FDA guidelines. Therefore, this study sought to (1) examine overall anemia management trends (ESA, intravenous iron, and blood transfusion) in non-dialysis patients with CKD from 2006 to 2015, and (2) to specifically evaluate the impact of TREAT's study results (October 2009) and FDA's (June 2011) safety warnings and guidelines on the use of ESA therapy in the current treatment of anemia.

Methods

Data source

We conducted a retrospective cohort study using the Truven Health Analytic Marketscan Commercial database and the Medicare Supplemental database (January 2005 through September 2015). The Commercial Database contains records on employer-sponsored insurance covering 15–50 million individuals annually. The Medicare Supplemental database contains records on retired employees and their spouses who are enrolled in Medicare with supplemental insurance paid for by their former employers, representing ~ 2.5 million covered individuals annually. The Medicare Supplemental Database include both the Medicare covered and employer-paid portions of healthcare encounters utilization, and cost information. Institutional review board approval was obtained from the University of Florida.

Study population

To conduct a trend analysis, we established monthly cohorts of patients who met the inclusion criteria from January 2006–September 2015 (116 months of study =116 cohorts). 2005 data was used to ensure at least 12-months of baseline period. Patients entered the cohort if they: 1) were at least 18 years of age; 2) had at least two outpatient claims or one inpatient claim for CKD, defined as International Classification of Diseases, Ninth Revision, 585.3 (stage 3), 585.4 (stage 4), 585.5 (stage 5) within 1-year period, or at least one specific (585.3–585.5) and one unspecific claim (585.9) for CKD; and 3) were continuously enrolled for at least 1-year before they entered the cohort. Among CKD patients, if a least one claim carried a CKD stage code during the 1-year baseline period that defined CKD, the code for the highest stage was used each month. Patients were excluded if they had a diagnosis code(s) for any malignancy as ESAs are also used to treat anemic cancer patients undergoing chemotherapy. Patients were censored when they began dialysis, received a kidney transplant, end of enrollment, or 30 September, 2015, whichever came first. For each monthly cohort, denominator was calculated as the number of patients who were alive and were not censored the entire month; and numerator was calculated as the number of patients who received anemia care (defined below).

To examine the association between the publication of TREAT (October 2009), FDA safety warning on ESAs

(June 2011) and anemia therapy in CKD patients, the study period was divided into three periods. Specifically, the first period, the pre-TREAT period, covers the 45 months from January 2006 to September 2009 before the TREAT study was published. The second period, the post-TREAT period, encompassed the 20 months after the TREAT study was published and ended right before the June 2011 new FDA guidelines were released (from October 2009 through May 2011). The third period, the post-FDA warning period, included the 51 months from the publication of the FDA ESA guidelines to the end of the study (from June 2011 through September 2015).

The use of ESA, intravenous iron, and blood transfusions
ESA therapy was defined as the receipt of darbepoietin alfa and/or epoetin alfa. ESA therapy was identified using Healthcare Common Procedure Coding System (HCPCS) for the inpatient and outpatient settings, and National Drug Code (NDC) for the outpatient pharmacy claims. Receipt of intravenous iron was identified using HCPCS codes. Blood transfusions was identified using Clinical Procedural Terminology (CPT), HCPCS codes, or ICD-9 procedure codes. (see Additional file 1: Table S1 for a complete list of codes). We calculated the monthly anemia treatment rates as the proportion of patients with at least one prescription claim of ESA, intravenous iron or blood transfusions divided by the total number of CKD patients each month.

Covariates
Baseline patient characteristics were obtained from the 12-month period prior to the entrance of cohort each month, including demographic characteristics (i.e., age, gender, region), the Charlson comorbidity Index (CCI), presence of chronic diseases (i.e., diabetes mellitus, hypertension, heart failure, cardiovascular disease, peripheral artery disease, chronic obstructive pulmonary disease (COPD), and the involvement of a nephrologist (> = 2 visits in the previous 12 months). The presence of chronic diseases was defined as the presence of one inpatient or two outpatient claims within 12-month period before the cohort.

Statistical analysis
Patient characteristics were grouped into one of the three time periods (pre-TREAT, post-TREAT, post-FDA warning period) previously described. We then tabulated and plotted receipt of each category of anemia treatment by insurance type (Medicare and commercial insurance) and by CKD stages for ESA use only. To describe the general trend in anemia management from January 2006 – September 2015, we used Autoregressive Integrated Moving Average (ARIMA) model. ARIMA is a well-established modeling strategy for time series data with repeated

observations. Since the series were not stationary, first-order differences in proportion of patients receiving treatment were used for modeling to achieve stationarity. The autocorrelation and partial autocorrelation functions of the complete differenced series were used to identify the ARIMA models. We included autoregressive (AR) terms, moving average (MA) terms, and seasonality in the model and used Akaike Infomration Criteria (AIC) to select the most parsimonious model.

To explore the association of the publication of TREAT and/or FDA safety warnings with anemia management in CKD, we used a Generalized Estimating Equation (GEE) model with a binominal distribution and logit-link function. The GEE model with autoregressive correlation structure was employed to account for patient-level factors for ESA prescribing, intravenous iron prescribing, and blood transfusions as well as repeated measurement. The GEE model estimated the probability of receiving anemia treatment on a monthly basis during the post-TREAT and post-FDA safety waning periods compared to the pre-TREAT period. All statistical analyses were 2-tailed, with an a priori significance level of $\alpha = 0.05$. All analyses were conducted using SAS 9.4 (SAS Institute Inc., Cary, NC) and STATA version 14 (Stata Corp., College Station, TX).

Results
Patient characteristics
We identified 157,293 Medicare and 361,385 commercially insured unique patients between 2006 January and September 2015 who had CKD and were not on dialysis. Table 1 summarizes the baseline demographic and clinical characteristics of the study population during the three study periods using the median month of each study period. Medicare patients were older, more likely to be women, and more likely to have CKD stages 4 and 5, and a higher CCI score relative to commercially insured patients. Patient demographics including age and gender were comparable in the three periods. Compared to the pre-TREAT period, patients in the post-TREAT and post-FDA warning periods tended to have more comorbidities including hypertension, heart failure, peripheral artery disease, and COPD but less advanced CKD diseases.

Autoregressive integrated moving average (ARIMA) model
Additional file 1 : Table S2 shows ARIMA model results for ESA, intravenous iron supplementation, and blood transfusion. (See : Additional file 1: Tables S3 and S4 for crude monthly rate)

Monthly ESA use
Monthly ESA use are shown in Fig. 1 separately for CKD stages 3–5 in Medicare and commercially insured

Table 1 Demographic and clinical characteristics of the study populations

	Medicare			Commercial Insurance		
	Pre-TREAT [a]	Post-TREAT [b]	Post- FDA warning [c]	Pre-TREAT [a]	Post-TREAT [b]	Post- FDA warning [c]
No. unique patients	48,614	64,694	117,452	103,980	127,054	244,191
No. patients in the median month of each period	12,806	29,594	39,310	22,559	50,433	55,218
Male (%)	52.1	49.8	49.4	55.2	55.6	56.3
Age 19–44 (%)	0	0	0	13.3	12.1	11.4
Age 45–64 (%)	1.2	1.0	1.2	85.6	85.1	84.9
Age > =65 (%)	98.8	99.0	98.8	1.1	2.8	3.6
CKD stage 3	43.4	49.0	51.0	70.0	76.5	80.8
CKD stage 4	49.6	45.8	44.2	24.3	19.5	15.9
CKD stage 5	7.0	5.2	4.9	5.7	4	3.4
Diabetes mellitus (%)	43.8	47.7	51.2	43.9	42.6	41.8
Hypertension (%)	52.7	73.2	85.9	62.9	73.1	73.1
Heart Failure (%)	10.1	17.4	21.2	5.2	6.2	6.4
Cerebrovascular disease (%)	14.7	16.9	18.4	5.5	5.5	5.0
Peripheral Artery Disease (%)	8.8	13.5	16.2	4.2	4.9	4.3
Chronic obstructive pulmonary disease (%)	16.3	19.7	23.1	6.8	8.3	8.1
Nephrologist involvement (%)	46.8	45.3	39.0	49.0	48.0	44.8
Charlson Comorbidity Index, mean (SD)	4.2 (1.8)	4.6 (2.0)	4.9 (2.1)	3.7 (1.8)	3.7 (1.8)	3.7 (1.8)

[a] January 2006 through October 2009; November 2007 cohort was used to summarize demographics and clinical characteristics of CKD patients during the pre-TREAT periods
[b] November 2009 through June 2011; August 2010 cohort was used to summarize demographics and clinical characteristics of CKD patients during the post-TREAT periods
[c] July 2011 through September 2015; August 13 cohort was used to summarize demographics and clinical characteristics of CKD patients during the post-FDA warning periods

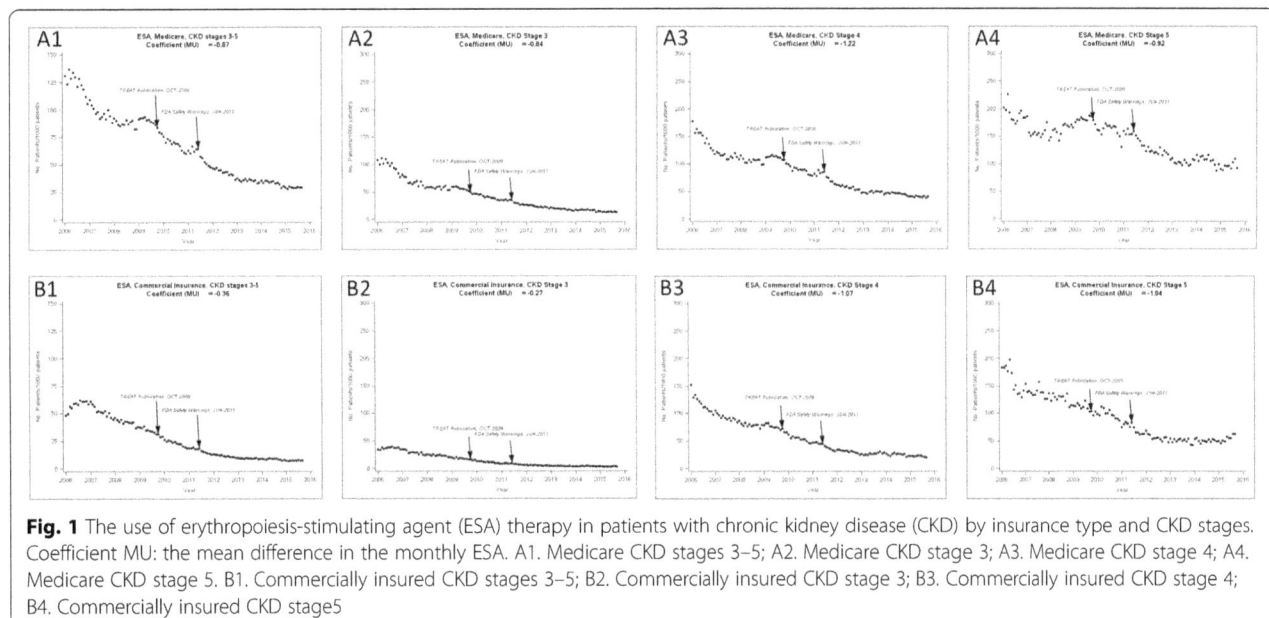

Fig. 1 The use of erythropoiesis-stimulating agent (ESA) therapy in patients with chronic kidney disease (CKD) by insurance type and CKD stages. Coefficient MU: the mean difference in the monthly ESA. A1. Medicare CKD stages 3–5; A2. Medicare CKD stage 3; A3. Medicare CKD stage 4; A4. Medicare CKD stage 5. B1. Commercially insured CKD stages 3–5; B2. Commercially insured CKD stage 3; B3. Commercially insured CKD stage 4; B4. Commercially insured CKD stage5

patients. Overall ESA use was 130.8 per 1000 Medicare patients in January 2006. After adjustment for seasonality, the mean difference (MU) in the monthly ESA use in Medicare patients was $-0.87‰$ ($p < 0.001$), indicating on average, the ESA use decreased at a rate of 0.87 per 1000 patients per month over the study period, reaching 29.3 per 1000 patients in September 2015. Overall ESA prescribing prevalence was 48.3 per 1000 commercially insured patients in January 2006 and continuously decreased at a rate of 0.36 individuals per 1000 patients per month (MU $= -0.36‰$; $p < 0.05$), reaching 7.1 per 1000 patients in September 2015.

Monthly ESA use by CKD stages

We stratified our analysis for ESA use by CKD stages. The mean differences in monthly ESA use (MU) in Medicare patients showed that patients with CKD stage 4 had the largest decrease rate in the ESA use- CKD stages 3, 4 and 5 MU were $-0.84‰$, $-1.21‰$ and $-0.92‰$, respectively. The mean differences in monthly ESA use in commercially insured patients showed patients with CKD stages 3 and 4 experienced a smaller decrease in the rate of ESA use than Medicare patients- CKD stages 3, 4, and 5 MU were $-0.27‰$, $-1.07‰$ and $-1.04‰$, respectively.

Monthly intravenous Iron use

Monthly intravenous iron supplementation and blood transfusion use are shown in Fig. 2 The mean of the monthly intravenous iron difference (MU) in Medicare patients was $0.01‰$ ($p = 0.435$), indicating on average, the intravenous iron use increased, but this was not statistically significant and the rate was low (0.01 individuals per 1000 patients per month). Similarly, the mean of the monthly intravenous iron difference in commercially insured patients was $0.005‰$ ($p = 0.720$).

Monthly blood transfusion use

The mean of the monthly blood transfusion use difference (MU) in Medicare patients was $0.03‰$ ($p = 0.120$), indicating on average, the prevalence of blood transfusion in a latter month was not significantly different from a former month. The mean of the monthly blood transfusion difference in commercially insured patients was $-0.002‰$ but this difference was not statistically significant ($p = 0.957$).

Interrupted time series analysis using GEE model

Table 2 displays the probability of prescribing ESA, intravenous iron, and blood transfusions per month during the post-TREAT and post-FDA safety warning periods compared to the pre-TREAT period. After adjustment, the probabilities of prescribing ESA in the post-TREAT and post-FDA warning periods were 31% (odds ratio (OR) = 0.69, 95% confidence interval (CI): 0.67, 0.72) and 59% (OR = 0.41, 95% CI: 0.40, 0.42) lower

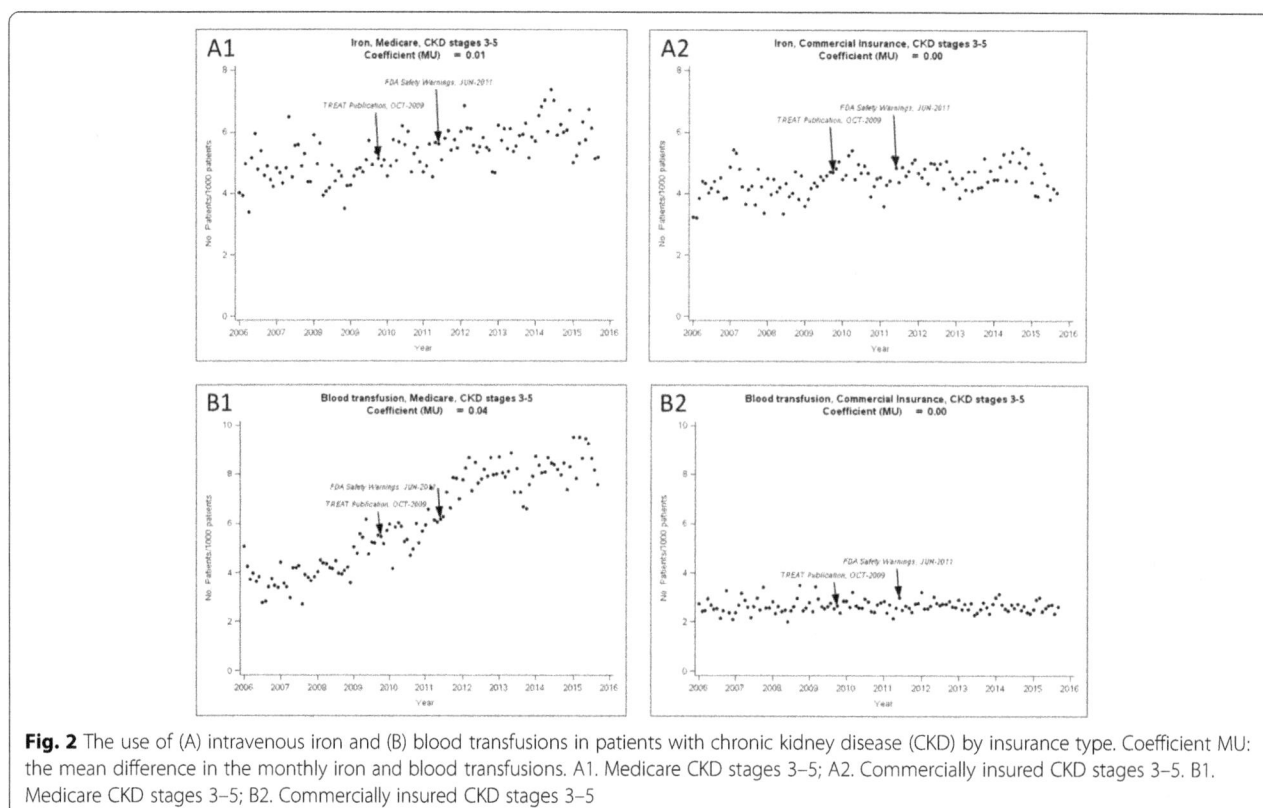

Fig. 2 The use of (A) intravenous iron and (B) blood transfusions in patients with chronic kidney disease (CKD) by insurance type. Coefficient MU: the mean difference in the monthly iron and blood transfusions. A1. Medicare CKD stages 3–5; A2. Commercially insured CKD stages 3–5. B1. Medicare CKD stages 3–5; B2. Commercially insured CKD stages 3–5

Table 2 Probability of prescribing erythropoiesis-stimulating agent (ESA) and intravenous iron therapy, and blood transfusions during post-FDA safety warnings (June 2011–September 2015) vs pre-FDA warnings (January 2009–May 2011)

	ESA			Intravenous iron			Blood transfusions		
	Adjusted odds ratio	95% CI		Adjusted odds ratio	95% CI		Adjusted odds ratio	95% CI	
Medicare									
After TREAT published	0.69	0.67	0.72	1.03	0.94	1.12	1.14	1.06	1.23
After FDA warning	0.41	0.40	0.42	1.11	1.03	1.19	1.31	1.22	1.39
Female (vs male)	1.27	1.24	1.30	1.12	1.06	1.18	0.97	0.93	1.02
Age	1.01	1.01	1.01	0.99	0.99	0.99	1.01	1.01	1.02
CKD stage 4 (vs stage 3)	1.50	1.46	1.54	1.17	1.11	1.24	1.10	1.06	1.15
CKD stage 5 (vs stage 3)	2.22	2.13	2.31	1.39	1.25	1.54	1.41	1.30	1.53
Diabetes mellitus	1.22	1.19	1.27	0.93	0.87	1.00	0.79	0.75	0.83
Hypertension	0.90	0.88	0.92	1.01	0.94	1.10	1.00	0.95	1.06
Heart failure	0.90	0.88	0.93	1.12	1.05	1.19	1.35	1.29	1.42
Cerebrovascular disease	0.90	0.87	0.92	0.91	0.86	0.98	0.94	0.89	0.99
Peripheral artery disease	1.00	0.97	1.03	1.10	1.03	1.18	1.10	1.05	1.16
Chronic obstructive pulmonary disease	0.90	0.88	0.93	1.10	1.03	1.17	1.22	1.17	1.28
Charlson Comorbidity Index	1.00	1.00	1.01	1.09	1.07	1.11	1.17	1.15	1.18
Nephrologist involvement	1.33	1.31	1.37	1.00	0.95	1.06	0.97	0.93	1.01
Commercial insurance									
After TREAT published	0.55	0.53	0.57	1.04	0.98	1.10	0.93	0.87	1.00
After FDA warning	0.26	0.25	0.27	1.06	1.00	1.11	0.94	0.89	1.00
Female (vs male)	2.21	2.14	2.29	1.57	1.51	1.63	1.49	1.42	1.56
Age	1.00	1.00	1.01	0.99	0.99	0.99	0.99	0.99	1.00
CKD stage 4 (vs stage 3)	2.75	2.67	2.84	1.24	1.18	1.29	1.81	1.71	1.90
CKD stage 5 (vs stage 3)	4.34	4.15	4.56	1.40	1.29	1.54	2.12	1.92	2.34
Diabetes mellitus	1.39	1.34	1.45	0.96	0.91	1.00	0.71	0.67	0.76
Hypertension	1.01	0.98	1.04	0.98	0.94	1.03	1.06	1.00	1.13
Heart failure	1.05	1.00	1.10	1.10	1.03	1.18	1.79	1.68	1.91
Cerebrovascular disease	0.84	0.80	0.89	0.89	0.83	0.96	1.00	0.93	1.08
Peripheral artery Disease	0.97	0.92	1.03	1.16	1.08	1.24	1.27	1.18	1.37
Chronic obstructive pulmonary disease	0.87	0.84	0.91	1.31	1.24	1.39	1.10	1.04	1.18
Charlson Comorbidity Index	1.12	1.11	1.14	1.18	1.17	1.20	1.37	1.36	1.39
Nephrologist involvement	1.43	1.39	1.47	1.08	1.04	1.12	1.01	0.97	1.06

than the pre-TREAT period for Medicare patients. After adjusting for covariates, the probability of prescribing intravenous iron was increased in the post-FDA warning period (OR = 1.11, 95% CI: 1.03–1.19). The probabilities of prescribing blood transfusion were increased by 14% (OR = 1.14, 95% CI: 1.06–1.23) and 31% (OR = 1.31, 95% CI: 1.22–1.39), respectively, during the post-TREAT and post-FDA warning periods compared to the pre-warning period.

For Medicare patients, characteristics associated with the increased likelihood of ESA prescribing included advanced CKD stages, female, diabetes mellitus, and involvement of a nephrologist. Variables associated with the administration of intravenous iron included advanced CKD stages, female, heart failure, and higher CCI score. Older age, advanced CKD stages, heart failure, peripheral artery disease, COPD, and higher CCI scores were associated with an increased probability of receiving blood transfusions.

Similar results were observed in the commercially insured CKD patients. The probabilities of prescribing ESAs were 45 and 74% lower (OR = 0.55, 95% CI: 0.53–0.57 and OR = 0.26, 95% CI: 0.25–0.27) in the post-TREAT and post-FDA warning periods. The probabilities of prescribing intravenous iron were increased (OR = 1.04, 95% CI: 0.98–1.10 and OR = 1.06, 95% CI:

1.00–1.11). The probabilities of blood transfusions were 7% (OR = 0.93, 95% CI: 0.87–1.00) and 6% (OR = 0.94, 95% CI: 0.89–1.00) lower, respectively, during the post-TREAT and post-FDA warning periods compared to the pre-TREAT period. However, these changes were not statistically significant. Characteristics associated with the increased likelihood of prescribing ESA in this group included advanced CKD stages, being female, having diabetes mellitus, having a higher CCI score, and involvement of a nephrologist. Factors associated with an increased likelihood of prescribing intravenous iron included: being female, advanced CKD stages, having peripheral artery disease, COPD, a higher CCI score, and involvement of a nephrologist. Variables associated with associated with an increased probability of prescribing blood transfusions included: being female, advanced CKD stages, having heart failure, peripheral artery disease, COPD, and a higher CCI score.

Discussion

The purposes of this study were to examine overall anemia management trends (ESA, intravenous iron and blood transfusion) in non-dialysis patients with CKD from 2006 to 2015, and to evaluate the impact of TREAT's study results (October 2009) and FDA's (June 2011) safety warnings and guidelines on the use of ESA therapy in the current treatment of anemia. We found that the use of ESA treatment in CKD non-dialysis patients decreased considerably from 2006 until 2015 (from 13 to 3% in Medicare patients; from 5 to 0.7% in commercially insured patients) in addition to finding a small increase in the use of intravenous iron supplementation (from 0.40 to 0.52% in Medicare patients; from 0.32 to 0.40% in commercially insured patients). We also found that the use of blood transfusions increased in Medicare patients (from 0.51 to 0.76% in Medicare patients) but not in commercially insured patients.

Interestingly, results of our time-series analysis indicated a steady decline in the use of EPO agents such that less than one fifth of patients received ESA in 2015 compared to 2005, with the trend starting as early as 2006, and the most significant changes occurring from 2006 to 2009. Notably, the initial decline in the use of ESA occurred with publication of the first randomized trials, CHOIR [5] and CREATE [6] in which investigators reported a higher prevalence of cardiovascular and cancer events in patients who received ESA agents [5, 6]. In addition, following closely after the publication of these two trial results, the KDOQI anemia guidelines were revised in 2007 to include an evidence-based warning to avoid hemoglobin levels above 13 g/dl when CKD patients are treated with ESAs [11]. The release of the 2007 recommendations corresponded with the largest drop in the use of ESA's seen in this study and

substantiate a previous study which also observed significant declines in the percentage of patients receiving ESAs between 2005 and 2009 [12].

Although we found slightly increase in the use of intravenous iron supplementation over the 10 years of the study, the proportion of patients who received intravenous iron remained small, at roughly 0.4–0.5% in 2015. In addition, we found that there was increase in the use of blood transfusions but the proportion of patients who received at least one transfusion remained relatively low, at 0.3–0.8% in 2015. Though there still remains questions as to when to initiate blood transfusions in patients with non-dialysis CKD, there is agreement that blood transfusions should be avoided in potential transplant candidates and used judiciously in all other patients [11]. As such, this would explain the very low rate of transfusions in this group of patients and only those that were older and sicker with advanced CKD were administered blood products. This finding is significant because there are concerns about an increase in blood transfusion as consequence of avoidance of ESAs. Transfusion avoidance is especially important in patients with advanced CKD because receipt of blood transfusions significantly increases the risk of developing allo-sensitization which may prolong the time on the kidney transplant waiting list and possibly jeopardize the kidney transplant outcome if one were to be transplanted [13, 14].

Similar to a previous study [15], our study found that after adjusting for clinical variables and co-morbidities using regression analyses, the proportion of CKD patients receiving at least one ESA decreased significantly after the publication of TREAT in 2009. After controlling for covariates, Medicare patients were significantly more likely to receive blood transfusions whereas there were no significant changes in commercially insured patients. We also explored anemia treatment patterns after the FDA warnings in 2011. To the best of our knowledge, no study has provided the impact of FDA actions yet. Similar to the trend after the TREAT publication, we found that the proportion of CKD patients treated with ESA's continued to decrease significantly while there was an increase in the use of intravenous iron supplementations after the FDA warnings. Blood transfusion continued to increase significantly in Medicare patients while it remained stable in commercially insured patients after controlling for covariates.

These results suggest that in Medicare patients, the use of iron and blood transfusions substituted the use of ESAs to treat anemia associated with CKD. Interestingly, in our study, although changes in the use of ESAs were substantial, the use of iron and blood transfusions did not increase significantly in commercially-insured patients. Although the reason for this difference is unclear, it could reflect differences in clinical practice for elderly CKD patients with cardiovascular comorbidities as well as differences in insurance coverage for intravenous versus oral medications in addition to lower prevalence of anemia treatment in younger commercially-insured patients compared to older Medicare patients. It is worth noting that in 2012, the Center for Medicare and Medicaid Services (CMS) implemented changes to the prospective payment system, including ESA administration, became part of a capitated payment, incentivizing providers to administer minimum yet adequate amounts of expensive treatments while striving to provide quality care and improve patient outcomes [16]. Although this reimbursement change may have impacted on Medicare dialysis patients, it may influence providers' practice for non-dialysis dependent CKD patients. A recent study reported that ESA use remained stable between 2006 and 2010, and then substantial declines in ESA use and hemoglobin levels occurred among patients on hemodialysis in the U.S. from 2010 to 2013, which reflects efforts in response to changes in FDA warning and reimbursement policy [17].

A striking finding was that among both groups of patients, the likelihood of receiving an ESA agent was greater if nephrologist was involved in the case (33–43% more likely to be prescribed ESA therapy). In contrast, a previous study found that that involvement of a nephrologist was associated with 18% lower likelihood of being prescribed ESA therapy during 2007–2011 [15]. Possible explanations for these discrepant findings could be differences in study populations and study periods. The previous study included cancer patients who receive ESA therapy due to cancer-related anemia [15]. Studies have shown that oncologists and hematologists were more likely than any other physician specialist including nephrologists to prescribe ESA [18, 19]. Our study, however, excluded patients with any cancer diagnosis to focus on CKD patients and their anemia management and was conducted for 2006–2015. However, the receipt of blood transfusions was not associated with being seen by a nephrologist. This may be due to better appreciation of the importance of transfusion avoidance by nephrologists.

A major strength of our study is the rigorous statistical analysis we used to determine the trends of anemia management overtime. The ARIMA model for estimating the monthly utilization patterns is popular because of the Box-Jenkins methodology in the modeling process which controls for secular trend (e.g, autocorrelation and seasonality) [20]. Specifically, the many events that occurred over the 10 year timespan of this study [CKD patients' clinco-demographics, publication of a landmark clinical study (TREAT), and changes in FDA's safety warnings for use of ESA's], we used the interrupted

time-series analysis GEE regression model that accounts for repeated measurement for the same patient adjusting for pertinent covariates- a valuable study design for evaluating longitudinal effects of population level interventions that have been implemented at a defined point in time [21–23].

There are also several study limitations. The first is the lack of hemoglobin data to determine whether the changes in practice led to changes in hemoglobin levels, to what extent, and if specific treatments were related to the severity of anemia. The revised EPO label provides more conservative dosing recommendations; however, we were unable to evaluate changes in EPO dose as information about EPO dose was no available in data. Oral iron was not included as it has variable coverage by insurance plans and is often purchased over the counter. In addition, this study included patients who had either commercial insurance or commercial plus Medicare supplemental insurance as their primary coverage. Thus, these results may not be generalizable to patients who are covered only by Medicare. This study is also limited by using ICD-9 codes, HCPCS, CPT, and revenue codes as recorded on administrative claims. It is possible that incomplete, missing, or miscoded claims impacted the study findings; however, coding errors are likely equally distributed across study periods and groups. Because we used the highest CKD stage during the 1-year baseline period for those who changed CKD stages over the study period, it is also possible that we might underestimate the lower stage and overestimate the higher stage. We also lacked patient clinical outcomes to determine how these prescribing patterns translated into patient outcomes. However, since there remains a lack of clarity and consensus within the current guidelines on how each of these therapeutic interventions should be used to treat anemia in CKD patients, interpretation of any findings would be difficult. But, it is clear from the data presented that physician prescribing patterns to correct anemia in CKD patients have changed with a noted decrease in the use of ESA's and an increase in the use of intravenous iron supplementation and blood transfusions. These are important changes to debate because as healthcare providers, we need to weigh the possible benefits of using ESAs to avoid the need for blood transfusions against the increased risks for serious cardiovascular events. However, more work is clearly needed to better understand how these changes translate into patient and budgetary outcomes as well as to establish clear guidelines to help manage anemia in CKD patients.

Conclusions

Over 10 years of study, there has been a marked decline in the number of CKD patients receiving ESA therapy, and consequently, a modest increase in the number of individuals receiving intravenous iron supplement and blood transfusions in patients with non-dialysis-dependent CKD. After the FDA warnings in 2011, ESA use continued to decrease and the iron supplement continued to increase. Blood transfusion continued to increase in Medicare patients but seemed to plateau in commercially-insured patients. Further studies are needed to evaluate the impact of these significant changes in anemia management on patient outcomes to include mortality, cardiovascular events, patient reported anemia symptoms and quality of life.

Abbreviations
AIC: Akaike Infomration Criteria; AR: Autoregressive; ARIMA: Autoregressive Integrated Moving Average; CCI: Charlson comorbidity Index; CDC: Centers for Disease Prevention and Control; CHOIR: Correction of Hemoglobin and Outcomes in Renal Insufficiency; CKD: Chronic kidney disease; CMS: Center for Medicare and Medicaid Services; COPD: Chronic obstructive pulmonary disease; CPT: Clinical Procedural Terminology; CREATE: Cardiovascular Risk Reduction by Early Anemia Treatment with Epoetin Beta; ESAs: Erythropoiesis stimulating agents; FDA: Food and Drug Administration; GEE: Generalized Estimating Equation; HCPCS: Healthcare Common Procedure Coding System; KDOQI: National Kidney Disease Outcomes Quality Initiative; MA: Moving average; NDC: National Drug Code; TREAT: Trial to Reduced Cardiovascular Events with Ananesp Therapy

Acknowledgements
Not applicable.

Funding
This study was not funded.

Authors' contributions
Research idea and study design: HP, XL, LH, JH, ER; data acquisition: HP, XL; data analysis/interpretation: XL, HP, LH, ER; statistical analysis: HP, XL, JH. Each author contributed important intellectual content during manuscript drafting or revision and accepts accountability for the overall work. All authors read and approved the final manuscript.

Competing interests
The authors declare that they have no competing interests.

Author details
[1]Department of Pharmaceutical Outcomes and Policy, University of Florida College of Pharmacy, HPNP Building Room 3325, 1225 Center Drive, Gainesville, FL 32610, USA. [2]Department of Behavioral Sciences and Social Medicine, Florida State University, College of Medicine, Tallahassee, FL 32306, USA. [3]Department of Internal Medicine, University of Central Florida, College of Medicine, Orlando, FL 32827, USA.

References
1. Centers for Disease Control and Prevention. 2017 National Chronic Kidney Disease Fact Sheet. Available at: https://www.cdc.gov/diabetes/pubs/pdf/kidney_factsheet.pdf. Accessed January 25, 2018.
2. Eschbach JW, Adamson JW. Anemia of end-stage renal disease (ESRD). Kidney Int. 1985;28(1):1–5.
3. Obrador GT, Macdougall IC. Effect of red cell transfusions on future kidney transplantation. Clin J Am Soc Nephrol. 2013;8(5):852–60.
4. National Kidney Foundation -Dialysis Outcomes Quality Initiative (NKF-DOQI). Clinical practice guidelines for the treatment of anemia of chronic renal failure. Am J Kidney Dis. 1997;30(4 Suppl 3):S192–240.
5. Singh AK, Szczech L, Tang KL, et al. Correction of anemia with epoetin alfa in chronic kidney disease. N Engl J Med. 2006;355(20):2085–98.
6. Drueke TB, Locatelli F, Clyne N, et al. Normalization of hemoglobin level in patients with chronic kidney disease and anemia. N Engl J Med. 2006; 355(20):2071–84.
7. Pfeffer MA, Burdmann EA, Chen CY, et al. A trial of darbepoetin alfa in type 2 diabetes and chronic kidney disease. N Engl J Med. 2009;361(21):2019–32.
8. Singh AK. Resolved: Targeting a higher hemoglobin is associated with greater risk in patients with CKD anemia: pro. J Am Soc Nephrol. 2009;20(7):1436–41.
9. U.S. Food and Drug Administration (FDA). FDA Drug Safety Communication: modified dosing recommendations to improve the safe use of erythropoiesis-stimulating agents (ESAs) in chronic kidney disease. 2011. Available at: https://www.fda.gov/Drugs/DrugSafety/ucm259639.htm. Accessed 25 Jan 2018.
10. Kidney Disease Improving Global Outcomes (KDIGO) Anemia Work Group. KDIGO Clinial practice guideline for anemia in chronic kidney disease. Kidney Int Suppl. 2012;2:279–335.
11. Kliger AS, Foley RN, Goldfarb DS, Goldstein SL, Johansen K, Singh A. Szczech L. KDOQI US commentary on the 2012 KDIGO clinical practice guideline for Anemia in CKD. Am J Kidney Dis. 2013;62(5):849–59.
12. Regidor D, McClellan WM, Kewalramani R, Sharma A, Bradbury BD. Changes in erythropoiesis-stimulating agent (ESA) dosing and haemoglobin levels in US non-dialysis chronic kidney disease patients between 2005 and 2009. Nephrol Dial Transplant. 2011;26(5):1583–91.
13. Thamer M, Zhang Y, Kshirsagar O, Cotter DJ, Kaufman JS. Erythropoiesis-stimulating agent use among non-Dialysis-dependent CKD patients before and after the trial to reduce cardiovascular events with Aranesp therapy (TREAT) using a large US health plan database. Am J Kidney Dis. 2014;64(5):706–13.
14. Center for Medicare & Medicaid services (CMS). Medicare program; end-stage renal disease prospective payment system and quality incentive program; ambulance fee schedule: durable medical equipment; and competitive acquisition of certain durable medical equipment, prosthetics, orthotics an supplies: final rule. Fed Regist 2011:70228–316.
15. Cardarelli F, Pascual M, Tolkoff-Rubin N, et al. Prevalence and significance of anti-HLA and donor-specific antibodies long-term after renal transplantation. Transpl Int. 2005;18(5):532–40.
16. Macdougall IC, Obrador GT. How important is transfusion avoidance in 2013? Nephrol Dial Transplant. 2013;28(5):1092–9.
17. Fuller DS, Bieber BA, Pisoni RL, Li Y, Morgenstern H, Akizawa T, Jacobson SH, et al. International comparisons to assess effects of payment and regulatory changes in the United States on Anemia practice in patients on hemodialysis: the Dialysis outcomes and practice patterns study. J Am Soc Nephrol. 2016;27:2205–15.
18. Collins AJ, Guo H, Gilbertson DT, Bradbury BD. Predictors of ESA use in the non-dialysis chronic kidney disease population with anemia. Nephron Clinical practice. 2009;111(2):c141–8.
19. Siegel J, Jorgenson J, Johnson PE, et al. Use and prescribing patterns for erythropoiesis-stimulating agents in inpatient and outpatient hospital settings. Am J Health Syst Pharm. 2008;65(18):1711–9.
20. Zhang X, Zhang T, Young AA, Li X. Applications and comparisons of four time series models in epidemiological surveillance data. PLoS One. 2014;9(2):e88075.
21. Lopez Bernal J, Cummins S, Gasparrini A. Interrupted time series regression for the evaluation of public health interventions: a tutorial. Int J Epidemiol. 2017;46(1):348–55.
22. Wagner AK, Soumerai SB, Zhang F, Ross-Degnan D. Segmented regression analysis of interrupted time series studies in medication use research. J Clin Pharm Ther. 2002;27(4):299–309.
23. Bernal JL. Interrupted time series regression for the evaluation of public health interventions: a tutorial. Int J Epidemiol. 2017;46(1):348–55.

19

Early predictors of one-year mortality in patients over 65 presenting with ANCA-associated renal vasculitis: a retrospective, multicentre study

Dimitri Titeca-Beauport[1]*[iD], Alexis Francois[1], Thierry Lobbedez[2,3], Dominique Guerrot[4,5], David Launay[6,7,8,9,10], Laurence Vrigneaud[11], Maité Daroux[12], Celine Lebas[13], Boris Bienvenu[14,15], Eric Hachulla[6,7,8,9,10], Momar Diouf[16] and Gabriel Choukroun[1]

Abstract

Background: The risk of early death is particularly high in patients over the age of 65 presenting with antineutrophil cytoplasmic antibody (ANCA)-associated renal vasculitis. We hypothesized that by combining disease severity markers, a comorbidity index and serious adverse event reports, we would be able to identify early predictors of one-year mortality in this population.

Methods: We performed a multicentre, retrospective study in the nephrology and internal medicine departments of six tertiary hospitals in northern France. A total of 149 patients (median [interquartile range (IQR)] age: 72.7 [68.5–76.8] years) presenting with ANCA-associated vasculitis and renal involvement were included between January 2002 and June 2015. The primary endpoint was the one-year mortality rate.

Results: Renal function was severely impaired at presentation (median [IQR] peak serum creatinine (SCr): 337 [211–522] μmol/l), and 45 patients required dialysis. The Five-Factor Score (FFS, scored as + 1 point for each poor prognostic factor (age > 65 years, cardiac symptoms, gastrointestinal involvement, SCr ≥150 μmol/L, and the absence of ear, nose, and throat involvement)) was ≥3 in 120 cases. The one-year mortality rate was 19.5%. Most of the deaths occurred before month 6, and most of these were related to severe infections. In a univariate analysis, age, a high comorbidity index, a performance status of 3 or 4, a lack of co-trimoxazole prophylaxis, early severe infection, and disease activity parameters (such as the albumin level, haemoglobin level, peak SCr level, dialysis status, and high FFS) were significantly associated with one-year mortality. In a multivariable analysis, the best predictors were a high FFS (relative risk (RR) [95% confidence interval (CI)] = 2.57 [1.30–5.09]; $p = 0.006$) and the occurrence of a severe infection during the first month (RR [95%CI] = 2.74 [1.27–5.92]; $p = 0.01$).

Conclusions: When considering various disease severity markers in over-65 patients with ANCA-associated renal vasculitis, we found that an early, severe infection (which occurred in about a quarter of the patients) is a strong predictor of one-year mortality. A reduction in immunosuppression, the early detection of infections, and co-trimoxazole prophylaxis might help to reduce mortality in this population.

Keywords: ANCA, Elderly, Glomerulonephritis, Infection, Mortality

* Correspondence: titeca.dimitri@chu-amiens.fr
[1]Department of Nephrology, Dialysis and Transplantation, Amiens University Hospital, F-80054 Amiens, France
Full list of author information is available at the end of the article

Background

Antineutrophil cytoplasmic antibody (ANCA)-associated vasculitis (AAV) is a systemic form of small vessel polyangiitis. Over 75% of patients with granulomatosis with polyangiitis (GPA), microscopic polyangiitis (MPA) or eosinophilic granulomatosis with polyangiitis are positive for circulating ANCA [1, 2].

AAV is primarily a disease of the elderly, with a mean age at diagnosis of 63 for patients with GPA and 66 for patients with MPA [3]. The incidence peaks at between 65 and 74 years of age, with 52.9 cases per million in the general population [4]. Renal involvement (characterized by focal, necrotizing, pauci-immune glomerulonephritis) is seen in over 70% of patients with AAV [5].

In patients over the age of 65, myeloperoxidase (MPO) ANCAs are preponderant. Renal function is generally severely impaired, and renal replacement therapy is frequently required. However, the clinical presentation is much the same as in younger patients [3]. Most deaths occur within the first year after diagnosis, and the two factors that best predict a poor prognosis in AAV are severe renal failure and age over 65 [6].

Patients over 65 with renal impairment at time of diagnosis are therefore particularly at risk of early death, since they have a higher risk of infection and reduced tolerance to immunosuppressive agents [7].

The objective of the present study was thus to identify early predictors for one-year mortality in a high-risk population of patients over 65 presenting with AAV and renal involvement.

Patients and methods

Study design

We performed a multicentre, retrospective study in the nephrology and internal medicine departments of four university hospitals and two tertiary hospitals in northern France. Patients aged 65 or more and presenting with AAV and inaugural renal involvement from January 2002 to June 2015 were included on the basis of registry data in the different centres.

The diagnosis of AAV with renal involvement was defined by acute renal impairment with proteinuria (> 300 mg/day) and/or haematuria (> 10/mm^3) a positive ANCA assay (indirect immunofluorescence and/or an antigen-specific immunoassay), and (if available) a renal biopsy confirming the presence of pauci-immune glomerulonephritis. The time of diagnosis was defined as the date of the first ANCA-positive assay.

Data collection

Patients were entered into the study from when a diagnosis of AAV with renal involvement was established. All data concerning the patients' diagnosis and follow-up were extracted retrospectively from medical records.

At presentation, each patient's age, gender, bodyweight and any history of hypertension, diabetes mellitus, chronic pulmonary disease, cardiovascular disease, malignancy and/or other comorbid conditions were recorded. The Charlson Comorbidity Index (CCI) was calculated from each patient's data [8]. Baseline general condition (ECOG Performance Status, weight loss, fever, etc.), extrarenal manifestations, the Birmingham Vasculitis Activity Score (BVAS) were recorded. The 2009 Five-Factor Score (FFS) was calculated for each patient, with + 1 point for each poor prognostic factor (age > 65 years, cardiac symptoms, gastrointestinal involvement, stabilized peak serum creatinine (SCr) ≥150 μmol/L, and the absence of ear, nose, and throat (ENT) involvement) [9]. Clinical biochemistry data such as the serum C-reactive protein and albumin levels, the leukocyte count, the haemoglobin level, the baseline peak SCr level (in a pre-dialysis sample, in cases of dialysis), the urine protein-to-creatinine ratio, haematuria, and the type (proteinase 3 (PR3)/MPO) and level of ANCAs were recorded at diagnosis. Induction treatments of AAV (including steroids, cyclophosphamide (CYC), rituximab (RTX) and plasma exchange) were recorded. When performed, renal biopsies were rated according to Berden et al.'s prognostic classification [10].

During the study period, we recorded the glomerular filtration rate (calculated with the Modification of Diet in Renal Disease equation), dialysis, specific treatments and their dose levels, anti-infectious prophylaxis, the number and types of severe infection (defined as infections requiring hospitalization or intravenous antibiotics), leukopenia, cardiovascular events, and the above-mentioned clinical biochemistry parameters at month (M)1, M6, M12 and M24.

Remission was defined as the disappearance of clinically active disease and a stabilization of (or improvement in) renal function for at least 4 weeks. Relapse was defined as the reappearance of clinical symptoms and/or organ involvement prompting the intensification of immunosuppressive therapy. The time of first relapse was defined as the date when the immunosuppressive therapy was intensified. The last follow-up corresponded to the patient's death or the last visit before the end of the study (June 30th, 2016). Hence, all included patients participated in the study for at least 12 months. The study protocol was approved by the local independent ethics committee (Amiens, France; reference: TB/LR/2016–88).

Study endpoints

The primary endpoint was the one-year mortality rate. The secondary endpoints were the onset of end-stage renal disease (ESRD) and relapse.

Statistical analysis

The patients' characteristics were summarized as the frequency (%) for categorical variables and as the median and interquartile range [IQR] for continuous variables. Risk factors for one-year mortality were evaluated using univariate and multivariable log-binomial regression models, and the results were expressed as the relative risk (RR) [95% confidence interval (CI)] and the p value. Survival was assessed using the Kaplan–Meier method. The median follow-up time was calculated using the reverse Kaplan-Meier method. Risk factors for relapse and ESRD were investigated with univariate and multivariable competing-risks regression models by applying Fine and Gray's method and calculating the hazard ratio (HR) [95%CI]. The cumulative incidence curves for ESRD and relapse were analysed in a competing risks regression model. The threshold for statistical significance was set to $p < 0.05$ in all univariate and multivariable analyses. All statistical analyses were performed using SAS software (version 9.4, SAS Institute Inc., Cary, NC) and R software (version 3.2.3, URL http://www.R-project.org/).

Results

The study population

Overall, 149 patients were included in the study and analyzed. The median [IQR] age at diagnosis was 72.7 [68.5–76.8], and 54 (36%) patients were over the age of 75. MPO-ANCAs were detected in 101 (68%) patients, and PR3-ANCAs were detected in 46 (31%) patients. Two patients had non-specific ANCAs. Eighty (54%) patients were diagnosed with MPA, 60 (40%) were diagnosed with GPA, and 9 (6%) were diagnosed with renal limited vasculitis (according to the Chapel Hill Consensus Conference nomenclature) [2]. The median [IQR] peak SCr level was 337 µmol/l [211–522], and 45 (30%) patients required dialysis at presentation. Renal biopsies were available for 131 patients. Pulmonary disease was the most common extrarenal manifestation and affected 67 (45%) patients, including 36 cases with diffuse alveolar haemorrhage. The median [IQR] BVAS was 18 [14–22], and 120 (81%) patients had an FFS ≥3. The baseline demographic and clinical data are summarized in Table 1.

Treatments

One hundred and forty-six patients received oral high-dose induction corticosteroids (1 mg/kg/day), and 117 of these received a median of 3 methylprednisolone pulses. One hundred and thirteen patients (76%) received CYC (intravenously in 96% of cases). The mean initial and one-month cumulative doses of CYC were respectively 11.0 ± 3.1 mg/kg/pulse and 25.6 ± 12.2 mg/kg. When considering the remaining patients, 11 (7.4%) received RTX, 20 (14.8%) received corticosteroids alone, one received azathioprine (AZA) and another

Table 1 Baseline demographic and clinical data

Age (years)	72.7 [68.5–76.8]
Female	72 (48)
Comorbidities	
Hypertension	99 (66)
Diabetes mellitus	18 (12)
Cardiovascular diseases	21 (14)
Malignancy	16 (11)
Charlson Comorbidity Index	4 [3–5]
Performance Status	
0–2	129 (87)
3–4	20 (13)
AAV type	
MPO/PR3	101/46
GPA	60 (40)
MPA	80 (54)
RVL	9 (6)
Renal involvement	
Peak SCr (µmol/l)	337 [221–522]
uPCR (g/day)	1.8 [0.9–2.6]
Dialysis	45 (30)
Renal biopsy	131 (88)
Focal	31
Crescentic	38
Mixed	36
Sclerotic	26
Inflammatory parameters	
C-reactive protein (mg/l)	88 [19–151]
Serum albumin (g/l)	28 [22–32]
Leukocyte count ($\times 10^9$/l)	9.2 [7.1–12.9]
Haemoglobin (g/dl)	9.4 [8.3–10.5]
Organ involvement	
Cutaneous	12 (8)
Ocular	8 (5.3)
Ear, nose, throat	27 (18)
Pulmonary	67 (45)
Cardiac	8 (5.3)
Gastrointestinal	11 (7.3)
Musculoskeletal	41 (27.5)
Nervous system	27 (18)
BVAS	18 [14–22]
Five-Factor Score ≥ 3	120 (81)

Data are quoted as n (%) median and interquartile range. *AAV* anti-neutrophil cytoplasmic antibody, *ANCA* associated vasculitis, *MPO* myeloperoxidase, *PR3* proteinase 3, *MPA* microscopic polyangiitis, *GPA* granulomatosis with polyangiitis, *RVL* renal-limited vasculitis, *SCR* serum creatinine, *uPCR* urinary protein to creatinine ratio, *BVAS* Birmingham Vasculitis Activity Score

received mycophenolate mofetil (MMF). Plasmapheresis was performed in 40 cases, including 18 individuals with pulmonary-renal syndrome. Prophylaxis with co-trimoxazole (CTZ) was administered in only 85 cases. Corticosteroids were progressively tapered after the first month, with a mean daily dose at M6 of 13.7 ± 9.1 mg. Of the 120 patients alive after 12 months, 109 were receiving maintenance treatment. Ninety-seven patients were still on oral steroids (mean daily dose: 8.8 ± 5.9 mg). The most commonly prescribed immunosuppressant was AZA (in 41 patients), followed by MMF (in 24) and RTX (in 19). Other drugs were administered much less frequently (e.g. methotrexate in 4 patients and CYC in 4 patients).

Complications and patient survival

Eight patients were lost to follow-up after a median (range) time period of 76.9 months (24–127). The estimated median [95%CI] follow-up time was 69.3 months [53.4–76.0]. In all, 52 patients died, with 29 (56%) deaths related to infection, 7 (13%) related to cardiovascular disease, 4 related to malignancies and 4 directly related to active vasculitis. The estimated one, three and five-year survival rates [95%CI] were respectively 80% [74–87], 76% [70–84] and 74% [67–82].

Sixteen (11%) patients displayed leukopenia (< 4000 cells/mm^3), and thirty-nine (26%) patients experienced a severe infection at some point during the first month of care. In total, 42% of the study population experienced at least one serious infectious complication during the first six months of care. The lungs, urinary tract, and abdomen were the most common infection sites, and Gram-negative bacteria and staphylococci were predominant.

Overall, 29 patients died during the first year of care, giving a one-year mortality rate of 19.5%. Twenty-four of these deaths occurred during the first six months, and 19 (70.3%) were related to infectious disease (mostly septic shock; for details, see Additional file 1: Table S1). In a univariate analysis, age, the CCI, a performance status of 3 or 4, a lack of CTZ prophylaxis, and disease activity parameters (such as albuminaemia, haemoglobin level, peak SCr level, and dialysis status) were significantly associated with one-year mortality (Table 2). In the multivariable model, a high FFS (RR [95%CI] = 2.57 [1.30–5.09]; p = 0.006) and the occurrence of a severe infection during the first month of care (RR [95%CI] = 2.74 [1.27–5.92] p = 0.01) were the best predictors of one-year mortality (Table 3). The estimated survival median [IQR] time was 112 months [102–138]. Data on five-year patient survival (as a function of the two independent predictors of one-year mortality) are presented in Fig. 1.

Renal survival and relapses

After treatment initiation, the number of dialysed subjects fell from 45 at inclusion M0 to 22 after one month of care

Table 2 Univariate analysis for one-year mortality

Variable	RR [95%CI]	p value
Age	1.34 [1.01–1.68][a]	0.03
Female	1.10 [0.94–1.28]	0.20
Diabetes mellitus	1.90 [0.90–4.02]	0.10
CCI	1.32 [1.02–1.71]	0.04
PS 3–4 vs. 0–2	2.90 [1.55–5.45]	< 0.001
PR3 vs. MPO	0.75 [0.31–1.78]	0.50
Peak SCr	1.13 [1.02–1.24][b]	0.01
Dialysis	2.40 [1.26–4.55]	0.007
Serum albumin	0.94 [0.89–0.99]	0.02
Haemoglobin	0.67 [0.52–0.86]	0.002
Leukocyte	0.98 [0.89–1.07]	0.62
CRP	0.99 [0.95–1.04]	0.79
BVAS	1.04 [1.00–1.09]	0.05
FFS	3.48 [2.10–5.79]	< 0.001
CYC	0.50 [0.22–1.12]	0.09
MP pulses	0.83 [0.32–2.16]	0.70
PLEX	1.66 [0.75–3.66]	0.21
Co-trimoxazole	0.40 [0.20–0.84]	0.02
Infection at M1	3.47 [1.84–6.54]	< 0.001
Leukopenia at M1	2.05 [0.76–5.56]	0.15

RR relative risk, *CI* confidence interval, *CCI* Charlson Comorbidity Index, *PS* Performance Status, *PR3* proteinase 3, *MPO* myeloperoxidase, *SCr* serum creatinine, *CRP* C-reactive protein, *FFS* Five-Factor Score, *CYC* cyclophosphamide, *MP* methylprednisolone, *PLEX* plasma exchange
[a]per 5 years
[b]per 100 µmol/l

(21 patients had been weaned off dialysis, and 3 had died). Only two patients were weaned off dialysis after one month of care. At one year, 102 patients had conserved a degree of renal function, with a mean SCr level of 159 ± 67 µmol/l and a mean eGFR of 39.8 ± 16.7 ml/min/1.73 m² (Fig. 2). The estimated proportion [95%CI] of patients on dialysis at 1, 3 and 5 years was 19% [12.6–25.0], 22% [15.2–28.8] and 27% [19.3–34.5], respectively. At baseline, the peak SCr concentration (HR [95%CI] = 1.27 [1.16–1.38]; p < 0.001), dialysis (HR [95%CI] = 2.66 [1.34–5.28]; p = 0.005) and the CCI (HR [95%CI] = 1.37 [1.11–1.68]; p = 0.002) were all independently associated with the risk of ESRD (Additional file 2: Table S2).

During the follow-up, a total of 43 (29%) patients relapsed. Thirty-two were major relapses, of which 29 involved the kidney (67%) and 4 involved the lungs. Eleven were minor relapses (ENT, joints, and eyes). Twenty-seven (63%) of these relapses occurred after the withdrawal of immunosuppression. The estimated median [95%CI] relapse-free survival time was 39.7 months [32.9–72.3]. In a multivariable analysis, PR3-ANCA was an independent risk factor for relapse (HR [95%CI] = 2.10 [1.15–3.82]; p = 0.01). Conversely, a high CCI (HR [95%CI] = 0.75

Table 3 Multivariable analysis for one-year mortality

Third variable added to the model	AIC	AUC	RR [95%CI]	p value
Infection at M1	122.1	0.799	FFS 2.57 [1.30; 5.09]	0.006
			Infection 2.74 [1.27; 5.92]	0.01
			Age 1.05 [0.99; 1.12]	0.09
PS 3–4 vs. 0–2	129.0	0.781	FFS 3.09 [1.51; 6.27]	0.002
			PS 1.92 [0.84; 4.35]	0.12
			Age 1.05 [0.99; 1.12]	0.13
Haemoglobin	126.7	0.761	FFS 3.06 [1.46; 6.40]	0.003
			Hg 0.82 [0.63; 1.06]	0.13
			Age 1.05 [0.99; 1.12]	0.09
Serum creatinine	130.1	0.759	FFS 2.98 [1.45; 6.13]	0.003
			SCr 1.09 [0.97; 1.22]	0.15
			Age 1.05 [0.99; 1.12]	0.07
Dialysis	130.2	0.758	FFS 2.96 [1.44; 6.08]	0.003
			Dialysis 1.66 [0.76; 3.60]	0.20
			Age 1.05 [0.99; 1.12]	0.10
Co-trimoxazole	127.5	0.752	FFS 2.98 [1.40; 6.34]	0.004
			CTZ 0.53 [0.23; 1.20]	0.13
			Age 1.04 [0.98; 1.11]	0.20
CCI	132.4	0.749	FFS 3.43 [1.71; 6.89]	0.0005
			CCI 1.12 [0.80; 1.57]	0.51
			Age 1.04 [0.97; 1.11]	0.22

Given the limited number of events for the primary endpoint (29 deaths) and Peduzzi et al.'s recommendations [26], we built several multivariable models with three variables (including age and the Five-Factor Score (FFS)) known to be prognostic factors. Next, each of the other candidate variables with a univariate $p < 0.05$ was added as the third variable. Even though age is included in the FFS score, we selected it because all patients were aged 65 or over. The best multivariable model was considered to be that with the lowest Akaike information criterion (AIC) and highest area under the curve (AUC)

RR relative risk, *CI* confidence interval, *PS* performance status, *Hg* haemoglobin, *CTZ* Co-trimoxazole, *CCI* Charlson comorbidity index

[0.59–0.96]; $p = 0.02$) and dialysis dependency (HR [95%CI] = 0.11 [0.01–1.17]; $p = 0.07$) were associated with a lower risk of relapse (Additional file 3: Table S3).

Discussion

Our present results confirmed the severity of ANCA-associated renal vasculitis in older patients; the observed one-year mortality rate of 19.5% was much higher than the value of 2.6% recorded in the age-matched general population [11]. In agreement with the literature data, we found that most of the deaths occurred within the first six months and were primarily related to infectious diseases [6, 7]. Hence, when seeking to identify early predictors of death, we focused on baseline demographic characteristics and the first month of care. As reported previously, we found that disease severity markers (such as hypoalbuminemia, anaemia, a high FFS and altered renal function) are linked to "hard" outcomes [6, 9]. We (as others) found that the severity of renal disease at presentation correlated with the risk of ESRD [3, 12, 13]. Overall, 19% of the patients still had ESRD or had progressed to ESRD at one year. Lastly, 43 patients relapsed after a median of 40 months. Most of these relapses

involved the kidney, and occurred after immunosuppression had been withdrawn. Hence, the presence of severe renal disease in the present study (as in the literature) was associated with a reduced risk of relapse [14, 15].

Our present results highlighted the impact of early infections on mortality. About 40% of the patients experienced a severe infection during the first 6 months of care - almost twice as many as the 24% reported by Little et al. at 12 months in a large cohort of AAV patients [7]. About a quarter of the patients developed a severe infection within the first month, and this event was independently associated with one-year mortality. Mc Gregor et al. have already shown that (i) the risk of death increases with the number of infections, and (ii) patients who experience a severe infection have a four-fold greater risk of death within 12 months [16]. Although we failed to show a statistically significant link between the therapeutic strategy and early mortality, it is clear that our study population (given the older age and the altered renal function) presented a higher risk of adverse drug reactions. Furthermore, the infection rate was highest during the first month and fell after the discontinuation of CYC and the steroid dose reduction.

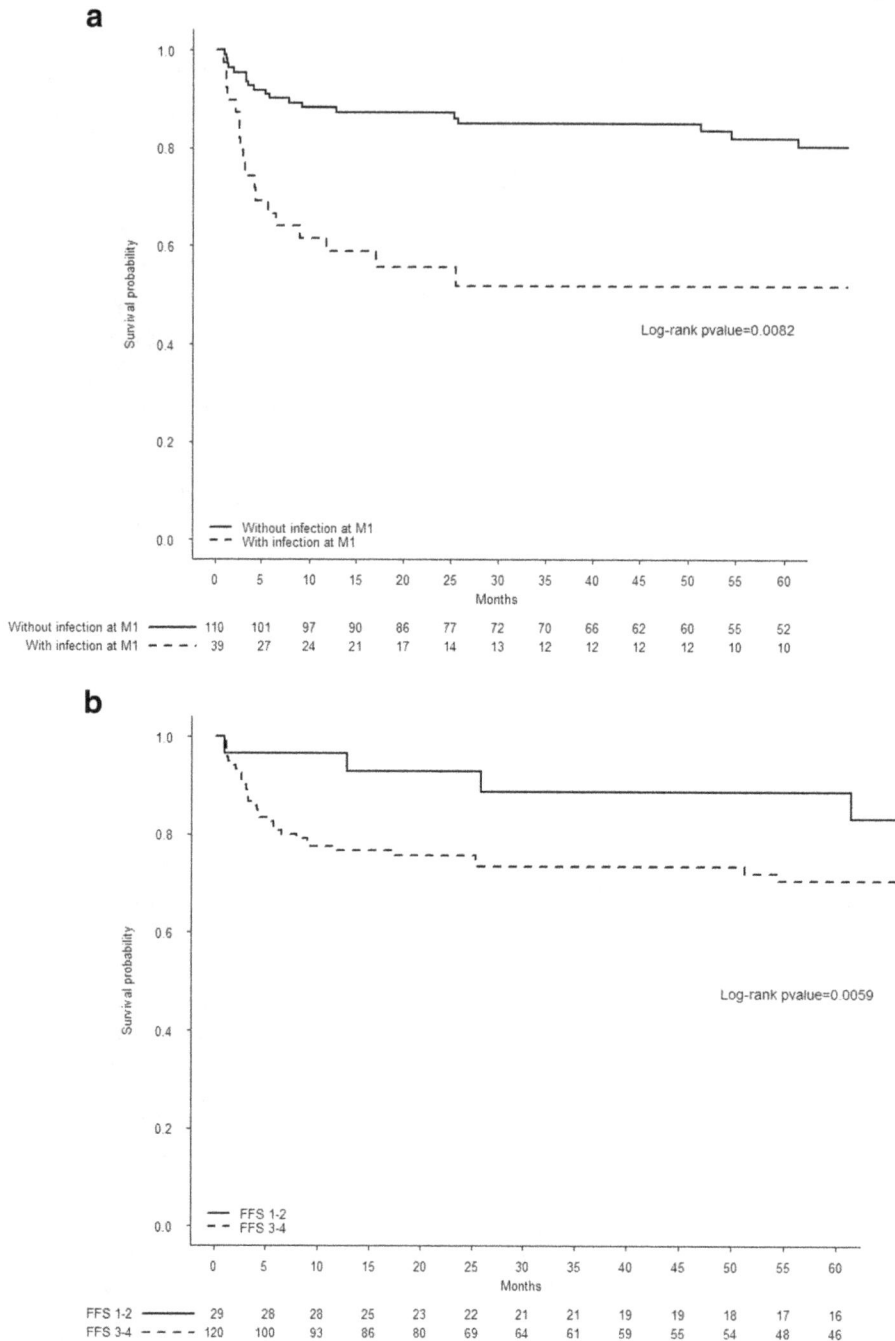

Fig. 1 Kaplan-Meier curves for five-year survival, as a function of the independent predictors of a poor one-year outcome: **a** infections during the first month of care, and **b** the Five-Factor Score

The beneficial effect of immunosuppression on survival and ESRD was proved decades ago, and the response rate to immunosuppression is the same in elderly patients as it is in younger patients [17, 18]. However, the expected benefit of aggressive treatment is counterbalanced by the individual risk of adverse events and disease manifestations. For example, dialysis dependency after 1 month was associated with a low probability of renal recovery or disease relapse.

Hence, in the absence of other organ-threating manifestations, the risk-benefit ratio should prompt a drastic reduction in the intensity of immunosuppressive therapy. In this respect, the KDIGO guidelines suggest discontinuing CYC after 3 months of dialysis dependency [19]. Given the early occurrence of infectious complications and deaths, it might be judicious to consider the early reduction or withdrawal of immunosuppressive therapy in some cases.

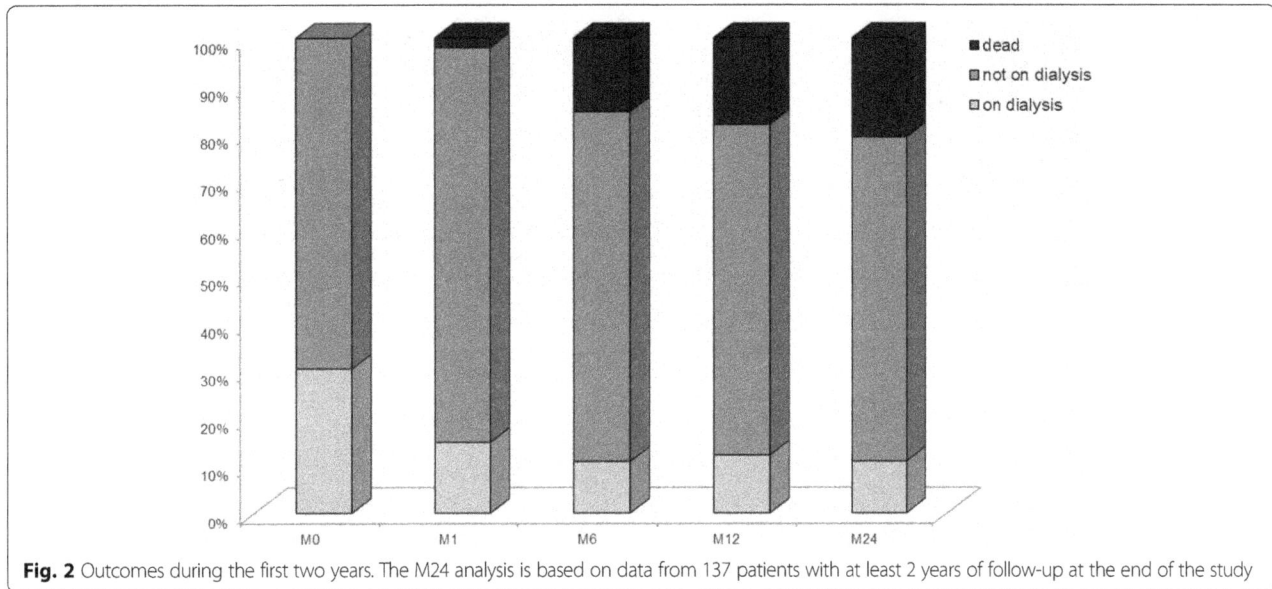

Fig. 2 Outcomes during the first two years. The M24 analysis is based on data from 137 patients with at least 2 years of follow-up at the end of the study

Reducing immunosuppression-related toxicity has been a constant concern over the last few decades. The association between corticosteroid exposure and infection is well established [20, 21], and the putative benefit of a reduced-dose glucocorticoid regimen in vasculitis is being tested in many ongoing randomized trials. A possible way forward has been addressed by the CORTAGE randomized trial of 140 over-65 patients with a mean baseline SCr of 233 μmol/l; treatment with low-dose corticosteroids and a fixed 500 mg IV pulse of CYC was associated with (i) a significant, early reduction in the adverse event rate and (ii) the same efficacy as a standard protocol [22]. These results confirm the importance of immunosuppressant-sparing strategies for improving the management of vasculitis in the elderly.

In parallel, strategies for preventing infection by the most common pathogens (comprehensive lung examinations, dipstick screening for urinary tract infection, the removal of non-essential intravascular catheters, etc.) might also help to reduce the incidence of severe infections. Given the study's retrospective design and the long study period, it was difficult to clearly identify the specific reasons for the limited use of CTZ. Despite similar renal presentations, the attitude to prophylaxis varied from one centre to another. The use of CTZ was associated with a reduction in the early infection and one-year mortality rates, independently of the baseline serum creatinine level. Given the low rate of pneumocystis pneumonia (a single case), this result can be partly explained by CTZ's ability to prevent bacterial infections [23] - suggesting a benefit of bacterial infection prophylaxis during the induction phase.

Our results also suggest that other patient-specific factors (such as the baseline ECOG Performance Status and the CCI) contribute to reduced tolerance of immunosuppression. Some previous studies have also found that comorbidity is correlated with lower patient and renal survival rates [24, 25].

Our study had several limitations. Firstly, the retrospective design may have introduced information and recall bias. However, the most important data were recorded during first month of care - a period during which the data collection was more reliable and clinical practice was relatively similar in the six centres. We found a one-year mortality rate of 19.5%, which is lower than the values of around 30% reported by previous studies of similar populations [3, 18]; this finding suggests that our study might not have been large enough to detect all the risk factors. Nevertheless, our demographic data and baseline presentations are similar to those observed in other series, and few patients were lost to follow-up. Cases of ANCA-negative pauci-immune glomerulonephritis were not included in the present study, which limits the extension of the present results to this population.

In conclusion, we found that over-65 patients presenting with AAV and renal involvement have a high mortality rate during the first months of care. Nevertheless, patients who survive the first year conserve a relatively good overall prognosis. When considering a variety of disease severity markers, an early-onset, severe infection (which affected about a quarter of the patients) was a strong predictor of one-year mortality. This finding should be taken into account during the initial steps in patient management. A reduction in immunosuppression, the early detection of infections, and systematic CTZ prophylaxis might help to reduce mortality in this population.

Abbreviations
AAV: ANCA-associated vasculitis; AZA: Azathioprine; BVAS: Birmingham Vasculitis Activity Score; CCI: Charlson Comorbidity Index; CRP: C-reactive protein; CTZ: Co-trimoxazole; CYC: Cyclophosphamide; ECOG: Eastern Cooperative Oncology Group; eGFR: Estimated glomerular filtration rate; ESRD: End stage renal disease; FFS: 2009 Five-Factor Score; GPA: Granulomatosis with polyangiitis; MMF: Mycophenolate mofetil; MPA: Microscopic polyangiitis; MPO: Myeloperoxidase; PR3: Proteinase 3; RTX: Rituximab; SCr: Serum creatinine

Acknowledgments
The authors thank Joelle Gracia, Audrey Sultan and Magaly Parsy for the help with collecting the data.

Funding
None to declare

Authors' contributions
DTB, AF and GC participated in the study design. DTB and AF acquired the data. DTB and MD analysed the data. DTB and GC participated in the manuscript preparation. All authors read and approved the final manuscript.

Competing interests
The authors declare that they have no competing interests.

Author details
[1]Department of Nephrology, Dialysis and Transplantation, Amiens University Hospital, F-80054 Amiens, France. [2]Department of Nephrology, Caen University Hospital, Caen, France. [3]Registre de Dialyse Péritonéale de Langue Française, Pontoise, France. [4]Department of Nephrology, Rouen University Hospital, Rouen, France. [5]INSERM, U1096 Rouen, France. [6]University of Lille, U995 Lille, France. [7]Lille Inflammation Research International Center (LIRIC), Lille, France. [8]Inserm, U995 Lille, France. [9]Département de Médecine Interne et Immunologie Clinique, CHU Lille, Lille, France. [10]Centre national de Référence Maladies Systémiques et Auto-immunes Rares (Sclérodermie Systémique), Lille, France. [11]Department of Nephrology and Internal Medicine, Valenciennes General Hospital, Valenciennes, France. [12]Department of Nephrology, Duchenne Hospital, Boulogne-sur-Mer, France. [13]Department of Nephrology, Calmette Hospital, Lille University Hospital, Lille, France. [14]Department of Internal Medicine, Caen, France. [15]Normandie Univ, UNICAEN, INSERM, COMETE, Caen, France. [16]Clinical Research and Innovation Directorate, Amiens University Hospital, Amiens, France.

References
1. Jennette JC, Falk RJ, Bacon PA, Basu N, Cid MC, Ferrario F, et al. 2012 revised international Chapel Hill consensus conference nomenclature of Vasculitides. Arthritis Rheum. 2013;65:1–11.
2. Guillevin L, Durand-Gasselin B, Cevallos R, Gayraud M, Lhote F, Callard P, et al. Microscopic polyangiitis: clinical and laboratory findings in eighty-five patients. Arthritis Rheum. 1999;42:421–30.
3. Harper L, Savage CO. ANCA-associated renal vasculitis at the end of the twentieth century--a disease of older patients. Rheumatology (Oxford). 2005; 44:495–501.
4. Watts RA, Lane SE, Bentham G, Scott DG. Epidemiology of systemic vasculitis: a ten-year study in the United Kingdom. Arthritis Rheum. 2000;43:414–9.
5. Franssen CF, Stegeman CA, Kallenberg CG, Gans RO, De Jong PE, Hoorntje SJ, et al. Antiproteinase 3- and antimyeloperoxidase-associated vasculitis. Kidney Int. 2000;57:2195–206.
6. Flossmann O, Berden A, de Groot K, Hagen C, Harper L, Heijl C, et al. Long-term patient survival in ANCA-associated vasculitis. Ann Rheum Dis. 2011;70:488–94.
7. Little MA, Nightingale P, Verburgh CA, Hauser T, De Groot K, Savage C, et al. Early mortality in systemic vasculitis: relative contribution of adverse events and active vasculitis. Ann Rheum Dis. 2010;69:1036–43.
8. Charlson ME, Pompei P, Ales KL, MacKenzie CR. A new method of classifying prognostic comorbidity in longitudinal studies: development and validation. J Chronic Dis. 1987;40:373 83.
9. Guillevin L, Pagnoux C, Seror R, Mahr A, Mouthon L, Le Toumelin P. The five-factor score revisited: assessment of prognoses of systemic necrotizing vasculitides based on the French Vasculitis study group (FVSG) cohort. Medicine (Baltimore). 2011;90:19–27.
10. Berden AE, Ferrario F, Hagen EC, Jayne DR, Jennette JC, Joh K, et al. Histopathologic classification of ANCA-associated glomerulonephritis. J Am Soc Nephrol. 2010;21:1628–36.
11. Aboua A, Eb M, Rey G, Pavillon G, Jougla E. Mortality data in France, the main causes of death in 2008 and trends since 2000. BEH. 2011;22:249–55.
12. Chen M, Yu F, Zhang Y, Zhao MH. Antineutrophil cytoplasmic autoantibody-associated vasculitis in older patients. Medicine (Baltimore). 2008;87:203–9.
13. Lee T, Gasim A, Derebail VK, Chung Y, McGregor JG, Lionaki S, et al. Predictors of treatment outcomes in ANCA-associated vasculitis with severe kidney failure. Clin J Am Soc Nephrol. 2014;9:905–13.
14. Walsh M, Flossmann O, Berden A, Westman K, Höglund P, Stegeman C, et al. Risk factors for relapse of antineutrophil cytoplasmic antibody-associated vasculitis. Arthritis Rheum. 2012;64:542–8.
15. Lionaski S, Hogan SL, Jennette CEHY, Hamra JB, Jennette JC, et al. The clinical course of ANCA small-vessel vasculitis on chronic dialysis. Kidney Int. 2009;76:644–51.
16. McGregor JG, Negrete-Lopez R, Poulton CJ, Kidd JM, Katsanos SL, Goetz L, et al. Adverse events and infectious burden, microbes and temporal outline from immunosuppressive therapy in antineutrophil cytoplasmic antibody-associated vasculitis with native renal function. Nephrol.Dial. Transplantation. 2015;30:i171–i18.
17. Fauci AS, Katz P, Haynes BF, Wolff SM. Cyclophosphamide therapy of severe systemic necrotizing vasculitis. N Engl J Med. 1979;301:235–8.
18. Weiner M, Goh SM, Mohammad AJ, Hruskova Z, Tanna A, Bruchfeld A, et al. Outcome and treatment of elderly patients with ANCA-associated vasculitis. Clin J Am Soc Nephrol. 2015;10:1128–35.
19. Kidney Disease. Improving Global Outcomes (KDIGO) Glomerulonephritis Work Group. KDIGO Clinical Practice Guideline for Glomerulonephritis. Kidney inter. Suppl. 2012;2:139–274.
20. Franklin J, Lunt M, Bunn D, Symmons D, Silman A. Risk and predictors of infection leading to hospitalisation in a large primary-care-derived cohort of patients with inflammatory polyarthritis. Ann Rheum Dis. 2007;66:308–12.
21. McGregor JG, Hogan SL, Hu Y, et al. Glucocorticoids and relapse and infection rates in anti-neutrophil cytoplasmic antibody disease. Clin J Am Soc Nephrol. 2012;7:240–7.
22. Pagnoux C, Quéméneur T, Ninet J, Diot E, Kyndt X, de Wazières B, et al. Treatment of systemic necrotizing vasculitides in patients aged sixty-five years or older: results of a multicenter, open-label, randomized controlled trial of corticosteroid and cyclophosphamide-based induction therapy. Arthritis Rheumatol. 2015;67:1117–27.
23. van de Wetering MD, de Witte MA, Kremer LC, Offringa M, Scholten RJ, Caron HN. Efficacy of oral prophylactic antibiotics in neutropenic afebrile oncology patients: a systematic review of randomised controlled trials. Eur J Cancer. 2005 Jul;41(10):1372–82.
24. Haris Á, Polner K, Arányi J, Braunitzer H, Kaszás I, Mucsi I. Clinical outcomes of ANCA-associated vasculitis in elderly patients. Int Urol Nephrol. 2014;46:1595–600.
25. Ofer-Shiber S, Molad Y. Association of the Charlson comorbidity index with renal outcome and all-cause mortality in antineutrophil cytoplasmatic antibody-associated vasculitis. Medicine (Baltimore). 2014;93:e152.
26. Peduzzi P, Concato J, Kemper E, Holford TR, Feinstein AR. A simulation study of the number of events per variable in logistic regression analysis. J Clin Epidemiol. 1996 Dec;49(12):1373–9.

20

Autologous arteriovenous fistula is associated with superior outcomes in elderly hemodialysis patients

Eunjin Bae[1], Hajeong Lee[2,3], Dong Ki Kim[2,3], Kook-Hwan Oh[2], Yon Su Kim[2,3], Curie Ahn[2,3], Jin Suk Han[2,3], Sang-Il Min[4], Seung-Kee Min[4], Hyo-Cheol Kim[5] and Kwon Wook Joo[2,3,6*]

Abstract

Background: The number of elderly patients with end-stage renal disease is increasing rapidly. The higher prevalence of comorbidities and shorter life expectancy in these patients make it difficult to decide on the type of vascular access (VA). We explored the optimal choice for VA in elderly hemodialysis patients.

Methods: We included elderly patients (> 65 years) visiting our VA clinic and divided them into three groups as follows: radiocephalic arteriovenous fistula (AVF), brachiocephalic AVF, and prosthetic arteriovenous graft (AVG). The primary outcomes were VA abandonment and all-cause mortality. The secondary outcome was maturation failure (MF).

Results: Of 529 patients, 61.2% were men. The mean age was 73.6 ± 6.0 years. The VA types were as follows: 49.9% radiocephalic AVF, 31.8% brachiocephalic AVF, and 18.3% AVG. Patients with an AVG tended to be older, female, and have a lower body mass index. More than half of patients (n = 302, 57.1%) started dialysis with central catheters, but the proportion of predialysis central catheter placement was not different among the VA types. Radiocephalic AVF was significantly superior to AVG in terms of VA abandonment (P = 0.005) and all-cause mortality (P < 0.001) in spite of a higher probability of MF. Brachiocephalic AVF was associated with a shorter time to the first needling and fewer interventions before maturation than radiocephalic AVF.

Conclusions: Autologous AVF was suggested as the preferred VA choice in terms of long-term outcomes in elderly patients.

Keywords: Elderly, Hemodialysis, Vascular access type, Vascular access abandonment, All-cause mortality

Background

The number of aging patients with end-stage renal disease (ESRD) is rapidly increasing. According to the United States Renal Data System report, the prevalence of ESRD increased from 4156 per million in 2000 to 6223 per million in 2015 in people aged > 65 years [1]. Similarly, the proportion of elderly ESRD patients aged > 65 years has increased over time, reaching 45.9% in 2016 in Korea [2, 3]. Dialysis initiation in elderly patients with a higher burden of age-related problems is associated with a variety of concerns, including the selection of vascular access (VA).

The current Kidney Disease Outcomes Quality Initiative guidelines support the Fistula First Initiative for all HD patients. Autologous arteriovenous fistulas (AVFs) have been preferred VA for the past decade [4–6] because AVFs have the lowest risk of infectious complications, the longest patency, and superior survival rate despite difficulties with maturation. However, the optimal VA strategy in elderly dialysis patients remains unclear because of their relatively shorter life expectancy, higher prevalence of comorbidities, and difficulty in VA maturation. In recent years, some studies have presented different opinions on the Fistula First Initiative in elderly patients. Some studies have suggested that insertion of an AVG in the predialysis period could be beneficial in elderly patients by sparing transient catheter insertion and related

* Correspondence: junephro@gmail.com
EB and HL are contributed equally and co-first authors.
[2]Department of Internal Medicine, Seoul National University Hospital, Seoul, South Korea
[3]Kidney Reasearch Institute, Seoul National University College of Medicine, Seoul, South Korea
Full list of author information is available at the end of the article

complications [7–9]. Another study suggested a catheter as the main form of dialysis access in very elderly patients needing dialysis in terms of maturation failure (MF) [10]. However, there are concerns about catheter-related blood-stream infections and shorter survival. In elderly patients, few studies have compared the survival rates following AVF and AVG creation for VA. Some studies showed longer survival for AVFs [11–14], whereas other studies showed similar or shorter survival for AVFs compared with AVGs [15–17].

Most previous studies compared one outcome, such as MF, VA abandonment, or patient survival rate, between patients receiving an AVF or AVG rather than comparing the different VA subtypes. With this in mind, the aim of this study was to evaluate which VA type is better for each clinical outcome in elderly Koreans.

Methods

Study population

We retrospectively enrolled outpatients visiting Seoul National University Hospital Vascular Access Clinic between January 2008 and March 2014 [18].

Elderly patients aged > 65 years who were maintained on HD were included. Patients who 1) had no VA, 2) visited our clinic only during an emergency, or 3) had undergone intervention or surgical treatment for VA within

Table 1 Patient characteristics by the vascular access type

	Total (N = 529)	RC AVF (N = 264)	BC AVF (N = 168)	AVG (N = 97)	P
Age (years)	73.6 ± 6.0	72.9 ± 5.8	74.2 ± 6.0	74.9 ± 6.4	0.007
Men (N, %)	324 (61.2)	176 (66.7)	92 (54.8)	56 (57.7)	0.087
BMI (kg/m²)	23.1 ± 3.3	23.5 ± 3.1	22.8 ± 3.5	22.7 ± 3.3	0.043
SBP (mmHg)	130.0 ± 19.5	131.0 ± 18.6	128.7 ± 18.1	129.2 ± 24.0	0.473
DBP (mmHg)	69.3 ± 10.8	69.7 ± 10.7	68.4 ± 10.3	70.0 ± 12.1	0.466
Hemoglobin (g/dL)	10.2 ± 1.4	10.1 ± 1.4	10.0 ± 1.4	10.5 ± 1.4	0.039
Albumin (g/dL)	3.5 ± 0.5	3.5 ± 0.5	3.5 ± 0.6	3.4 ± 0.4	0.126
Total chol. (g/dL)	153.4 ± 39.2	151.7 ± 37.5	153.7 ± 38.8	158.1 ± 44.8	0.428
Calcium (mg/dL)	8.5 ± 0.7	8.5 ± 0.7	8.4 ± 0.7	8.6 ± 0.7	0.222
Phosphorus (mg/dL)	4.2 ± 1.1	4.2 ± 1.1	4.1 ± 1.0	4.1 ± 1.2	0.614
Glucose (mg/dL)	123.7 ± 56.6	126.1 ± 57.4	117.2 ± 51.0	128.7 ± 62.8	0.206
PTH (pg/mL)	168.5 ± 149.1	170.8 ± 149.5	173.4 ± 142.6	147.0 ± 169.6	0.670
Uric Acid (mg/dL)	6.7 ± 2.1	6.8 ± 2.1	6.6 ± 2.4	6.2 ± 1.7	0.031
hs-CRP (mg/dL)	2.4 ± 4.3	2.1 ± 3.8	2.4 ± 4.8	3.1 ± 4.6	0.254
Follow up duration (month)	67.1 ± 44.6	71.0 ± 46.5	66.0 ± 41.3	58.1 ± 43.8	0.048
Etiology of ESRD					0.538
DM (N, %)	247 (45.7)	126 (47.7)	74 (44.0)	42 (43.3)	
HTN (N, %)	40 (7.6)	20 (7.6)	13 (7.7)	7 (7.2)	
GN (N, %)	35 (6.6)	18 (6.8)	8 (4.8)	9 (9.3)	
Others (N, %)	61 (11.3)	22 (8.3)	24 (14.3)	14 (14.4)	
Unknown (N, %)	152 (28.7)	78 (29.5)	49 (29.2)	25 (25.6)	
Comorbidities					
DM (N, %)	304 (57.5)	157 (59.5)	93 (55.4)	54 (55.7)	0.648
HTN (N, %)	419 (79.2)	218 (82.6)	131 (78.0)	70 (72.2)	0.087
CAD (N, %)	120 (22.7)	60 (22.7)	32 (19.0)	28 (28.9)	0.184
PVD (N, %)	26 (4.9)	9 (3.4)	11 (6.5)	6 (6.2)	0.276
CVD (N, %)	106 (20.0)	53 (20.1)	27 (16.1)	26 (26.8)	0.110
CHF (N, %)	77 (14.6)	32 (12.1)	31 (18.5)	14 (14.4)	0.191
Malignancy (N, %)	98 (18.3)	75 (17.2)	23 (23.2)	98 (18.3)	0.161

Values are presented as number (%) or mean ± standard deviation

AVF arteriovenous fistula, AVG arteriovenous graft, BMI body mass index, BC brachiocephalic, CAD coronary artery disease, CVD cerebrovascular disease, CHF congestive heart failure, DBP diastolic blood pressure, DM diabetes mellitus, ESRD end stage renal disease, GN glomerular nephritis, hs-CRP high-sensitivity C-reactive protein, HTN hypertension, PTH parathyroid hormone, PVD peripheral vascular disease, SBP systolic blood pressure, RC radiocephalic

the last month were excluded. After exclusion, we stratified the remaining patients into three groups according to VA types, as follows: radiocephalic (RC) AVF, brachiocephalic (BC) AVF, and AVG.

Clinical data collection

We retrospectively reviewed the demographic and clinical data. Body mass index (BMI) was calculated as weight in kg divided by height in m^2. Laboratory data and etiology of ESRDwere obtained at the time of VA creation. We gathered information from these pre-operative surveillance techniques. We also examined VA duplex ultra-sonography (DUS) findings at the time of the first visit. After surgery for VA creation, we regularly followed-up VA maturation status with a 2–4-week interval until the VA had matured sufficiently. We collected data on the time to the first VA use and whether patients received percutaneous transluminal angioplasty (PTA) due to poor maturation of the VA.

Outcome assessment

The primary endpoints were VA abandonment and all-cause mortality. VA abandonment was defined as an access that could no longer be used for 1- or 2-needle dialysis as it might be unable to provide adequate flow and/or be deemed unsafe for the patient if the associated problem could not be corrected by medical, surgical, or radiological interventions or rest [18]. For patients who withdrew from the study, we ascertained the mortality data from both an electronic medical record review and Statistics Korea [19].

The secondary endpoint was MF. MF was defined as a VA that could not be used successfully for dialysis from 90 days following its creation, despite radiological or surgical intervention [20].

Statistical analysis

Differences among the three groups were analyzed using the chi-square test for categorical variables and the analysis of variance t-test for continuous variables. The data are presented as mean ± standard deviation, median with range, or frequency (count and percentage). To explore the association between VA type and primary endpoints, a Kaplan-Meier curve was plotted according to VA types. Survival differences were compared using the log-rank test. To explore the association between VA types and Primary endpoints, multivariate Cox proportional hazards regression analysis using backward stepwise process was applied. Variables that showed a significant association ($P < 0.10$) in univariate analysis or were of considerable theoretical relevance were entered into the multivariate Cox proportional hazards regression models.

To assess the relationship between MF and VA types, we excluded patients who died within 90 days or follow up loss, and performed multivariate logistic regression analysis.

Statistical analyses were performed using SPSS version 21.0 for Windows (SPSS Inc., Chicago, IL, USA). Statistical significance was defined as a P-value < 0.05.

Results
Baseline patient characteristics

A total of 529 patients were included in the final analysis. Among them, 432 (81.7%) patients received an AVF, including 264 (61.1%) RC and 168 (38.9%) BC fistulas. AVGs were placed in 97 (18.3%) patients. The mean age was 73.6 ± 6.0 years and 61.2% of patients were men. Table 1 compares the baseline characteristics of the three VA groups. Patients receiving an AVG were older and had a lower BMI than those who received an RC AVF but were similar to those who received a BC AVF. Furthermore, their hemoglobin levels were higher but serum uric acid (UA) levels were lower than those of patients with AVFs.

Table 2 Analysis of the clinical characteristics before first use of vascular access according to vascular access type

		Total (N = 529)	RC AVF (N = 264)	BC AVF (N = 168)	AVG (N = 97)	P
CVC	None	227 (42.9)	121 (45.8)	69 (41.1)	37 (38.1)	0.358
	IJC	3 (0.6)	2 (0.8)	0 (0)	1 (1.0)	
	Permanent catheter	299 (56.5)	141 (53.4)	99 (58.9)	59 (60.0)	
CVC duration (days)		113.4 ± 73.5	115.3 ± 68.7	112.7 ± 63.7	109.3 ± 101.4	0.891
Preoperative surveillance	None	192 (36.4)	123 (46.8)	53 (31.5)	16 (16.5)	< 0.001
	Duplex ultrasonography	207 (39.2)	102 (38.8)	85 (50.6)	20 (20.6)	
	Venography	60 (11.4)	17 (6.5)	19 (13.3)	24 (24.7)	
	Both	69 (13.1)	21 (8.0)	11 (6.5)	37 (38.1)	
Time to 1st use (days)		64.0 (14.0–124.0)	75.0 (12.0–138.0)	65.5 (8.8–122.3)	35.0 (5.0–65.0)	0.001
PTA before maturation		112 (21.2)	70 (26.5)	27 (16.1)	15 (15.5)	0.011

Values are presented as number (%), mean ± standard deviation, or median with range
AVF arteriovenous fistula, *AVG* arteriovenous graft, *BA* brachial artery, *BC* brachiocephalic, *CVC* central vein catheter, *IJC* internal jugular catheter, *PSV* peak systolic velocity, *PTA* percutaneous transluminal angioplasty, *RC* radiocephalic

Table 3 Analysis of the duplex ultrasonography findings before first use of vascular access

		Total (N = 529)	RC AVF (N = 264)	BC AVF (N = 168)	AVG (N = 97)	P
Duplex ultrasonography	BA diameter (cm)	5.7 ± 3.7	5.7 ± 4.4	5.7 ± 3.5	5.6 ± 1.1	0.955
	BA flow (ml/min)	1009.6 ± 610.3	860.8 ± 477.8	1226.6 ± 743.7	1005.6 ± 535.0	< 0.001
	BA PVS (cm/sec)	207.0 ± 84.7	188.1 ± 68.1	238.9 ± 99.2	195.0 ± 76.8	< 0.001
	Cephalic vein diameter	5.7 ± 6.1	4.9 ± 3.0	6.6 ± 6.7	6.0 ± 10.2	< 0.001
	Cephalic vein flow	911.8 ± 664.8	726.5 ± 505.3	1153.2 ± 788.3	1008.8 ± 672.9	< 0.001
	Cephalic vein PSV	161.7 ± 73.3	146.3 ± 64.6	167.7 ± 72.6	194.2 ± 85.2	0.032

Values are presented as number (%), mean ± standard deviation, or median with range
AVF arteriovenous fistula, AVG arteriovenous graft, BA brachial artery, BC brachiocephalic, PSV peak systolic velocity, RC radiocephalic

Otherwise, there were no significant differences according to VA types with respect to blood pressure, laboratory tests, etiology of ESRD, and co-morbidities.

Preoperative VA-related characteristics
More than half of patients (n = 302, 57.1%) started their HD using a CVC. The mean duration of CVC use was 113.6 ± 73.2 days. Of these, 27 (9.0%) had VA abandonment, 30 (9.9%) died, 57 (22.4%) could not use their VA due to MF, 94 (33%) received PTA and 24 (8.4%) received 2nd or revision operation. Before access creation, 337 (63.7%) patients received preoperative surveillance for artery and vein status. Among them, 207 (61.4%) patients were evaluated by DUS, 60 (17.8%) by venography, and 69 (20.5%) by both DUS and venography. A total of 112 (21.2%) patients received PTA before maturation. The median time to the first use of the VA was 64.0 (14.0–124.0) days.

Table 2 compares the preoperative VA-related clinical characteristics according to VA types. There was no difference in CVC placement proportion and duration according to VA types. Patients who underwent AVG placement tended to receive more aggressive preoperative surveillance, although their maturation time was shorter and proportion of vascular intervention before maturation was lower than in patients who received AVFs. Patients with an RC AVF had the lowest proportion of preoperative vascular surveillance. However, their rate of PTA before maturation was highest and their time to needling was longest among all of the VA types assessed. The proportion of patients with a BC AVF receiving intervention before maturation was

much lower than that of patients with an RC AVF but similar to that of patients with an AVG.

DUS findings
Table 3 compares the DUS findings at the time of the first use according to VA types. The diameter of the brachial artery (BA) was not different according to the type of VA. BA flow and peak systolic velocity (PSV) was highest in BC fistulas. In addition, needling-site cephalic venous flow was highest in BC AVFs. PSV of the cephalic vein was highest in AVGs.

Outcomes according to VA types
During a mean follow-up of 66.9 ± 44.5 months, VA abandonment occurred in 8.2% (n = 43) and death by any cause occurred in 24.2% (n = 128) of elderly dialysis patients. Table 4 presents the clinical outcomes according to VA types. Figure 1 shows the VA abandonment and all-cause mortality rates according to VA types obtained using the Kaplan-Meier method. The VA abandonment rate was highest in AVGs, followed by RC AVFs and BC AVFs (P = 0.005). In terms of all-cause mortality, patients with an AVG showed the worst results, followed by those with a BC AVF and RC AVF (P < 0.001).

Table 5 summarizes the results of multivariate Cox regression analysis for outcomes. In multivariate Cox regression analysis, AVGs significantly elevated the VA abandonment risk (adjusted HR 2.77, 95% CI 1.22–6.27, P = 0.033) compared with RC AVFs. Additionally, hemoglobin level (HR 1.41, 95% CI 1.11–1.81,

Table 4 Clinical outcomes of the elderly hemodialysis patients according to VA Types

	Total (N = 302)	RC AVF (N = 143)	BC AVF (N = 99)	AVG (N = 60)	P
VA abandonment (n, %)	43 (8.2)	22 (8.4)	8 (4.8)	13 (13.5)	0.043
All-cause mortality (n, %)	44 (8.3)	17 (6.4)	11 (6.5)	16 (16.5)	0.005
Maturation failure (n, %)	136 (33.0)	84 (40.0)	43 (31.6)	9 (13.6)	< 0.001
PTA before maturation (n, %)	112 (21.2)	70 (26.5)	27 (16.1)	15 (15.5)	0.011
Secondary operation (n, %)	30 (6.1)	8 (3.3)	12 (7.7)	10 (11.2)	0.018

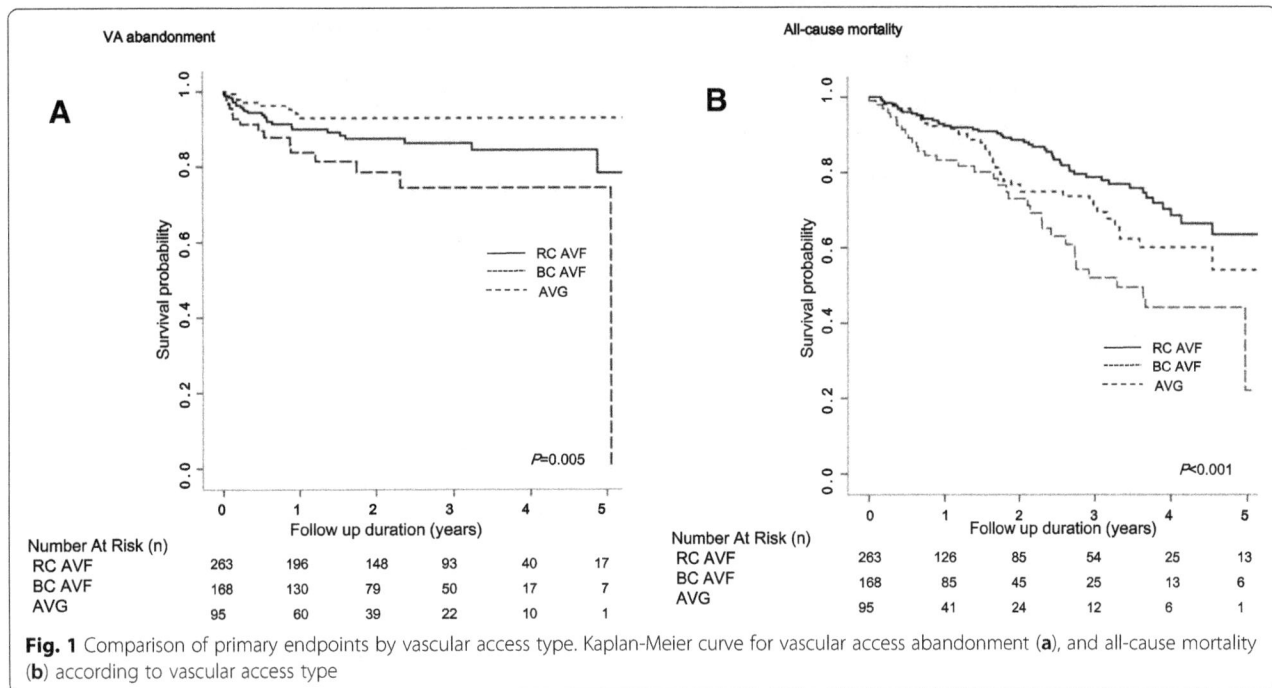

Fig. 1 Comparison of primary endpoints by vascular access type. Kaplan-Meier curve for vascular access abandonment (**a**), and all-cause mortality (**b**) according to vascular access type

$P = 0.006$) and BA diameter (HR 0.59, 95% CI 0.37–0.93, $P = 0.024$) were significantly associated with VA abandonment. In terms of all-cause mortality, AVGs were an independent risk factor for mortality (adjusted HR 2.65, 95% CI 1.52–4.63, $P = 0.003$). Age (adjusted HR 1.08, 95% CI 1.05–1.12, $P < 0.001$) and peripheral vascular disease (adjusted HR 2.39, 95% CI 1.13–5.06, $P = 0.023$) were significantly associated with all-cause mortality.

MF was observed in 33.0% ($n = 136$) of patients. The rate was highest for RC AVFs ($n = 84$, 40.0%), followed by BC AVFs ($n = 43$, 31.6%) and AVGs ($n = 9$, 13.3%). When we explored the factors associated with MF, AVGs were associated with significantly lower risks of MF than

RC fistulas (adjusted odds ratio 0.24, 95% CI 0.09–0.60, $P = 0.002$). BC fistulas tended to have a lower MF risk than RC fistulas, although this difference was not statistically significant.

Outcomes according to VA types in very elderly patients

We identified the outcomes associated with different VA types in very elderly patients (≥ 80 years). Figure 2b shows the VA abandonment rate in patients aged > 80 years determined using the Kaplan Meier method. There was no statistically significant relationship and no inferiority of AVFs compared to AVGs. In addition, AVFs were significantly superior to AVGs in terms of all-cause mortality.

Table 5 Hazard ratios of primary endpoints in elderly patients

	VA abandonment		All-cause mortality		Maturation failure	
	HR (95% CI)	P value	HR (95% CI)	P value	OR (95% CI)	P value
Age	–	–	1.08 (1.05–1.12)	< 0.001		
Hemoglobin	1.41 (1.11–1.81)	0.006	–	–		
Albumin	–	–	–	–	2.61 (1.6.0–4.25)	< 0.001
VA type (ref. RC AVF)		0.033		0.003		0.010
BC AVF	0.97 (0.35–2.68)	0.955	1.54 (0.92–2.57)	0.102	0.81 (0.47–1.42)	0.464
AVG	2.77 (1.22–6.27)	0.015	2.65 (1.52–4.63)	0.001	0.24 (0.09–0.60)	0.002
PVD	–	–	2.39 (1.13–5.06)	0.023		
BA diameter	0.59 (0.37–0.93)	0.024	–	–		

Adjusted for age, sex, BMI, systolic pressure, Hemoglobin, cholesterol, albumin, calcium, phosphorus, DM, CAD, PVD, CVD, CHF, VA type, history of CVC, duplex U/S findings (Brachial a. diameter, Brachial a. flow, Needling site diameter, Needling site flow)

VA vascular access, *BMI* body mass index, *CHF* congestive heart failure, *BA* brachial artery, *SBP* systolic blood pressure, *PVD* peripheral vascular disease, *HR* hazard ratio, *CI* confidence index, *OR* odds ratio

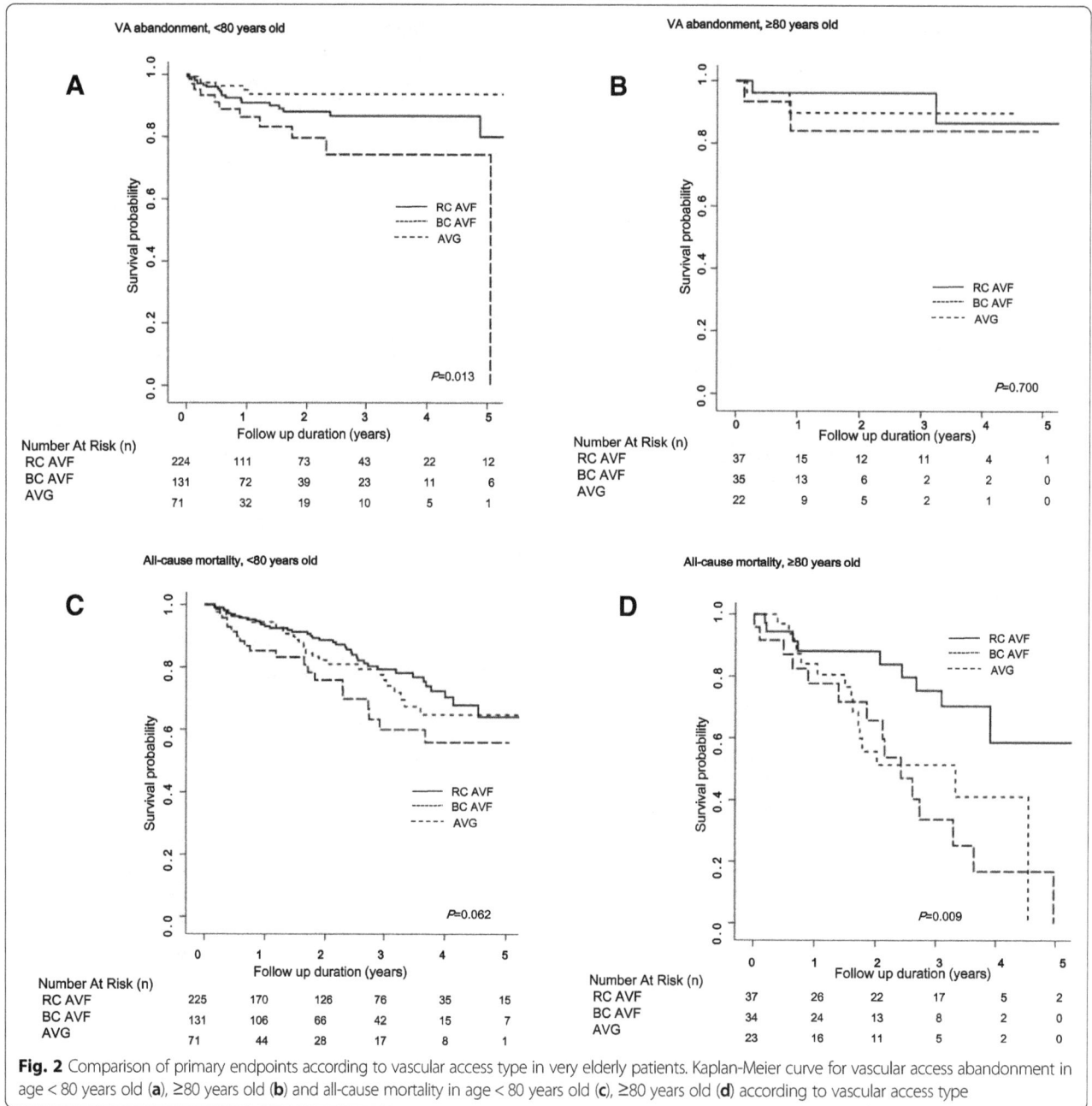

Fig. 2 Comparison of primary endpoints according to vascular access type in very elderly patients. Kaplan-Meier curve for vascular access abandonment in age < 80 years old (**a**), ≥80 years old (**b**) and all-cause mortality in age < 80 years old (**c**), ≥80 years old (**d**) according to vascular access type

Table 6 shows the effect of VA type on outcomes in patients aged > 80 years. In very elderly patients, RC AVFs were associated with lower risks of all-cause mortality than BC AVFs and AVGs. VA types did not have a significant effect on other outcomes, such as VA abandonment and MF.

Discussion

In this study, we investigated baseline characteristics, DUS findings, and outcomes according VA types in elderly HD patients. Our aim was to determine the optimal VA type

in elderly patients. We found that AVFs were superior to AVGs with respect to all-cause mortality and VA abandonment, although AVFs were associated with a higher risk of MF in elderly HD patients. Among AVFs, BC fistulas showed similar benefits to RC fistulas in terms of VA abandonment, all-cause mortality, and MF risk. However, BC fistulas had a lower intervention rate than RC fistulas. Moreover, DUS findings were more favorable for BC fistulas than RC fistulas. Consequently, BC fistulas might be a VA type that is not inferior to RC fistulas for elderly dialysis patients.

Table 6 Hazard ratios of vascular access type on endpoints according to age

	VA abandonment		All-cause mortality		Maturation failure	
	HR (95% CI)	P value	HR (95% CI)	P value	OR (95% CI)	P value
Age < 80 years						
VA type (ref. RC AVF)		0.019				0.015
BC AVF	0.55 (0.18–1.70)	0.299			0.68 (0.39–1.20)	0.184
AVG	2.71 (1.09–6.73)	0.032			0.23 (0.09–0.65)	0.005
Age ≥ 80 years						
VA type (ref. RC AVF)				0.002		
BC AVF			3.47 (1.34–9.01)	0.011		
AVG			6.30 (2.29–17.35)	< 0.001		

Adjusted for age, sex, BMI, systolic blood pressure, Hemoglobin, cholesterol, albumin, calcium, phosphorus, DM, CAD, PVD, CVD, CHF, VA type, history of CVC, duplex U/S findings (BA diameter, BA flow, Cephalic vein diameter, Cephalic vein flow)

AVF arteriovenous fistula, *AVG* arteriovenous graft, *BA* brachial artery, *BMI* body mass index, *BC* brachiocephalic, *CAD* coronary artery disease, *CVC* central vein catheter, *CVD* cerebrovascular disease, *CHF* congestive heart failure, *DM* diabetes mellitus, *PVD* peripheral vascular disease, *PSV* peak systolic velocity, *PTA* percutaneous transluminal angioplasty, *RC* radiocephalic, *U/S* ultrasonography, *HR* hazard ratio, *CI* confidence index, *OR* odds ratio

Inadequate VA leads to recurrent PTA, re-operation, and CVC insertion, which increase the risk of infection and mortality. In addition, inadequate VA is related to poor quality of life. Researchers have investigated various aspects of VA, such as timing, placement, and type. Some previous studies compared RC and BC AVFs. In terms of patency, BC AVFs have advantages over RC AVFs [7, 13, 21–23], whereas BC AVFs are associated with more steal syndrome than RC AVFs [24]. The present study demonstrated that AVFs are superior to AVGs in terms of all-cause mortality and VA abandonment but not MF. In patients aged 65–80 years, BC AVFs showed no significant difference in all-cause mortality compared to RC AVFs and favorable outcomes in terms of VA abandonment and MF. In patients aged > 80 years, BC AVFs showed inferior outcomes to RC AVFs in terms of all-cause mortality. BC AVFs were associated with less PTA before maturation and better DUS findings than RC AVFs. In view of these findings, AVFs should be considered as the first-choice VA rather than AVGs in elderly patients. Furthermore, it is not necessary to insist on RC AVFs. Rather, the choice between BC and RC AVFs should be determined based on blood vessel status.

In this study, RC AVFs accounted for the largest proportion of AVFs at 61.1% in elderly patients, showing a large proportion of RC AVFs were placed compared to other studies. Other previous studies showed that 24.7% to 60.7% patients received RC AVFs in AVFs [13, 21–23]. It might be following reasons; skilled surgical technique, recently enrolled patients could have better vascular condition than the patients in the previous studies. There were no significant differences in gender or age between our study and previous studies.

The results of this study should be interpreted with caution. Although all patients were elderly, patients with RC AVFs had better vascular status and fewer co-

morbidities than patients with other BC AVFs or AVGs. In this study, patients in the RC AVF group were the youngest and their BMI and UA level were higher than those of patients in the other VA type groups. The higher BMI and UA level could reflect the good nutritional status of patients in the RC AVF group in this study. Although, we adjusted for nutritional status and co-morbidities, the relationship between all-cause mortality and RC AVF should be interpreted as a surrogate marker rather than as an effect of RC AVF itself.

The present study investigated details related to VA in elderly dialysis patients, such as methods of VA surveillance before the first dialysis, DUS findings, interventions, first dialysis methods, MF, and VA abandonment. Previous studies mainly focused on outcome-related factors, whereas this study evaluated the overall characteristics associated with VA, such as the process of creating a VA and outcomes during the follow-up period.

We analyzed DUS findings, which were associated with the clinical outcomes of VA creation. Among the DUS findings, only BA diameter was significantly associated with VA abandonment. One previous study [25] showed that BA diameter was positively correlated with AVF success. Other studies [26, 27] reported good BA flow rate consequent to RC wrist AVF maturation. As such, the BA represents an ideal site for studying distal AVFs. As yet, there is no definite DUS finding that can predict VA outcomes. However, the results of this study could represent evidence that the BA is relatively important in DUS findings, especially in elderly patients.

The present study had some limitations. First, the study was retrospective in nature. As such, it was difficult to infer causal relationships and selection bias cannot be completely ruled out. Second, since most of the study population was Asian, the data cannot be generalized to other races. Third, DUS was performed by well-trained specialists but not by the same person, which could have led to differences in the DUS results. To overcome these limitations, well-planned prospective, multicenter studies are needed.

Conclusions

In conclusion, the fistula first strategy could also be applied to elderly HD patients with respect to VA abandonment and all-cause mortality. BC AVFs could be considered as the first-choice VA depending on the patient's condition.

Abbreviations
AVF: Autologous arteriovenous fistula; AVG: Arteriovenous graft; BA: Brachial artery; BC: Brachiocephalic; BMI: Body mass index; CI: Confidence interval; CVC: Central venous catheter; DUS: Duplex ultra-sonography; ESRD: End-stage renal disease; HD: Hemodialysis; HR: hazard ratio; PSV: Peak systolic velocity; PTA: Percutaneous transluminal angioplasty; RC: Radiocephalic; VA: Vascular access

Acknowledgements
Not applicable

Funding
No funding exits regarding this manuscript.

Authors' contributions
Research idea and study design: EB, HL, KO, KWJ; acquisition of data: EB, HL, KO, YSK, JSH, SiM, SkM, HK; data analysis/interpretation: EB, HL, SiM, SkM, CA; statistical analysis: EB, HL, DKK, JSH; writing the manuscript: EB, HL, YSK, HK, KWJ; review, revision, and final approval: all authors. All the authors read and approved the final version of the manuscript to be published.

Competing interests
The authors declare that they have no competing interests.

Author details
[1]Department of Internal Medicine, Gyeongsang National University Changwon Hospital, Changwon, South Korea. [2]Department of Internal Medicine, Seoul National University Hospital, Seoul, South Korea. [3]Kidney Reasearch Institute, Seoul National University College of Medicine, Seoul, South Korea. [4]Department of Surgery, Seoul National University College of Medicine, Seoul, South Korea. [5]Department of Radiology, Seoul National University College of Medicine, Seoul, South Korea. [6]Department of Internal Medicine, Seoul National University College of Medicine, 101 Daehak-Ro, Jongno-Gu, Seoul 03080, Republic of Korea.

References
1. (USRDS) USRDS: Usrds 2016 annual data report: Atlas of chronic kidney disease and end-stage renal disease in the united states, 2016,
2. Jin DC, Yun SR, Lee SW, Han SW, Kim W, Park J, Kim YK. Current characteristics of dialysis therapy in Korea: 2016 registry data focusing on diabetic patients. Kidney Res Clin Pract. 2018;37:20–9.
3. Committee ER: Current renal replacement therapy in Korea 2016., 2016,
4. Lok CE, Foley R. Vascular access morbidity and mortality: trends of the last decade. Clin J Am Soc Nephrol. 2013;8:1213–9.
5. Dhingra RK, Young EW, Hulbert-Shearon TE, Leavey SF, Port FK. Type of vascular access and mortality in u.S. hemodialysis patients. Kidney Int. 2001;60:1443–51.
6. Daugirdas JT, Depner TA, Inrig J, Mehrotra R, Rocco MV, Suri RS, Weiner DE, Greer N, Ishani A, MacDonald R, Olson C, Rutks I, Slinin Y, Wilt TJ, Rocco M, Kramer H, Choi MJ, Samaniego-Picota M, Scheel PJ, Willis K, Joseph J, Brereton L. Kdoqi clinical practice guideline for hemodialysis adequacy: 2015 update. Am J Kidney Dis. 2015;66:884–930.
7. DeSilva RN, Patibandla BK, Vin Y, Narra A, Chawla V, Brown RS, Goldfarb-Rumyantzev AS. Fistula first is not always the best strategy for the elderly. J Am Soc Nephrol. 2013;24:1297–304.
8. Lee T, Thamer M, Zhang Y, Zhang Q, Allon M. Outcomes of elderly patients after predialysis vascular access creation. J Am Soc Nephrol. 2015;26:3133–40.
9. Leake AE, Yuo TH, Wu T, Fish L, Dillavou ED, Chaer RA, Leers SA, Makaroun MS. Arteriovenous grafts are associated with earlier catheter removal and fewer catheter days in the United States renal data system population. J Vasc Surg. 2015;62:123–7.
10. Diandra JC, Lo ZJ, Ang WW, Feng JF, Narayanan S, Tan GWL, Chandrasekar S. A review of arteriovenous fistulae creation in octogenarians. Ann Vasc Surg. 2018;46:331–6.
11. Xue JL, Dahl D, Ebben JP, Collins AJ. The association of initial hemodialysis access type with mortality outcomes in elderly medicare esrd patients. Am J Kidney Dis. 2003;42:1013–9.
12. Woo K, Goldman DP, Romley JA. Early failure of dialysis access among the elderly in the era of fistula first. Clin J Am Soc Nephrol. 2015;10:1791–8.
13. Lok CE, Oliver MJ, Su J, Bhola C, Hannigan N, Jassal SV. Arteriovenous fistula outcomes in the era of the elderly dialysis population. Kidney Int. 2005;67: 2462–9.
14. Lee T, Thamer M, Zhang Q, Zhang Y, Allon M. Vascular access type and clinical outcomes among elderly patients on hemodialysis. Clin J Am Soc Nephrol. 2017;12:1823–30.
15. Drew DA, Lok CE, Cohen JT, Wagner M, Tangri N, Weiner DE. Vascular access choice in incident hemodialysis patients: a decision analysis. J Am Soc Nephrol. 2015;26:183–91.
16. Yuo TH, Chaer RA, Dillavou ED, Leers SA, Makaroun MS. Patients started on hemodialysis with tunneled dialysis catheter have similar survival after arteriovenous fistula and arteriovenous graft creation. J Vasc Surg. 2015;62: 1590–7 e1592.
17. Park HS, Kim WJ, Kim YK, Kim HW, Choi BS, Park CW, Kim YO, Yang CW, Kim YL, Kim YS, Kang SW, Kim NH, Jin DC. Comparison of outcomes with arteriovenous fistula and arteriovenous graft for vascular access in hemodialysis: a prospective cohort study. Am J Nephrol. 2016;43:120–8.
18. Kim HJ, Lee H, Kim DK, Oh KH, Kim YS, Ahn C, Han JS, Min SK, Min SI, Kim HC, Joo KW. Recurrent vascular access dysfunction as a novel marker of cardiovascular outcome and mortality in hemodialysis patients. Am J Nephrol. 2016;44:71–80.
19. Korean statistical information service, 2014. Available at: www.kosis.kr/. Accessed 30 Dec 2014.
20. Lee T, Mokrzycki M, Moist L, Maya I, Vazquez M, Lok CE. Standardized definitions for hemodialysis vascular access. Semin Dial. 2011;24:515–24.
21. Olsha O, Hijazi J, Goldin I, Shemesh D. Vascular access in hemodialysis patients older than 80 years. J Vasc Surg. 2015;61:177–83.
22. Renaud CJ, Pei JH, Lee EJ, Robless PA, Vathsala A. Comparative outcomes of primary autogenous fistulas in elderly, multiethnic asian hemodialysis patients. J Vasc Surg. 2012;56:433–9.
23. Staramos DN, Lazarides MK, Tzilalis VD, Ekonomou CS, Simopoulos CE, Dayantas JN. Patency of autologous and prosthetic arteriovenous fistulas in elderly patients. Eur J Surg. 2000;166:777–81.
24. Goh MA, Ali JM, Iype S, Pettigrew GJ. Outcomes of primary arteriovenous fistulas in patients older than 70 years. J Vasc Surg. 2016;63:1333–40.
25. Gibyeli Genek D, Tuncer Altay C, Unek T, Sifil A, Secil M, Camsari T. Can primary failure of arteriovenous fistulas be anticipated? Hemodial Int. 2015;19:296–305.
26. Lomonte C, Casucci F, Antonelli M, Giammaria B, Losurdo N, Marchio G, Basile C. Is there a place for duplex screening of the brachial artery in the maturation of arteriovenous fistulas? Semin Dial. 2005;18:243–6.
27. Wiese P, Nonnast-Daniel B. Colour doppler ultrasound in dialysis access. Nephrol Dial Transplant. 2004;19:1956–63.

21

Assessing the effect of oral activated vitamin D on overall survival in hemodialysis patients: a landmark analysis

Jo-Yen Chao[1,2], Hsu-Chih Chien[2], Te-Hui Kuo[1,3], Yu-Tzu Chang[1,4], Chung-Yi Li[3], Ming-Cheng Wang[1,2] and Yea-Huei Kao Yang[2]* [ID]

Abstract

Background: Patients with end stage renal disease have a high all-cause and cardiovascular mortality. Secondary hyperparathyroidism and vitamin D deficiency are considered part of the mechanism for the excess mortality observed. We aimed to evaluate the relationship between vitamin D use and all-cause mortality.

Methods: In this retrospective cohort study, we included all incident patients who started hemodialysis in Taiwan between 2001 and 2009. Patients were followed from landmark time, i.e., the 360th day from hemodialysis initiation, through the end of 2010 or death. We evaluated the association between activated vitamin D use or not before landmark time and all-cause mortality using conditional landmark analysis with Cox regression. We used group-based trajectory model to categorize high-dose versus average-dose users to evaluate dose-response relationships.

Results: During the median follow-up of 1019 days from landmark time, vitamin D users had a lower crude mortality rate than non-users (8.98 versus 12.93 per 100 person-years). Compared with non-users, vitamin D users was associated with a lower risk of death in multivariate Cox model (HR 0.91 [95% CI, 0.87–0.95]) and after propensity score matching (HR 0.94 [95% CI, 0.90–0.98]). High-dose vitamin D users had a lower risk of death than conventional-dose users, HR 0.75 [95% CI, 0.63–0.89]. The association of vitamin D treatment with reduced mortality did not alter when we re-defined landmark time as the 180th day or repeated analyses in patients who underwent hemodialysis in the hospital setting.

Conclusions: Our findings supported the survival benefits of activated vitamin D among incident hemodialysis patients.

Keywords: Hemodialysis, Activated vitamin D, Prescribing pattern, Mortality, End-stage renal disease (ESRD)

Background

Cardiovascular disease is an important cause of death in patients with chronic kidney disease (CKD) [1, 2]. Apart from diabetes, dyslipidemia, and atherosclerosis, non-traditional risk factors, especially secondary hyperparathyroidism, vascular calcification, and heart failure, all play important roles in patients with CKD and end stage renal disease (ESRD) [3–6]. In addition, vitamin D insufficiency and deficiency, which result from malnutrition, reduced 1α-hydroxylase activity, and increased fibroblast growth factor-23, are highly prevalent in advanced CKD and contribute to secondary hyperparathyroidism and adverse cardiovascular outcomes [7].

In the literature, low 25-hydroxyvitamin D and 1, 25-dihydroxyvitamin D levels are associated with increased all-cause and cardiovascular mortality in the general population, CKD, and uremic patients [8–14]. Pleiotropic effects of activated vitamin D include improving endothelial function, inhibition of vascular smooth muscle proliferation and vascular calcification, suppression of renin production, and modification of inflammatory response [15–18]. Treatment with activated vitamin D is associated with lower incidence of left ventricular hypertrophy, myocardial fibrosis, and pulmonary congestion [17, 19, 20].

* Correspondence: yhkao@mail.ncku.edu.tw
[2]Institute of Clinical Pharmacy and Pharmaceutical Sciences, College of Medicine, National Cheng Kung University, Tainan, Taiwan
Full list of author information is available at the end of the article

Findings from observational studies have suggested that administration of activated vitamin D was associated with reduced mortality and improved cardiovascular outcome in advanced CKD and ESRD patients [21–25]. Results from one study had ever suggested that patients treated with oral activated vitamin D had a 45% reduction in mortality but the survival benefit was inversely related to the vitamin D dose [22]. Findings from another meta-analysis of randomized controlled trials had suggested that treatment of vitamin D compounds was associated with increased risk of hypercalcemia and hyperphosphatemia while inconsistently reducing parathyroid hormone (PTH) levels. The potential beneficial effect on mortality was unproven and underpowered to be evaluated because only few studies reported clinical hard outcomes [26].

In clinical practice, concerns about hypercalcemia and potential vascular calcification have confined treatment of vitamin D in patients with elevated PTH and with relatively low calcium levels. Besides, patients prescribed vitamin D are generally younger and healthier, implying unmeasured confounders that could not be removed by statistical adjustment, which could have biased the findings from previous studies [22, 27, 28].

In Taiwan, the prevalence of ESRD reached 2584 per million in 2010, while rates of 2260 and 1870 were reported in Japan and the United States [29]. Given the potential benefits of activated vitamin D mentioned above, we hypothesized that prescription of activated vitamin D should improve overall outcome in ESRD patients. Regarding the universal coverage of health care and bundled payment for dialysis in Taiwan, the National Health Insurance Research Database (NHIRD) can be employed to examine the effect of activated vitamin D in the real world setting and establish the domestic evidence for clinical practice.

Using NHIRD, we aimed to determine the prevalence of activated vitamin D prescriptions, including calcitriol and alfacalcidol, in incident hemodialysis patients in Taiwan and the association of vitamin D use with potential effect on all-cause mortality.

Methods

Data sources

Taiwan National Health Insurance (NHI) provides comprehensive health care service to over 23 million residents, covering more than 99% of the population in Taiwan since 1995. The NHIRD is established from the de-identified claims data of NHI, which comprise demographic data of enrollees, information of healthcare professionals, medical facilities, and service claims from ambulatory care, hospital admission, and contracted pharmacies.

The registry of catastrophic illness patients is a subset of NHIRD that covers patients with specific severe disease conditions that require close and costly medical care. Because patients with catastrophic illness certificate (CIC) are exempted from co-payment for related medical services, this registry is representative of most, if not all, patients with medically qualified diseases. In Taiwan, ESRD patients with uremia and dialysis dependence are eligible for CIC when they initiate maintenance dialysis, which is reviewed and approved by nephrologists in the National Health Insurance Administration.

All diagnoses in the NHIRD were coded according to the International Classification of Disease, 9th revision, Clinical Modification (ICD-9-CM).

Study design, population and outcome

We included all incident uremic patients that initiated hemodialysis between January 1, 2001 and June 30, 2009. Patients who were younger than 20 years or had past history of malignancy were excluded. Those who had kidney transplant graft failure and re-initiated dialysis were also excluded due to a very small number of patients and different patient characteristics regarding chronic kidney disease and mineral bone disorders. The diagnosis of uremia and long-term dialysis dependence was confirmed using the database of catastrophic illnesses.

The date of the first hemodialysis treatment was defined as the cohort entry date. Concerning that hemodialysis patients had a highest mortality rate during the first year following dialysis initiation [30], we applied landmark design and patients were followed from the 360th day after cohort entry until death or the end of 2010. The study protocol was approved by the Institutional Review Board (IRB) of National Cheng Kung University Hospital (IRB number: A-EX-104-037).

Baseline information and covariates

Baseline information including age, sex, vascular access type, baseline comorbidities, and medications were showed in Table 1. Information of baseline comorbidities were retrieved using diagnostic codes from the claims data of ambulatory care or hospital admission within 90 days prior to or after the date of cohort entry, i.e. the baseline period. We applied the diagnostic codes modified from the Elixhauser comorbidity index to define comorbidities (Additional file 1: Appendix S1) [31]. Co-medications including antiplatelets, warfarin, anti-diabetic agents, statins, angiotensin-converting enzyme inhibitors/Angiotensin II receptor blockers, beta-blockers, diuretics, and erythropoiesis-stimulating agents (Additional file 1: Appendix S2) were retrieved as well during the baseline period. Information of vascular access type (Additional file 1: Appendix S3) were retrieved using procedure codes from claims data of ambulatory care or hospital admission within 360 days prior to or 180 days after the hemodialysis initiation.

Table 1 Baseline characteristics of activated vitamin D users versus non-users according to status by landmark time, before and after propensity score (PS) matching

	Entire cohort			After PS match		
	Vitamin D users	Non-users	d^a	Vitamin D users	Non-users	d^a
N (%)	8151 (15.5)	44,606 (84.5)		7232 (25.0)	21,696 (75.0)	
Age, year	58.9 (14.1)	62.5 (13.3)	0.26	60.7 (13.5)	60.8 (13.7)	< 0.01
< 53	2847 (34.9)	10,949 (24.6)	0.25	1933 (26.7)	5967 (27.5)	0.02
≥ 53 and < 64	2128 (26.1)	11,653 (26.1)		1932 (26.7)	5728 (26.4)	
≥ 64 and < 73	1749 (21.5)	11,325 (25.4)		1776 (24.6)	5123 (23.6)	
≥ 73	1427 (17.5)	10,679 (23.9)		1591 (22.0)	4878 (22.5)	
Gender (male)	3680 (45.2)	22,619 (50.7)	0.11	3540 (48.9)	10,647 (49.7)	< 0.01
Comorbidities						
DM	3327 (40.8)	26,616 (59.7)	0.38	3325 (46.0)	10,032 (46.2)	< 0.01
CHF	2200 (27.0)	15,195 (34.1)	0.15	2136 (29.5)	6438 (29.7)	< 0.01
MI	1932 (23.7)	13,868 (31.1)	0.17	1896 (26.2)	5574 (25.7)	0.01
PVD	259 (3.2)	1509 (3.4)	0.01	242 (3.4)	687 (3.2)	0.01
CVD	774 (9.5)	7095 (15.9)	0.19	774 (10.7)	2388 (11.0)	0.01
COPD	14 (0.2)	128 (0.3)	0.02	14 (0.2)	40 (0.2)	< 0.01
CTD	176 (2.2)	1021 (2.3)	< 0.01	163 (2.3)	498 (2.3)	< 0.01
PUD	1344 (16.5)	8023 (18.0)	0.04	1252 (17.3)	3605 (16.6)	0.02
Neoplasia	10 (0.1)	56 (0.1)	< 0.01	9 (0.1)	30 (0.1)	< 0.01
Chronic liver diseases	1001 (12.3)	5353 (12.0)	< 0.01	917 (12.7)	2643 (12.2)	0.02
Vascular access type			0.15			0.06
AVF	6372 (78.2)	34,240 (76.7)		5811 (80.4)	17,145 (79.2)	
AVG	617 (7.6)	4308 (9.7)		585 (8.1)	1833 (8.5)	
Permanent catheter	116 (1.4)	1097 (2.5)		110 (1.5)	443 (2.0)	
Double lumen catheter	539 (6.6)	3219 (7.2)		389 (5.4)	1392 (6.4)	
Unknown	507 (6.2)	1742 (3.9)		337 (4.7)	883 (4.1)	
Medications						
Antiplatelets[b]	3929 (48.2)	24,796 (55.6)	0.15	3687 (50.9)	10,900 (50.2)	0.01
Aspirin / Clopidogrel	2324 (28.5)	15,600 (35.0)	0.14	2189 (30.3)	6567 (30.3)	< 0.01
Cilostazol	154 (1.9)	1146 (2.6)	0.05	147 (2.0)	440 (2.0)	< 0.01
Warfarin	143 (1.8)	988 (2.2)	0.03	140 (1.9)	387 (1.8)	0.01
Statins	1373 (16.8)	9535 (21.4)	0.12	1303 (18.0)	3820 (17.6)	0.01
Insulin	1615 (19.8)	12,898 (28.9)	0.21	1604 (22.2)	4825 (22.2)	< 0.01
OAD	1812 (22.2)	16,003 (35.9)	0.30	1809 (25.0)	5579 (25.7)	0.02
Metformin	179 (2.2)	1857 (4.2)	0.11	179 (2.5)	530 (2.4)	< 0.01
Sulfonylurea	917 (11.3)	8041 (18.0)	0.19	917 (12.7)	2893 (13.3)	0.02
α-glucosidase inhibitors	148 (1.8)	1478 (3.3)	0.09	148 (2.1)	458 (2.1)	< 0.01
TZD	81 (1.0)	684 (1.5)	0.05	80 (1.1)	253 (1.2)	< 0.01
DPP-4 inhibitors	2 (0.02)	5 (0.01)	0.01	0 (0.00)	1 (0.00)	< 0.01
Meglitinides	485 (6.0)	3938 (8.8)	0.11	485 (6.7)	1444 (6.7)	< 0.01
ACEI / ARB	3972 (48.7)	23,726 (53.2)	0.09	3569 (49.4)	10,730 (49.5)	< 0.01
Beta-blockers	4173 (51.2)	24,243 (54.4)	0.06	3764 (52.1)	11,205 (51.7)	0.01
Diuretics	5737 (70.4)	34,377 (77.1)	0.15	5229 (72.3)	15,793 (72.8)	0.01
ESA	1887 (23.2)	10,133 (22.7)	0.01	1691 (23.4)	5011 (23.1)	0.01

Note:
(1) The landmark time is the 360th day of initiation of hemodialysis
(2) Values for categorical variables are given as numbers (percent); for continuous variables, as means (standard deviation)
Abbreviations: *DM* diabetes mellitus, *CHF* congestive heart failure, *MI* myocardial infarction, *PVD* peripheral vascular disease, *CVD* cerebrovascular disease, *COPD* chronic obstructive pulmonary disease, *CTD* connective tissue disease including rheumatoid arthritis, systemic lupus erythematosus, etc, *PUD* peptic ulcer disease; Chronic liver diseases: chronic viral hepatitis, cirrhosis and its complications, *AVF* arteriovenous fistula, *AVG* arteriovenous graft, *PS* propensity score, *OAD* oral antidiabetic drugs, *TZD* thiazolidinediones, *DPP-4 inhibitors* dipeptidyl peptidase 4 inhibitors, *ACEI / ARB* angiotensin converting enzyme inhibitors/angiotensin II receptor blockers, *ESA* erythropoiesis-stimulating agents
[a]Standardized difference (*d*): statistically significantly different between two comparison groups if *d* > 0.10
[b]Antiplatelets included aspirin, clopidogrel, cilostazol, dipyridamole and ticlopidine

Exposure of oral activated vitamin D and landmark design

Records of oral activated vitamin D, including calcitriol and alfacalcidol, during each hemodialysis session, ambulatory care, and hospital admission were collected. Considering the relatively late initiation of activated vitamin D in uremic patients in Taiwan and high mortality rate especially in the first year of dialysis initiation, we chose the 360th day after cohort entry as the landmark time in order to obtain more patients prescribed vitamin D (180th day as an alternative in the sensitivity analysis) to recruit as many patients in the analysis as possible [32, 33]. Patients were classified as vitamin D users or non-users according to whether they were prescribed vitamin D before the landmark time, regardless of subsequent changes in vitamin D status [34]. Patients who died or were lost to follow-up before the landmark date were excluded. This study design helps to eliminate immortal time bias or "time-to-treatment" bias.

Statistical analyses

For baseline characteristics, we used standardized difference (d) to compare the difference between vitamin D users and non-users, where less than 0.10 indicates a negligible difference between treatment groups [35, 36].

We reported crude mortality rate and estimated overall survival using Kaplan-Meier method. Conditional landmark analysis with Cox proportional hazards regression was used to evaluate mortality hazard ratios (HR) in relation to activated vitamin D use, adjusting for potential confounders. The covariates of the model included age, sex, vascular access type, baseline comorbidities, and medications.

All statistical analyses were conducted using SAS version 9.4 (SAS Institute Inc., Cary, NC).

Propensity score method

To minimize potential confounding, we calculated propensity score (PS) of oral activated vitamin D prescriptions using age, sex, vascular access type, baseline comorbidities, and co-medications. PS trimming and inverse probability treatment weighting (IPTW) were applied to estimate population average treatment effects. Greedy algorithm was employed to match vitamin D users to non-users on PS with a ratio of 1:3 [37]. Mortality hazard ratio was estimated using PS trimming, IPTW weighting, and PS matching.

Trajectory model

To examine the dose gradient between vitamin D use and clinical outcomes, we calculated cumulative dosage in three 120-day periods within the first 360 days of hemodialysis initiation. Only those who survived 360 days were included in the analysis. In dialysis patients, the initiation and titration dosage of calcitriol or alfacalcidol are mostly 0.25 μg per day or every other day [38, 39]. We thus defined 0.25 μg as the single dosage unit for activated vitamin D for ease of reference.

For the dynamic nature of vitamin D prescription over time, we modeled the three 120-day cumulative dosage as the longitudinal outcome and used logistic regression for the group-based trajectory models [40]. Patients were classified into high-dose and average-dose users. We evaluated where the dose-response relationship existed.

Sensitivity analyses

Two sensitivity analyses were performed. It has been noted that a high incidence of drug record discrepancies existed in out-patient hemodialysis [41]. One of the most common medication-related problems is "indication without drug therapy" [42, 43]. To solve this, we performed the first sensitivity analysis by analyzing patients who received maintenance hemodialysis in hospital-based dialysis units from the 345th through 375th day of hemodialysis initiation. The urbanization of city/township where the hospital was located and the hospital accreditation level were incorporated into the Cox and PS models [44].

Using the landmark design, the patient selection was conditioned on the survival time [34]. Based on the study of the primary analysis, we included patients who survived more than 360 days to ensure adequate observation periods for vitamin D observation. However, the design limited the generalizability of our finding. We performed the second sensitivity analysis by change the landmark time to the 180th day of cohort entry to justify the robustness of our finding.

Results

Between Jan 1, 2001 and June 30, 2009, there were 83,433 incident uremic patients who had undergone hemodialysis treatment for more than 90 days. After exclusion of those who were not eligible for CIC ($n = 21,380$) either due to renal function recovery or non-continuation of dialysis therapy, those registered "dead" but with missing death date ($n = 350$), and those with date of vitamin D prescription later than the last recorded date of dialysis therapy ($n = 218$), a total of 61,485 patients were included (Fig. 1). Patients who were not eligible for CIC were healthier and had fewer comorbidities (data not shown).

Of these 61,485 patients, 15,793 (25.7%) patients had ever been prescribed oral activated vitamin D during the follow-up period. The median duration of vitamin D use were 354 days (IQR 89–973 days). Among these patients, 8867 (56.1%) received vitamin D in the first

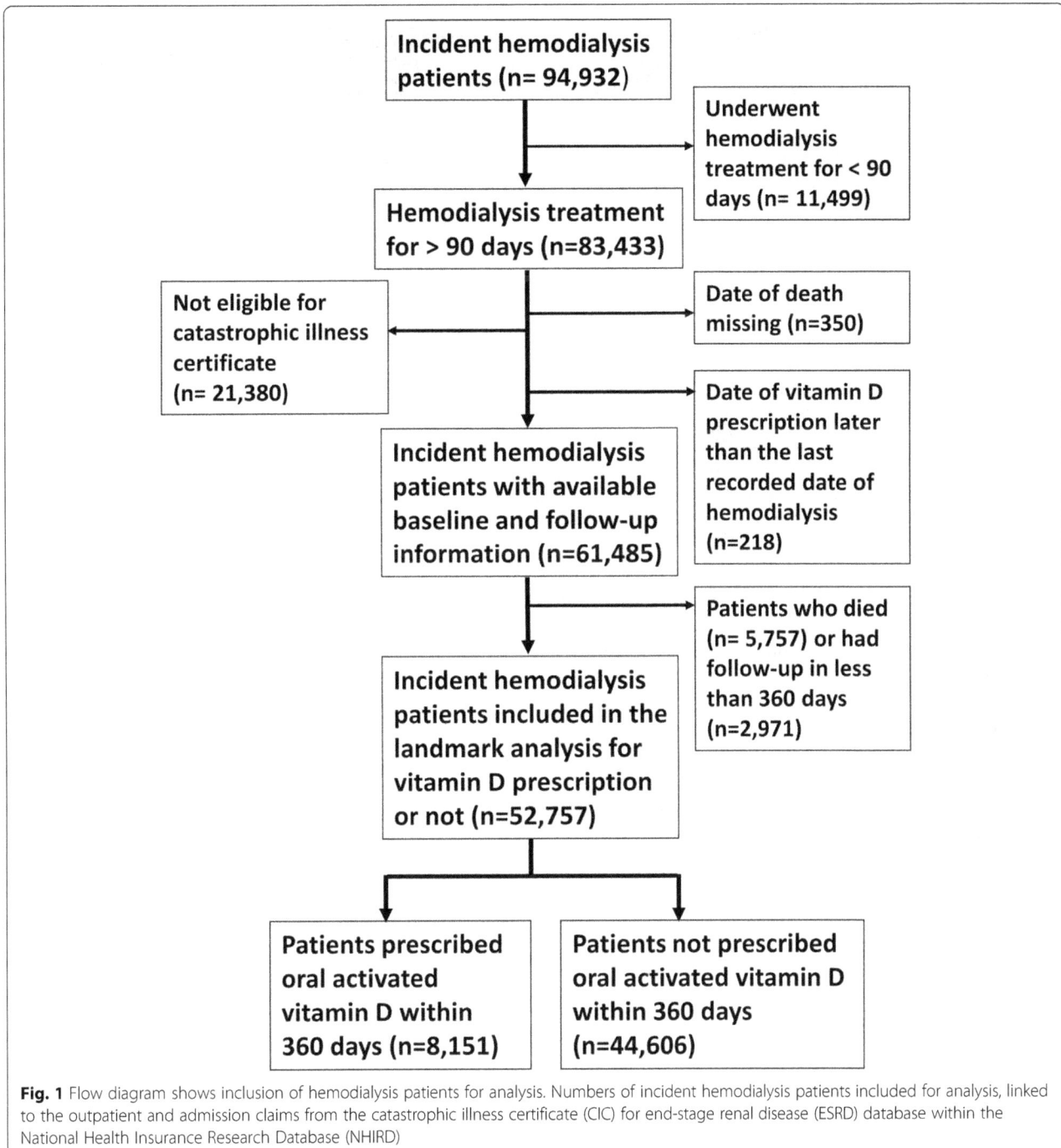

Fig. 1 Flow diagram shows inclusion of hemodialysis patients for analysis. Numbers of incident hemodialysis patients included for analysis, linked to the outpatient and admission claims from the catastrophic illness certificate (CIC) for end-stage renal disease (ESRD) database within the National Health Insurance Research Database (NHIRD)

360 days after hemodialysis initiation (Additional file 1: Table S1).

Patients who died (n = 5757) or had follow-up less than 360 days (n = 2971) were excluded from analysis (Fig. 1). Vitamin D users (n = 8151) were significantly younger and healthier than non-users (n = 44,606), with less prevalence of diabetes and accompanying past histories of myocardial infarction or stroke. Vitamin D users also had more prevalent use of arteriovenous fistula and less use of graft or permanent catheters as long-term vascular access (Table 1).

By the end of the follow-up from the landmark time (median 1019, IQR 473–1777 days), there were 2619 deaths during 29,158.6 person-years of observation (crude mortality rate 8.98 per 100 person-years) among vitamin D users, as compared with 18,482 deaths during 142,948.7 person-years follow-up (12.93 per 100 person-years) among non-users (Additional file 1: Table S2). The survival curve of activated vitamin D users and non-users was shown (Fig. 2). Vitamin D users were less likely to die compared to non-users in unadjusted (HR

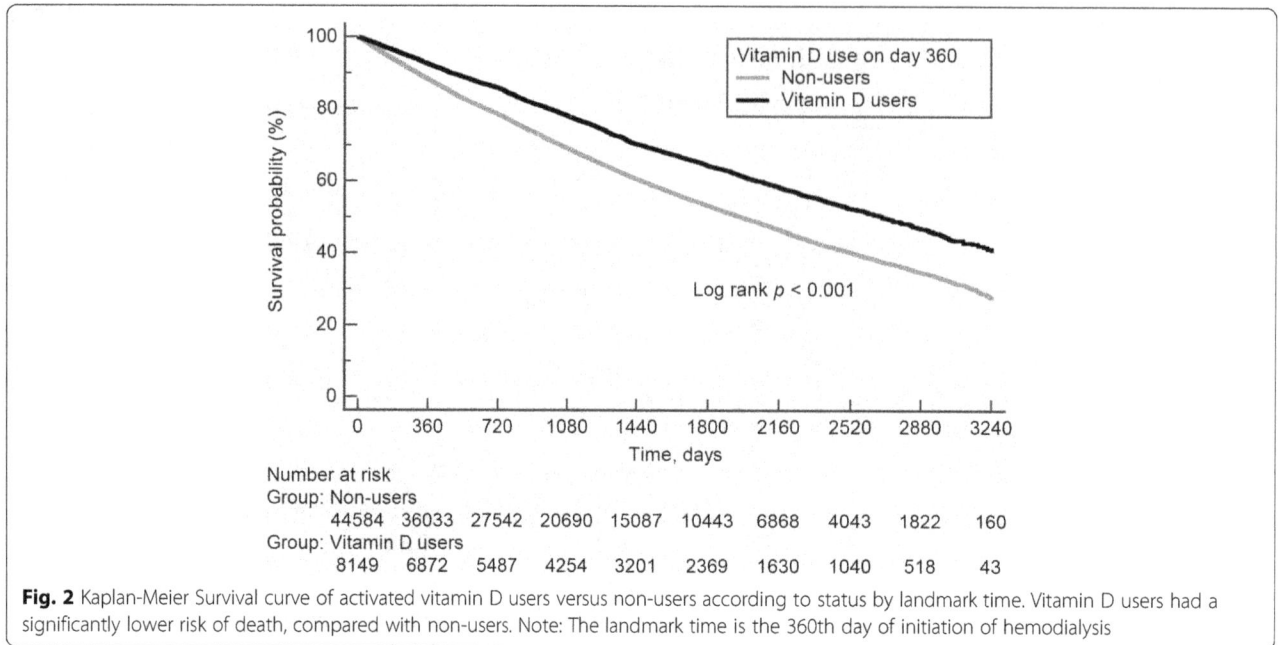

Fig. 2 Kaplan-Meier Survival curve of activated vitamin D users versus non-users according to status by landmark time. Vitamin D users had a significantly lower risk of death, compared with non-users. Note: The landmark time is the 360th day of initiation of hemodialysis

0.69 [95% CI, 0.66–0.72]) and multivariate adjusted model (HR 0.91 [95% CI, 0.87–0.95]) (Table 2).

After propensity score method employed and matching, the baseline covariates were balanced between vitamin D users and non-users (Table 1). The overlap of the distribution of propensity score across vitamin D users and non-users were displayed, before and after PS matching (Additional file 1: Figures S1 and S2), respectively. Vitamin D users still had a lower risk of death with the method of PS trimming (HR 0.71 [95% CI, 0.68–0.74]), IPTW (HR 0.94 [95% CI, 0.92–0.96]), and PS matching (HR 0.94 [95% CI, 0.90–0.98]) (Table 2). We

had further performed a matched pairs analysis from which vitamin D users still had a lower risk of death (HR 0.91 [95% CI, 0.86–0.96]), compared with non-users.

To evaluate prescribing pattern and examine the dose response relationship, ambulatory claims for activated vitamin D prescriptions were collected in the first 360 days after hemodialysis initiation. Using 0.25 µg as dosage unit, the median (IQR) cumulative dosage were 80 (35–168), 60 (30–112) and 60 (30–112) units in three 120-day intervals, respectively (Additional file 1: Table S3).

Table 2 Multivariate Cox proportional hazards models examining activated vitamin D treatment as compared with no treatment by landmark time

Model	HR (95% CI)
Unadjusted	0.69 (0.66–0.72)
Adjusted	
Age and sex	0.79 (0.76–0.82)
Age, sex, and comorbidities	0.90 (0.86–0.94)
Age, sex, vascular access type, and comorbidities	0.90 (0.87–0.94)
Age, sex, comorbidities, and medications	0.90 (0.87–0.94)
Age, sex, vascular access type, comorbidities and medications	0.91 (0.87–0.95)
Propensity score (PS) method	
PS trimming (1–99%)	0.71 (0.68–0.74)
PS trimming + IPTW	0.94 (0.92–0.96)
PS matching	0.94 (0.90–0.98)

Note: The landmark time is the 360th day of initiation of hemodialysis
Propensity score (PS): PS was calculated with logistic regression using covariates of age, sex, vascular access type, baseline comorbidities, and medications. The PS matched methods we employed compared vitamin D users versus non-users without further adjustment of baseline covariates
Abbreviation: *HR* hazard ratio, *CI* confidence intervals, *PS* propensity score, *IPTW* inverse probability treatment weighting

In the trajectory analysis (Additional file 1: Appendix S4), 326 (6.2%) patients were noted to have been given higher than average doses, while the remaining 6849 (93.8%) were prescribed the conventional daily dosage (Fig. 3). Whether high dose or conventional dose vitamin D users, they were prescribed higher dose in the first 120 days. After adjustments of potential confounders, we observed a significant survival benefit in patients receiving conventional dose (HR 0.88 [95% CI, 0.84–0.92]) and high dose activated vitamin D (HR 0.66 [95% CI, 0.55–0.78]) (Table 3). Compared with conventional dosage group, the high dose group still had a lower risk of death (HR 0.75 [95% CI, 0.63–0.89]).

We did sensitivity analyses by analyzing patients who had regular hemodialysis in hospital-based dialysis units. The activated vitamin D users ($n = 5449$) were still younger (58.7 versus 62.1 years) and had fewer baseline comorbidities than non-users ($n = 23,245$). The crude mortality rate was lower in vitamin D users compared with non-users (8.60 versus 12.36 per 100 person-years) (Additional file 1: Table S2). After adjustment for age, sex, vascular access type, comorbidities, medications, urbanization, and hospital levels, vitamin D users were still associated with a lower risk of death (HR 0.91 [95% CI, 0.87–0.96]). Using PS matching, vitamin D users still had a lower risk of death (HR 0.95 [95% CI, 0.89–1.00]) (Table 4).

Additionally, we compared 6848 vitamin D users with 50,921 non-users, using the 180th day after hemodialysis

initiation as the landmark time. Vitamin D users were noted to have a lower risk of death in the multivariate adjusted (HR 0.87 [95% CI, 0.84–0.91]) and PS matched model (HR 0.94 [95% CI, 0.90–0.98]), compared with non-users. After trajectory analysis and adjustment of potential confounders, high-dose vitamin D users still had a lower risk of death, compared with non-users (HR 0.64 [95% CI, 0.55–0.74]) and conventional dose users (HR 0.76 [95% CI, 0.65–0.89]), respectively.

Discussion

In this cohort of 61,485 incident hemodialysis patients between 2001 and 2010, patients treated with oral activated vitamin D in the first 360 days after dialysis initiation had a survival advantage compared with those not treated, even after adjustment for potential confounders. The result was significant in the entire cohort using a different landmark time and subgroup of hospital-based hemodialysis patients. The presence of dose-response relationship further supported the potential benefit of activated vitamin D prescription in these patients.

According to the Dialysis Outcomes and Practice Pattern Study (DOPPS), intravenous vitamin D was most common in the United States but oral administration was more prevalent in all other countries. The percentage of patients on vitamin D were 33% in France, 66% in the United States, and 39% in Japan in the DOPPS III (2005–2006) [27]. In the Current Management of Secondary hyperparathyroidism – a multicenter Observational Study

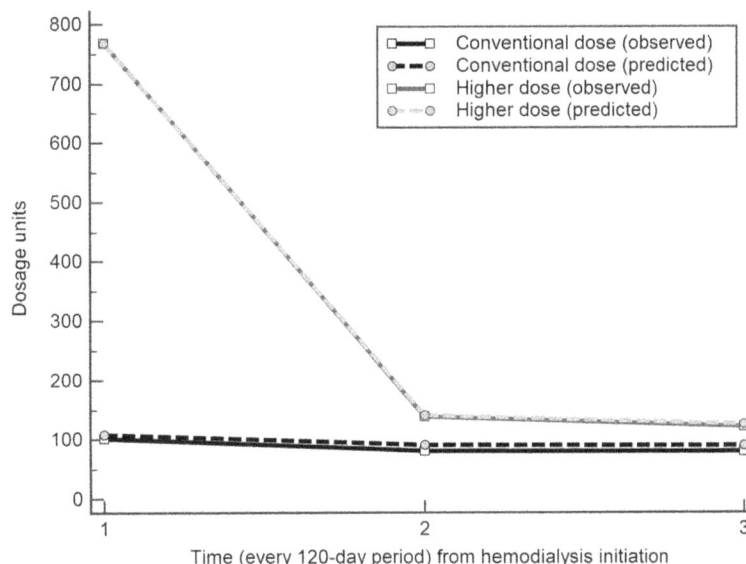

Fig. 3 Result of group-based trajectory analysis. Trajectory of vitamin D dosage grouping from initiation of hemodialysis in the first 360 days. Trajectory model using 2 groups. Every 0.25 μg of calcitriol or alfacalcidol was defined as one dosage unit. The predicted dosage unit in each group is plotted with dotted lines. The observed proportion of individuals in each group are plotted in solid lines. After exclusion of the patients with upper 99th percentile dosage ($n = 196$) and application of trajectory analysis, the majority (dark black line) of vitamin D users ($n = 6849$) received a median of 110 (IQR 45–220) dosage units, while the remaining 326 patients (grey line) received higher cumulative dosages, median 805 (IQR 635–1080) dosage units, in the first 360 days

Table 3 Crude mortality rate and multivariate adjusted hazard ratio for mortality according to the different dosage categories of oral activated vitamin D based on trajectory analysis

	N (%)	Follow-up (person-years)	Death (%)	Crude mortality rate (per 100 person-year)	Adjusted HR[b] (95% CI)
Non-users	45,386 (86.0)	145,396.7	18,853 (41.5)	12.97	Reference
Conventional dose vitamin D	6849 (13.0)	24,398.0	2112 (30.8)	8.66	0.88 (0.84–0.92)
High dose vitamin D users[a]	522 (1.0)	2312.6	136 (26.1)	5.88	0.66 (0.55–0.78)
Overall	52,757 (100)	172,107.3	21,101 (40.0)	12.26	

Abbreviations: HR hazard ratio, *CI* confidence intervals
[a]The high dose vitamin D users consisted of the upper 99th percentile of dosage prescriptions (*n* = 196) that were previously excluded from trajectory analysis plus the minority of higher dose vitamin D users (*n* = 326) in the trajectory analysis
[b]The Cox model was adjusted by covariates including age, sex, vascular access type, baseline comorbidities, and medications

(COSMOS), 48% of prevalent hemodialysis patients in Europe were using activated vitamin D, mostly calcitriol and alfacalcidol [45].

In Taiwan, oral route but not intravenous administration of activated vitamin D is reimbursed by the NHI. In our study, we found that only 25.7% of patients had ever been prescribed activated vitamin D, exclusively in oral form. The prescription of activated vitamin D in Taiwan was not as prevalent or as early as those in the United States and European countries [24, 27, 45]. This may result from the different indications between vitamin D supplementation and suppression of parathyroid hyperplasia [46]. Higher geographic latitude or dark skin may be associated with a higher prevalence of vitamin D deficiency, higher PTH levels, and more prescriptions of activated vitamin D [47]. In Taiwan, the widespread use of inexpensive calcium-containing phosphate binders may lead to reduced PTH levels, which contributed to fewer prescriptions of vitamin D. In addition, the level of vitamin D was rarely tested in ESRD patients in Taiwan and

activated vitamin D was often prescribed for secondary hyperparathyroidism, which often developed in the later dialysis vintage. The median time to the first prescription was 252 (IQR 31–919) days after hemodialysis initiation, obviously later than that in the DOPPS, although the exact indications and levels of PTH were not available from the NHIRD.

In the literature, oral calcitriol use was associated with lower all-cause mortality in CKD stage 3–4 patients. In these non-dialyzed CKD studies, patients given calcitriol were older, having higher PTH level and lower glomerular filtration rate, and more were diabetics [21, 23]. In contrast, evidence from observational studies of hemodialysis patients have shown that patients prescribed activated vitamin D were younger and healthier [22, 24]. Different from the above studies, our study did not choose time-dependent exposure to assess vitamin D effect because the concept of time-dependent has been thought of as more focused on the "state of exposure" on the outcome rather than the effect of early

Table 4 Multivariate Cox proportional hazard models examining activated vitamin D treatment as compared with no treatment by landmark time in hospital-setting hemodialysis patients

Model	HR (95% CI)
Unadjusted	0.69 (0.66–0.73)
Adjusted	
Urbanization and hospital level	0.72 (0.68–0.76)
Age and sex	0.78 (0.74–0.82)
Age, sex, urbanization, and hospital level	0.80 (0.76–0.84)
Age, sex, vascular access type, and comorbidities	0.89 (0.85–0.94)
Age, sex, comorbidities, and baseline medications	0.90 (0.85–0.95)
Age, sex, urbanization, hospital level, vascular access, comorbidities, and baseline medications	0.91 (0.87–0.96)
Propensity score (PS) method	
PS trimming (1–99%)	0.70 (0.67–0.74)
PS trimming + IPTW	0.95 (0.92–0.97)
PS matching (1: 3)	0.95 (0.89–1.00)

Propensity score (PS): PS was calculated with logistic regression using covariates of age, sex, vascular access type, baseline comorbidities, medications, and levels of hospital and urbanization. The PS matched methods was employed compared vitamin D users versus non-users without further adjustment of baseline covariates
Abbreviations: HR hazard ratio, *CI* confidence intervals, *PS* propensity score, *IPTW* inverse probability treatment weighting

vitamin D supplement or exposure on the long-term outcome. We also did not use marginal structural model (MSM) to deal with time-varying covariates because of lack of laboratory data and detailed comorbidity information in claims data of hemodialysis treatment in the NHI. Instead, we retrieved not only diagnostic codes but comprehensive medication use and vascular access type obtained from claims data of all medical services during baseline periods, which were deemed reliable for input in PS to adjust for imbalance between vitamin D users versus non-users.

Survival benefits of oral calcitriol have been found, in those receiving mean daily doses of less than 1 μg [22]. However, the author also found that the lower the vitamin D dose, the lower the risk of death. Using MSM, Miller et al. [48]. have found that higher dose paricalcitol was associated with greater survival in hemodialysis patients but failed to confirm this using conventional Cox model or PS matched method. However, patients taking paricalcitol represented a small proportion of the hemodialysis population in the U.S., and thus, the result could not be extrapolated to populations in other countries [48]. Concerning the high cost, paricalcitol is not reimbursed in the NHI and thus rarely used in Taiwan practically.

Randomized controlled trials comparing activated vitamin D use versus placebo are unacceptable ethically. Thus, observational studies still have a role in leading the trend of clinical practice.

The strength of this study is the large real-life cohort with detailed information of comorbidities and co-medications and a long follow-up duration up to 10 years. In addition, the inclusion of incident hemodialysis patients with utilization of landmark design reduced immortal time bias [49]. Although the design of landmark analysis introduced misclassification bias when some vitamin D users were categorized into non-users, as may underestimate the effect of vitamin D, the true beneficial effect must be even greater since we found a lower risk of mortality in vitamin D users. Despite lack of active comparators, we adopted PS matching and reduced the imbalance between users and non-users.

Additionally, our study had illustrated trajectories of vitamin D prescription dosage and to highlighted the temporal changes in the first 360 days of dialysis initiation. It is straightforward to use trajectories to classify different dosage groups which may help us to determine the dose exposure patterns. The positive association of higher dose calcitriol or alfacalcidol and reduced all-cause mortality in our analysis further supported the beneficial effect of activated vitamin D in hemodialysis patients. Reducing use of calcium-based phosphate binders should be considered to trade off for more

activated vitamin D prescriptions to avoid the risk of hypercalcemia, inadequately suppressed PTH levels, or low bone turnover disease. Further study may be needed.

One major limitation of our study is that there were no laboratory data such as calcium, phosphorus, PTH, hemoglobin, smoking status, and markers of inflammatory status available from Taiwan NHI medical claims.

We conducted a stratified analysis in only female patients to minimize the potential confounding by smoking since the prevalence of smoking is very low (4.3%) among female population in Taiwan [50]. Compared with non-users, vitamin D users were associated with a lower all-cause mortality risk (HR 0.89 [95% CI, 0.84–0.94]) in females who were largely non-smokers. Such reduced effect observed in females was also similarly observed in male patients (HR 0.93 [95% CI, 0.87–0.98]), who had a smoking prevalence of 46.8%. This sex-stratified analyses provided further reassurance that the potential of confounding by smoking is very small in our study.

The overall mortality in this hemodialysis cohort in Taiwan was substantially lower than that in other countries, as may result from different race, life style, or fewer cardiovascular events and better medical accessibility due to comprehensive health insurance coverage [30, 51]. The observation from our study implies that using inexpensive activated vitamin D may bring about significant survival benefit, even though newer vitamin D analogs with fewer hypercalcemic side effects were not prescribed extensively in Taiwan.

Conclusions

In incident hemodialysis patients, treatment of oral calcitriol or alfacalcidol was associated with lower risks of death. There was no excess risk for death in patients receiving higher doses of vitamin D. Therefore, our data supports the prescription of activated vitamin D in these patients unless contraindicated.

Additional file

Additional file 1: Table S1. The frequency in incident hemodialysis patients according to first-time prescription of activated vitamin D. **Table S2.** Events of death and crude mortality rates by status of vitamin D use on the landmark time in the entire cohort and subgroup of patients in hospital-based hemodialysis setting. **Table S3.** Cumulative and average dosage units of vitamin D use in each 120-day period of the first 360 days of hemodialysis initiation. **Appendix S1.** Details of diagnostic codes to retrieve comorbidity information from baseline period. **Appendix S2.** Details of prescribed medication during baseline period. **Appendix S3.** Details of procedure codes of vascular access type. **Appendix S4.** Details of trajectory model for vitamin D dosage category. **Figures S1 and S2.** The distribution of propensity score across vitamin D users and non-users before and after propensity score matching (DOCX 86 kb)

Abbreviations
ACEI / ARB: angiotensin converting enzyme inhibitors/angiotensin II receptor blockers; AVF: Arteriovenous fistula; AVG: Arteriovenous graft; CHF: Congestive heart failure; Chronic liver diseases: Chronic viral hepatitis, cirrhosis and its complications; CIC: Catastrophic illness certificate; CKD: Chronic kidney disease; COPD: Chronic obstructive pulmonary disease; CTD: Connective tissue disease including rheumatoid arthritis, systemic lupus erythematosus, etc.; CVD: Cerebrovascular disease; DM: Diabetes mellitus; DPP-4 inhibitors: Dipeptidyl peptidase 4 inhibitors; ESA: Erythropoiesis-stimulating agents; ESRD: End stage renal disease; IPTW: Inverse probability treatment weighting; MI: Myocardial infarction; NHI: National Health Insurance; NHIRD: National Health Insurance Research Database; OAD: Oral antidiabetic drugs; PS: Propensity score; PTH: Parathyroid hormone; PUD: Peptic ulcer disease; PVD: Peripheral vascular disease; TZD: Thiazolidinediones

Acknowledgements
Not applicable

Funding
This work was supported by grants from National Cheng Kung University Hospital, College of Medicine, National Cheng Kung University, Tainan, Taiwan (NCKUH-10503018). http://crc.hosp.ncku.edu.tw/upload/insidePlan/files/105.pdf
The funders had no role in study design, data collection and analysis, decision to publish, or preparation of the manuscript.

Authors' contributions
JYC the design of study, data collection and statistical analysis, interpretation, critical appraisal of the paper, and drafting of the work. HCC the design of the study, interpretation, critical appraisal of the paper, and editing of the work. THK the design of the study, statistical analysis, and critical appraisal of the paper. YTC the interpretation and critical appraisal of the paper. MCW the interpretation, critical appraisal of the paper, and editing of the work. CYL the interpretation, critical appraisal of the paper, and editing of the work. YHKY - the interpretation, critical appraisal of the paper, and editing of the work. All authors contributed to the development of the manuscript, and approved the final version.

Competing interests
The authors declare that they have no competing interests.

Author details
[1]Division of Nephrology, Department of Internal Medicine, National Cheng Kung University Hospital, College of Medicine, National Cheng Kung University, No.1, University Road, Tainan 70101, Taiwan. [2]Institute of Clinical Pharmacy and Pharmaceutical Sciences, College of Medicine, National Cheng Kung University, Tainan, Taiwan. [3]Department of Public Health, College of Medicine, National Cheng Kung University, Tainan, Taiwan. [4]Graduate Institute of Clinical Medicine, College of Medicine, National Cheng Kung University, Tainan, Taiwan.

References
1. Sarnak MJ, Levey AS, Schoolwerth AC, Coresh J, Culleton B, Hamm LL, McCullough PA, Kasiske BL, Kelepouris E, Klag MJ, et al. Kidney disease as a risk factor for development of cardiovascular disease: a statement from the American Heart Association councils on kidney in cardiovascular disease, high blood pressure research, clinical cardiology, and epidemiology and prevention. Circulation. 2003;108(17):2154–69.
2. Gutiérrez OM, Mannstadt M, Isakova T, Rauh-Hain JA, Tamez H, Shah A, Smith K, Lee H, Thadhani R, Jüppner H, et al. Fibroblast growth factor 23 and mortality among patients undergoing hemodialysis. New Engl J Med. 2008;359(6):584–92.
3. Kidney Disease: Improving Global Outcomes (KDIGO) CKD-MBD Work Group. KDIGO clinical practice guideline for the diagnosis, evaluation, prevention, and treatment of chronic kidney disease - mineral and bone disorder (CKD-MBD). Kidney Int. 2009;76(Suppl 113):S1–130.
4. Barreto DV, Barreto FC, Liabeuf S, Temmar M, Boitte F, Choukroun G, Fournier A, Massy ZA. Vitamin D affects survival independently of vascular calcification in chronic kidney disease. Clin J Am Soc Nephrol. 2009;4(6): 1128–35.
5. National Kidney. F. KDOQI clinical practice guideline for hemodialysis adequacy: 2015 update. Am J Kidney Dis. 2015;66(5):884–930.
6. Garcia-Canton C, Bosch E, Ramirez A, Gonzalez Y, Auyanet I, Guerra R, Perez MA, Fernandez E, Toledo A, Lago M, et al. Vascular calcification and 25-hydroxyvitamin D levels in non-dialysis patients with chronic kidney disease stages 4 and 5. Nephrol Dial Transplant. 2011;26(7):2250–6.
7. Gutierrez OM. Fibroblast growth factor 23 and disordered vitamin D metabolism in chronic kidney disease: updating the "trade-off" hypothesis. Clin J Am Soc Nephrol. 2010;5(9):1710–6.
8. Kendrick J, Cheung AK, Kaufman JS, Greene T, Roberts WL, Smits G, Chonchol M, Investigators HS. Associations of plasma 25-hydroxyvitamin D and 1,25-dihydroxyvitamin D concentrations with death and progression to maintenance dialysis in patients with advanced kidney disease. Am J Kidney Dis. 2012;60(4):567–75.
9. Navaneethan SD, Schold JD, Arrigain S, Jolly SE, Jain A, Schreiber MJ Jr, Simon JF, Srinivas TR, Nally JV Jr. Low 25-hydroxyvitamin D levels and mortality in non-dialysis-dependent CKD. Am J Kidney Dis. 2011;58(4): 536–43.
10. Pilz S, Iodice S, Zittermann A, Grant WB, Gandini S. Vitamin D status and mortality risk in CKD: a meta-analysis of prospective studies. Am J Kidney Dis. 2011;58(3):374–82.
11. Melamed ML, Michos ED, Post W, Astor B. 25-Hydroxyvitamin D levels and the risk of mortality in the general population. Arch Intern Med. 2008; 168(15):1629–37.
12. Wolf M, Shah A, Gutierrez O, Ankers E, Monroy M, Tamez H, Steele D, Chang Y, Camargo CA Jr, Tonelli M, et al. Vitamin D levels and early mortality among incident hemodialysis patients. Kidney Int. 2007;72(8):1004–13.
13. Lavie CJ, Lee JH, Milani RV. Vitamin D and Cardiovascular disease - will it live up to its hype? J Am Coll Cardiol. 2011;58(15):1547–56.
14. Wang TJ, Pencina MJ, Booth SL, Jacques PF, Ingelsson E, Lanier K, Benjamin EJ, D'Agostino RB, Wolf M, Vasan RS. Vitamin D deficiency and risk of cardiovascular disease. Circulation. 2008;117(4):503–11.
15. Mathew S, Lund RJ, Chaudhary LR, Geurs T, Hruska KA. Vitamin D receptor activators can protect against vascular calcification. J Am Soc Nephrol. 2008; 19(8):1509–19.
16. Reddy Vanga S, Good M, Howard PA, Vacek JL. Role of vitamin D in cardiovascular health. Am J Cardiol. 2010;106(6):798–805.
17. Panizo S, Barrio-Vazquez S, Naves-Diaz M, Carrillo-Lopez N, Rodriguez I, Fernandez-Vazquez A, Valdivielso JM, Thadhani R, Cannata-Andia JB. Vitamin D receptor activation, left ventricular hypertrophy and myocardial fibrosis. Nephrol Dial Transplant. 2013;28(11):2735–44.
18. London GM, Guerin AP, Verbeke FH, Pannier B, Boutouyrie P, Marchais SJ, Metivier F. Mineral metabolism and arterial functions in end-stage renal disease: potential role of 25-hydroxyvitamin D deficiency. J Am Soc Nephrol. 2007;18(2):613–20.
19. Sueta S, Morozumi K, Takeda A, Horike K, Otsuka Y, Shinjo H, Murata M, Kato Y, Goto K, Inaguma D, et al. Ability of vitamin D receptor activator to prevent pulmonary congestion in advanced chronic kidney disease. Clin Exp Nephrol. 2015;19(3):371–8.
20. Wang AY, Fang F, Chan J, Wen YY, Qing S, Chan IH, Lo G, Lai KN, Lo WK, Lam CW, et al. Effect of paricalcitol on left ventricular mass and function in CKD--the OPERA trial. J Am Soc Nephrol. 2014;25(1):175–86.
21. Kovesdy CP, Ahmadzadeh S, Anderson JE, Kalantar-Zadeh K. Association of activated vitamin D treatment and mortality in chronic kidney disease. Arch Intern Med. 2008;168(4):397–403.
22. Naves-Diaz M, Alvarez-Hernandez D, Passlick-Deetjen J, Guinsburg A, Marelli C, Rodriguez-Puyol D, Cannata-Andia JB. Oral active vitamin D is associated with improved survival in hemodialysis patients. Kidney Int. 2008;74(8):1070–8.
23. Shoben AB, Rudser KD, de Boer IH, Young B, Kestenbaum B. Association of oral calcitriol with improved survival in nondialyzed CKD. J Am Soc Nephrol. 2008;19(8):1613–9.
24. Teng M, Wolf M, Ofsthun MN, Lazarus JM, Hernan MA, Camargo CA Jr, Thadhani R. Activated injectable vitamin D and hemodialysis survival: a historical cohort study. J Am Soc Nephrol. 2005;16(4):1115 25.
25. Zheng Z, Shi H, Jia J, Li D, Lin S. Vitamin D supplementation and mortality risk in chronic kidney disease: a meta-analysis of 20 observational studies. BMC Nephrol. 2013;14:199.
26. Palmer SC, McGregor DO, Macaskill P, Craig JC, Elder GJ, Strippoli GFM. Meta-analysis: vitamin D compounds in chronic kidney disease. Ann Intern Med. 2007;147(12):840–53.

27. Tentori F, Albert JM, Young EW, Blayney MJ, Robinson BM, Pisoni RL, Akiba T, Greenwood RN, Kimata N, Levin NW, et al. The survival advantage for haemodialysis patients taking vitamin D is questioned: findings from the Dialysis outcomes and practice patterns study. Nephrol Dial Transplant. 2009;24(3):963–72.

28. Thadhani R. Is calcitriol life-protective for patients with chronic kidney disease? J Am Soc Nephrol. 2009;20(11):2285–90.

29. United States Renal Data Registry: International Comparison. Accessed https://www.usrds.org/2012/view/v2_12.aspx Feb 16, 2017.

30. United States Renal Data Systems (USRDS) 2015 Annual Data Report, National Institute of Health, National Institute of Diabetes, Digestive, and Kidney Diseases, Bethesda, MD. 2015. https://www.usrds.org/2015/view/v2_06.aspx.

31. Elixhauser A, Steiner C, Harris DR, Coffey RM. Comorbidity measures for use with administrative data. Med Care. 1998;36(1):8–27.

32. Dafni U. Landmark analysis at the 25-year landmark point. Circ Cardiovasc Qual Outcomes. 2011;4(3):363–71.

33. United States Renal Data Registry: Mortality Accessed https://www.usrds.org/2016/view/v2_06.aspx Apr 23, 2017.

34. Mi X, Hammill BG, Curtis LH, Lai EC, Setoguchi S. Use of the landmark method to address immortal person-time bias in comparative effectiveness research: a simulation study. Stat Med. 2016;35(26):4824–36.

35. Cohen J. Statistical power analysis for the behavioral sciences. Toronto: Academic Press, Inc.; 1977. [chapter 2]

36. Austin PC. An introduction to propensity score methods for reducing the effects of confounding in observational studies. Multivariate Behav Res. 2011;46(3):399–424.

37. Lori S. Parsons ORG, Seattle, Washington. Performing a 1:N Case-Control Match on Propensity Score. http://www2.sas.com/proceedings/sugi29/165-29.pdf.

38. Fernandez E, Llach F. Guidelines for dosing of intravenous calcitriol in dialysis patients with hyperparathyroidism. Nephrol Dial Transplant. 1996;11(Suppl 3):96–101.

39. National Kidney Foundation. K/DOQI Clinical Practice Guidelines for Bone Metabolism and Disease in Chronic Kidney Disease. Am J Kidney Dis. 2003;42(Suppl 3):S1–S201.

40. Franklin JM, Shrank WH, Pakes J, Sanfe'lix-Gimeno G, Matlin OS, Brennan TA, Choudhry NK. Group-based trajectory models -- a new approach to classifying and predicting long-term medication adherence. Med Care. 2013;51(9):789–96.

41. Manley HJ, Drayer DK, McClaran M, Bender W, Muther RS. Drug record discrepancies in an outpatient electronic medical record: frequency, type, and potential impact on patient Care at a Hemodialysis Center. PHARMACOTHERAPY. 2003;23(2):231–9.

42. Ong SW, Fernandes OA, Cesta A, Bajcar JM. Drug-related problems on hospital admission: relationship to medication information transfer. Ann Pharmacother. 2006;40(3):408–13.

43. Pai AB, Cardone KE, Manley HJ, St Peter WL, Shaffer R, Somers M, Mehrotra R. Dialysis advisory Group of American Society of N. medication reconciliation and therapy management in dialysis-dependent patients: need for a systematic approach. Clin J Am Soc Nephrol. 2013;8(11):1988–99.

44. Liu CH, Chuang YT, Chen YL, Weng YJ, Liu WS, Liang JS, Incorporating Development KY. Stratification of Taiwan townships into sampling Design of Large Scale Health Interview Survey. J Health Manag. 2006;4(1):1–22.

45. Fernandez-Martin JL, Carrero JJ, Benedik M, Bos WJ, Covic A, Ferreira A, Floege J, Goldsmith D, Gorriz JL, Ketteler M, et al. COSMOS: the dialysis scenario of CKD-MBD in Europe. Nephrol Dial Transplant. 2013;28(7):1922–35.

46. Wolf M. Should activated vitamin D be used in patients with end-stage renal disease and low levels of parathyroid hormone? Semin Dial. 2011;24(4):428–30.

47. Wolf M, Betancourt J, Chang Y, Shah A, Teng M, Tamez H, Gutierrez O, Camargo CA Jr, Melamed M, Norris K, et al. Impact of activated vitamin D and race on survival among hemodialysis patients. J Am Soc Nephrol. 2008;19(7):1379–88.

48. Miller JE, Molnar MZ, Kovesdy CP, Zaritsky JJ, Streja E, Salusky I, Arah OA, Kalantar-Zadeh K. Administered paricalcitol dose and survival in hemodialysis patients: a marginal structural model analysis. Pharmacoepidemiol Drug Saf. 2012;21(11):1232–9.

49. Mi X, Hammill BG, Curtis LH, Greiner MA, Setoguchi S. Impact of immortal person-time and time scale in comparative effectiveness research for medical devices: a case for implantable cardioverter-defibrillators. J Clin Epidemiol. 2013;66(8 Suppl):S138–44.

50. Wen CP, Levy DT, Cheng TY, Hsu CC, Tsai SP. Smoking behaviour in Taiwan. 2001 Tob Control. 2005;14(Suppl 1):i51–5.

51. Wu MS, Wu IW, Hsu KH. Survival Analysis of Taiwan Renal Registry Data System (TWRDS) 2000-2009. Acta Nephrologica. 2012;26(2):104–8.

22

Elevated preoperative Galectin-3 is associated with acute kidney injury after cardiac surgery

Moritz Wyler von Ballmoos[1], Donald S. Likosky[2,3], Michael Rezaee[4], Kevin Lobdell[5], Shama Alam[6], Devin Parker[6], Sherry Owens[6], Heather Thiessen-Philbrook[7], Todd MacKenzie[6,8] and Jeremiah R. Brown[6,8,9*]

Abstract

Background: Previous research suggests that novel biomarkers may be used to identify patients at increased risk of acute kidney injury following cardiac surgery. The purpose of this study was to evaluate the relationship between preoperative levels of circulating Galectin-3 (Gal-3) and acute kidney injury after cardiac surgery.

Methods: Preoperative serum Gal-3 was measured in 1498 patients who underwent coronary artery bypass graft (CABG) surgery and/or valve surgery as part of the Northern New England Biomarker Study between 2004 and 2007. Preoperative Gal-3 levels were measured using multiplex assays and grouped into terciles. Univariate and multinomial logistic regression was used to assess the predictive ability of Gal-3 terciles and AKI occurrence and severity.

Results: Before adjustment, patients in the highest tercile of Gal-3 had a 2.86-greater odds of developing postoperative KDIGO Stage 2 or 3 ($p < 0.001$) and 1.70-greater odds of developing KDIGO Stage 1 ($p = < 0.001$), compared to the first tercile. After adjustment, patients in the highest tercile had 2.95-greater odds of developing KDIGO Stage 2 or 3 ($p < 0.001$) and 1.71-increased odds of developing KDIGO Stage 1 ($p = 0.001$), compared to the first tercile. Compared to the base model, the addition of Gal-3 terciles improved discriminatory power compared to without Gal-3 terciles (test of equality = 0.042).

Conclusion: Elevated preoperative Gal-3 levels significantly improves predictive ability over existing clinical models for postoperative AKI and may be used to augment risk information for patients at the highest risk of developing AKI and AKI severity after cardiac surgery.

Keywords: Acute kidney injury (AKI), Galectin-3 (Gal-3), Cardiac surgery, Prediction, Biomarkers

Background

Acute kidney injury (AKI) is a well recognized complication following cardiac surgery, and significantly affects morbidity and mortality [1, 2]. Up to 40% of patients develop AKI after cardiac surgery and places patients at 5-fold higher risk of death during hospitalization [3]. AKI has also been associated with hospital readmissions following cardiac surgery and hospitalization for heart failure or acute myocardial infarction (MI) [4–8].

* Correspondence: jbrown@dartmouth.edu; jeremiah.r.brown@dartmouth.edu
[6]The Dartmouth Institute for Health Policy and Clinical Practice, Geisel School of Medicine, Lebanon, NH, USA
[8]Department of Biomedical Data Science, HB 7505 Dartmouth-Hitchcock Medical Center, Lebanon, NH NH 03756, USA
Full list of author information is available at the end of the article

Conventional metrics used to define and monitor the progression of AKI, such as serum creatinine and blood urea nitrogen levels, are insensitive, nonspecific and change notably only after significant kidney injury [8]. Identifying patients at increased risk of AKI prior to surgery is critical to take preventative measures and counsel patients on potential outcomes after cardiac surgery. A timely diagnosis would allow for earlier clinical intervention, greater care management prior to surgery, improved patient engagement and could improve patient outcomes.

New biomarkers allow a diagnosis to be made earlier than conventional measures, and allows kidney injury to be diagnosed even in the absence of concurrent or subsequent dysfunction. Biomarkers have been utilized to investigate AKI and augment the prediction of AKI risk and other complications following cardiac surgery [9–12]. A specific and sensitive marker of AKI risk could improve risk stratification, potentially identify patients that will benefit from greater care management prior to surgery and alert clinicians to individuals that will need earlier interventions to prevent AKI. Current risk prediction models for AKI following cardiac surgery have been developed on patient and disease characteristics alone. The addition of a specific protein biomarker may improve predictive ability over existing clinical models and may augment risk information for patients at higher risk of AKI after surgery.

Galectin-3 (Gal-3) is a beta-galactoside-binding lectin that has emerged as a key regulator of inflammation and tissue fibrosis [13]. Experimental studies in models of cancer, congestive heart failure and inflammatory disease have demonstrated that Gal-3 expression is elevated in these pathologic conditions [9]. In animal models, Gal-3 is acutely up-regulated in the kidneys in response to ischemic and toxic injury and is associated with renal fibrosis [14–17]. In humans, elevated levels of circulating Gal-3 have been found to be associated with increased risk of incident chronic kidney disease (CKD) and loss of kidney function over time [11, 18]. Gal-3 therefore can be considered a marker of both acute and chronic inflammatory processes in the kidneys, even in the absence of traditional clinical markers of renal injury.

There is an urgent need to analyze the predictive utility of Gal-3 to identify patients at greater risk of developing postoperative AKI. To date, Gal-3 has not been investigated as a potential biomarker for AKI in humans. The purpose of this study was to evaluate the assocation between preoperative Gal-3 and postoperative AKI in a large cohort of cardiac surgical patients.

Methods

NNE biomarker study

This study expands on the experience of Northern New England Cardiovascular Disease Study Group (NNECDSG), a regional collaborative consortium founded in 1987. All eight hospitals in this consortium submit data on cases with validation of procedure numbers and mortality conducted every 2 years. The NNECDSG registry contains data on patient characteristics, procedural indications, clinical variables and in-hospital outcomes. Data are periodically validated to ensure that all procedures and endpoints included in the registry have been accurately assessed. The NNECDSG has extensive experience in risk prediction in CABG surgery [4, 5]. The Northern New England (NNE) Biomarker Study is an initiative designed to assess the role of biomarkers in cardiac surgery.

Patient, procedural and outcome data were collected from patients undergoing coronary CABG surgery.

Those undergoing CABG incidental to heart valve repair or replacement, resection of a ventricular aneurysm, or other surgical procedure were not included. Only patients that had biomarker levels collected were retained in the final analyses ($n = 1498$). For the present study, the sample included patients undergoing emergent, urgent and non-urgent CABG surgeries. Investigators and patients were blinded to the collected biomarker levels. The Committee for the Protection of Human Subjects at Dartmouth College (Institutional Review Board) approved this study for both the prospective cohort with patient consent and the linkage of readmission and mortality events.

Galectin-3

Preoperative levels of Gal-3 was the main exposure of interest for this study. Blood samples were preoperatively collected prior to incision at each participating site in a 10-mL serum tube. Preoperative biomarker levels were measured using custom made multiplex ELISA assays (Meso Scale Discovery, Rockville, MD). Blood was allowed to clot at room temperature for 20 min to separate out the red blood cells, the tubes were centrifuged at 3500 rpm for 20 min, and the sera stored at the respective medical centers below – 80 degree Celcius until transportation on dry ice to the Laboratory for Clinical and Biomedical Research in Colchester, Vermont where they were stored at – 80 degree Celcius until measurement. Frozen serum was analyzed at a central laboratory, at the same time for biomarker measurement. Biomarkers were linked to the NNECDSG cohort to conduct the preoperative risk prediction modeling. Biomarkers were evaluated as continuous variables, natural log-transformed, and as terciles.

Acute kidney injury

The primary outcome of this study was the development of AKI after cardiac surgery. The last serum creatinine (SCr) prior to cardiac surgery and highest postoperative SCr prior to discharge were used to classify the stage of AKI. AKI stages were defined by the Kidney Disease: Improving Global Outcomes (KDIGO) definition as follows [19]: Stage 1: increase in SCr by ≥ 0.3 mg/dL within 48 h or ≥ 1.5 times baseline within 7 days; Stage 2: increase in SCr to 2 to 2.9-fold baseline; and Stage 3: increase in SCr to 3.0 times baseline or increase in SCr to ≥ 4.0 mg/dL or initiation of renal replacement therapy. Due to the small proportion of patients in KDIGO stage 2 and 3, we bundled stage 2 or 3 patients' outcomes in this report.

Statistical analysis

We evaluated the Gal-3 measurements to determine the association with the primary outcome (AKI) using univariate and multinomial logistic regression. Postoperative outcomes were compared using chi-squared tests, and continuous data were compared using the ANOVA test with the Bonferroni correction. Adjustment was carried out using variables from the Society of Thoracic Surgeons (STS) readmission model (Appendix) [20].To evaluate the association of the biomarker with AKI outcomes, we divided the cohort into terciles on the basis of Gal-3 values, where the lowest tercile is the reference group. We included indicator variables for the middle and highest terciles. We applied the mean imputation replacement method to account for variables with missing values. All biomarker values below the assay's lower quantitative limit were assigned the lower limit of detection. The performance of the risk model was assessed by measuring the total area under the receiver operating characteristic curve (AUC or c-statistic). Standard errors and 95% confidence intervals were estimated for the c-statistic using a bootstrap method. All analyses were conducted using Stata 13.1 College Station, TX).

Secondary Analyes

We compared the incremental value of Gal-3 to preoperative eGFR, a traditional risk marker of AKI. We adjusted the model using the STS readmission model and used the test of equality of ROC areas to assess differences in model performance. We calculated the Net Reclassification Improvement (NRI) and Integrated Discrimination Improvement (IDI) indices for risk models including Gal-3 and eGFR values.

Finally, we also created an alternative final model including both preoperative N-terminal pro b-type natriuretic peptide (NT-proBNP) values and preoperative Gal-3, in addition to the base STS readmission prediction model, to assess the predictive power using

a combination of biomarkers. We compared model performance using the test of equality of ROC areas.

Results

Overall, 1489 patients were included in the study. 481 (32.1%) developed AKI within KDIGO Stage 1 (26.3%) and 87 (5.8%) experienced KDIGO Stage 2 or 3 (Fig. 1). Patient and procedural characteristics are summarized in Table 1. Patient and procedural characteristics and the association with Gal-3 tercile measurements are summarized in Table 2. Gal-3 sample measurements ranged from 1.38 to 102.35 ng/mL with a median (Q1, Q3) value of 10.30 ng/mL (6.96 to 14.67 ng/mL).

Among patients studied, there was a significant difference between postoperative AKI incidence for older patients and patients with a higher BMI, history of smoking, atrial fibrillation, congestive heart failure (CHF), diabetes, ejection fraction < 40, prior MI, vascular disease, received transfused blood, and red blood cells transfused postoperatively. There is a significant relationship between elevated Gal-3 measurements and increased AKI severity ($p < 0.001$). For patients in the lowest tercile of Gal-3, 22.9% experienced KDIGO Stage 1 compared to 31.6% in the highest biomarker tercile. Similarly, for patients in the highest Gal-3 tercile, 1.8% of patients experienced KDIGO Stage 3 compared to 1.2% in the lowest tercile.

Table 3 describes the unadjusted and adjusted results for the AKI risk model and Gal-3 biomarker terciles. Before adjustment, patients in the highest tercile of Gal-3 had a 2.86-greater odds of developing postoperative KDIGO Stage 2 or 3 AKI ($p < 0.001$) and 1.70-greater odds of developing KDIGO Stage 1 ($p < 0.001$). After adjustment, patients in the highest tercile had 2.95-greater odds of developing KDIGO Stage 2 or 3

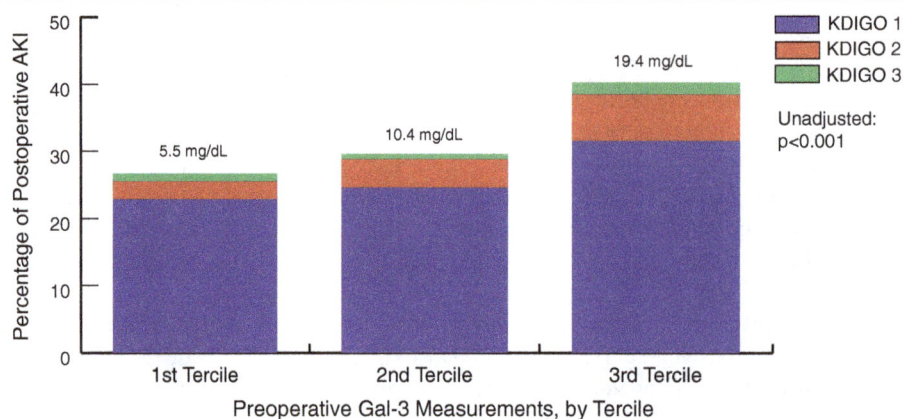

Fig. 1 Association of preoperative Galectin-3 and postoperative AKI severity after coronary artery bypass graft surgery, by Galectin-3 tercile. The mean Galectin-3 measurement for each tercile increases stepwise with postoperative AKI severity. There is a significant relationship between elevated preoperative Galectin-3 and AKI severity by KDIGO

Table 1 Patient and procedural characteristics and postoperative AKI occurrence

	No AKI (N = 1017)	AKI (N = 481)	p value
Age*	64.02 ± 9.99	68.08 ± 9.90	0.000
Female	23.8%	23.0%	0.740
BMI*	29.22 ± 5.17	30.35 ± 6.07	0.000
BSA*	2.03 ± 0.24	2.04 ± 0.26	0.200
Smoker	26.1%	16.6%	0.000
Atrial fibrillation	5.2%	9.3%	0.003
CHF	8.4%	13.5%	0.002
Pre-operative creatinine*	1.08 ± 1.02	1.15 ± 0.43	0.108
Diabetes	32.8%	43.3%	0.000
EF < 40	8.9%	14.0%	0.003
Hypertension	80.2%	81.7%	0.503
Pre-operative IABP	3.2%	5.7%	0.019
Prior MI			0.004
None	59.7%	49.8%	
< 24 h preop	1.5%	1.9%	
> 24 h & < 7 days	17.7%	21.9%	
> 7 & < 365 days	8.4%	12.5%	
> 365 days	12.7%	13.9%	
VAD	24.5%	32.5%	0.001
Unstable angina	55.3%	56.0%	0.780
COPD	12.4%	14.3%	0.321
LM stenosis	33.3%	35.0%	0.520
Prior CABG	1.8%	3.3%	0.064
Prior PCI	20.3%	18.4%	0.396
Priority			0.297
Emergency or emergent salvage	1.5%	2.7%	
Urgent	67.6%	67.9%	
Non-urgent	30.9%	29.5%	
Received transfused blood	29.1%	54.9%	0.000
pRBCs transfused pre-operatively			0.385
0	98.5%	97.3%	
1	0.4%	1.0%	
2	0.7%	1.3%	
3 or more	0.4%	0.4%	
pRBCs transfused post-operatively			0.000
0	77.8%	57.9%	
1	5.9%	9.1%	
2	10.7%	16.8%	
3 or more	5.7%	16.2%	
Pump time (mean, SD)	100.88 ± 32.01	112.44 ± 37.43	0.000

AKI acute kidney injury, *BMI* body mass index (kg/m^2), *BSA* body surface area (m^2), *CABG* coronary artery bypass graft, *CHF* congestive heart failure, *COPD* chronic obstructive pulmonary disease, *IABP* intra-operative balloon pump, *MI* myocardial infarction, *PCI* percutaneous coronary intervention, *RBC* red blood cell, *SD* standard deviation
*signifies continuous variables

($p < 0.001$) and 1.71-increased odds of developing KDIGO Stage 1 ($p = 0.001$). When preoperative levels of NT-proBNP were added to the risk prediction model, we observed similar results. Patients in the highest tercile of Gal-3 had 2.85-greater odds of developing KDIGO Stage 2 or 3 AKI ($p = 0.001$) and patients in the lowest tercile at 1.65-greater odds of KDIGO Stage 1 AKI ($p = 0.003$).

The base and augmented models are summarized in Table 4. The base model yielded a c-statistic of 0.69 (95% CI: 0.66–0.71). The base model with the addition of preoperative Gal-3 terciles yielded a c-statistic of 0.70 (95% CI: 0.67–0.72) and has a significant ROCCOMP p value of 0.042 compared to the base model alone. With the addition of Gal-3 and NT-proBNP terciles to the base model, the c-statistic remains at 0.70 (95% CI: 0.68 0.73) and is significantly improved from the base model alone (ROCCOMP p value = 0.005).

In an exploratory analysis where we compared preoperative Gal-3 terciles to preoperative eGFR values, we did not find an appreciable difference between the two makers and risk of developing AKI. Models comparing preoperative Gal-3 tercile values to continuous eGFR values are reported in Table 5.

Discussion

We are the first to demonstrate a significant relationship between the inflammatory biomarker Gal-3 and AKI in a multi-site, prospectively enrolled cohort of patients undergoing cardiac surgery. We found Gal-3 concentrations increased concurrently with decreasing kidney function. In our study, patients in the highest tercile of preoperative Gal-3 levels had 1.7 times the adjusted odds of KDIGO Stage 1 AKI compared to patients in the lowest tercile of Gal-3. Patients in the highest tercile of preoperative Gal-3 also had 2.9 times the adjusted odds of KDIGO Stage 2 or 3 AKI compared to the lowest tercile.

Gal-3 is a well-established biomarker for cardiac fibrosis, ventricular dysfunction, and poor prognosis in heart failure [21–23]. In addition, Gal-3 has demonstrated diagnostic and prognostic value in diseases of the kidney [9, 11, 18]. Drechsler et al. found a positive association between elevated levels of Gal-3 and adverse outcomes in patients with preexisting renal disease. Additionally, in the well recognized Framingham Heart Study, researchers demonstrated that elevated Gal-3 levels precede the development of CKD [10, 11]. Prior to our analysis, studies examining the relationship between Gal-3 and acute renal injury after surgery had been limited to animal models. Multiple animal studies have demonstrated that Gal-3 expression is up-regulated in the kidneys in response to ischemic and toxic injury and is associated with renal fibrosis [14–17].

Table 2 Patient and procedural characteristics and association with Gal-3 terciles

Patient characteristics	Overall	1st Tercile	2nd Tercile	3rd Tercile	p value
KDIGO					
No AKI	67.9%	73.4%	70.5%	59.6%	< 0.001
Stage 1	26.3%	22.9%	24.6%	31.6%	
Stage 2	4.5%	2.6%	4.2%	6.9%	
Stage 3	1.3%	1.2%	0.8%	1.8%	
Age[a]	65.7 ± 9.9	63.6 ± 10.0	65.5 ± 9.6	66.8 ± 10.6	0.464
Female	22.7%	18.2%	20.6%	32.0%	< 0.001
BMI[a]	29.6 ± 5.5	29.6 ± 5.2	29.6 ± 5.5	29.8 ± 5.9	0.464
BSA[a]	2.0 ± 0.2	2.0 ± 0.3	2.1 ± 0.2	2.0 ± 0.3	0.464
Smoker	21.4%	24.4%	22.2%	21.4%	0.488
Atrial fibrillation	6.5%	5.4%	6.2%	8.7%	0.082
CHF	11.2%	7.3%	8.7%	15.9%	< 0.001
Last pre-op serum creatinine (mean, SD)	1.1 ± 0.6	1.1 ± 0.5	1.1 ± 1.4	1.3 ± 1.0	0.464
Diabetes	38.0%	34.6%	33.9%	43.8%	0.001
Ejection fraction < 40%	12.1%	10.6%	10.0%	12.3%	0.508
Hypertension	81.0%	79.2%	80.1%	83.0%	0.273
IABP pre-op	3.8%	4.6%	4.8%	2.7%	0.165
Prior MI					
No	54.6%	57.3%	57.4%	53.7%	0.098
< 24 h pre-op	1.5%	1.4%	1.5%	2.1%	
> 24 h & < 7 days pre-op	20.5%	18.7%	19.6%	18.0%	
> 7 days & < 365 days pre-op	9.8%	7.9%	8.45%	13.6%	
> 365 days pre-op	13.6%	14.7%	12.7%	12.6%	
Vascular disease	27.8%	26.1%	25.2%	30.2%	0.154
Unstable angina	58.2%	53.7%	55.0%	58.1%	0.347
COPD	12.6%	11.2%	12.1%	15.5%	0.095
Left main, ≥50% stenosis	31.5%	33.0%	35.3%	33.0%	0.669
Prior CABG	2.4%	2.3%	2.8%	1.8%	0.566
Prior PCI	19.6%	20.5%	18.7%	20.0%	0.760
Priority					
Emergent	1.5%	2.5%	1.7%	1.6%	0.815
Urgent	70.1%	68.0%	67.4%	67.8%	
Non-urgent	28.3%	29.5%	30.8%	30.6%	
Received pRBC units		30.4%	35.5%	48.6%	< 0.001
Number of pRBC units given pre-op					
0	97.9%	99.4%	97.5%	97.1%	0.142
1 or more	2.1%	0.6%	2.5%	2.9%	

[a](Mean, SD)
AKI acute kidney injury, *KDIGO* Kidney Disease: Improving Global Outcomes, *BMI*, body mass index (kg/m²), *BSA* body surface area (m²), *CABG* coronary artery bypass graft, *CHF* congestive heart failure, *COPD* chronic obstructive pulmonary disease, *IABP* intra-operative balloon pump, *MI* myocardial infarction, *PCI* percutaneous coronary intervention, *RBC* red blood cell, *SD* standard deviation

In the kidney, Gal-3 has multiple functions including regulating the inflammatory response and cell growth, proliferation, and differentiation [24, 25]. Gal-3 has been proposed to be a marker of combined cardiac and renal fibrosis in the chronic setting [24, 25]. The prognostic value of baseline impaired cardiac and renal functional reserve may predict risk of AKI after cardiac surgery [26]. A 15% change from baseline has been associated with significantly more heart failure hospitalizations and

Table 3 Unadjusted and STS adjusted model evaluating preoperative Gal-3 measurements and association with KDIGO stage severity

	KDIGO Stage 1			KDIGO Stage 2 or 3		
	OR	95% CI	p value	OR	95% CI	p value
Unadjusted						
Preoperative	1.03	1.01–1.04	0.000	1.04	1.02–1.06	0.000
Natural log	1.47	1.19–1.81	0.000	2.03	1.40–2.94	0.000
Tertiles						
1	1.00	1.00–1.00		1.00	1.00–1.00	
2	1.12	0.83–1.50	0.456	1.36	0.74–2.52	0.322
3	1.70	1.28–2.27	0.000	2.86	1.63–5.01	0.000
Preoperative above median	1.36	1.08–1.72	0.009	2.44	1.53–3.89	0.000
STS Readmission Prediction Model[a]						
Preoperative	1.03	1.01–1.04	0.002	1.03	1.00–1.06	0.005
Natural log	1.40	1.10–1.78	0.006	1.87	1.23–2.86	0.004
Tertiles						
1	1.00	1.00–1.00		1.00	1.00–1.00	
2	1.08	0.79–1.48	0.625	1.37	0.73–2.56	0.329
3	1.71	1.24–2.37	0.001	2.95	1.63–5.34	0.000
Preoperative above median	1.30	1.00–1.68	0.046	2.31	1.39–3.85	0.001
STS Readmission Prediction Model + NT-pro BNP						
Preoperative	1.02	1.01–1.04	0.005	1.03	1.00–1.06	0.007
Natural log	1.31	1.03–1.68	0.028	1.73	1.13–2.65	0.012
Tertiles						
1	1.00	1.00–1.00		1.00	1.00–1.00	
2	1.08	0.79–1.48	0.631	1.36	0.72–2.57	0.337
3	1.65	1.19–2.29	0.003	2.85	1.57–5.16	0.001
Preoperative above median	1.28	0.99–1.66	0.060	2.26	1.35–3.76	0.002

[a]Model adjusts for variables included in the STS readmission prediction model
KDIGO Kidney Disease: Improving Global Outcomes, *CI* confidence interval, *OR* odds ratio, *STS* Society of Thoracic Surgeons

increased mortality compared with lower and decreasing levels [21]. In addition, Gal-3 has been shown to stimulate macrophages to release pro-inflammatory cytokines (e.g. MCP-1, IL-6, and IL-1B) and produce reactive oxygen species, enhancing the inflammatory response in the kidney [17]. Knocking-out the Gal-3 gene or directly inhibiting the Gal-3 protein is known to inhibit renal fibrosis and lessen renal injury in AKI [16, 27, 28].

We have demonstrated that preoperative levels of circulating Gal-3 are associated with AKI and AKI severity after cardiac surgery. Patients with higher levels of circulating Gal-3 may be predisposed to excessive inflammatory processes. Preoperative Gal-3 levels could also be acting as a marker for early CKD, identifying patients more susceptible to AKI because of underlying kidney disease. Further, preoperative Gal-3 may be serving as an indicator of heart failure (HF) and those patients at risk of AKI due to ischemic renal injury secondary to pump failure. Preoperative measurement of Gal-3 may provide a means to evaluate AKI risk due to multiple etiologies.

Multiple preoperative biomarkers have been evaluated for their ability to predict AKI after cardiac surgery. Cystatin C (CysC) is a circulating protease inhibitor and correlates with the glomerular filtration

Table 4 Model comparison statistics evaluating the discriminatory power of the base regression model and the additive value of preoperative Gal-3 terciles and preoperative NT-proBNP terciles

	C-statistic (95% CI)	ROCCOMP p value[a]
STS Readmission Prediction Model	0.69 (0.66–0.71)	
STS model + Gal-3 preoperative terciles	0.70 (0.67–0.72)	0.042
STS model + combined Gal-3 and NT-pro BNP preoperative terciles	0.70 (0.68–0.73)	0.005

[a]ROC comparison against base model

Table 5 Model evaluation Gal3 & eGFR

	STS Readmission Prediction Model + Risk Marker					
	C-statistic (95% CI)	NRI	NRI P	IDI	IDI P	Test of Equality P[b]
STS Readmission Model	0.69 (0.66–0.71)					
Preoperative Gal-3 terciles	0.70 (0.67–0.72)	0.03	0.067	0.01	0.000	0.042
Preoperative eGFR[a] (mL/min/1.73 m^2)	0.69 (0.66–0.72)	0.02	0.124	0.00	0.010	0.302

P represents the statistical p value.
[a]Estimated glomerular filtration rate (eGFR)
[b]ROC comparison against base model
NRI Net Reclassification Improvement index, IDI Integrated Discrimination Improvement index

rate (GFR) [13]. Its preoperative values have been shown to independently associate with AKI following cardiac surgery [29, 30]. Similarly, prior research has demonstrated a relationship between brain natriuretic peptide (BNP), NT-proBNP and Gal-3 with elevation in both markers related to outcomes [31]. Preoperative BNP, a polypeptide released by the ventricles in response to volume overload, has been shown to predict postoperative development of AKI [29, 32]. The inclusion of NT-proBNP in our study resulted in only a moderate difference from our adjusted prediction model. Compared to the adjusted model, the above median preoperative Gal3 measurements were non-signfiicant for those developing KDIGO Stage 1 in augmented model with NT-proBNP. The inclusion of BNP in our prediction model could provide important inferences on cardiac-surgery associated with AKI and heart failure, but further evaluation is needed. Given the varying kinetics and characteristics of individual biomarkers, it is likely that the measurement of multiple biomarkers, in addition to Gal-3, is necessary to accurately perform preoperative risk assessment for AKI [29, 33].

The primary strength of this study is its large sample size comprised of patients who underwent cardiac surgery at eight hospitals across Maine, Vermont and New Hampshire. Studies on preoperative biomarker levels and prediction of AKI have been previously conducted with small cohorts, in single-center settings and lacked defined, explicit outcomes [34]. In this study, we leveraged the NNECDSG registry, which is comprehensive in the patient and procedural data that it contains. The completeness and quality of this data also helps ensure that adequate adjustment was carried out.

Study limitations
There are limitations to this study to consider. First, we lacked detailed information on some conditions known to affect the incidence of AKI including cardiopulmonary bypass times, hemodynamics or the use of inotropic and vasoactive drugs in the

perioperative period. Therefore, residual confounding of the demonstrated association of Gal-3 with AKI can not be excluded. Gal-3 has been found to be correlated with pre-existing renal disease and heart failure. Medical support to maintain blood pressure arguably would be more aggressive in patients with higher Gal-3 values, and our results would more likely be biased towards the null-hypothesis. Secondly, we also used creatinine-based definitions for AKI which are relatively insensitive and non-specific in the period directly following insults to the kidney [35]. Thirdly, we were also unable to evaluate long-term outcomes such as major adverse renal and cardiac events (MARCE). Fourthly, given the unique patient characteristics associated with the CABG patient population, there may be reproducibility limitations with a more heterogeneous population. Finally, the mean imputation method used to address missing data may influence the overall composition and performance of the prediction model.

Conclusion
Improving the predictive ability of AKI risk prior to surgery is critical to take preventative measures and counsel patients on potential outcomes after cardiac surgery. Elevated preoperative Gal-3 levels may be used to augment risk information for patients at greatest risk of developing AKI and AKI severity after cardiac surgery. If Gal-3 is elevated, there are several AKI mitigation strategies to employ including avoiding surgery on the same day as cardiac catherization, limiting transfusion, remote ischemic preconditioning prior to surgery and stopping angiotensin-converting enzymes inhibitors (ACEIs) and angiotensin receptor blockers (ARBs) for 2 days after surgery.

We are the first to demonstrate a significant association between the inflammatory and fibrosis biomarker Gal-3 and AKI in patients undergoing cardiac surgery. Our findings suggest that preoperative Gal-3 levels could be used to identify patients at the highest risk of developing AKI after cardiac surgery.

Appendix

Table 6 STS Model Variables and NNE Registry Data

STS	NNE
1. We were unable to adjust for chronic lung disease or prior myocardial infarction in the same way as the investigators did in the STS preoperative readmission model.	
STS registry had data on the severity of chronic lung disease (none, mild, moderate, severe)	NNE registry only contains information on whether or not members of our patient cohort had chronic obstructive pulmonary disease (COPD) or not.
2. The STS and NNE registries also categorize prior myocardial infarctions in different ways.	
STS uses four different categories (no recent MI, MI between one and 21 days ago, MI more than six and less than 24 h ago, and MI less than or equal to 6 h ago)	NNE registry instead uses five categories for our cohort (no prior MI, MI less than 24 h prior to operation, MI more than 24 h but less than 7 days prior to operation, MI more than 7 days but less than 1 year prior to operation, and MI more than 0 year prior to operation)
3. We were unable to adjust for immunosuppressive treatment at all, since the NNE registry did not collect that information for our cohort.	
4. Our final NNE version of the STS preoperative readmission risk adjustment model included 30 covariates.	

This table describes the differences in variables between the STS model and variables available in the NNE registry dataset

Abbreviations
ACEIs: Angiotensin-converting enzymes inhibitors; AKI: Acute kidney injury; AKIN: Acute Kidney Injury Network; AMI: Acute myocardial infarction; ARB: Angiotensin receptor blockers; BMI: Body mass index; BSA: Body surface area; CABG: Coronary artery bypass graft; CHF: Chronic heart failure; CI: Confidence interval; COPD: Chronic obstructive pulmonary disease; IABP: Intra-aortic balloon pump; IL-1: Interleukin-1; KDIGO: Kidney Disease: Improving Global Outcomes; MARCE: Major adverse renal and cardiac events; MI: Myocardial infarction; NNE: Northern New England; NNECDSG: Northern New England Cardiovascular Disease Study Group; OR: Odds ratio; PCI: Percutaneous coronary intervention; pRBC: Packed red blood cells; ST2: Serum soluble ST2; STS: Society of Thoracic Surgeons; VAD: Ventricular assist device

Acknowledgements
Not applicable.

Funding
This research is supported by the National Heart Lung and Blood Institute R01HL119664 (PI: Brown). All authors are research staff or investigators on the grant.

Authors' contributions
MWB, DL, MR, and KL made substantial contributions to conception and design and analysis and interpretation of the data. SO, HTP and TA was involved in the drafting and revising and critical to the analysis and interpretation of the data. SA and DP made substantial contributions to conception and design, was involved in the drafting and revising it critically for important intellectual content. JR made significant contributions to conception and design, was involved in the drafting and revising, acquired the data, and was critical in the analysis and interpretation of the data. All authors read and approved the final manuscript.

Competing interests
The authors declare that they have no competing interests.

Author details
[1]Division of Cardiovascular and Thoracic Surgery, Duke University Medical Center, Durham, NC, USA. [2]Institute for Healthcare Policy and Innovation, University of Michigan, Ann Arbor, MI, USA. [3]Section of Health Services Research and Quality, Department of Cardiac Surgery, University of Michigan, Ann Arbor, MI, USA. [4]Section of Urology, Department of Surgery, Dartmouth-Hitchcock Medical Center, Lebanon, NH, USA. [5]Carolinas HealthCare System, Charlotte, NC, USA. [6]The Dartmouth Institute for Health Policy and Clinical Practice, Geisel School of Medicine, Lebanon, NH, USA. [7]Division of Nephrology, Department of Medicine, Johns Hopkins University, Baltimore, MD, USA. [8]Department of Biomedical Data Science, HB 7505 Dartmouth-Hitchcock Medical Center, Lebanon, NH NH 03756, USA. [9]Department of Epidemiology, Geisel School of Medicine, Lebanon, NH, USA.

References
1. Schaub JA, Parikh CR. Biomarkers of acute kidney injury and associations with short- and long-term outcomes. F1000Res. 2016;5.
2. Rosner MH, Okusa MD. Acute kidney injury associated with cardiac surgery. Clin J Am Soc Nephrol. 2006;1(1):19–32.
3. O'Neal JB, Shaw AD, Billings FT. Acute kidney injury following cardiac surgery: current understanding and future directions. Crit Care. 2016;20(1): 187.
4. Brown JR, Malenka DJ, DeVries JT, Robb JF, Jayne JE, Friedman BJ, Hettleman BD, Niles NW, Kaplan AV, Schoolwerth AC, Thompson CA. Transient and persistent renal dysfunction are predictors of survival after percutaneous coronary intervention: insights from the Dartmouth Dynamic Registry. Catheter Cardiovasc Interv. 2008;72(3):347-54.
5. Brown JR, Parikh CR, Ross CS, et al. Impact of perioperative acute kidney injury as a severity index for thirty-day readmission after cardiac surgery. Ann Thorac Surg. 2014;97(1):111–7.
6. Goldenberg I, Chonchol M, Guetta V. Reversible acute kidney injury following contrast exposure and the risk of long-term mortality. Am J Nephrol. 2009;29(2):136–44.
7. Thakar CV, Parikh PJ, Liu Y. Acute kidney injury (AKI) and risk of readmissions in patients with heart failure. Am J Cardiol. 2012;109(10):1482–6.
8. Vaidya VS, Ferguson MA, Bonventre JV. Biomarkers of acute kidney injury. Annu Rev Pharmacol Toxicol. 2008;48:463–93.
9. Drechsler C, Delgado G, Wanner C, et al. Galectin-3, renal function, and clinical outcomes: results from the LURIC and 4D studies. J Am Soc Nephrol. 2015;26(9):2213–21.
10. Ho JE, Liu C, Lyass A, et al. Galectin-3, a marker of cardiac fibrosis, predicts incident heart failure in the community. J Am Coll Cardiol. 2012;60(14):1249–56.
11. O'Seaghdha CM, Hwang SJ, Ho JE, Vasan RS, Levy D, Fox CS. Elevated galectin-3 precedes the development of CKD. J Am Soc Nephrol. 2013;24(9): 1470–7.
12. Parikh CR, Coca SG, Thiessen-Philbrook H, et al. Postoperative biomarkers predict acute kidney injury and poor outcomes after adult cardiac surgery. J Am Soc Nephrol. 2011;22(9):1748–57.
13. Dharnidharka VR, Kwon C, Stevens G. Serum cystatin C is superior to serum creatinine as a marker of kidney function: a meta-analysis. Am J Kidney Dis. 2002;40(2):221–6.
14. Nishiyama J, Kobayashi S, Ishida A, et al. Up-regulation of galectin-3 in acute renal failure of the rat. Am J Pathol. 2000;157(3):815–23.

15. Henderson NC, Mackinnon AC, Farnworth SL, et al. Galectin-3 expression and secretion links macrophages to the promotion of renal fibrosis. Am J Pathol. 2008;172(2):288–98.

16. Kolatsi-Joannou M, Price KL, Winyard PJ, Long DA. Modified Citrus pectin reduces Galectin-3 expression and disease severity in experimental acute kidney injury. PLoS One. 2011;6(4):e18683.

17. Fernandes Bertocchi AP, Campanhole G, Wang PH, et al. A role for galectin-3 in renal tissue damage triggered by ischemia and reperfusion injury. Transplant international : official journal of the European Society for Organ Transplantation. 2008;21(10):999–1007.

18. Ji F, Zhang S, Jiang X, et al. Diagnostic and prognostic value of galectin-3, serum creatinine, and cystatin C in chronic kidney diseases. *Journal of clinical laboratory analysis*. 2017;31:5.

19. Kidney Disease. Improving Global Outcomes (KDIGO) Acute Kidney Injury Work Group. KDIGO Clinical Practice Guideline for Acute Kidney Injury. *Kidney inter, Suppl*. 2012;2:1–138.

20. Shahian DM, He X, O'Brien SM, Grover FL, Jacobs JP, Edwards FH, Welke KF, Suter LG, Drye E, Shewan CM, Han L, Peterson E. Development of a clinical registry-based 30-day readmission measure for coronary artery bypass grafting surgery. Circulation. 2014;130(5):399–409.

21. de Boer RA, Yu L, van Veldhuisen DJ. Galectin-3 in cardiac remodeling and heart failure. Current Heart Failure Reports. 2010;7(1):1–8.

22. de Boer RA, van Veldhuisen DJ, Gansevoort RT, et al. The fibrosis marker galectin-3 and outcome in the general population. J Intern Med. 2012; 272(1):55–64.

23. Shah RV, Chen-Tournoux AA, Picard MH, van Kimmenade RRJ, Januzzi JL. Galectin-3, cardiac structure and function, and long-term mortality in patients with acutely decompensated heart failure. Eur J Heart Fail. 2010; 12(8):826–32.

24. Chen SC, Kuo PL. The role of Galectin-3 in the kidneys. Int J Mol Sci. 2016; 17(4):565.

25. Desmedt V, Desmedt S, Delanghe JR, Speeckaert R, Speeckaert MM. Galectin-3 in renal pathology: more than just an innocent bystander. Am J Nephrol. 2016;43(5):305–17.

26. Hundae A, McCullough PA. Cardiac and renal fibrosis in chronic cardiorenal syndromes. Nephron Clin Pract. 2014;127(1-4):106-12.

27. Varrier M, Forni LG, Ostermann M. Long-term sequelae from acute kidney injury: potential mechanisms for the observed poor renal outcomes. Crit Care. 2015;19(1):102.

28. Calvier L, Martinez-Martinez E, Miana M, et al. The impact of galectin-3 inhibition on aldosterone-induced cardiac and renal injuries. JACC Heart failure. 2015;3(1):59–67.

29. Koyner JL, Parikh CR. Clinical utility of biomarkers of AKI in cardiac surgery and critical illness. Clin J Am Soc Nephrol. 2013;8(6):1034–42.

30. Shlipak MG, Coca SG, Wang Z, et al. Presurgical serum cystatin C and risk of acute kidney injury after cardiac surgery. American journal of kidney diseases : the official journal of the National Kidney Foundation. 2011;58(3): 366–73.

31. McCullough PA, Olobatoke A, Vanhecke TE. Galectin-3: a novel blood test for the evaluation and management of patients with heart failure. Rev Cardiovasc Med. 2011;12(4):200–10.

32. Patel UD, Garg AX, Krumholz HM, et al. Preoperative serum brain natriuretic peptide and risk of acute kidney injury after cardiac surgery. Circulation. 2012;125(11):1347–55.

33. de Geus HR, Betjes MG, Bakker J. Biomarkers for the prediction of acute kidney injury: a narrative review on current status and future challenges. Clin Kidney J. 2012;5(2):102–8.

34. O'Brien SM, Clarke DR, Jacobs JP, et al. An empirically based tool for analyzing mortality associated with congenital heart surgery. J Thorac Cardiovasc Surg. 2009;138(5):1139–53.

35. Moran SM, Myers BD. Course of acute renal failure studied by a model of creatinine kinetics. Kidney Int. 1985;27(6):928–37.

23

Female sex reduces the risk of hospital-associated acute kidney injury: a meta-analysis

Joel Neugarten*[iD] and Ladan Golestaneh*

Abstract

Background: Female sex has been included as a risk factor in models developed to predict the development of AKI. In addition, the commentary to the Kidney Disease Improving Global Outcomes Clinical Practice Guideline for AKI concludes that female sex is a risk factor for hospital-acquired AKI. In contrast, a protective effect of female sex has been demonstrated in animal models of ischemic AKI.

Methods: To further explore this issue, we performed a meta-analysis of AKI studies published between January, 1978 and April, 2018 and identified 83 studies reporting sex-stratified data on the incidence of hospital-associated AKI among nearly 240,000,000 patients.

Results: Twenty-eight studies (6,758,124 patients) utilized multivariate analysis to assess risk factors for hospital-associated AKI and provided sex-stratified ORs. Meta-analysis of this cohort showed that the risk of developing hospital-associated AKI was significantly greater in men than in women (OR 1.23 (1.11,1.36). Since AKI is not a single disease but instead represents a heterogeneous group of disorders characterized by an acute reduction in renal function, we performed subgroup meta-analyses. The association of male sex with AKI was strongest among studies of patients who underwent non-cardiac surgery. Male sex was also associated with AKI in studies which included unselected hospitalized patients and in studies of critically ill patients who received care in an intensive care unit. In contrast, cardiac surgery-associated AKI and radiocontrast-induced AKI showed no sexual dimorphism.

Conclusions: Our meta-analysis contradicts the established belief that female sex confers a greater risk of AKI and instead suggests a protective role.

Keywords: Acute kidney injury, Gender, Meta-analysis, Systematic review, Acute renal failure

Background

Sexual dimorphism is a well-established feature of chronic progressive kidney disease [1]. Although less well recognized, sexual dimorphism has also been established in the development of ischemic acute kidney injury (AKI) [2]. Animal models have consistently demonstrated that female sex is protective in the development of AKI after ischemia-reperfusion injury [2–14]. Despite these experimental observations, it has been suggested that the direction of sexual dimorphism is reversed in humans with AKI. Female sex has been included as a risk factor in models developed to predict the risk of

AKI associated with cardiac surgery, aminoglycoside nephrotoxicity, rhabdomyolysis and radio-contrast administration [15–18]}. The commentary to the Kidney Disease Improving Global Outcomes (KDIGO) Clinical Practice Guideline for Acute Kidney Injury (arguably the most authoritative commentary in the field) states that female sex is among the "shared susceptibility factors" that confer a higher risk of AKI [19]. This conclusion is based on observations that female sex is associated with a higher risk for AKI after cardiac surgery and after the administration of radio-contrast or aminoglycosides. On this basis, the commentary concludes that, "contrary to most chronic kidney disease disorders, it is the female gender that carries a higher risk for AKI." This conclusion, however, is qualified by the observation that

* Correspondence: jneugart@montefiore.org; lgolesta@montefiore.org
Department of Medicine, Nephrology Division, Montefiore Medical Center, Albert Einstein College of Medicine, 111 E. 210 St, Bronx, NY 10467, USA

males predominate in reports of AKI complicating infections with HIV, malaria, leptospirosis and other community-acquired forms of AKI.

We have previously challenged the generally held consensus that female sex is an independent risk factor for cardiac surgery-associated AKI and for aminoglycoside nephrotoxicity [18, 20]. In the present study, we sought to explore the relationship between sex and hospital-associated AKI (HAAKI) in greater detail by performing a systematic review and meta-analysis of studies published between January, 1978 and April, 2018 which report the sex-stratified incidence of HAAKI.

Methods

Search strategy and selection criteria

We conducted a systematic review and meta-analysis of the English literature to evaluate the reported incidence of acute kidney injury in hospitalized women versus hospitalized men. Our analysis was conducted according to the Preferred Reporting Items for Systematic Reviews and Meta-analyses protocol [21].

We searched PubMed for English-language articles published between January 1, 1978 and April 1, 2018. The following medical subject heading terms were used: male, female, sex, gender, acute kidney injury, and acute renal failure. EMBASE was also queried with the terms sex difference, acute kidney injury and acute renal failure. Titles and abstracts of articles found in the database search were reviewed to identify eligible studies. Full text versions of selected studies were analyzed in detail. We also examined the bibliographies of recovered articles for additional resources. Any case control or cohort study of 10,000 or more hospitalized patients in which

the sex-stratified incidence of AKI was reported was eligible for inclusion (Fig. 1). To determine study quality, the studies were assessed using the Newcastle Ottawa Score for cohort and case control studies [22].

Definition of AKI

Hospital-associated AKI was defined as AKI that developed in hospitalized patients. This definition included patients who developed AKI within the first 48 h of admission to the hospital (community-acquired AKI) and patients who developed AKI later during their hospital course (hospital-acquired). We accepted studies that defined AKI by investigator-created, creatinine-based criteria, Acute Kidney Injury Network (AKIN) criteria, Kidney Disease: Improving Global Outcomes (KDIGO) criteria, Risk, Injury, Failure, Loss of kidney function, End-stage kidney disease (RIFLE) criteria, or by the requirement for renal replacement therapy (AKI-D) [19, 23, 24].

Data extraction

All studies were examined for duplication of data. Attention was given to the reporting clinical centers, years covered, and overlap with larger regional or national databases. In the case of overlap, a weighting factor was assigned to the smaller study that was inversely proportional to the degree of overlap. If the weighted number of patients fell below 10,000, the study was excluded. We also excluded studies with less than 25 AKI events among either of the sexes.

We separated the selected studies in to 2 groups. The first group included studies in which the investigators utilized multivariate analysis and reported adjusted odds ratios. The second group included studies in which unadjusted data was reported.

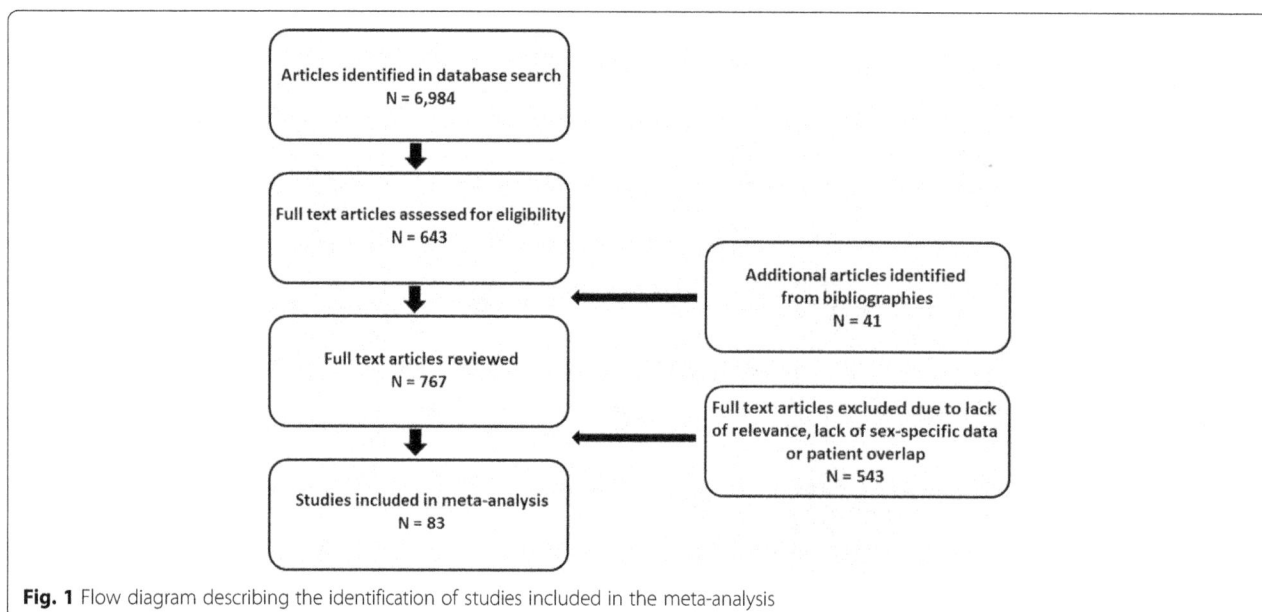

Fig. 1 Flow diagram describing the identification of studies included in the meta-analysis

We analyzed separately studies restricted to patients who underwent radio-contrast procedures (percutaneous coronary interventions or computerized axial tomography) but which failed to specify whether the procedure was performed in an ambulatory care setting or was associated with an in-patient hospital stay. In this regard, most computerized axial tomography procedures are performed in an out-patient rather than in an in-patient setting and percutaneous coronary interventions have moved from an exclusively in-patient procedure to a predominantly ambulatory procedure over the last decade (0% ambulatory in 2009 to 77% ambulatory in 2015) [25].

Statistical analysis

Data were analyzed using a random effects model with RevMan Version 5.3, The Cochrane Collaboration 2014. Meta-regression analysis and sub-group meta-analysis were performed with OpenMetaAnalyst 2016 [26].

Results

Adjusted analyses

Twenty-eight studies (6,758,124 patients; 2,313,202 women and 4,444,922 men) utilized multivariate analysis to assess risk factors for hospital-associated AKI and provided sex-stratified ORs (Fig. 2) [27–53]. Eight studies included only hospitalized patients who underwent cardiac surgery, 10 studies included only hospitalized patients who underwent predominantly non-cardiac surgery, 3 studies included only critically ill patients who received care in an intensive care unit, 6 studies included unselected hospitalized patients, whereas the remaining study included only hospitalized patients with a diagnosis of acute decompensated heart failure. AKI was defined by KDIGO criteria in 10 studies, by RIFLE criteria in 1 study, by AKIN criteria in 2 studies, by the need for renal replacement therapy in 7 studies, and by investigator-created, creatinine-based criteria in the remaining 8 studies. Nearly all studies that utilized RIFLE, AKIN or KDIGO criteria to define AKI relied solely on serum creatinine criteria rather than urine output criteria.

Meta-analysis of this cohort showed that men were significantly more likely to develop HAAKI than women (OR 1.23 (1.11,1.36), n = 28 studies, 6,758,124 patients).

We observed a high degree of statistical heterogeneity in the meta-analysis (I^2 = 98.0%, $p < 0.001$). This is not surprising since AKI is not a single disease but instead represents a heterogeneous group of disorders characterized by an acute reduction in renal function. To evaluate the source of statistical heterogeneity, we performed a regression meta-analysis and subgroup analyses.

We found that statistical heterogeneity was related to the criteria used to select the study cohort and to the

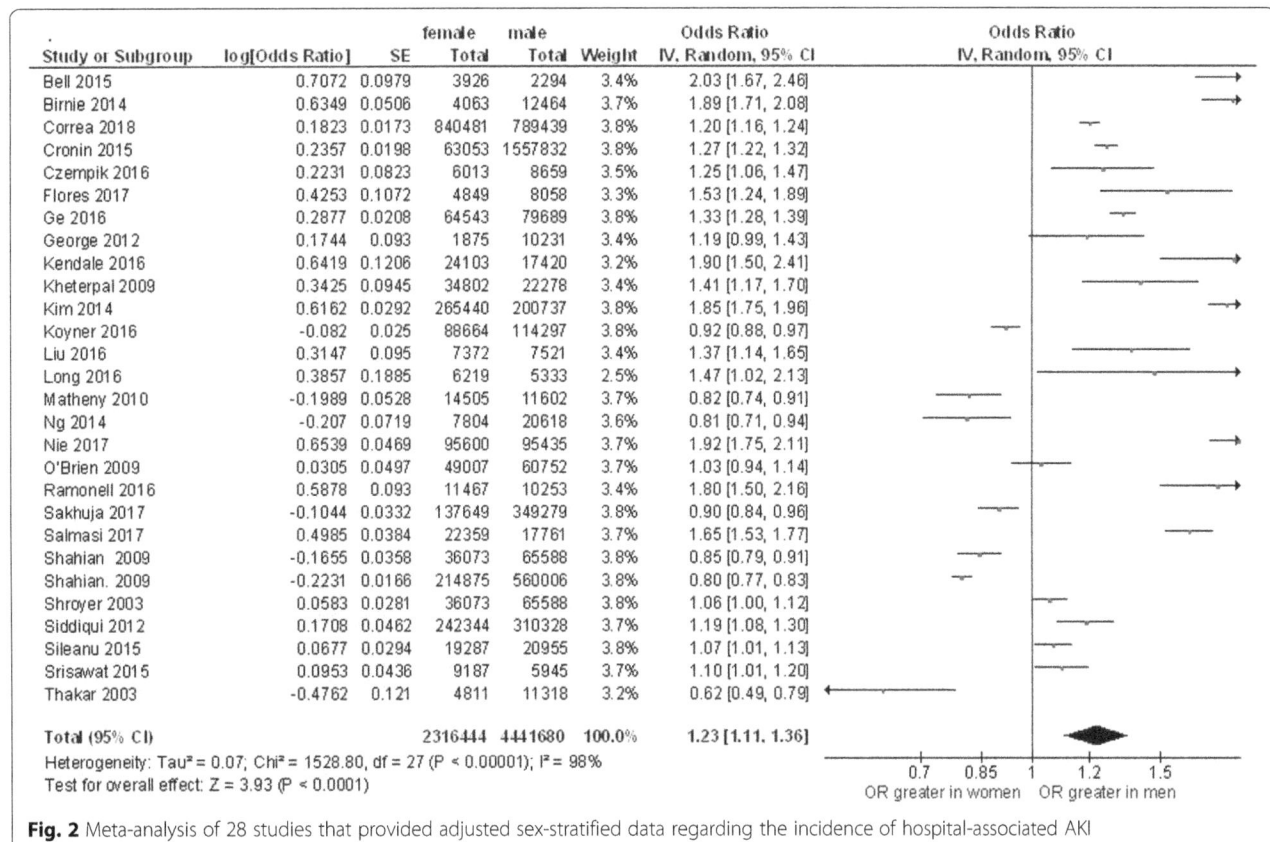

Study or Subgroup	log[Odds Ratio]	SE	female Total	male Total	Weight	Odds Ratio IV, Random, 95% CI
Bell 2015	0.7072	0.0979	3926	2294	3.4%	2.03 [1.67, 2.46]
Birnie 2014	0.6349	0.0506	4063	12464	3.7%	1.89 [1.71, 2.08]
Correa 2018	0.1823	0.0173	840481	789439	3.8%	1.20 [1.16, 1.24]
Cronin 2015	0.2357	0.0198	63053	1557832	3.8%	1.27 [1.22, 1.32]
Czempik 2016	0.2231	0.0823	6013	8659	3.5%	1.25 [1.06, 1.47]
Flores 2017	0.4253	0.1072	4849	8058	3.3%	1.53 [1.24, 1.89]
Ge 2016	0.2877	0.0208	64543	79689	3.8%	1.33 [1.28, 1.39]
George 2012	0.1744	0.093	1875	10231	3.4%	1.19 [0.99, 1.43]
Kendale 2016	0.6419	0.1206	24103	17420	3.2%	1.90 [1.50, 2.41]
Kheterpal 2009	0.3425	0.0945	34802	22278	3.4%	1.41 [1.17, 1.70]
Kim 2014	0.6162	0.0292	265440	200737	3.8%	1.85 [1.75, 1.96]
Koyner 2016	-0.082	0.025	88664	114297	3.8%	0.92 [0.88, 0.97]
Liu 2016	0.3147	0.095	7372	7521	3.4%	1.37 [1.14, 1.65]
Long 2016	0.3857	0.1885	6219	5333	2.5%	1.47 [1.02, 2.13]
Matheny 2010	-0.1989	0.0528	14505	11602	3.7%	0.82 [0.74, 0.91]
Ng 2014	-0.207	0.0719	7804	20618	3.6%	0.81 [0.71, 0.94]
Nie 2017	0.6539	0.0469	95600	95435	3.7%	1.92 [1.75, 2.11]
O'Brien 2009	0.0305	0.0497	49007	60752	3.7%	1.03 [0.94, 1.14]
Ramonell 2016	0.5878	0.093	11467	10253	3.4%	1.80 [1.50, 2.16]
Sakhuja 2017	-0.1044	0.0332	137649	349279	3.8%	0.90 [0.84, 0.96]
Salmasi 2017	0.4985	0.0384	22359	17761	3.7%	1.65 [1.53, 1.77]
Shahian 2009	-0.1655	0.0358	36073	65588	3.8%	0.85 [0.79, 0.91]
Shahian. 2009	-0.2231	0.0166	214875	560006	3.8%	0.80 [0.77, 0.83]
Shroyer 2003	0.0583	0.0281	36073	65588	3.8%	1.06 [1.00, 1.12]
Siddiqui 2012	0.1708	0.0462	242344	310328	3.7%	1.19 [1.08, 1.30]
Sileanu 2015	0.0677	0.0294	19287	20955	3.8%	1.07 [1.01, 1.13]
Srisawat 2015	0.0953	0.0436	9187	5945	3.7%	1.10 [1.01, 1.20]
Thakar 2003	-0.4762	0.121	4811	11318	3.2%	0.62 [0.49, 0.79]
Total (95% CI)			2316444	4441680	100.0%	1.23 [1.11, 1.36]

Heterogeneity: Tau² = 0.07; Chi² = 1528.80, df = 27 (P < 0.00001); I² = 98%
Test for overall effect: Z = 3.93 (P < 0.0001)

Odds Ratio IV, Random, 95% CI
0.7 0.85 1 1.2 1.5
OR greater in women   OR greater in men

Fig. 2 Meta-analysis of 28 studies that provided adjusted sex-stratified data regarding the incidence of hospital-associated AKI

criteria used to define AKI, but was not related to year of publication, number of AKI events or total number of patients studied. The association of male sex with the development of AKI was strongest among studies restricted to patients who underwent predominantly non-cardiac surgery (OR 1.56 (1.37,1.77), n = 10 studies, 1,225418 patients, 606,881 women and 618,537 men). Male sex was also associated with AKI in studies of unselected hospitalized patients (OR 1.22 (1.01,1.49), n = 6 studies, 2,196,772 patients, 332,584 women and 2,196,772 men), and in studies of critically ill patients who received care in an intensive care unit (OR 1.10 (1.03,1.18), n = 3 studies, 70,046 patients, 34,487 women and 35,559 men). In contrast, cardiac surgery-associated AKI showed no sexual dimorphism (OR 0.95 (0.80,1.13), n = 8 studies, 1,635,968 patients, 490,355 women and 1,145,613 men).

The sex-stratified incidence of HAAKI also varied according to the criteria used to define AKI. Men were more likely to develop HAAKI than were women when AKI was identified by KDIGO criteria (OR 1.38 (1.19,1.59), n = 10 studies, 2,263,679 patients, 361,914 women and 1,901,765 men), and by AKIN criteria (OR 1.69 (1.52,1.88), n = 2 studies, 81,643 patients, 46,462 women and 35,181 men). There was no difference in the incidence of HAAKI between the sexes when AKI was identified by the need for renal replacement therapy (OR 1.05 (0.92, 1.10), n = 7 studies, 2,822,186 patients, 1,282,180 females and 1,540,006 men) or by investigator-created, creatinine-based criteria (1.19 (0.91, 1.55), n = 8 studies, 1,564,509 patients, 611,383 women and 953,126 men).

In a separate analysis, the incidence of AKI among adjusted studies of patients who underwent percutaneous coronary interventions or computerized axial tomography was equivalent in men and women (OR 1.05 (0.79,1.40), n = 3 studies, 1,087,879 patients, 347,811 women and 740,068 men) [54–56].

Unadjusted analyses
The unadjusted cohort consisted of 68 studies which included 232,586,252 patients (130,605,382 women and 101,970,870 men (Figs. 3 and 4) [29, 31–34, 36, 38, 42, 43, 45, 47, 57–112]. Studies could be divided into 7 distinct categories. Twenty-four studies included unselected hospitalized patients, 11 studies included only hospitalized patients who underwent cardiac surgery, 13 studies included only hospitalized patients who underwent predominantly non-cardiac surgery, 11 studies included only critically ill patients who received care in an intensive care unit, whereas the remaining 9 studies included hospitalized patients selected based on their underlying disease (liver disease, cerebrovascular disease, human immunodeficiency virus infection, congestive heart failure, or atrial fibrillation). AKI was defined by RIFLE criteria in 5 studies, by AKIN criteria in 11 studies, by KDIGO criteria in

17 studies, by the need for renal replacement therapy in 20 studies, and by investigator-created, creatinine-based criteria in the remaining 15 studies. Nearly all studies that utilized RIFLE, AKIN or KDIGO criteria to define AKI relied solely on serum creatinine criteria rather than urine output criteria.

Meta-analysis of the entire cohort of unadjusted studies showed that men were significantly more likely to develop HAAKI than women (OR 1.29 (1.18,1.42), n = 68 studies, 232,586,252 patients). We observed a high degree of statistical heterogeneity in this analysis (I^2 = 99.6%, p < 0.001). This is not surprising since AKI is not a single disease but instead represents a heterogeneous group of disorders characterized by an acute reduction in renal function. To evaluate the source of statistical heterogeneity, we performed a regression meta-analysis and subgroup analyses. We found that statistical heterogeneity was related to the criteria used to select the study cohort and to the criteria used to define AKI, but was not related to year of publication, number of AKI events or total number of patients.

The association of male sex with the development of AKI was strongest among studies reporting unadjusted data from patients undergoing predominantly non-cardiac surgery (OR 1.63 (1.34,1.97), n = 13 studies, 556,647 patients, 246,136 women and 310,511 men) and among studies of unselected hospitalized patients (OR 1.52 (1.34,1.70), n = 24 studies, 224,740,578 patients, 127,168,880 women and 97,571,698 men). Male sex was also associated with AKI among studies in which patients were selected based on a disease-specific diagnosis (1.31 (1.04,1.65), n = 9 studies, 4,055,606 patients, 1,919,721 women and 2,135,885 men). In contrast, among unadjusted studies of cardiac surgery-associated AKI, AKI was less frequent in men than in women (OR 0.82 (0.74, 0.91), n = 11 studies, 1,413,349 patients, 398,205 women and 1,015,144 men). The incidence of AKI among critically ill patients who received care in an intensive care unit was similar in men and women (OR 1.05 (0.89,1.25), n = 11 studies, 1,774,707 patients, 846,347 women and 928,460 men).

The unadjusted sex-stratified incidence of HAAKI also varied according to the criteria used to define AKI. Men were more likely to develop HAAKI than were women when AKI was identified by KDIGO criteria (OR 1.34 (1.20,1.51), n = 17 studies, 1,804,815 patients, 868,140 women and 936,675 men), or by the need for renal replacement therapy (OR 1.33 (1.17,1.50), n = 20 studies, 217,375,505 patients, 128,841,628 women and 98,533,877 men). In contrast, men were less likely to develop HAAKI than were women when AKI was identified by RIFLE criteria (OR 0.89 (0.82,0.96), n = 5 studies, 260,132 patients, 112,564 women and 157,568 men). There was no significant difference in the incidence of HAAKI between the sexes when AKI was identified by AKIN criteria (OR 1.23 (0.98,1.54), n = 11 studies, 1,783,778 patients, 286,062

Studies	Estimate (95% C.I.)	Ev/Trt	Ev/Ctrl
Al-Jaghbeer 2018	1.640 (1.613, 1.668)	34881/228586	29631/299522
Gao 2015	0.938 (0.696, 1.264)	95/69182	79/53943
Ge 2016	1.242 (1.200, 1.286)	8909/79689	5937/64543
Hatakeyema 2016	1.408 (1.350, 1.469)	5218/57105	4371/65548
Heung 2016	1.592 (1.459, 1.736)	16456/99413	593/5351
Hsu 2016	1.541 (1.420, 1.672)	1237/17620	1214/25991
Hsu 2008	1.837 (1.671, 2.019)	1029/260909	735/341675
Hsu 2015	1.869 (1.844, 1.894)	51248/9903232	38503/13871509
Jannot 2017	1.406 (1.344, 1.472)	5291/69301	3188/57434
Kashani 2017	1.416 (1.332, 1.504)	2251/21700	2300/30430
Neugarten 2018	2.192 (2.158, 2.227)	41644/84061275	24869/109999724
Koulourridis 2015	1.164 (1.081, 1.252)	1679/10338	1666/11663
Koyner 2016	1.139 (1.105, 1.175)	8537/88664	9004/105293
Koyner 2018	1.256 (1.217, 1.297)	8911/55857	8571/65301
LaFrance 2010	1.709 (1.653, 1.768)	130527/1075937	3789/50699
Long 2016	0.986 (0.937, 1.036)	5389/13126	5030/12148
Nie 2017	2.133 (1.934, 2.353)	1254/95600	591/95435
Omotoso 2016	1.289 (0.994, 1.672)	163/7044	90/4988
Pannu 2013	1.213 (1.140, 1.290)	2117/74508	1994/84695
Shema 2009	0.947 (0.850, 1.055)	673/11610	727/11917
Waiker 2007	1.979 (1.892, 2.069)	4454/1264625	3399/1906524
Wang 2013	1.298 (1.211, 1.391)	2322/9876	1794/9370
Warnock 2015	4.002 (3.851, 4.158)	15028/27114	5563/23466
Zeng 2014	2.171 (2.050, 2.299)	2947/11280	2898/20687
Subgroup HA	**1.519 (1.356, 1.701)**	**352260/97613591**	**156536/127217856**
Bagshaw 2008	0.818 (0.799, 0.838)	24469/71461	18926/48662
Bagshaw 2007	0.942 (0.861, 1.030)	1246/24424	846/15669
Chao 2012	0.746 (0.695, 0.802)	1863/18951	1556/12208
Czempik 2016	1.265 (1.121, 1.429)	790/8659	442/6013
Gammelager 2013	1.333 (1.237, 1.436)	1946/61381	1116/46556
Horkan 2015	0.881 (0.841, 0.923)	4664/37024	3525/25072
Kane-Gil 2015	0.992 (0.952, 1.033)	14234/22660	10886/17276
Liborio 2015	0.831 (0.784, 0.881)	5605/10434	4648/7976
Mansuri 2017	1.446 (1.414, 1.479)	17452/555182	13690/623729
Rimes 2015	1.143 (1.084, 1.204)	3842/57994	2429/41551
Thakar 2009	1.573 (1.367, 1.810)	13347/60290	235/1535
Subgroup ICU	**1.054 (0.889, 1.250)**	**89458/928460**	**58299/846247**
Bahar 2005	1.139 (0.804, 1.614)	125/10376	43/4061
Chakar 2017	0.939 (0.748, 1.179)	197/11456	123/6726
Mehta 2016	0.665 (0.596, 0.741)	835/66954	545/29244
Mehta 2013	0.854 (0.729, 1.000)	464/9437	251/4397
Ng 2014	0.952 (0.853, 1.064)	1176/20618	466/7804
Ryden 2014	1.085 (0.996, 1.182)	2972/23082	749/6248
Sakhuja 2017	0.691 (0.640, 0.746)	1795/285566	1041/114708
Shahian 2009	0.780 (0.760, 0.800)	19402/560006	9455/214875
Thakar 2003	0.575 (0.499, 0.663)	488/11888	350/5054
Van Straten 2010	0.920 (0.792, 1.069)	799/7797	254/2301
Wijeysundera 2007	0.704 (0.493, 1.005)	93/7964	46/2787
Subgroup CSAKI	**0.820 (0.736, 0.913)**	**28346/1015144**	**13323/398205**
Chan	1.177 (0.992, 1.397)	270/231882	255/257793
Correa 2018	1.364 (1.318, 1.411)	7595/789439	5943/840481
Fox 2012	0.745 (0.713, 0.779)	5725/39000	3934/20970
Kate 2016	1.232 (1.129, 1.344)	1154/10791	1101/12426
Kociol 2010	2.604 (2.435, 2.785)	7249/8793	7249/11270
Li 2012	1.289 (1.036, 1.603)	6544/43718	93/774
Nadkarni 2016	1.323 (1.261, 1.389)	5277/424250	2438/258593
Nadkarni 2016.	1.067 (1.025, 1.111)	6542/299241	3860/188181
Nadkarni 2015	1.611 (1.432, 1.813)	665/288771	471/329233
Subgroup Disease	**1.309 (1.041, 1.645)**	**41021/2135885**	**25344/1919721**
Cram 2018	2.000 (1.246, 3.211)	40/40575	30/60834
Flores 2017	1.349 (1.106, 1.646)	324/8058	146/4849
George 2012	2.849 (2.368, 3.429)	503/6657	152/5451
Grams 2016	1.916 (1.657, 2.216)	9311/77611	199/2996
Jamsa 2017	1.275 (0.758, 2.147)	25/6925	33/11650
Kheterpal 2009	2.075 (1.754, 2.454)	319/22278	242/34802
Kheterpal 2007	1.199 (0.836, 1.720)	68/7811	53/7291
Nadkarni 2017	1.165 (1.033, 1.314)	831/37017	400/20698
Ozrazgat-Baslani 2016	1.198 (1.156, 1.242)	11131/26201	8894/23321
Ramonell 2016	1.852 (1.493, 2.296)	221/10253	136/11567
Salmasi 2017	2.176 (1.993, 2.375)	1403/17761	848/22359
Tong 2014	2.138 (1.777, 2.572)	343/16643	171/17545
Subgroup General Surgery	**1.707 (1.388, 2.100)**	**24519/277790**	**11304/223353**
Overall (I^2=99.61 % , P=0.000)	**1.293 (1.180, 1.417)**	**535604/101970870**	**264806/130605382**

0.49   0.99 1.29   2.47   4.16
Odds Ratio (log scale)

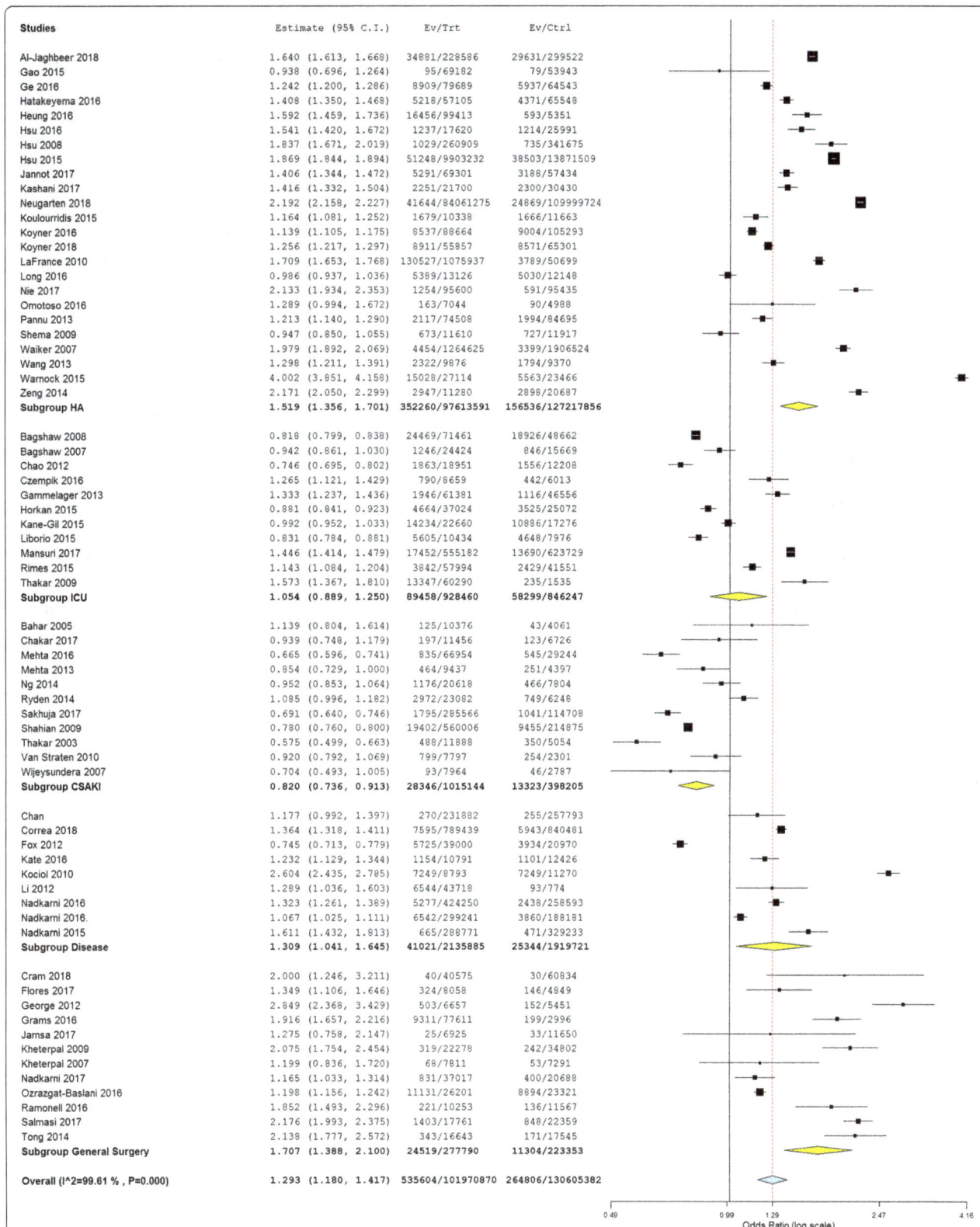

Fig. 3 Subgroup meta-analysis of 68 studies that provided unadjusted sex-stratified data regarding the incidence of hospital-associated AKI. Abbreviations used: *ICU* Intensive care unit; *HA* Hospital-associated AK; *CSAKI* Cardiac surgery-associated AKI

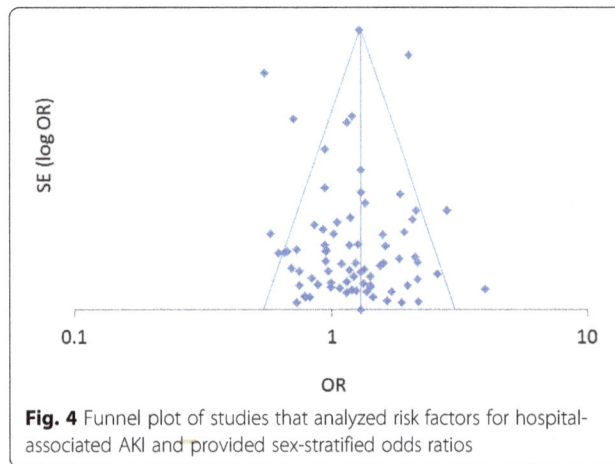

Fig. 4 Funnel plot of studies that analyzed risk factors for hospital-associated AKI and provided sex-stratified odds ratios

women and 1,497,716 men) or by investigator-created, creatinine-based criteria (OR 1.37 (0.92, 2.03), n = 15 studies, 1,306,657 patients, 470,795 women and 835,862 men).

In a separate analysis of unadjusted studies, radio-contrast-induced AKI in patients undergoing computerized axial tomography or percutaneous coronary interventions was less frequent in men than in women (OR 0.79 (0.69,0.90), n = 9 studies, 1,516,807 patients, 478,719 women and 1,038,088 men).

Discussion

Sexual dimorphism is a well-recognized feature of chronic progressive kidney disease [1]. Although less well recognized, sexual dimorphism has also been clearly established in AKI [2]. In contrast to CKD, where female sex is reno-protective, the direction of sexual dimorphism has been reported to be reversed in hospital-acquired AKI with female sex being associated with the development of AKI [19]. Moreover, female sex has been included as a risk factor in models developed to predict the risk of AKI associated with cardiac surgery, aminoglycoside nephrotoxicity, rhabdomyolysis and radio-contrast administration [15–18]. On the basis of these observations, the commentary to the KDIGO Clinical Practice Guideline for Acute Kidney Injury concludes that female sex is a risk factor for hospital-acquired AKI, while recognizing that male sex predominates in certain forms of community-acquired AKI. In the present study, we clearly show that it is male sex, not female sex, that is a risk factor for HAAKI, although we cannot determine whether this sexual dimorphism is driven by community-acquired or hospital-acquired AKI or both.

There is strong experimental basis to support our hypothesis that female sex is reno-protective in AKI [2–14, 20, 113]. Sexual dimorphism in AKI may be mediated by effects of sex hormones on cellular processes instrumental in the pathogenesis of AKI, analogous to our suggestion that sex hormones mediate sexual dimorphism in chronic kidney disease [1]. In experimental models of ischemic AKI, females show less severe renal functional impairment and less histologic damage after ischemia-reperfusion injury [2–14]. Numerous hypotheses have been proposed to explain these observations [2, 8, 113]. Sex-related differences in the generation of nitric oxide, in the synthesis and vascular response to endothelin-1, and in the renal hemodynamic response to angiotensin II have been demonstrated in experimental models and in human patients [2, 8]. Cellular responses to ischemia-reperfusion injury have also been shown to differ between the sexes. In response to ischemia-reperfusion, Na + -K+ ATPase enzyme activity is greater in females than in males and transcellular translocation of Na + -K+ ATPase is reduced [4]. Females subjected to ischemia-reperfusion injury maintain a reno-protective profile compared to their male counterparts with respect to heat shock protein HSP72, anti-oxidants such as superoxide dismutase, caspases and proteases involved in apoptosis, metalloproteinases such as meprin, inflammatory cytokines and members of signaling pathways that mediate pro-inflammatory responses [2–14, 113].

While our meta-analysis of adjusted studies demonstrated that, overall, female sex was associated with protection from HAAKI, our subgroup analysis revealed a relationship between the etiology of HAAKI and the presence or absence of sexual dimorphism. This is not surprising insofar as AKI is not a single disease but instead represents a heterogeneous group of disorders characterized by an acute reduction in renal function.

The association between female sex and protection from HAAKI was stronger among studies of hospitalized patients who underwent non-cardiac surgery than in the entire cohort of adjusted studies. Studies of critically ill patients receiving care in an intensive care unit and studies of unselected hospitalized patients also showed a higher incidence of AKI in men than in women. In this regard, unselected hospitalized patients better reflect the true relationship between sex and HAAKI as compared to studies in which patients were selected based on the etiology of AKI. In contrast, among studies of cardiac surgery-associated AKI, our meta-analysis demonstrated no difference between the sexes.

We have previously suggested that the association between female sex and cardiac surgery-associated AKI in unadjusted analyses reflects the greater burden of preexisting comorbidities among women undergoing cardiac surgery and does not indicate a greater intrinsic susceptibility of women to develop AKI under these circumstances [18]. This conclusion is reinforced by our demonstration in the present study that the sexual dimorphism associated with cardiac surgery-associated AKI in unadjusted analyses disappeared after adjustment for confounding factors.

It has been repeatedly demonstrated in unadjusted analyses and accepted by most authorities, including the commentary to the KDIGO Clinical Practice Guideline for AKI, that the incidence of contrast-induced nephropathy is greater in women than in men. However, some investigators have suggested that the association of contrast-induced nephropathy with female sex may merely reflects a higher dose of contrast administered to women compared to men [18]. Women generally have a lower body surface area than men, and accordingly the volume of administered contrast, when expressed as the volume of contrast administered per body surface area, has frequently been reported to be greater in women than in men. This hypothesis is consistent with our data which show that female sex was associated with contrast-induced nephropathy in unadjusted analyses, but that this association did not survive multivariate analysis.

We were surprised to find that only a modest, albeit significant, association of male sex with HAAKI in adjusted analyses of critically ill patients requiring care in an intensive care unit. Ischemic acute tubular necrosis is frequently the etiology of AKI in this setting and it is this form of renal injury that is most analogous to experimental ischemia-reperfusion injury, a model in which the reno-protection afforded by female sex is most robust [2–14].

A major limitation of our analysis relates to the inherent difficulty in defining AKI in men relative to women in light of sex-related differences in creatinine kinetics and the relationship of these differences to established criteria that define AKI. Waiker and Bonventre [114] assessed creatinine kinetics in patients with underlying chronic kidney disease and superimposed AKI. They identified differences in the sensitivity of absolute increases in serum creatinine levels versus relative increases in serum creatinine levels in identifying AKI in this population. They also emphasized the importance of the observation time in detecting threshold changes in serum creatinine levels. These observations are also relevant to comparisons of AKI incidence in men versus women. Since differences in the rate of generation and elimination of creatinine and in its volume of distribution exist between men and women with AKI, different criteria to define AKI might result in different sex-stratified incidence rates. Where AKI is defined by a percent change in the level of serum creatinine, the absolute change in creatinine needed to qualify as an AKI event is lower in women than in men since women generally have lower baseline serum creatinine levels. In contrast, where AKI is defined by an absolute increase in serum creatinine level, the percent change is serum creatinine required to qualify as an AKI event is greater in women than in men.

Also relevant to this issue are data reported by Srisawat et al. [52], which showed that the incidence of AKI was greater in men than in women when KDIGO criteria were used to define AKI, but that sex-related differences in the incidence of AKI disappeared when RIFLE criteria were used. These findings suggest that KDIGO criteria identify relatively more men than women with AKI compared to RIFLE criteria. Thus, it is possible that use of RIFLE criteria to define AKI, relative to KDIGO criteria, may mask the effect on female sex on the incidence of AKI, or conversely, that use of KDIGO criteria may magnify the effect. Consistent with this suggestion, our subgroup analysis shows that female sex was more likely to be associated with protection from AKI in those studies which utilized KDIGO criteria than in those that utilized RIFLE criteria. However, this conclusion is limited by the fact that our analysis, unlike the Srisawat data [52], compares outcomes based on differing definitions of AKI among different studies but not within an individual study.

We did not include in our meta-analysis 24 studies which utilized diagnosis codes to identify patients with non-dialysis-requiring AKI in the absence of corroborating biochemical data. Although Grams et al. [115] found a similar sensitivity and specificity for diagnosis codes in identifying AKI in men versus women, Waikar et al. [116] reported that the sensitivity was greater in men than in women. Were Waikar's data to apply, any conclusions about the relationship between sex and AKI identified by diagnosis codes would be placed in serious jeopardy. Incidentally, the incidence of AKI was greater in men than in women in nearly all of these studies.

In contrast, we included studies that relied on AKI-D data identified by diagnosis and procedure codes. Numerous studies have established the high sensitivity, specificity, positive predictive value and negative predictive value of diagnostic codes to identify AKI-D in a variety of administrative databases [115–119]. These indices generally exceeded 90% in all studies except that reported by Grams et al. [115]. Not only do diagnostic codes to identify AKI-D have a greater accuracy than those to identify AKI, they are also unlikely to be subject to miscoding based on the sex of the patient. Yet the fact remains that, despite the objective basis for dialysis coding, the actual decision to initiate dialysis by the clinician is a subjective one.

We recently performed a systematic review of dialysis practices in AKI and found no evidence that dialysis is initiated more often or earlier in men than in women with AKI of identical severity [120]. In fact, data exist to indicate the opposite, i.e. that dialysis is more aggressively pursued in women than in men despite identical severity of AKI. After propensity score matching of patients with AKI, Wilson et al. [121] reported that dialysis was more likely to be initiated in women than in men. Similarly, Chou et al. [122] utilized propensity matching of patients with sepsis and AKI treated in surgical intensive care units and found that female sex was associated with earlier initiation of dialysis. Moreover, data from the North American Consortium for the Study of End-Stage Liver Disease indicates that hospitalized cirrhotic women are nearly twice as likely as men to receive renal replacement therapy despite similar median delta creatinine levels [123]. Thus, these studies suggest that the subjectivity inherent in the decision to initiate dialysis creates a bias that operates counter to our hypothesis, thereby strengthening our conclusion that the incidence of severe AKI requiring RRT is more common in men than in women.

Conclusions

A meta-analysis of studies providing sex-stratified incidence of HAAKI demonstrates that female sex is associated with protection from AKI. This finding undermines the established belief that female sex is a significant risk factor for AKI. On the contrary, and consistent with observations in animal models, it is male sex that is associated with HAAKI.

Abbreviations
AKI: Acute kidney injury; AKI-D: Acute kidney injury requiring dialysis; AKIN: Acute Kidney Injury Network; HAAKI: Hospital-associated acute kidney injury; KDIGO: Kidney Disease: Improving Global Outcomes; RIFLE: Risk, Injury, Failure, Loss of kidney function, End-stage kidney disease (RIFLE); RRT: Renal replacement therapy

Acknowledgements
None.

Funding
None.

Authors' contribution
All authors participated in the design and execution of the study and in drafting the manuscript. Both authors read and approved the final version.

Competing interests
The authors declare that they have no competing interests.

References
1. S.R. NJS, Golestaneh L. Gender and kidney disease. In: Amsterdam BBM, editor. Brenner and Rector's The Kidney. Edn. Netherlands: Elsevier; 2008. p. 674–80.
2. Hutchens MP, Dunlap J, Hurn PD, Jarnberg PO. Renal ischemia: does sex matter? Anesth Analg. 2008;107(1):239–49.
3. Fekete A, Vannay A, Ver A, Rusai K, Muller V, Reusz G, Tulassay T, Szabo AJ. Sex differences in heat shock protein 72 expression and localization in rats following renal ischemia-reperfusion injury. Am J Physiol Renal Physiol. 2006;291(4):F806–11.
4. Fekete A, Vannay A, Ver A, Vasarhelyi B, Muller V, Ouyang N, Reusz G, Tulassay T, Szabo AJ. Sex differences in the alterations of Na(+), K(+)-ATPase following ischaemia-reperfusion injury in the rat kidney. J Physiol. 2004;555(Pt 2):471–80.
5. Hutchens MP, Fujiyoshi T, Komers R, Herson PS, Anderson S. Estrogen protects renal endothelial barrier function from ischemia-reperfusion in vitro and in vivo. Am J Physiol Renal Physiol. 2012;303(3):F377–85.
6. Kang KP, Lee JE, Lee AS, Jung YJ, Kim D, Lee S, Hwang HP, Kim W, Park SK. Effect of gender differences on the regulation of renal ischemia-reperfusion-induced inflammation in mice. Mol Med Rep. 2014;9(6):2061–8.
7. Kher A, Meldrum KK, Wang M, Tsai BM, Pitcher JM, Meldrum DR. Cellular and molecular mechanisms of sex differences in renal ischemia-reperfusion injury. Cardiovasc Res. 2005;67(4):594–603.
8. Metcalfe PD, Meldrum KK. Sex differences and the role of sex steroids in renal injury. J Urol. 2006;176(1):15–21.
9. Muller V, Losonczy G, Heemann U, Vannay A, Fekete A, Reusz G, Tulassay T, Szabo AJ. Sexual dimorphism in renal ischemia-reperfusion injury in rats: possible role of endothelin. Kidney Int. 2002;62(4):1364–71.
10. Park KM, Kim JI, Ahn Y, Bonventre AJ, Bonventre JV. Testosterone is responsible for enhanced susceptibility of males to ischemic renal injury. J Biol Chem. 2004;279(50):52282–92.
11. Rodriguez F, Nieto-Ceron S, Fenoy FJ, Lopez B, Hernandez I, Martinez RR, Soriano MJ, Salom MG. Sex differences in nitrosative stress during renal ischemia. Am J Physiol Regul Integr Comp Physiol. 2010;299(5):R1387–95.
12. Satake A, Takaoka M, Nishikawa M, Yuba M, Shibata Y, Okumura K, Kitano K, Tsutsui H, Fujii K, Kobuchi S, et al. Protective effect of 17beta-estradiol on ischemic acute renal failure through the PI3K/Akt/eNOS pathway. Kidney Int. 2008;73(3):308–17.
13. Takayama J, Takaoka M, Sugino Y, Yamamoto Y, Ohkita M, Matsumura Y. Sex difference in ischemic acute renal failure in rats: approach by proteomic analysis. Biol Pharm Bull. 2007;30(10):1905–12.
14. Tanaka R, Tsutsui H, Kobuchi S, Sugiura T, Yamagata M, Ohkita M, Takaoka M, Yukimura T, Matsumura Y. Protective effect of 17beta-estradiol on ischemic acute kidney injury through the renal sympathetic nervous system. Eur J Pharmacol. 2012;683(1–3):270–5.
15. Mehran R, Aymong ED, Nikolsky E, Lasic Z, Iakovou I, Fahy M, Mintz GS, Lansky AJ, Moses JW, Stone GW, et al. A simple risk score for prediction of contrast-induced nephropathy after percutaneous coronary intervention: development and initial validation. J Am Coll Cardiol. 2004;44(7):1393–9.
16. Moore RD, Smith CR, Lipsky JJ, Mellits ED, Lietman PS. Risk factors for nephrotoxicity in patients treated with aminoglycosides. Ann Intern Med. 1984;100(3):352–7.
17. McMahon GM, Zeng X, Waikar SS. A risk prediction score for kidney failure or mortality in rhabdomyolysis. JAMA Intern Med. 2013;173(19):1821–8.
18. Neugarten J, Sandilya S, Singh B, Golestaneh L. Sex and the risk of AKI following cardio-thoracic surgery: a meta-analysis. Clin J Am Soc Nephrol. 2016;11(12):2113–22.
19. KDIGO Clinical Practice Guideline for Acute Kidney Injury. Kidney Int 2012, 2(Supplement 1):1–138; Online Appendices A-F.
20. Neugarten J, Golestaneh L. The effect of gender on aminoglycoside-associated nephrotoxicity. Clin Nephrol. 2016;86(10):183–9.
21. Hutton B, Salanti G, Caldwell DM, Chaimani A, Schmid CH, Cameron C, Ioannidis JP, Straus S, Thorlund K, Jansen JP, et al. The PRISMA extension statement for reporting of systematic reviews incorporating network meta-analyses of health care interventions: checklist and explanations. Ann Intern Med. 2015;162(11):777–84.
22. Wells GA SB, O'Connell D, Peterson J, Welch V, Losos M, Tugwell P:: The Newcastle-Ottawa Scale (NOS) for assessing the quality of nonrandomised studies in meta-analyses. [http://www.ohrica/programs/clinical_epidemiology/oxfordasp].
23. Bellomo R, Ronco C, Kellum JA, Mehta RL, Palevsky P. Acute Dialysis quality initiative w: acute renal failure - definition, outcome measures, animal models, fluid therapy and information technology needs: the second international consensus conference of the acute Dialysis quality initiative (ADQI) group. Crit Care. 2004;8(4):R204–12.
24. Mehta RL, Kellum JA, Shah SV, Molitoris BA, Ronco C, Warnock DG, Levin A. Acute kidney injury N: acute kidney injury network: report of an initiative to improve outcomes in acute kidney injury. Crit Care. 2007;11(2):R31.

25. Valle JA, McCoy LA, Maddox TM, Rumsfeld JS, Ho PM, Casserly IP, Nallamothu BK, Roe MT, Tsai TT, Messenger JC. Longitudinal risk of adverse events in patients with acute kidney injury after percutaneous coronary intervention: insights from the National Cardiovascular Data Registry. Circ Cardiovasc Interv. 2017;10(4).

26. Wallace BC, Schmid CH, Lau J, Trikalinos TA. Meta-analyst: software for meta-analysis of binary, continuous and diagnostic data. BMC Med Res Methodol. 2009;9:80.

27. Bell S, Dekker FW, Vadiveloo T, Marwick C, Deshmukh H, Donnan PT, Van Diepen M. Risk of postoperative acute kidney injury in patients undergoing orthopaedic surgery--development and validation of a risk score and effect of acute kidney injury on survival: observational cohort study. BMJ. 2015;351:h5639.

28. Birnie K, Verheyden V, Pagano D, Bhabra M, Tilling K, Sterne JA, Murphy GJ, Collaborators UAiCS. Predictive models for kidney disease: improving global outcomes (KDIGO) defined acute kidney injury in UK cardiac surgery. Crit Care. 2014;18(6):606.

29. Correa A, Patel A, Chauhan K, Shah H, Saha A, Dave M, Poojary P, Mishra A, Annapureddy N, Dalal S, et al. National Trends and outcomes in Dialysis-requiring acute kidney injury in heart failure: 2002-2013. J Card Fail. 2018;24(7):442–50.

30. Cronin RM, VanHouten JP, Siew ED, Eden SK, Fihn SD, Nielson CD, Peterson JF, Baker CR, Ikizler TA, Speroff T, et al. National Veterans Health Administration inpatient risk stratification models for hospital-acquired acute kidney injury. J Am Med Inform Assoc. 2015;22(5):1054–71.

31. Czempik P, Ciesla D, Knapik P, Krzych LJ. Risk factors of acute kidney injury requiring renal replacement therapy based on regional registry data. Anaesthesiol Intensive Ther. 2016;48(3):185–90.

32. Flores E, Lewinger JP, Rowe VL, Woo K, Weaver FA, Shavelle D, Clavijo L, Garg PK. Increased risk of mortality after lower extremity bypass in individuals with acute kidney injury in the vascular quality initiative. J Vasc Surg. 2017;65(4):1055–61.

33. Ge S, Nie S, Liu Z, Chen C, Zha Y, Qian J, Liu B, Teng S, Xu A, Bin W, et al. Epidemiology and outcomes of acute kidney injury in elderly chinese patients: a subgroup analysis from the EACH study. BMC Nephrol. 2016;17(1):136.

34. George TJ, Arnaoutakis GJ, Beaty CA, Pipeling MR, Merlo CA, Conte JV, Shah AS. Acute kidney injury increases mortality after lung transplantation. Ann Thorac Surg. 2012;94(1):185–92.

35. Kendale SM, Lapis PN, Melhem SM, Blitz JD. The association between pre-operative variables, including blood pressure, and postoperative kidney function. Anaesthesia. 2016;71(12):1417–23.

36. Kheterpal S, Tremper KK, Heung M, Rosenberg AL, Englesbe M, Shanks AM, Campbell DA Jr. Development and validation of an acute kidney injury risk index for patients undergoing general surgery: results from a national data set. Anesthesiology. 2009;110(3):505–15.

37. Kim M, Brady JE, Li G. Variations in the risk of acute kidney injury across intraabdominal surgery procedures. Anesth Analg. 2014;119(5):1121–32.

38. Koyner JL, Adhikari R, Edelson DP, Churpek MM. Development of a multicenter Ward-based AKI prediction model. Clin J Am Soc Nephrol. 2016;11(11):1935–43.

39. Liu X, Ye Y, Mi Q, Huang W, He T, Huang P, Xu N, Wu Q, Wang A, Li Y, et al. A predictive model for assessing surgery-related acute kidney injury risk in hypertensive patients: a retrospective cohort study. PLoS One. 2016;11(11):e0165280.

40. Long TE, Helgason D, Helgadottir S, Palsson R, Gudbjartsson T, Sigurdsson GH, Indridason OS, Sigurdsson MI. Acute kidney injury after abdominal surgery: incidence, risk factors, and outcome. Anesth Analg. 2016;122(6):1912–20.

41. Matheny ME, Miller RA, Ikizler TA, Waitman LR, Denny JC, Schildcrout JS, Dittus RS, Peterson JF. Development of inpatient risk stratification models of acute kidney injury for use in electronic health records. Med Decis Mak. 2010;30(6):639–50.

42. Ng SY, Sanagou M, Wolfe R, Cochrane A, Smith JA, Reid CM. Prediction of acute kidney injury within 30 days of cardiac surgery. J Thorac Cardiovasc Surg. 2014;147(6):1875–83 1883 e1871.

43. Nie S, Feng Z, Tang L, Wang X, He Y, Fang J, Li S, Yang Y, Mao H, Jiao J, et al. Risk factor analysis for AKI including laboratory indicators: a Nationwide multicenter study of hospitalized patients. Kidney Blood Press Res. 2017;42(5):761–73.

44. O'Brien SM, Shahian DM, Filardo G, Ferraris VA, Haan CK, Rich JB, Normand SL, DeLong ER, Shewan CM, Dokholyan RS, et al. The Society of Thoracic Surgeons 2008 cardiac surgery risk models: part 2--isolated valve surgery. Ann Thorac Surg. 2009;88(1 Suppl):S23–42.

45. Ramonell KM, Fang S, Perez SD, Srinivasan JK, Sullivan PS, Galloway JR, Staley CA, Lin E, Sharma J, Sweeney JF, et al. Development and validation of a risk calculator for renal complications after colorectal surgery using the National Surgical Quality Improvement Program Participant use Files. Am Surg. 2016;82(12):1244–9.

46. Sakhuja A, Kashani K, Schold J, Cheungpasitporn W, Soltesz E, Demirjian S. Hospital procedure volume does not predict acute kidney injury after coronary artery bypass grafting-a nationwide study. Clin Kidney J. 2017;10(6):769–75.

47. Salmasi V, Maheshwari K, Yang D, Mascha EJ, Singh A, Sessler DI, Kurz A. Relationship between intraoperative hypotension, defined by either reduction from baseline or absolute thresholds, and acute kidney and myocardial injury after noncardiac surgery: a retrospective cohort analysis. Anesthesiology. 2017;126(1):47–65.

48. Shahian DM, O'Brien SM, Filardo G, Ferraris VA, Haan CK, Rich JB, Normand SL, DeLong ER, Shewan CM, Dokholyan RS, et al. The Society of Thoracic Surgeons 2008 cardiac surgery risk models: part 3--valve plus coronary artery bypass grafting surgery. Ann Thorac Surg. 2009;88(1 Suppl):S43–62.

49. Shroyer AL, Coombs LP, Peterson ED, Eiken MC, DeLong ER, Chen A, Ferguson TB Jr, Grover FL, Edwards FH. Society of Thoracic S: the Society of Thoracic Surgeons: 30-day operative mortality and morbidity risk models. Ann Thorac Surg. 2003;75(6):1856–64 discussion 1864-1855.

50. Siddiqui NF, Coca SG, Devereaux PJ, Jain AK, Li L, Luo J, Parikh CR, Paterson M, Philbrook HT, Wald R, et al. Secular trends in acute dialysis after elective major surgery--1995 to 2009. CMAJ. 2012;184(11):1237–45.

51. Sileanu FE, Murugan R, Lucko N, Clermont G, Kane-Gill SL, Handler SM, Kellum JA. AKI in low-risk versus high-risk patients in intensive care. Clin J Am Soc Nephrol. 2015;10(2):187–96.

52. Srisawat N, Sileanu FE, Murugan R, Bellomod R, Calzavacca P, Cartin-Ceba R, Cruz D, Finn J, Hoste EE, Kashani K, et al. Variation in risk and mortality of acute kidney injury in critically ill patients: a multicenter study. Am J Nephrol. 2015;41(1):81–8.

53. Thakar CV, Liangos O, Yared JP, Nelson D, Piedmonte MR, Hariachar S, Paganini EP. ARF after open-heart surgery: influence of gender and race. Am J Kidney Dis. 2003;41(4):742–51.

54. Aubry P, Brillet G, Catella L, Schmidt A, Benard S. Outcomes, risk factors and health burden of contrast-induced acute kidney injury: an observational study of one million hospitalizations with image-guided cardiovascular procedures. BMC Nephrol. 2016;17(1):167.

55. Brown JR, DeVries JT, Piper WD, Robb JF, Hearne MJ, Ver Lee PM, Kellet MA, Watkins MW, Ryan TJ, Silver MT, et al. Serious renal dysfunction after percutaneous coronary interventions can be predicted. Am Heart J. 2008;155(2):260–6.

56. Khanal S, Attallah N, Smith DE, Kline-Rogers E, Share D, O'Donnell MJ, Moscucci M. Statin therapy reduces contrast-induced nephropathy: an analysis of contemporary percutaneous interventions. Am J Med. 2005;118(8):843–9.

57. Al-Jaghbeer M, Dealmeida D, Bilderback A, Ambrosino R, Kellum JA. Clinical decision support for in-hospital AKI. J Am Soc Nephrol. 2018;29(2):654–60.

58. Bagshaw SM, George C, Bellomo R, Committee ADM. Changes in the incidence and outcome for early acute kidney injury in a cohort of Australian intensive care units. Crit Care. 2007;11(3):R68.

59. Bagshaw SM, George C, Bellomo R, Committee ADM. Early acute kidney injury and sepsis: a multicentre evaluation. Crit Care. 2008;12(2):R47.

60. Bahar I, Akgul A, Ozatik MA, Vural KM, Demirbag AE, Boran M, Tasdemir O. Acute renal failure following open heart surgery: risk factors and prognosis. Perfusion. 2005;20(6):317–22.

61. Briggs A, Havens JM, Salim A, Christopher KB. Acute kidney injury predicts mortality in emergency general surgery patients. Am J Surg. 2018.

62. Chaker Z, Badhwar V, Alqahtani F, Aljohani S, Zack CJ, Holmes DR, Rihal CS, Alkhouli M. Sex differences in the utilization and outcomes of surgical aortic valve replacement for severe aortic stenosis. J Am Heart Assoc. 2017;6(9).

63. Chan L, Mehta S, Chauhan K, Poojary P, Patel S, Pawar S, Patel A, Correa A, Patel S, Garimella PS, et al. National Trends and impact of acute kidney injury requiring hemodialysis in hospitalizations with atrial fibrillation. J Am Heart Assoc. 2016;5(12).

64. Chao CT, Hou CC, Wu VC, Lu HM, Wang CY, Chen L, Kao TW. The impact of dialysis-requiring acute kidney injury on long-term prognosis of patients requiring prolonged mechanical ventilation: nationwide population-based study. PLoS One. 2012;7(12):e50675.

65. Cram P, Hawker G, Matelski J, Ravi B, Pugely A, Gandhi R, Jackson T. Disparities in knee and hip arthroplasty outcomes: an observational analysis of the ACS-NSQIP clinical registry. J Racial Ethn Health Disparities. 2018;5(1):151–61.

66. Fox CS, Muntner P, Chen AY, Alexander KP, Roe MT, Wiviott SD. Short-term outcomes of acute myocardial infarction in patients with acute kidney injury: a report from the national cardiovascular data registry. Circulation. 2012;125(3):497–504.

67. Gammelager H, Christiansen CF, Johansen MB, Tonnesen E, Jespersen B, Sorensen HT. Five-year risk of end-stage renal disease among intensive care patients surviving dialysis-requiring acute kidney injury: a nationwide cohort study. Crit Care. 2013;17(4):R145.

68. Gao J, Chen M, Wang X, Wang H, Zhuo L. Risk factors and prognosis of acute kidney injury in adult hospitalized patients: a two-year outcome. Minerva Urol Nefrol. 2015;67(3):179–85.

69. Grams ME, Sang Y, Coresh J, Ballew S, Matsushita K, Molnar MZ, Szabo Z, Kalantar-Zadeh K, Kovesdy CP. Acute kidney injury after major surgery: a retrospective analysis of veterans health administration data. Am J Kidney Dis. 2016;67(6):872–80.

70. Hatakeyama Y, Horino T, Kataoka H, Matsumoto T, Ode K, Shimamura Y, Ogata K, Inoue K, Taniguchi Y, Terada Y, et al. Incidence of acute kidney injury among patients with chronic kidney disease: a single-center retrospective database analysis. Clin Exp Nephrol. 2017;21(1):43–8.

71. Heung M, Steffick DE, Zivin K, Gillespie BW, Banerjee T, Hsu CY, Powe NR, Pavkov ME, Williams DE, Saran R, et al. Acute kidney injury recovery pattern and subsequent risk of CKD: an analysis of veterans health administration data. Am J Kidney Dis. 2016;67(5):742–52.

72. Horkan CM, Purtle SW, Mendu ML, Moromizato T, Gibbons FK, Christopher KB. The association of acute kidney injury in the critically ill and postdischarge outcomes: a cohort study. Crit Care Med. 2015;43(2):354–64.

73. Hsu CY, Hsu RK, Yang J, Ordonez JD, Zheng S, Go AS. Elevated BP after AKI. J Am Soc Nephrol. 2016;27(3):914–23.

74. Hsu CY, Ordonez JD, Chertow GM, Fan D, McCulloch CE, Go AS. The risk of acute renal failure in patients with chronic kidney disease. Kidney Int. 2008; 74(1):101–7.

75. Hsu RK, McCulloch CE, Heung M, Saran R, Shahinian VB, Pavkov ME, Burrows NR, Powe NR, Hsu CY, Centers for disease C, et al. Exploring potential reasons for the temporal trend in Dialysis-requiring AKI in the United States. Clin J Am Soc Nephrol. 2016;11(1):14–20.

76. Jamsa P, Jamsen E, Lyytikainen LP, Kalliovalkama J, Eskelinen A, Oksala N. Risk factors associated with acute kidney injury in a cohort of 20,575 arthroplasty patients. Acta Orthop. 2017;88(4):370–6.

77. Jannot AS, Burgun A, Thervet E, Pallet N. The diagnosis-wide landscape of hospital-acquired AKI. Clin J Am Soc Nephrol. 2017;12(6):874–84.

78. Kane-Gill SL, Sileanu FE, Murugan R, Trietley GS, Handler SM, Kellum JA. Risk factors for acute kidney injury in older adults with critical illness: a retrospective cohort study. Am J Kidney Dis. 2015;65(6):860–9.

79. Kashani K, Shao M, Li G, Williams AW, Rule AD, Kremers WK, Malinchoc M, Gajic O, Lieske JC. No increase in the incidence of acute kidney injury in a population-based annual temporal trends epidemiology study. Kidney Int. 2017;92(3):721–8.

80. Kate RJ, Perez RM, Mazumdar D, Pasupathy KS, Nilakantan V. Prediction and detection models for acute kidney injury in hospitalized older adults. BMC Med Inform Decis Mak. 2016;16:39.

81. Kheterpal S, Tremper KK, Englesbe MJ, O'Reilly M, Shanks AM, Fetterman DM, Rosenberg AL, Swartz RD. Predictors of postoperative acute renal failure after noncardiac surgery in patients with previously normal renal function. Anesthesiology. 2007;107(6):892–902.

82. Kociol RD, Greiner MA, Hammill BG, Phatak H, Fonarow GC, Curtis LH, Hernandez AF. Long-term outcomes of medicare beneficiaries with worsening renal function during hospitalization for heart failure. Am J Cardiol. 2010;105(12):1786–93.

83. Koulouridis I, Price LL, Madias NE, Jaber BL. Hospital-acquired acute kidney injury and hospital readmission: a cohort study. Am J Kidney Dis. 2015;65(2):275–82.

84. Koyner JL, Carey KA, Edelson DP, Churpek MM. The development of a machine learning inpatient acute kidney injury prediction model. Crit Care Med. 2018.

85. Lafrance JP, Miller DR. Defining acute kidney injury in database studies: the effects of varying the baseline kidney function assessment period and considering CKD status. Am J Kidney Dis. 2010;56(4):651–60.

86. Li Y, Shlipak MG, Grunfeld C, Choi AI. Incidence and risk factors for acute kidney injury in HIV infection. Am J Nephrol. 2012;35(4):327–34.

87. Liborio AB, Leite TT, Neves FM, Teles F, Bezerra CT. AKI complications in critically ill patients: association with mortality rates and RRT. Clin J Am Soc Nephrol. 2015;10(1):21–8.

88. Long TE, Sigurdsson MI, Sigurdsson GH, Indridason OS. Improved long-term survival and renal recovery after acute kidney injury in hospitalized patients: a 20 year experience. Nephrology (Carlton). 2016;21(12):1027–33.

89. Mansuri U, Patel A, Shah H, Chauhan K, Poojary P, Saha A, Dave M, Hazra A, Mishra T, Annapureddy N, et al. Trends and outcomes of sepsis hospitalizations complicated by acute kidney injury requiring hemodialysis. J Crit Care. 2017;38:353–5.

90. Mehta RH, Castelvecchio S, Ballotta A, Frigiola A, Bossone E, Ranucci M. Association of gender and lowest hematocrit on cardiopulmonary bypass with acute kidney injury and operative mortality in patients undergoing cardiac surgery. Ann Thorac Surg. 2013;96(1):133–40.

91. Mehta RH, Grab JD, O'Brien SM, Bridges CR, Gammie JS, Haan CK, Ferguson TB, Peterson ED. Society of Thoracic Surgeons National Cardiac Surgery Database I: bedside tool for predicting the risk of postoperative dialysis in patients undergoing cardiac surgery. Circulation. 2006;114(21):2208–16 quiz 2208.

92. Nadkarni GN, Chauhan K, Patel A, Saha A, Poojary P, Kamat S, Patel S, Ferrandino R, Konstantinidis I, Garimella PS, et al. Temporal trends of dialysis requiring acute kidney injury after orthotopic cardiac and liver transplant hospitalizations. BMC Nephrol. 2017;18(1):244.

93. Nadkarni GN, Patel A, Simoes PK, Yacoub R, Annapureddy N, Kamat S, Konstantinidis I, Perumalswami P, Branch A, Coca SG, et al. Dialysis-requiring acute kidney injury among hospitalized adults with documented hepatitis C virus infection: a nationwide inpatient sample analysis. J Viral Hepat. 2016; 23(1):32–8.

94. Nadkarni GN, Patel AA, Konstantinidis I, Mahajan A, Agarwal SK, Kamat S, Annapureddy N, Benjo A, Thakar CV. Dialysis requiring acute kidney injury in acute cerebrovascular accident hospitalizations. Stroke. 2015;46(11):3226–31.

95. Nadkarni GN, Simoes PK, Patel A, Patel S, Yacoub R, Konstantinidis I, Kamat S, Annapureddy N, Parikh CR, Coca SG. National trends of acute kidney injury requiring dialysis in decompensated cirrhosis hospitalizations in the United States. Hepatol Int. 2016;10(3):525–31.

96. Neugarten J, Golestaneh L, Kolhe NV. Sex differences in acute kidney injury requiring dialysis. BMC Nephrol. 2018;19(1):131.

97. Omotoso BA, Abdel-Rahman EM, Xin W, Ma JZ, Scully KW, Arogundade FA, Balogun RA. Dialysis requirement, long-term major adverse cardiovascular events (MACE) and all-cause mortality in hospital acquired acute kidney injury (AKI): a propensity-matched cohort study. J Nephrol. 2016;29(6):847–55.

98. Ozrazgat-Baslanti T, Thottakkara P, Huber M, Berg K, Gravenstein N, Tighe P, Lipori G, Segal MS, Hobson C, Bihorac A. Acute and chronic kidney disease and cardiovascular mortality after major surgery. Ann Surg. 2016;264(6):987–96.

99. Pannu N, James M, Hemmelgarn B, Klarenbach S, Alberta kidney disease N. Association between AKI, recovery of renal function, and long-term outcomes after hospital discharge. Clin J Am Soc Nephrol. 2013;8(2):194–202.

100. Rimes-Stigare C, Frumento P, Bottai M, Martensson J, Martling CR, Bell M. Long-term mortality and risk factors for development of end-stage renal disease in critically ill patients with and without chronic kidney disease. Crit Care. 2015;19:383.

101. Ryden L, Sartipy U, Evans M, Holzmann MJ. Acute kidney injury after coronary artery bypass grafting and long-term risk of end-stage renal disease. Circulation. 2014;130(23):2005–11.

102. Sakhuja A, Kumar G, Gupta S, Mittal T, Taneja A, Nanchal RS. Acute kidney injury requiring Dialysis in severe Sepsis. Am J Respir Crit Care Med. 2015; 192(8):951–7.

103. Shahian DM, O'Brien SM, Filardo G, Ferraris VA, Haan CK, Rich JB, Normand SL, DeLong ER, Shewan CM, Dokholyan RS, et al. The Society of Thoracic Surgeons 2008 cardiac surgery risk models: part 1--coronary artery bypass grafting surgery. Ann Thorac Surg. 2009;88(1 Suppl):S2–22.

104. Shema L, Ore L, Geron R, Kristal B. Hospital-acquired acute kidney injury in Israel. Isr Med Assoc J. 2009;11(5):269–74.

105. Thakar CV, Christianson A, Freyberg R, Almenoff P, Render ML. Incidence and outcomes of acute kidney injury in intensive care units: a veterans administration study. Crit Care Med. 2009;37(9):2552–8.

106. Tong BC, Kosinski AS, Burfeind WR Jr, Onaitis MW, Berry MF, Harpole DH Jr, D'Amico TA. Sex differences in early outcomes after lung cancer resection: analysis of the Society of Thoracic Surgeons general thoracic database. J Thorac Cardiovasc Surg. 2014;148(1):13–8.

107. van Straten AH, Hamad MA, van Zundert AA, Martens EJ, Schonberger JP, de Wolf AM. Risk factors for deterioration of renal function after coronary artery bypass grafting. Eur J Cardiothorac Surg. 2010;37(1):106–11.

108. Waikar SS, Curhan GC, Ayanian JZ, Chertow GM. Race and mortality after acute renal failure. J Am Soc Nephrol. 2007;18(10):2740–8.

109. Wang HE, Jain G, Glassock RJ, Warnock DG. Comparison of absolute serum creatinine changes versus kidney disease: improving global outcomes consensus definitions for characterizing stages of acute kidney injury. Nephrol Dial Transplant. 2013;28(6):1447–54.

110. Warnock DG, Powell TC, Donnelly JP, Wang HE. Categories of hospital-associated acute kidney injury: time course of changes in serum creatinine values. Nephron. 2015;131(4):227–36.

111. Wijeysundera DN, Karkouti K, Dupuis JY, Rao V, Chan CT, Granton JT, Beattie WS. Derivation and validation of a simplified predictive index for renal replacement therapy after cardiac surgery. JAMA. 2007;297(16):1801–9.

112. Zeng X, McMahon GM, Brunelli SM, Bates DW, Waikar SS. Incidence, outcomes, and comparisons across definitions of AKI in hospitalized individuals. Clin J Am Soc Nephrol. 2014;9(1):12–20.

113. Dubey RK, Jackson EK. Estrogen-induced cardiorenal protection: potential cellular, biochemical, and molecular mechanisms. Am J Physiol Renal Physiol. 2001;280(3):F365–88.

114. Waikar SS, Bonventre JV. Creatinine kinetics and the definition of acute kidney injury. J Am Soc Nephrol. 2009;20(3):672–9.

115. Grams ME, Waikar SS, MacMahon B, Whelton S, Ballew SH, Coresh J. Performance and limitations of administrative data in the identification of AKI. Clin J Am Soc Nephrol. 2014;9(4):682–9.

116. Waikar SS, Wald R, Chertow GM, Curhan GC, Winkelmayer WC, Liangos O, Sosa MA, Jaber BL. Validity of international classification of diseases, ninth revision, clinical modification codes for acute renal failure. J Am Soc Nephrol. 2006;17(6):1688–94.

117. Quinn RR, Laupacis A, Austin PC, Hux JE, Garg AX, Hemmelgarn BR, Oliver MJ. Using administrative datasets to study outcomes in dialysis patients: a validation study. Med Care. 2010;48(8):745–50.

118. Romano PS, Mark DH. Bias in the coding of hospital discharge data and its implications for quality assessment. Med Care. 1994;32(1):81–90.

119. Vlasschaert ME, Bejaimal SA, Hackam DG, Quinn R, Cuerden MS, Oliver MJ, Iansavichus A, Sultan N, Mills A, Garg AX. Validity of administrative database coding for kidney disease: a systematic review. Am J Kidney Dis. 2011;57(1):29–43.

120. Blush J, Lei J, Ju W, Silbiger S, Pullman J, Neugarten J. Estradiol reverses renal injury in Alb/TGF-beta1 transgenic mice. Kidney Int. 2004;66(6):2148–54.

121. Wilson FP, Yang W, Machado CA, Mariani LH, Borovskiy Y, Berns JS, Feldman HI. Dialysis versus nondialysis in patients with AKI: a propensity-matched cohort study. Clin J Am Soc Nephrol. 2014;9(4):673–81.

122. Chou YH, Huang TM, Wu VC, Wang CY, Shiao CC, Lai CF, Tsai HB, Chao CT, Young GH, Wang WJ, et al. Impact of timing of renal replacement therapy initiation on outcome of septic acute kidney injury. Crit Care. 2011;15(3):R134.

123. O'Leary JG, Wong F, Reddy KR, Garcia-Tsao G, Kamath PS, Biggins SW, Fallon MB, Subramanian RM, Maliakkal B, Thacker L, et al. Gender-specific differences in baseline, peak, and Delta serum creatinine: the NACSELD experience. Dig Dis Sci. 2017;62(3):768–76.

Permissions

All chapters in this book were first published in NEPHROLOGY, by BioMed Central; hereby published with permission under the Creative Commons Attribution License or equivalent. Every chapter published in this book has been scrutinized by our experts. Their significance has been extensively debated. The topics covered herein carry significant findings which will fuel the growth of the discipline. They may even be implemented as practical applications or may be referred to as a beginning point for another development.

The contributors of this book come from diverse backgrounds, making this book a truly international effort. This book will bring forth new frontiers with its revolutionizing research information and detailed analysis of the nascent developments around the world.

We would like to thank all the contributing authors for lending their expertise to make the book truly unique. They have played a crucial role in the development of this book. Without their invaluable contributions this book wouldn't have been possible. They have made vital efforts to compile up to date information on the varied aspects of this subject to make this book a valuable addition to the collection of many professionals and students.

This book was conceptualized with the vision of imparting up-to-date information and advanced data in this field. To ensure the same, a matchless editorial board was set up. Every individual on the board went through rigorous rounds of assessment to prove their worth. After which they invested a large part of their time researching and compiling the most relevant data for our readers.

The editorial board has been involved in producing this book since its inception. They have spent rigorous hours researching and exploring the diverse topics which have resulted in the successful publishing of this book. They have passed on their knowledge of decades through this book. To expedite this challenging task, the publisher supported the team at every step. A small team of assistant editors was also appointed to further simplify the editing procedure and attain best results for the readers.

Apart from the editorial board, the designing team has also invested a significant amount of their time in understanding the subject and creating the most relevant covers. They scrutinized every image to scout for the most suitable representation of the subject and create an appropriate cover for the book.

The publishing team has been an ardent support to the editorial, designing and production team. Their endless efforts to recruit the best for this project, has resulted in the accomplishment of this book. They are a veteran in the field of academics and their pool of knowledge is as vast as their experience in printing. Their expertise and guidance has proved useful at every step. Their uncompromising quality standards have made this book an exceptional effort. Their encouragement from time to time has been an inspiration for everyone.

The publisher and the editorial board hope that this book will prove to be a valuable piece of knowledge for researchers, students, practitioners and scholars across the globe.

List of Contributors

Xiajing Che, Xiaoqian Yang, Jiayi Yan, Yanhong Yuan, Qing Ma, Minfang Zhang, Qin Wang, Zhaohui Ni and Shan Mou
Department of Nephrology, Molecular Cell Laboratory for Kidney Disease, Renji Hospital, School of Medicine, Shanghai Jiao Tong University, 160 Pujian Road, Shanghai 200127, China

Ming Zhang and Liang Ying
Transplantation Center of Ren Ji Hospital, School of Medicine, Shanghai Jiao Tong University, 160 Pujian Road, Shanghai 200127, China

Alaa A Ali and Michael D Hughson
Department of Pathology, Shorsh General Hospital, Qirga Road, Sulaimaniyah, Kurdistan, Iraq

Dana A Sharif
Department of Medicine, Sulaimaniyah University, Sulaimaniyah, Iraq

Safa E Almukhtar
Hawler University College of Medicine, Erbil, Iraq

Kais Hasan Abd and Zana Sidiq M Saleem
Dohuk University, Dohuk, Iraq

Bancha Satirapoj and Rattanawan Dispan
Division of Nephrology, Department of Medicine, Phramongkutklao Hospital and College of Medicine, Bangkok, Thailand

Piyanuch Radinahamed and Chagriya Kitiyakara
Division of Nephrology, Department of Medicine, Faculty of Medicine Ramathibodi Hospital, Mahidol University, 270 Rama 6 Rd, Bangkok 10400, Thailand

Suguru Yamamoto
Division of Clinical Nephrology and Rheumatology, Niigata University Graduate School of Medical and Dental Sciences, 1-757 Asahimachi-dori, Niigata 951-8510, Japan

Angelo Karaboyas, Ronald L. Pisoni, Bruce M. Robinson and Brian A. Bieber
Arbor Research Collaborative for Health, Ann Arbor, MI, USA

Masafumi Fukagawa and Hirotaka Komaba
Division of Nephrology, Endocrinology and Metabolism, Tokai University School of Medicine, Isehara, Japan

Masatomo Taniguchi
Fukuoka Renal Clinic, Fukuoka, Japan

Takanobu Nomura
Medical Affairs Department, Kyowa Hakko Kirin Co. Ltd., Tokyo, Japan

Patricia De Sequera
University Hospital Infanta Leonor, Madrid, Spain

Anders Christensson
Department of Nephrology, Skåne University Hospital, Malmö-, Lund, Sweden

Mariette J Chartier, Randy Walld, Ina Koseva, Charles Burchill and Kari-Lynne McGowan
Manitoba Centre for Health Policy, Department of Community Health Sciences, University of Manitoba, Winnipeg, Canada

Navdeep Tangri and Paul Komenda
Chronic Disease Innovation Centre, Seven Oaks General Hospital, Department of Medicine and Community Health Sciences, Max Rady College of Medicine, University of Manitoba, Winnipeg, Canada

Allison Dart
Department of Pediatrics and Child Health, Section of Nephrology, University of Manitoba, Winnipeg, Canada

Andrea Corsonello, Silvia Bustacchini and Fabrizia Lattanzio
Italian National Research Center on Aging (INRCA), Ancona, Fermo and Cosenza, Italy

Lisanne Tap and Francesco Mattace-Raso
Section of Geriatric Medicine, Department of Internal Medicine, Erasmus University Medical Center Rotterdam, Rotterdam, The Netherlands

Regina Roller-Wirnsberger and Gerhard Wirnsberger
Department of Internal Medicine, Medical University of Graz, Auenbruggerplatz 15, 8036, Graz, Austria

Carmine Zoccali
CNR-IFC, Clinical Epidemiology and Pathophysiology of Hypertension and Renal Diseases, Ospedali Riuniti, Reggio Calabria, Italy

Tomasz Kostka and Agnieszka Guligowska
Department of Geriatrics, Healthy Ageing Research Centre, Medical University of Lodz, Lodz, Poland

Pedro Gil and Lara Guardado Fuentes
Department of Geriatric Medicine, Hospital Clinico San Carlos, Madrid, Spain

Itshak Meltzer
The Recanati School for Community Health Professions at the faculty of Health Sciences, Ben-Gurion University of the Negev, Beersheba, Israel

Ilan Yehoshua
Maccabi Healthcare Services Southern Region, Tel Aviv, Israel

Francesc Formiga-Perez and Rafael Moreno-González
Geriatric Unit, Internal Medicine Department and Nephrology Department, Bellvitge University Hospital – IDIBELL – L'Hospitalet de Llobregat, Barcelona, Spain

Christian Weingart and Ellen Freiberger
Department of General Internal Medicine and Geriatrics, Krankenhaus Barmherzige Brüder Regensburg and Institute for Biomedicine of Aging, Friedrich-Alexander-Universität Erlangen-Nürnberg, Erlangen, Germany

Johan Ärnlöv
Department of Medical Sciences, Uppsala University, Uppsala, Sweden
School of Health and Social Studies, Dalarna University, Falun, Sweden
Division of Family Medicine, Department of Neurobiology, Care Sciences and Society, Karolinska Institutet, Stockholm, Sweden

Axel C. Carlsson
Department of Medical Sciences, Uppsala University, Uppsala, Sweden
Division of Family Medicine, Department of Neurobiology, Care Sciences and Society, Karolinska Institutet, Stockholm, Sweden

Ayse Akcan Arikan
Department of Pediatrics, Renal Section, Baylor College of Medicine, Houston, TX, USA

Alyssa A. Riley
Department of Pediatrics, Renal Section, Baylor College of Medicine, Houston, TX, USA
Department of Pediatrics, Dell Medical School, The University of Texas at Austin, Austin, TX, USA

Mary Watson, Carolyn Smith and Helen Currier
Texas Children's Hospital, Houston, TX, USA
Department of Pediatrics, Dell Medical School, The University of Texas at Austin, Austin, TX, USA

Danielle Guffey and Charles G. Minard
Dan L. Duncan Institute for Clinical and Translational Research, Baylor College of Medicine, Houston, TX, USA

Erika De Sousa-Amorim, Frederic Cofán and Federico Oppenheimer
Department of Nephrology and Renal Transplantation, ICNU, Hospital Clinic, Barcelona, Spain

Gastón J Piñeiro, Pedro Ventura-Aguiar and David Cucchiari
Department of Nephrology and Renal Transplantation, ICNU, Hospital Clinic, Barcelona, Spain
Laboratori Experimental de Nefrologia i Trasplantament(LENIT), IDIBAPS, Barcelona, Spain

Ignacio Revuelta and Fritz Diekmann
Department of Nephrology and Renal Transplantation, ICNU, Hospital Clinic, Barcelona, Spain
Laboratori Experimental de Nefrologia i Trasplantament(LENIT), IDIBAPS, Barcelona, Spain

Josep M Campistol
Department of Nephrology and Renal Transplantation, ICNU, Hospital Clinic, Barcelona, Spain
Red de Investigación Renal (REDinREN), Madrid, Spain

Jordi Rovira
Laboratori Experimental de Nefrologia i Trasplantament(LENIT), IDIBAPS, Barcelona, Spain
Red de Investigación Renal (REDinREN), Madrid, Spain

Manel Solé
Department of Pathology, Hospital Clinic, Barcelona, Spain

José Ríos
Medical Statistics Core Facility, IDIBAPS, Hospital Clinic, Barcelona, Spain
Biostatistics Unit, Faculty of Medicine, Autonomous University of Barcelona, Barcelona, Spain

Joan Cid and Miguel Lozano
Apheresis Unit, Department of Hemotherapy and Hemostasis, IDIBAPS, Hospital Clinic, Barcelona, Spain

Eduard Palou
Department ofImmunology, Hospital Clinic, Barcelona, Spain

Paschal Ruggajo
Department of Internal Medicine, Muhimbili University of Health and Allied Sciences (MUHAS), Dar es Salaam, Tanzania

Department of Clinical Medicine, University of Bergen, Bergen, Norway

Einar Svarstad and Hans-Peter Marti
Department of Clinical Medicine, University of Bergen, Bergen, Norway
Department of Medicine, Haukeland University Hospital, Bergen, Norway

Sabine Leh
Department of Clinical Medicine, University of Bergen, Bergen, Norway
Department of Pathology, Haukeland University Hospital, Bergen, Norway

Bjørn Egil Vikse
Department of Clinical Medicine, University of Bergen, Bergen, Norway
Department of Medicine, Haugesund Hospital, Haugesund, Norway

Annekathrin Haase, Fabian Ludwig, Aniela Angelow, Maria Mahner and Jean-François Chenot
Department of General Practice, Institute for Community Medicine, University Medicine Greifswald, Fleischmannstr. 6, 17475 Greifswald, Germany

Gesine F C Weckmann
Department of General Practice, Institute for Community Medicine, University Medicine Greifswald, Fleischmannstr. 6, 17475 Greifswald, Germany
Faculty of Applied Health Sciences, European University of Applied Sciences, Rostock, Germany

Sylvia Stracke
Department of Internal Medicine A, Nephrology Dialysis and Hypertension, University Medicine Greifswald, Greifswald, Germany

Jacob Spallek
Department of Public Health, Brandenburg University of Technology Cottbus-Senftenberg, Senftenberg, Germany

Jetske M Emmelkamp
Department II – Cardiology, Clinic for Internal Medicine, Pulmonology and General Internal Medicine, DRK-Krankenhaus Teterow, Teterow, Germany

Stanford E. Mwasongwe
Jackson Heart Study, Jackson State University, 350 W. Woodrow Wilson Ave., Suite 701, Jackson, MS 39213, USA

Bessie Young
Division of Nephrology, Kidney Research Institute University of Washington, Seattle, WA, USA

Veterans Affairs Puget Sound Health Care System, Seattle, WA, USA

Mario Sims, Adolfo Correa and Solomon K. Musani
Department of Medicine, University of Mississippi Medical Center, Jackson, MS, USA

Aurelian Bidulescu
Department of Epidemiology and Biostatistics, School of Public Health, Indiana University, Bloomington, IN, USA

Michael J. Fischer
Center of Innovation for Complex Chronic Healthcare, Jesse Brown VA Medical Center, Chicago, IL, USA
Edward Hines Jr. VA Hospital, Hines, IL, USA
Department of Medicine, University of Illinois at Chicago, College of Medicine, Chicago, IL, USA

Swati Lederer
Center of Innovation for Complex Chronic Healthcare, Jesse Brown VA Medical Center, Chicago, IL, USA
Edward Hines Jr. VA Hospital, Hines, IL, USA
Department of Medicine, University of Illinois at Chicago, College of Medicine, Chicago, IL, USA
Department of Medicine, VA North Texas Healthcare System, 4500 South Lancaster Ave, MC 111G1, Dallas, TX 75216, USA

Jinsong Chen and James P. Lash
Department of Medicine, University of Illinois at Chicago, College of Medicine, Chicago, IL, USA

Nicole M. Sisen, Nancy Lepain and Kate Grubbs O'Connor
National Kidney Foundation of Illinois, Chicago, IL, USA

Yamin Wang
Community Health Sciences Division/Institute for Health Research and Policy, School of Public Health, University of Illinois at Chicago, Chicago, IL, USA

Laurie Ruggiero
Community Health Sciences Division/Institute for Health Research and Policy, School of Public Health, University of Illinois at Chicago, Chicago, IL, USA
Behavioral Health and Nutrition, College of Health Sciences, University of Delaware, Newark, DE, USA

Ai Katsuma, Yasuyuki Nakada, Izumi Yamamoto, Haruki Katsumata and Takashi Yokoo
Division of Nephrology and Hypertension, Department of Internal Medicine, The Jikei University School of Medicine, 3-25-8, Nishi-Shimbashi, Minato-ku, Tokyo 105-8461, Japan

Shigeru Horita
Department of Medicine, Kidney center, Tokyo Women's Medical University, Tokyo, Japan

Masayoshi Okumi, Hideki Ishida, Kazunari Tanabe, Miyuki Furusawa and Kohei Unagami
Department of Urology, Tokyo Women's Medical University, Tokyo, Japan

Claudia Sommerer and Martin Zeier
Department of Nephrology, University of Heidelberg, Im Neuenheimer Feld 162, 69120 Heidelberg, Germany

Oliver Witzke
Department of Infectious Diseases, University Duisburg-Essen, Essen, Germany

Frank Lehner
Department of General, Visceral and Transplantation Surgery, Hannover Medical School, Hannover, Germany

Wolfgang Arns
Department of Nephrology and Transplantation, Cologne Merheim Medical Center, Cologne, Germany

Petra Reinke
Department of Nephrology and Intensive Care, Charité Campus Virchow, Charité-Universitätsmedizin Berlin, Berlin, Germany

Ute Eisenberger and Bruno Vogt
Department of Nephrology and Hypertension, University of Bern, Inselspital, Bern, Switzerland

Katharina Heller and Johannes Jacobi
Department of Nephrology and Hypertension, University of Erlangen-Nuremberg, Erlangen, Germany

Markus Guba
Department of General-, Visceral- and Transplantation Surgery, Munich University Hospital, Campus Grosshadern, Munich, Germany

Rolf Stahl
Division of Nephrology, University Medical Center Hamburg-Eppendorf, Hamburg, Germany

Ingeborg A. Hauser
Med. Klinik III, Department of Nephrology, UKF, Goethe University, Frankfurt, Germany

Volker Kliem
Department of Internal Medicine and Nephrology, Kidney Transplant Center, Nephrological Center of Lower Saxony, Klinikum Hann, Münden, Germany

Rudolf P. Wüthrich
Division of Nephrology, University Hospital, Zürich, Switzerland

Anja Mühlfeld
Division of Nephrology and Immunology, University Hospital RWTH Aachen, Aachen, Germany

Barbara Suwelack
Department of Internal Medicine – Transplant Nephrology, University Hospital of Münster, Münster, Germany

Klemens Budde and Michael Duerr
Department of Nephrology, Charité Universitätsmedizin Berlin, Berlin, Germany

Martina Porstner and Eva-Maria Paulus
Novartis Pharma GmbH, Nürnberg, Germany

Paulo Ricardo Gessolo Lins, Wallace Stwart Carvalho Padilha and Marcelo Costa Batista
Discipline of Nephrology, Federal University of São Paulo, Rua Botucatu, 591 - 15 ° andar - Cj153 - Vila Clementino, São Paulo, SP 04023-062, Brazil

Aécio Flávio Teixeira de Gois and Carolina Frade Magalhaes Giradin Pimentel
Discipline of Medicine of Urgency and Evidence-Based Medicine from the Department of Medicine, Federal University of São Paulo, Rua Napoleão de Barros, 865 - Vila Clementino, São Paulo, SP 04023-090, Brazil

Tuyen Van Duong, Chi-Sin Wang, I-Hsin Tseng, Yi-Wei Feng and Tai-Yue Chang
School of Nutrition and Health Sciences, Taipei Medical University, No. 250 Wuxing Street, Taipei 110, Taiwan

Shwu-Huey Yang
School of Nutrition and Health Sciences, Taipei Medical University, No. 250 Wuxing Street, Taipei 110, Taiwan
Research Center of Geriatric Nutrition, Taipei Medical University, Taipei, Taiwan
Nutrition Research Center, Taipei Medical University Hospital, Taipei, Taiwan

Te-Chih Wong
Department of Nutrition and Health Sciences, Chinese Culture University, Taipei, Taiwan

Hsi-Hsien Chen
Department of Nephrology, Taipei Medical University Hospital, Taipei, Taiwan

School of Medicine, Taipei Medical University, Taipei, Taiwan

Tzen-Wen Chen
School of Medicine, Taipei Medical University, Taipei, Taiwan

Tso-Hsiao Chen
School of Medicine, Taipei Medical University, Taipei, Taiwan
Department of Nephrology, Taipei Medical University-Wan Fang Hospital, Taipei, Taiwan

Yung-Ho Hsu
School of Medicine, Taipei Medical University, Taipei, Taiwan
Division of Nephrology, Department of Internal Medicine, Taipei Medical University- Shuang Ho Hospital, Taipei, Taiwan

Sheng-Jeng Peng
Division of Nephrology, Cathay General Hospital, Taipei, Taiwan

Ko-Lin Kuo
Division of Nephrology, Taipei Tzu-Chi Hospital, Taipei, Taiwan

Hsiang-Chung Liu
Department of Nephrology, Wei Gong Memorial Hospital, Miaoli, Taiwan

En-Tzu Lin
Department of Nephrology, Lotung Poh-Ai Hospital, Yilan, Taiwan

Chien-Tien Su
School of Public Health, Taipei Medical University, Taipei, Taiwan
Department of Family Medicine, Taipei Medical University Hospital, Taipei, Taiwan

Lu Cai, Jianwen Yu, Jing Yu, Yuan Peng, Habib Ullah, Chunyan Yi, Jianxiong Lin and Xiao Yang
Department of Nephrology, The First Affiliated Hospital of Sun Yat-sen University, Guangzhou 510080, China
Key Laboratory of Nephrology, Ministry of Health and Guangdong Province, Guangzhou, China

Xueqing Yu
Department of Nephrology, The First Affiliated Hospital of Sun Yat-sen University, Guangzhou 510080, China
Key Laboratory of Nephrology, Ministry of Health and Guangdong Province, Guangzhou, China

Institute of Nephrology, Guangdong Medical University, Zhanjiang, China

Haesuk Park, Xinyue Liu and Linda Henry
Department of Pharmaceutical Outcomes and Policy, University of Florida College of Pharmacy, HPNP Building Room 3325, 1225 Center Drive, Gainesville, FL 32610, USA

Jeffrey Harman
Department of Behavioral Sciences and Social Medicine, Florida State University, College of Medicine, Tallahassee, FL 32306, USA

Edward A. Ross
Department of Internal Medicine, University of Central Florida, College of Medicine, Orlando, FL 32827, USA

Dimitri Titeca-Beauport, Alexis Francois and Gabriel Choukroun
Department of Nephrology, Dialysis and Transplantation, Amiens University Hospital, F-80054 Amiens, France

Thierry Lobbedez
Department of Nephrology, Caen University Hospital, Caen, France
Registre de Dialyse Péritonéale de Langue Française, Pontoise, France

Dominique Guerrot
Department of Nephrology, Rouen University Hospital, Rouen, France
INSERM, U1096 Rouen, France

David Launay and Eric Hachulla
University of Lille, U995 Lille, France
Lille Inflammation Research International Center (LIRIC), Lille, France
Inserm, U995 Lille, France
Département de Médecine Interne et Immunologie Clinique, CHU Lille, Lille, France
Centre national de Référence Maladies Systémiques et Auto-immunes Rares (Sclérodermie Systémique), Lille, France

Laurence Vrigneaud
Department of Nephrology and Internal Medicine, Valenciennes General Hospital, Valenciennes, France

Maité Daroux
Department of Nephrology, Duchenne Hospital, Boulogne-sur-Mer, France

Celine Lebas
Department of Nephrology, Calmette Hospital, Lille University Hospital, Lille, France

Boris Bienvenu
Department of Internal Medicine, Caen, France
Normandie Univ, UNICAEN, INSERM, COMETE,
Caen, France

Momar Diouf
Clinical Research and Innovation Directorate, Amiens
University Hospital, Amiens, France

Eunjin Bae
Department of Internal Medicine, Gyeongsang
National University Changwon Hospital, Changwon,
South Korea

Kook-Hwan Oh
Department of Internal Medicine, Seoul National
University Hospital, Seoul, South Korea

**Hajeong Lee, Dong Ki Kim, Yon Su Kim, Curie Ahn
and Jin Suk Han**
Department of Internal Medicine, Seoul National
University Hospital, Seoul, South Korea
Kidney Reasearch Institute, Seoul National University
College of Medicine, Seoul, South Korea

Kwon Wook Joo
Department of Internal Medicine, Seoul National
University Hospital, Seoul, South Korea
Kidney Reasearch Institute, Seoul National University
College of Medicine, Seoul, South Korea
Department of Internal Medicine, Seoul National
University College of Medicine, 101 Daehak-Ro,
Jongno-Gu, Seoul 03080, Republic of Korea

Sang-Il Min and Seung-Kee Min
Department of Surgery, Seoul National University
College of Medicine, Seoul, South Korea

Hyo-Cheol Kim
Department of Radiology, Seoul National University
College of Medicine, Seoul, South Korea

Jo-Yen Chao and Ming-Cheng Wang
Division of Nephrology, Department of Internal
Medicine, National Cheng Kung University Hospital,
College of Medicine, National Cheng Kung University,
No.1, University Road, Tainan 70101, Taiwan
Institute of Clinical Pharmacy and Pharmaceutical
Sciences, College of Medicine, National Cheng Kung
University, Tainan, Taiwan

Te-Hui Kuo
Division of Nephrology, Department of Internal
Medicine, National Cheng Kung University Hospital,
College of Medicine, National Cheng Kung University,
No.1, University Road, Tainan 70101, Taiwan
Department of Public Health, College of Medicine,
National Cheng Kung University, Tainan, Taiwan

Yu-Tzu Chang
Division of Nephrology, Department of Internal
Medicine, National Cheng Kung University Hospital,
College of Medicine, National Cheng Kung University,
No.1, University Road, Tainan 70101, Taiwan
Graduate Institute of Clinical Medicine, College of
Medicine, National Cheng Kung University, Tainan,
Taiwan

Hsu-Chih Chien and Yea-Huei Kao Yang
Institute of Clinical Pharmacy and Pharmaceutical
Sciences, College of Medicine, National Cheng Kung
University, Tainan, Taiwan

Chung-Yi Li
Department of Public Health, College of Medicine,
National Cheng Kung University, Tainan, Taiwan

Moritz Wyler von Ballmoos
Division of Cardiovascular and Thoracic Surgery,
Duke University Medical Center, Durham, NC, USA

Donald S. Likosky
Institute for Healthcare Policy and Innovation,
University of Michigan, Ann Arbor, MI, USA
Section of Health Services Research and Quality,
Department of Cardiac Surgery, University of
Michigan, Ann Arbor, MI, USA

Michael Rezaee
Section of Urology, Department of Surgery, Dartmouth-
Hitchcock Medical Center, Lebanon, NH, USA

Kevin Lobdell
Carolinas HealthCare System, Charlotte, NC, USA

Shama Alam, Devin Parker and Sherry Owens
The Dartmouth Institute for Health Policy and Clinical
Practice, Geisel School of Medicine, Lebanon, NH,
USA

Todd MacKenzie
The Dartmouth Institute for Health Policy and Clinical
Practice, Geisel School of Medicine, Lebanon, NH,
USA
Department of Biomedical Data Science, HB 7505
Dartmouth-Hitchcock Medical Center, Lebanon, NH
NH 03756, USA

Jeremiah R. Brown
The Dartmouth Institute for Health Policy and Clinical
Practice, Geisel School of Medicine, Lebanon, NH,
USA
Department of Biomedical Data Science, HB 7505
Dartmouth-Hitchcock Medical Center, Lebanon, NH
NH 03756, USA
Department of Epidemiology, Geisel School of
Medicine, Lebanon, NH, USA

Heather Thiessen-Philbrook
Division of Nephrology, Department of Medicine, Johns Hopkins University, Baltimore, MD, USA

Joel Neugarten and Ladan Golestaneh
Department of Medicine, Nephrology Division, Montefiore Medical Center, Albert Einstein College of Medicine, 111 E. 210 St, Bronx, NY 10467, USA

Index

www.ingramcontent.com/pod-product-compliance
Lightning Source LLC
Chambersburg PA
CBHW080506200326

41458CB00012B/4106